FUNCTIONAL MOVEMENT DEVELOPMENT

Across the Life Span

FUNCTIONAL MOVEMENT DEVELOPMENT

Across the Life Span

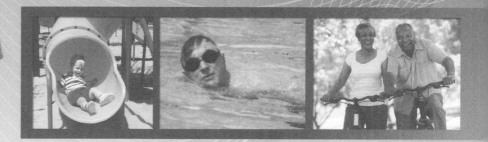

THIRD EDITION

Donna J. Cech, DHS, PT, PCS
Program Director and Professor
Physical Therapy Program
Midwestern University
Downers Grove, Illinois

Suzanne "Tink" Martin, MACT, PT
Professor
Department of Physical Therapy
University of Evansville
Evansville, Indiana

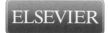

ELSEVIER

ELSEVIER
SAUNDERS

3251 Riverport Lane
St. Louis, Missouri 63043

FUNCTIONAL MOVEMENT DEVELOPMENT ACROSS THE LIFE SPAN,   978-1-4160-4978-4
THIRD EDITION

Notices

Knowledge and best practice in this field are constantly changing. As new research and
experience broaden our understanding, changes in research methods, professional practices,
or medical treatment may become necessary.

Practitioners and researchers must always rely on their own experience and knowledge in
evaluating and using any information, methods, compounds, or experiments described
herein. In using such information or methods they should be mindful of their own safety
and the safety of others, including parties for whom they have a professional responsibility.

With respect to any drug or pharmaceutical products identified, readers are advised to check
the most current information provided (i) on procedures featured or (ii) by the manufacturer
of each product to be administered, to verify the recommended dose or formula, the
method and duration of administration, and contraindications. It is the responsibility of
practitioners, relying on their own experience and knowledge of their patients, to make
diagnoses, to determine dosages and the best treatment for each individual patient, and
to take all appropriate safety precautions.

To the fullest extent of the law, neither the Publisher nor the authors, contributors, or
editors, assume any liability for any injury and/or damage to persons or property as a matter
of products liability, negligence or otherwise, or from any use or operation of any methods,
products, instructions, or ideas contained in the material herein.

978-1-4160-4978-4

Vice President and Publisher: Linda Duncan
Executive Editor: Kathryn Falk
Senior Developmental Editor: Christie M. Hart
Publishing Services Manager: Julie Eddy
Senior Project Manager: Andrea Campbell
Project Manager: Sivaraman Moorthy
Design Direction: Amy Buxton

Printed in the United States of America

Last digit is the print number: 9 8 7 6 5 4 3 2 1

To our three favorite fellows
Jim, Alec, and Terry

Contributors

Susan V. Duff, EdD, OTR/L, PT, CHT, BCP
Clinical Coordinator of the Upper Extremity and Limb
Deformities Centers of Excellence, Shriners Hospital
for Children, Philadelphia, Pennsylvania
Prehension

Timothy Hanke, PhD, PT
Associate Professor
Midwestern University
Downers Grove, Illinois
Posture and Balance; Locomotion

Preface

Movement is key to fully participating in meaningful life activities. It is necessary for safety, survival, mobility, occupation, leisure, health, and fitness. Functional movement plays a role throughout the span of everyone's life and contributes to our complete development. The ability to move changes across the life span—influenced by the development of muscular, skeletal, nervous, and cardiopulmonary systems. The motivation to move is innate, but the sociocultural environment and psychological development influence each person's development and functional movement. Each person's experiences in life are unique and affect development. This perspective reflects how important it is for a health care provider to integrate a thorough understanding of life course perspectives and the World Health Organizations model, the International Classification of Functioning, Disability, and Health (ICF), into the care provided to individuals across the life span.

The third edition of this text continues to be intended primarily for students of physical therapy, occupational therapy, and other professions that address movement dysfunction. This edition continues to emphasize normal development and focuses on the definitions of function and participation, how they are attained, and how participation is optimized across the life span. Development of functional movement and maintenance of functional skills throughout the life span are important to all individuals. For therapists to best support optimal participation for patients and clients, they must appreciate not only the developmental sequences of physical, social-emotional, and psychological development, but also bring a unique understanding of the normal development of the cellular and systems changes that begin in the embryo and continue throughout life. By understanding normal development of body structures and body functions, which contribute to functional movement across the life span, therapists can incorporate this knowledge into clinical decision making.

This book is organized into three units that will provide the reader with the background and tools necessary to understand the components of functional movement. Unit I reviews the biophysical, psychological, and sociocultural domains of development. This information assists the therapist in effectively communicating and working with patients. Students are also guided in integrating important theories of development into clinical decision making models. Chapters 3 and 4 have been revamped to bring students and clinicians the most current content on motor development, motor learning, and motor control, and their complex interrelationships. The content in Chapter 5 related to standardized assessment of function across the life span has been updated and expanded to include assessments at the activity and participation levels of the ICF. This information is important for therapists to consider as they include participation level outcomes in patient/client management.

Building on the foundation of Unit I, Unit II adds a comprehensive review of how body systems develop and affect functional movement from the prenatal period through older adulthood. Chapters focused on the skeletal system, the cardiovascular and pulmonary systems, and the nervous system have been rewritten with a stronger emphasis on information necessary for clinical decision making. Basic information on the anatomy, physiology, and histology of the systems has been condensed to identify only those aspects of body systems function and structure that change across the life span and influence functional mobility. More "Clinical Implications" sidebars have been added to the systems chapters to help students appreciate the importance of understanding each system's normal development within clinical practice.

The final unit, Unit III, focuses on functional outcomes key to mobility and participation in meaningful life activities. Age-related trends in balance, posture, locomotion, and prehension are presented. A key chapter on vital functions, such as sleep-wakefulness, eating, digestion, breathing, and elimination, also reviews endocrine function, which plays such an important role in a person's ability to participate in day-to-day activities. This chapter explores the influences vital functions have on functional mobility. In Unit III,

"Clinical Implications" sidebars again give the reader insights into the relationships between normal development and clinical practice. Finally, Chapter 15 discusses the issues of health and fitness, heightening awareness of the therapist's role in wellness and prevention issues across the life span.

The combined content of all 3 units of this text provides the reader with key information related to life span development, which when considered within clinical decision making, supports optimal development of function, participation, health, and quality of life of the patients served.

Donna J. Cech, DHS, PT, PCS
Downers Grove, Illinois

Suzanne "Tink" Martin, MACT, PT
Evansville, Indiana

Acknowledgments

We wish to thank the professional colleagues and many students who have provided feedback on our efforts and have offered encouragement not only for this third edition, but since the inception of this book. Special thanks go to coworkers at our respective universities for technical assistance and ongoing support. We appreciate the contributions of Susan Duff EdD, OTR/L, PT, CHT, BCP, over more than 20 years and all three editions of this book. Many thanks to Patrick Kitzman, PhD, for reviewing chapters. Jennifer Bottomley, PhD, PT, helped us better address issues related to older adulthood in the second edition. The contributions of Ann F. Vansant, PhD, PT, Patricia Wilder, PhD, PT, and Lori Quinn EdD, PT, to the first and second editions of the book have helped set the course for this book as it has developed and matured.

We also want to thank our friends and family for their continued support and encouragement. Terry, Jim, and Alec, your patience and understanding are so important to us. We acknowledge our parents for instilling in us the confidence that helped us to pursue a project of this scope, through all three editions.

Lastly, thank you to the many people in the publishing world who have supported and worked with us over the course of this project. These include the people we have worked with at Elsevier, for patiently waiting for our manuscript pages and for believing in the book. Our special regards go to Margaret Biblis for starting this entire process and her continued friendship and encouragement.

Donna J. Cech, DHS, PT, PCS
Downers Grove, Illinois

Suzanne "Tink" Martin, MACT, PT
Evansville, IN

Contents

UNIT 1   DEFINITION OF FUNCTIONAL MOVEMENT

1   Functional Independence: A Lifelong Goal   1

2   Theories Affecting Development   14

3   Motor Development   45

4   Motor Control and Motor Learning   68

5   Evaluation of Function, Activity, and Participation   88

UNIT II   BODY SYSTEMS CONTRIBUTING TO FUNCTIONAL MOVEMENT

6   Skeletal System Changes   105

7   Muscle System Changes   129

8   Cardiovascular and Pulmonary System Changes   151

9   Nervous System Changes   174

10   Sensory System Changes   213

UNIT III   FUNCTIONAL MOVEMENT OUTCOMES

11   Vital Functions   239

12   Posture and Balance   263   *Tim Hanke, Suzanne "Tink" Martin*

13   Locomotion   288   *Tim Hanke, Donna Cech*

14   Prehension   309   *Susan Duff*

15   Health and Fitness   335

Index   355

CHAPTER 1

Functional Independence: A Lifelong Goal

OBJECTIVES

After studying this chapter, the reader will be able to:

1. Define function as it relates to participation in life roles.
2. Appreciate the interrelationship of all domains of function in everyday life.
3. Discuss the relationship of functional abilities to health status.
4. Discuss factors contributing to participation in life roles within the framework of the International Classification of Functioning, Disability, and Health.
5. Appreciate life span issues related to participation and functional ability.
6. Identify the aspects of physical function that relate to quality of performance.

As humans, we strive to fully and actively participate in life roles and learn to exist within our environment. Throughout our life span, we constantly develop or adapt our abilities and skills to live our lives in a satisfying and meaningful manner. The capacity to exist within the environment is influenced by our ability to function, and the quality of our functional ability is related to all aspects of development: physical, social, emotional, and mental. In this book, we approach development as an ongoing, lifelong process and explore its influence on functional movement ability.

Improving our client's ability to fully participate in life roles is frequently our goal as health care professionals. Various health care professionals strive to help their clients optimize different aspects of function to realize the most satisfying and meaningful life possible. To meet this goal most effectively, we must understand the meaning of the word *function* within our respective disciplines. For example, physicians and nurses may focus primarily on the attainment and maintenance of good health as related to function, whereas social workers concentrate on an individual's ability to function within her social system. Occupational therapists work to improve the ability to function in daily life and to perform occupational tasks, whereas physical therapists structure programs to enhance physical function and mobility. All of these aspects of function are, of course, interdependent, and when considered as a conceptual whole, they help to reflect a person's ability to function or participate within our society and environment. The World Health Organization[1] defines the involvement of an individual in life situations as participation within the International Classification of Functioning, Disability, and Health.

FUNCTION

Widely accepted definitions of the word *function* include such phrases as "normal, characteristic actions," "purpose," and "group of related actions." More generally, function is a natural, required, or expected activity. The second edition of the *Guide to Physical Therapist Practice* identifies function as "those activities identified by an individual as essential to support physical, social, and psychological well-being and to create a personal sense of meaningful living.[2]" When related to the roles and activities of people, the term *function* can describe the action of an individual body part or the person as a whole. The heart functions to pump blood through the body, delivering nutrients to other organs and tissues. The legs function to support our body weight during standing and to propel us forward during walking. We gain mastery over the environment, functioning to complete roles and tasks important to everyday life.

Function as Related to Health

Function is very closely related to health. As globally defined by the World Health Organization (WHO), *health* is a state of complete physical, mental, and social well-being, not merely the absence of disease and infirmity.[3] This simple definition is difficult to use clinically because well-being is hard to measure and too broad a concept to accurately portray an individual's status. More specifically, health influences our ability to successfully complete the tasks expected by society. Without the necessary functional abilities, it is difficult to complete these tasks or to demonstrate a state of complete physical, mental, and social well-being. Well-being has been defined as "a subjective assessment of health which is less concerned with biological function than with feelings such as self-esteem and sense of belonging through social integration.[4]" From another perspective, well-being and functional ability can be disrupted as a result of poor health. Disease, infirmity, and illness interfere with our capacity to perform socially expected roles. It therefore is not difficult to understand why health professionals endeavor to improve how an individual functions.

International Classification of Functioning, Disability, and Health (ICF)

The ICF provides a model to describe the health of people as they function within their environment, highlighting the relationship between function and health. The ICF provides a framework from which to examine the relationships between the biological, personal, and social factors influencing health (Figure 1-1). How well a person functions and participates in socially expected roles is influenced by a person's health condition, body structure and function, and personal and environmental factors.

The ICF considers the biological construct of function through consideration of the body functions and structures. *Body functions* reflect the physiological processes that support a person's health and ability to participate in activities important to her. Anatomical support for health and function is reflected by consideration of *body structures*. The brain and all components of the nervous system are part of that support so that mental functions and sensory functions are included along with motor functions in this construct. Physical and psychological function are both supported by body functions and structures.

Personal factors also contribute to a person's overall health and ability to perform tasks related to her participation in life activities. In defining health, obvious personal factors such as sex, race, and age are considered. In addition, a person's lifestyle, level of fitness, social

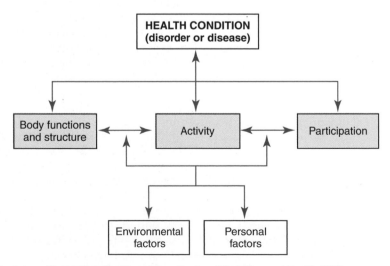

Figure 1-1 Model of the International Classification of Functioning, Disability, and Health (ICF).

background, culture, and value system are important personal characteristics that contribute to the definition of health. People who believe they have the ability to positively influence their own health and well-being are more likely to value advice from a health care professional and shift from risky behavior to healthy behavior. Promotion of health and wellness involves participation in positive health behaviors such as participation in an active lifestyle and self-management of chronic health conditions.

Similarly, health is certainly influenced by the environment in which one lives. In considering the environmental context of health, not only the physical environment, but also the social and attitudinal environments need to be considered. The *physical environment* includes consideration of basic factors such as climate and geography. Living in urban or rural settings also influence the physical environment in which a person functions. Similarly, where a person lives also helps define the person's social and attitudinal environment. *Social environment* includes a person's support system and social relationships. Family, friends, community, and civic groups are some of the many social relationships a person may have. Health professionals are part of the support system for a person with health issues. The *attitudinal environment* does not only reflect the general attitudes of society. The attitudinal environment also includes the programs provided within a community to support health and well-being, the policies that define these resources, and the systems in place within a community that support health and well-being. For example, availability of public education, parks and recreation facilities, and public transportation are services. Examples of local and national laws and policies include local ordinances banning smoking and national health insurance regulations such as Medicare. Health insurance availability and regulations also contribute to the attitudinal environment. The multiple facets of the environment impact significantly upon a person's health, functional abilities, and participation.

Client Assessment

To identify client needs and to develop interventions, health professionals must be able to measure an individual's health status. Health status can be measured by looking at three primary arenas: (1) physical manifestations, (2) client symptoms, and (3) functional status.[5] *Physical manifestations* are those aspects of body function that can be measured or observed, such as muscle strength, body temperature, blood pressure, and the presence of edema. *Client symptoms* reflect the client's impression of her health. The client may report a painful knee, weakness, fatigue, or generally feeling good. *Functional status* reflects how well the client

is able to perform day-to-day activities. Illness and injury, then, influence health status and can reduce one's ability to function. The impact of this reduction varies. Some people lose little ground in keeping up with their day-to-day tasks, whereas others may not be able to do the things they need to do. The reduction in function may also reflect where the person is on the developmental continuum. The amount of physiological reserve available to come back from an illness or injury lessens with older age. The terms *disability* and *handicap* are frequently used when daily tasks cannot be performed.

In general, *disability* refers to an individual's diminished functional capacity.[5] *Handicap* is a frame of reference defined by society; when individuals are no longer viewed as being able to perform the tasks expected by society, they are considered handicapped. However, the loss of functional ability does not necessarily result in disability or handicap. A person may lose some shoulder range of motion without incurring a problem with function, whereas the loss of a limb would be considered a disability and depending on architectural barriers may be a handicap. "*Disability* is the overarching term to connote impairments, activity limitations or restrictions in participation. Changes in health and functioning can take place at any time of life because of disease, disorder or injury and take place inevitably as we get older.[6]"

Health Status Models

Historically, several models were proposed to analyze the spectrum of status from functional independence to disability. These disablement models were thought to be helpful in identifying appropriate services and in planning treatment programs. Historically, the two most popular models included the International Classification of Impairments, Disabilities, and Handicaps (ICIDH) proposed by WHO[7] and the model of health status proposed by sociologist Saad Nagi.[8] These two models focused primarily on the negative aspects of illness and functional limitations to define health. Within these models, terms familiar to rehabilitation professionals were defined. The models reflected the relationships between pathology, impairment, disability, and handicap. *Impairment* was defined as any limitation or abnormality in anatomical, physiological, or psychological processes. The category of *functional limitation* described deficits occurring because of an impairment and affecting the ability to perform usual activities. *Disability* referred to a deficit in the performance of daily activities or the patterns of behavior that emerged when functional limitations were too great to allow successful completion of a task. *Handicap* was related to an individual's inability to perform expected social roles, leading to a diminished quality of life. These classification systems supported health care providers in identifying the most appropriate focus for patient interventions. The second edition of the *Guide to Physical Therapist Practice*[2] uses this model of disablement as a framework for the practice of physical therapy and to optimize client function.

The ICF[1] is similar to the Nagi model and the original ICIDH but focuses on the more positive aspect of ability and health. The terms *body functions* and *body structures* now describe either the physiological or psychological function and structure of the organs, limbs, and their components. Any problems with these body functions and structures that result in a deviation from the norm or a loss are referred to as *impairments*. The term *activity* refers to the execution of a task or action by an individual and *activity limitation* has replaced the term *disability* in the model and refers to difficulties in performance of activities by the individual. Finally, the term *participation* refers to participation in a life situation, and *participation restriction* has replaced the term *handicap,* referring to any problem the individual may have in participating in life situations.[1] The shift from the original ICIDH to the ICF is a shift from disablement to enablement. This shift is consistent with the view that health is more than the absence of disease. Health is a positive state in which differences in abilities still allow for function within society.

In the evaluation of the health status of individuals, health care providers need to understand each patient's life roles and optimal levels of participation. Such assessment allows the provider to focus on the issues most important to the client and to consider whether interventions can minimize an activity limitation or diminish participation restrictions. The ICF directs the provider to identify not only the impairments but also the personal and environmental factors that may be limiting performance of activities and participation in life roles. From this framework, an intervention approach can be designed that will focus on function rather than one solely directed to remediation of impairments. For example, work simplification may be as effective in improving function as a strengthening program for a person with chronic pain. Use of the ICF framework when working with patients helps the health care provider focus on assisting patients in maximizing participation in life situations and roles. Solutions are looked for within the social and attitudinal environments in which the person functions and within the person's physical environment.

In working with clients of different ages, it is also important to understand the role of development on the acquisition of functional skills and the ability to perform activities. Is the 3-year-old child who cannot tie her shoe disabled? Of course not. Developmentally, it is normal for a young child to require adult assistance with this task. By 8 years of age, the child usually has developed this skill and no longer needs adult assistance. If older adults with severe arthritis cannot put on their shoes because of limitations in hip flexion or finger mobility, are they disabled? Again, not necessarily. If that adult uses a long-handled shoehorn, she may be quite good at completing the task. Similarly, it is not uncommon for adults to use glasses or hearing aids to maximize ability to participate in life roles as they age. Developmental issues, social expectations, family attitudes, and adaptability of the environment are all issues that help determine whether limitations are present.[9]

Functional Activities Leading to Participation

Functional activities are those activities that contribute to an individual's physical, social, and psychological well-being.[2] These activities include self-care, household, vocational, and recreational tasks, allowing an individual to perform as independently as possible in all settings. Functional skills and activities not only support our biophysical and psychological well-being but also allow us to incorporate what we view as important into meaningful, everyday life. From early infancy to late adulthood, we must develop or adapt functional skills to best access the environment in which we live and to meet our own needs as independently as possible. The performance of functional activities not only depends on our physical abilities but also is affected by our emotional status, cognitive ability, and sociocultural expectations. These factors together define an individual's functional performance.

In general, certain categories of functional activities, such as eating, maintaining personal hygiene, dressing, ambulating, and grasping, are common to everyone. Other tasks related to our job or recreational activities vary from one person to the next. Within the health care model, personal care activities such as ambulating, feeding, bathing, dressing, grooming, maintaining continence, and toileting are referred to as *basic activities of daily living (BADL)*. Other important activities relate to how well we manage within the home setting and in the community. These activities are referred to as *instrumental activities of daily living (IADL)* and include tasks such as cooking, cleaning, handling finances, shopping, working, and using personal or public transportation. The health care provider often assesses BADL and IADL to define client status and to develop appropriate intervention programs (see Chapter 5). In addition to BADL and IADL, participation in life roles, social activities, and leisure activities is important to consider in defining a person's function and participation. Life roles may include going to school, performing a job, and parenting. Social activities include activities with friends and relatives, membership in a church, and participation in community activities. Leisure activities include hobbies, sports and recreation, and vacations.[10]

Function from a Life Span Perspective

Function defines mastery and competency over the environment. Throughout the life span, from conception until old age, we demonstrate varying abilities and levels of mastery over our environment. Initially, we are concerned with being able to survive and master a level of function concerned with the locus of self-need and control. Next, we learn to function well within the home environment, and finally we learn to function within the community (Figure 1-2). For example, to ensure survival, the infant learns to cry for food or when experiencing discomfort. She can also turn her head to keep her airway clear and can coordinate important tasks, such as breathing and swallowing. The toddler learns to function safely within her home: avoiding electrical outlets, climbing stairs, feeding herself, and using the toilet. The school-age child learns to safely cross the street on the way to school. These same levels of mastery are mirrored at all life stages as functional

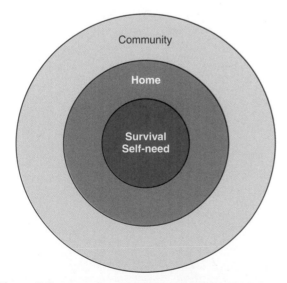

Figure 1-2 Acquisition of function. The concentric circles illustrate that acquisition of function begins with a focus on self, the locus of self-need and control, which evolves to increased levels of mastery over a broadening environment.

expectations change. The adult masters the self-care tasks of eating by shopping and cooking or dining out and provides shelter for herself and keeps it clean and warm. Finally, the adult masters functioning in a larger community, including the workplace.

From these examples, it is obvious that our functional ability is in part defined by age. As children become older, they are expected to gain independence in a wide variety of functional tasks and in an expanding environment. The 5-year-old child must meet the challenges of becoming competent within the new environment of school. Many 16-year-old youths assume the responsibilities of safely driving a car and functioning within their community. The functional expectations of adults expand as they have children and assume job responsibilities. Older adults may appear to be faced with fewer functional expectations as they retire and their children become independent. They may also be faced with challenges related to maintaining functional independence of even basic needs as they adapt to fixed incomes and declining physical abilities. Older adults, when asked to define successful aging, have emphasized the importance of being able to care for themselves and coping with challenges in their later years,[11] emphasizing the importance of functional independence and participation. It is clear that the definitions of function and functional independence change across the life span as our abilities change and the expectations of society vary.

Physical Growth and Function

In many ways, our functional abilities depend on physical abilities. Physical development not only influences the ability to perform physical activity but also affects our ability to interact with the environment. Movement has been related to cognitive development, social activity, and communication. Across the life span, the physical capacity of the individual changes and helps to define functional capacity.

During the embryonic development of a human, the first 7 to 8 weeks after conception are devoted to growth. Functional systems, although being formed, have not yet begun to work at their tasks. In the fetal period (8 weeks after conception until birth), the organ systems begin to function and the developing fetus becomes competent within the protective environment of the womb. After birth, the neonate must accommodate another environment, governed by the force of gravity. Infants attain functional skills in this new environment and systematically continue growing. The 1-year-old toddler may be very proud and excited about her ability to walk. Children who are 2 to 3 years old add important functional skills such as feeding and dressing themselves. Throughout childhood, physical growth occurs as the child becomes taller and stronger and demonstrates increasing endurance. The child actively explores her community on a bicycle or roller blades.

The balance between body growth and functional mastery continues until physical maturity is attained in young adulthood. Adults strive to attain and maintain functionally active lifestyles at home, in the workplace, and during leisure activities. The wear and tear that sometimes results from their functional activities can frequently be balanced by growth and the repair abilities of the body. By the time an adult reaches old age, growth and repair functions may be insufficient to maintain the optimal functional state of the body.

Wide variations in functional ability are seen among older adults. Most adults continue to live an active life, adapting as necessary to physical changes in their body systems. In other older adults, changes in strength, posture, or endurance may make efficient movement and physical function more demanding and difficult. Presence of chronic illnesses such as heart disease, arthritis, and diabetes also impact an older adult's functional ability. Age-related changes and presence of chronic illness may negatively impact the older adult's ability to participate in activities that are important to her, diminishing her ability to function and maintain a level of mastery over her environment.[12,13] The average life expectancy continues to increase in the United States and across the world. Many older adults will live into their 80s and 90s. In the United States, the number of older adults ages 85 years and older increased by 38% between 1990 and 2000.[14] The number of older adults in the United States, at least 100 years of age also increased from approximately 37,000 people to approximately 50,000 people.[14] A concomitant compression of the period of morbidity at the end of life has been demonstrated, most notably in older adults who have practiced good health behaviors (e.g., stress reduction, exercise, hydration, nutrition) throughout their life span.[15] Recent studies have shown that older adults who participate in exercise programs can improve levels of physical function, self-efficacy, and quality of life.[16,17]

Relationship Between Development and Function

Each individual develops throughout the life span. Development occurs not only as a result of physical changes within the body but also because of environmental influences. As we interact within family, community, social, and cultural contexts, our development is shaped and functional roles or tasks are defined. From this perspective, development and function are intertwined throughout the life span, much like a piece of cloth is woven.

Development is a lifelong process. Through childhood, growth of the body systems occurs, and various new tasks are learned. Through adulthood, the body systems maintain a steady state and the individual continues to learn new skills and develop new interests. Finally in older adulthood, participation in and development of skills and interests may continue, but biological "aging" may begin to impact physical function. *Senescence* is the progressive physiological decline that results in increasing vulnerability to stress and the progressing likelihood of death. Just like other phases of development, senescence is not a single process but rather many processes.

The *development of function* does not refer just to the growth process related to youth or to the decline often associated with senescence and aging. Similarly, it cannot necessarily be reflected linearly. Growth and development imply change, either positive or negative, which can be observed at any point within the life span. If the life span and functional development are considered two separate continuums, pleated onto one another to resemble the bellows of an accordion, their impact on each other is obvious (Figure 1-3). As adolescents experience growth spurts, attaining new height, they also experience losses in flexibility because muscle growth does not keep up with bone

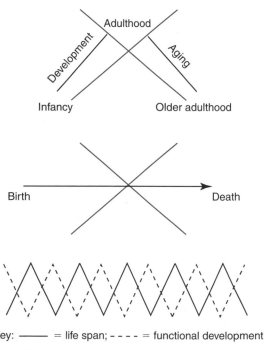

Key: —— = life span; - - - - = functional development

Figure 1-3 Interaction of life span and functional development.

growth. Adults may achieve new levels of productivity in the workplace but at a cost to family or social interactions. The life span approach to development and function appreciates all of the changes seen in an individual's abilities at any point in the life cycle, whether the changes reflect progression, regression, or reorganization.

Domains of Function

Functional activities with similar outcomes can be grouped together into categories or domains. We consider three domains of function here: biophysical domain, psychological domain, and sociocultural domain (Figure 1-4). The *biophysical domain* includes the sensorimotor skills needed to perform activities of daily living, such as dressing, ambulating, maintaining hygiene, and cooking. The *psychological domain* is influenced by intellectual activities. Motivation, concentration, problem solving, and judgment are all factors that contribute to psychological function, as well as affective function, which allows a person to cope with everyday stresses. The psychological domain also influences how we perceive our ability to function. Factors such as anxiety, depression, emotional well-being, self-awareness, and self-esteem influence affective function.[12] The *sociocultural domain* relates to our ability to interact with other people and to successfully complete social roles and obligations. Cultural norms or expectations help define social function.

These domains of function parallel domains of development discussed in Chapter 2, reinforcing the interrelationship of function and development. No one domain of function stands alone. Similarly, development within each domain is reflected by the progression of activities in each functional domain. For example, within the motor, psychological, and sociocultural domains of function, the young child focuses on learning motor skills such as walking, jumping, and running as she participates in play activities. Over time the child's functional skills expand into learning and being a student, then assuming job or career roles. Development of relationships with family members and friends begins in childhood and then expands as adults form intimate relationships with friends and life partners. Many sociocultural functions depend on our mobility and ability to physically manipulate objects. Likewise, our physical level of function can be easily influenced by emotional status, intellectual ability, or motivation. All three domains of function are interrelated and interdependent in meeting everyday challenges. Although all three domains of function are important, the primary focus of the rest of this chapter will be the domain of physical function.

PHYSICAL FUNCTION

Physical function can also be thought of as goal-directed movement. Function is the link between the physical actions we call movement and the environmental context in which they take place. For the act of reaching to be meaningful and therefore functional, it must take place when there is an object to reach for. Walking is functional because it is a means of moving from one place to another. People use movement every day as they interact with their environment. Goal-directed movement is important for an individual to survive, adapt, and learn within the environment. When our movement is inhibited, we may be less able to meet day-to-day needs. The young athlete with a broken leg suddenly must depend on crutches, making simple tasks such as walking to the bathroom or opening the door a challenge. As movement becomes less efficient, an individual may be faced with diminished functional independence. The individual with arthritis may not be able to quickly and efficiently button clothes. She may

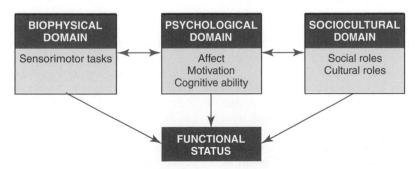

Figure 1-4 The three domains of function—biophysical, psychological, sociocultural—must operate independently as well as interdependently for human beings to achieve their best possible functional status.

also have difficulty picking up coins when paying for purchases in a store. As physical function becomes impaired, we frequently turn to health professionals for assistance.

Physical and occupational therapy intervention is frequently focused on improving physical function and maximizing an individual's ability to participate in life roles. Improved physical functioning also may be a positive influence on psychological and sociocultural functioning. After the therapist identifies a client's basic participation restrictions and activity limitations, additional assessment of sensory, cardiopulmonary, neurological, or musculoskeletal systems may then identify impairments that interfere with overall physical function. Such impairments may include anatomical or physiological changes such as limited range of motion or diminished strength. Therapeutic programs can then be devised to improve function. Therapy may focus on adapting a task or the environment in which the task takes place, or it may address an isolated impairment of body structure or function, which interferes with the patient's level of participation. The success of the therapeutic programs is measured based on the functional change demonstrated by the client, not on isolated changes in range of motion or strength impairments.

It is important for therapists to understand how biophysical function changes over time, the relationship of physical function to other domains of function, and the components of physical function that contribute to the quality and efficiency of movement. Knowledge of normal function of all body systems and how movement develops provides a means to detect movement dysfunction. With this knowledge, therapists can effectively create interventions that best meet a patient's individual need to be an active participant in life.

Development

How does physical function develop? What factors influence its development? Age, environment, and social expectations all contribute to a definition of normal biophysical function. Age not only defines size and biological capacity for movement but also reflects expectations about lifestyle.

During infancy and childhood, body size and the maturity of the body systems involved in movement limit and define functional abilities. For example, toddlers are able to walk, but because of their short legs, they have trouble keeping up with their parents. It is frequently more efficient and functional for them to be carried or pushed in a stroller. Young children may have trouble sitting at the table without fidgeting at a

meal, perhaps because their feet do not reach the floor and they cannot easily sit in the large chair provided for them. Functional limitations in these examples are closely related to the immaturity of the child's skeletal system, but the neuromuscular and cardiopulmonary systems are also undergoing rapid development during this time frame and affect the child's physical abilities. Fundamental motor skills such as postural control, locomotion, and prehension develop rapidly during childhood.

Functional expectations of the infant and child also influence their development of functional skills. A young infant's abilities are basically survival oriented. She can lift and turn her head; coordinate suck, swallow, and breathing; cry to indicate needs; and socially interact with her caregivers. As the infant begins to control her movement, the major job or task is to explore the environment. Through play, an infant learns about the world around her; as the toddler and young child associate play with functional activities, such as eating and dressing, caregivers begin to have higher expectations for functional independence.

Through childhood and adolescence, social roles and expectations continue to undergo constant change. Body growth and maturation of the body systems also continue. Once maturity is attained in adolescence or young adulthood, the systems of the body that contribute to motor performance have completed their development. At this point, these body systems are ready to operate at peak efficiency. Practice and motivation to excel contribute to our ability to learn and refine new motor tasks. Skills are refined as we try to improve performance through recreational activities such as baseball, ballet, and gymnastics.

Societal roles and lifestyle changes that accompany adulthood again redefine physical function and may result in decreased physical activity levels. Commuting time, combined with a full day at work, may limit time available for physically active recreational pursuits. As activity levels decrease, so does our level of fitness. Cardiopulmonary functioning and muscle strength may not be supported to full capacity, resulting in decreased endurance and weakness. Refinement of skills associated with job pursuits continues through adulthood. Some job skills may put repetitive stress on the musculoskeletal system, which can lead to injury. As the body systems are continually used in day-to-day activities, wear and tear, as well as ongoing developmental changes related to adulthood, may decrease the efficiency of the body in physical functioning. To optimize physical function across the life span, individuals of all ages are encouraged to maintain an active and healthy lifestyle.

In the older adult, biophysical functional ability may decline because of wear and tear on the body systems, normal development (senescence), and lifestyle changes. Retirement from a physically demanding job may result in a less active lifestyle. A common assumption made about older adults is that they have a diminished ability to perform physical activities. It is important to remember that much variation exists in the abilities and activity levels demonstrated by older adults. Each older adult has a unique history, experiences, and changes attributed to aging. When one considers the total population of older adults, the majority do not have significant functional limitations. They live independently and maintain a relatively active and satisfying lifestyle. Functional ability does decrease with age, but it is in the oldest populations (more than 85 years old) that physical disability is the greatest.[12] Numerous functional tasks are required of people who live independently, including BADL (self-care and mobility) and IADL (cooking, shopping, housekeeping, and transportation). Of these, housekeeping and

transportation difficulties were reported most often by older adults.[18] Figure 1-5 reflects the percentage of older adults in the United States indicating limitations in IADL and driving, confirming the percent of the population reporting limitations increases most for individuals 85 years of age and older.[19] Figure 1-6 demonstrates a similar trend of individuals over 85 years of age reporting the most difficulty with BADL.[19] Longitudinal studies of the functional status of adults older than 70 years report that many older adults remain functionally independent, but report difficulty in walking, doing heavy housework, and lower extremity function such as stooping.[20] Older adults who remain physically active maintain higher levels of physical function than their peers who are inactive.[21]

Components

"Efficient," "effective," "graceful," "fluid," and "smooth" are all adjectives frequently associated with movement. "Clumsy," "awkward," "disjointed," and "wasted" can

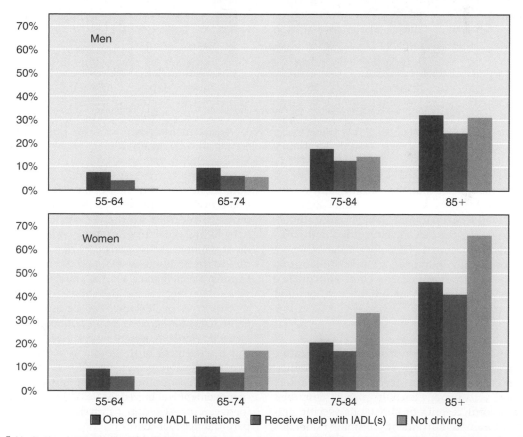

Figure 1-5 Limitation in Instrumental Activities of Daily Living, by age: 2002. (From National Institute on Aging: *Growing older in America: the health and retirement study*, Bethesda, MD:NIH Publication No. 07-5757, March, 2007.)

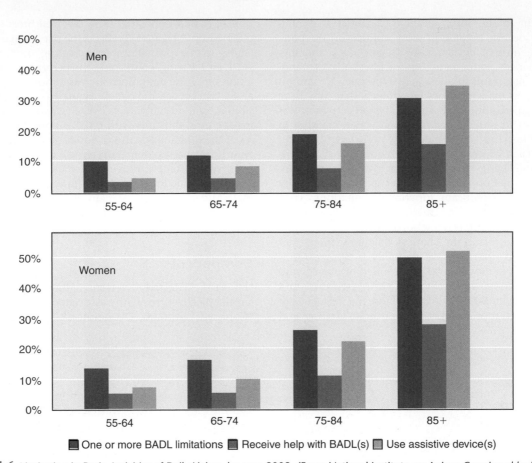

Figure 1-6 Limitation in Basic Activities of Daily Living, by age: 2002. (From National Institute on Aging: *Growing older in America: the health and retirement study*, Bethesda, MD:NIH Publication No. 07-5757, March, 2007.)

also describe movement, but these words paint a very different picture. Sports science, physical education, and physical and occupational therapy professionals have tried to define the factors that contribute to efficient, effective movement. Flexibility, balance, coordination, power, and endurance are some dimensions that affect the quality of physical function. Both quality and efficiency of movement are important to optimal physical function.

Flexibility

Flexibility is reflected by a person's ability to move through space without being restricted by the musculoskeletal system.[22] Most simply, *flexibility* refers to the capacity to bend. Flexibility can be described for a specific joint, a series of joints, or a specific person. Within human movement, flexibility depends on joint integrity, extensibility of the soft tissue (i.e., muscles, connective tissue, and skin) and joint

range of motion.[2] The tissues must maintain an appropriate resting length and pliability to allow the joint mobility necessary for the completion of activities of daily living. When a person has good flexibility, movement is more effective and efficient. Flexibility contributes to the ability to easily open the hand just enough to grasp a pencil or a glass, the ability to squat down to pick something up, and the ability to climb stairs.

Two types of flexibility can be assessed. *Static flexibility* refers to the range of motion available at a joint. *Dynamic flexibility* describes the resistance offered to active movement of the joint. As resistance increases, dynamic flexibility decreases. When optimal levels of resistance balance the motion around a joint, efficiency of movement is achieved. As flexibility increases, greater force can be exerted in a movement, and the speed of performance increases.[23]

Developmentally, flexibility is fairly stable in boys from age 5 to 8 years and then decreases slightly until age 12 to 13 years. After that time, it again increases slightly until age 18. In girls, flexibility is stable from age 5 to 11 years and then increases until age 14. After that time, flexibility reaches a plateau. At all ages, females are more flexible than males.[24] In older adults, flexibility may decrease because of cross-linkage of collagen fibers in connective tissue, inactivity, decreased muscle strength, and joint changes. Active older adults maintain greater levels of flexibility than do their more sedentary peers.[25,26]

Our flexibility is defined by the types of physical activities we pursue each day at work and engage in during recreational activities. Flexibility also influences health and physical function across the life span. The flexibility of the baseball pitcher's throwing arm is certainly greater than that of a typist's arm. A gymnast is probably more flexible than a football player. Levels of flexibility in adolescence have been shown to relate to decreased risk of neck problems in adulthood.[27] Flexibility exercises are also a component of most fall prevention programs for older adults, reinforcing the importance of flexibility for effective movement.[28,29]

Balance

Balance is related to a state of equilibrium and is an important component of skilled movement. Balance is achieved when we can maintain our center of gravity over our base of support, thereby maintaining equilibrium with gravity. Several factors contribute to the ability to balance, including efficient function of the nervous system, musculoskeletal system, and sensory systems. Balance is necessary during static activities such as standing still (*static balance*) and during movement (*dynamic balance*).[2,22]

Throughout childhood balance improves. Girls appear to perform better than boys in balance activities. In adolescence, both groups reach a plateau in balance skills; boys may perform slightly better than girls in this age group.[24] In older adulthood, poor balance is frequently reported as a problem and may be related to developmental changes or impairments in the body systems that contribute to balance. Some of these changes include impaired reflex activity, vestibular dysfunction, posture changes, deconditioning from disuse, medications, and dehydration.[30] Falling is also a problem related to balance issues in older adults.[29] Falls are a common problem in the community dwelling adult over the age of 65.[31] Falls can lead to fractures, hospitalization, and loss of function. Good balance is an important prerequisite skill for daily activities of living, and therefore balance activities are integral components of fall prevention and physical activity programs for older adults.[28,29,32,33]

Coordination

Coordination implies that various muscles are working together to produce a smooth and efficient movement. The right muscles must activate in the correct sequence and work at the right time, with the right intensity for the movement to be smooth, accurate, and efficient.[22] Coordination is needed to successfully crawl, skip, run to catch a bus, make a bed, or put on a pair of pants in the morning. Coordination develops over time in children as sensory and neuromotor systems develop. For example, reach and grasp coordination in 6-year-old children is variable, with improved coordination by age 8 years and an adult-like reach and grasp pattern at age 11 years.[34] In older adults, coordination decreases, negatively impacting motor performance.[35,36]

Power

Power refers to the rate at which work is done, the ability to exert force quickly. Related to movement, it is the rate at which a muscle can develop tension and produce a force, moving a body part through a range of motion.[37] Power is then related to both strength and speed. In childhood, power depends on size and maturity of the neurological and musculoskeletal systems. In particular, development of muscle fiber types able to work using anaerobic metabolism increases the power and force of the muscle contraction possible. Changes in muscle fiber types, specifically Type II muscle fibers, are reflected in variations in muscle power generated by individuals of different ages.[38,39] In older adults, as strength and speed decrease, power decreases.[38,40]

Power is important in the performance of activities such as walking, jumping, running, throwing, standing up from a chair, and climbing stairs. Decreased power generation negatively impacts the older adult's ability to perform everyday motor tasks. Research studies have shown that when older adults participate in power training programs, functional abilities such as stair climbing, rising from a chair, and walking speed improve.[16,17,41,42]

Endurance

Endurance is related to the ability to perform work over an extended period of time. Children, for example, can play actively for hours. We need endurance to perform repetitive activities of daily living, such as stirring food while cooking, using a blow dryer to dry our hair, or walking up steps. Recreational and job-related tasks also often require a high level of endurance.

Endurance can be affected by an individual muscle, a muscle group, or the total body. Total body endurance usually refers to cardiopulmonary endurance, reflecting the ability of the heart to deliver a steady supply of oxygen to working muscle. Muscle endurance reflects the ability to sustain repeated muscle contraction and is related to muscle strength. Developmentally, muscle endurance has been shown to increase linearly in boys between 5 and 13 years of age, after which a spurt is observed. A steady linear increase in muscle endurance is seen in girls.[24] Endurance decreases in older adults, with elite senior marathon runners demonstrating diminished endurance after the age of 50 years.[43,44]

SUMMARY

Human function is an elusive entity. We discuss function from a life span perspective and its relationship to the broader context of health. Optimal function contributes to an individual's well-being and is associated with biological health, but also the contribution of personal and environmental factors. The interactions and interdependence of the biophysical, psychological, and sociocultural domains are what define our ability to function. The domain of biophysical function requires in-depth understanding because this is the area that we, as physical and occupational therapists, hope to improve when working with our clients. The components that make movement efficient, effective, and, most important, functional have been reviewed. Using this knowledge base, we can assess how our clients are functioning and help them successfully meet their goals of improving function and maximizing their ability to participate in life roles.

REFERENCES

1. World Health Organization: *International classification of functioning, disability, and health*, Geneva, 2001, World Health Organization.
2. American Physical Therapy Association: *Guide to physical therapist practice*, ed 2, Alexandria, Va, 2001, American Physical Therapy Association.
3. World Health Organization: *The first ten years of the World Health Organization*, Geneva, 1958, World Health Organization.
4. Nutbeam D: Health promotion glossary, *Health Promot* 1(1):113–127, 1986.
5. Jette AM: State of the art in functional status assessment. In Rothstein J, editor: *Measurement in physical therapy*, New York, 1985, Churchill Livingstone, pp 137–168.
6. Nieuwenhuijsen ER, Zemper E, Miner KR, et al: Health behavior change models and theories: contributions to rehabilitation, *Disabil Rehabil* 28:245–256, 2006.
7. World Health Organization: *International classification of impairments, disabilities, and handicaps*, Geneva, 1980, World Health Organization.
8. Nagi SZ: Disability concepts revisited: implications for prevention. In Pope AM, Tarlov AR, editors: *Disability in America: toward a national agenda for prevention*, Washington, D.C., 1991, National Academy Press, pp 309–327.
9. Haley SM, Coster WJ, Ludlow LH, et al: *Pediatric evaluation of disability inventory (PEDI)*, Boston, 1992, New England Medical Center Hospital, Inc, PEDI Research Group.
10. Jette AM: Toward a common language for function, disability, and health, *Phys Ther* 86:726–744, 2006.
11. Phelan EA, Anderson LA, LaCroix AZ, et al: Older adults' view of "successful aging"—How do they compare with researchers' definitions? *J Am Geriatr Soc* 52:211–216, 2004.
12. Guccione AA: *Geriatric physical therapy*, ed 2, St Louis, 2000, Mosby.
13. Sinclair DC, Dangerfield P: *Human growth after birth*, ed 6, New York, 1998, Oxford University Press.
14. Hetzel L, Smith A: *The 65 years and over population: 2000: Census 2000 brief*, Washington, D.C., 2001, United States Census Bureau.
15. Blocker WP: Maintaining functional independence by mobilizing the aged, *Geriatrics* 47:42–56, 1992.
16. Henwood TR, Rick S, Taaffe DR: Strength versus muscle power-specific resistance training in community dwelling older adults, *J Gerontol A Biol Sci Med Sci* 63A(1):83–91, 2008.
17. Hazell T, Kenno K, Jakobi J: Functional benefit of power training for older adults, *J Aging Phys Act* 15:349–359, 2007.
18. Jackson OL, Lang RH: Comprehensive functional assessment of the elderly. In Jackson OL, editor: *Physical therapy of the geriatric patient*, ed 2 New York, 1989, Churchill Livingstone, pp 239–277.
19. National Institute on Aging: *Growing older in America: the health and retirement study*, Bethesda, Md.: NIH Publication No. 07-5757, March, 2007.
20. Wolinsky FD, Stump TE, Callahan CM: Consistency and change in functional status among older adults over time, *J Aging Health* 8:155–182, 1996.
21. Brach JS, Simonsick EM, Kritchevsky S, et al: The association between physical function and lifestyle activity and exercise in the health, aging and body composition study, *J Am Geriatr Soc* 52:502–509, 2004.
22. Kisner C, Colby LA: *Therapeutic exercise: foundations and techniques*, ed 5, Philadelphia, 2007, FA Davis.
23. Northrip JW, Logan GA, McKinney WC: *Introduction to biomechanic analysis of sport*, Dubuque, Iowa, 1974, William C Brown.
24. Malina RM, Bouchard C, Bar-or O: *Growth, maturation, and physical activity*, ed 2, Springfield, Ill, 2004, Human Kinetics Press.
25. Kaplan GA, Shawbridge WT, Camachs T, et al: Factors associated with change in physical functioning in the elderly, *J Aging Health* 5:140–153, 1993.
26. Walker JM, Sue D, Miles-Elkousy N: Active mobility of the extremities in older subjects, *Phys Ther* 64:919–923, 1984.
27. Millelsson LO, Nupponen H, Kaprio J, et al: Adolescent flexibility, endurance strength, and physical activity as predictors of adult tension neck, low back pain, and knee injury: a 25-year follow up study, *Br J Sports Med* 40:107–113, 2006.
28. Costello E, Edelstein JE: Update on falls prevention for community-dwelling older adults: review of single and multifactorial intervention programs, *J Rehabil Res Dev* 45(8):1135–1152, 2008.

29. Rubenstein LZ, Josephson KR: Falls and their prevention in elderly people: what does the evidence show? *Med Clin North Am* 90:807–824, 2006.

30. Lord SR, Clark RD, Webster IW: Physiological factors associated with falls in an elderly population, *J Am Geriatr Soc* 39:1194–1200, 1991.

31. Sturnieks DL, George R, Lord SR: Balance disorders in the elderly, *Clin Neurophysiol* 38:467–478, 2008.

32. Paterson DH, Jones GR, Rice CL: Ageing and physical activity: evidence to develop exercise recommendations for older adults, *Can J Public Health* 98(Suppl 2):S69–S108, 2007.

33. Sherrington C, Whitney JC, Lord SR, et al: Effective exercise for prevention of falls: a systematic review and meta-analysis, *J Am Geriatr Soc* S2:2234–2243, 2008.

34. Oliver I, Hay L, Bard C, et al: Age-related differences in the reaching and grasping coordination in children: unimanual and bimanual tasks, *Exp Brain Res* 179(1):17–27, 2007.

35. Fujiyama H, Garry MI, Levin O, et al: Age-related differences in inhibitory processes during interlimb coordination, *Brain Res* 1262:38–47, 2009.

36. Paquette C, Paquet N, Fung J: Aging affects coordination of rapid head motions with trunk and pelvis movements during standing and walking, *Gait Posture* 24(1):62–69, 2006.

37. Mangine R, Heckman TP, Eldridge VL: Improving strength, endurance and power. In Scully RM, Barnes MR, editors: *Physical therapy*, Philadelphia, 1989, JB Lippincott, pp 739–762.

38. Clemencon M, Hautier CA, Rahmani A, et al: Potential role of optimal velocity as a qualitative factor of physical functional performance in women aged 27 to 96 years, *Arch Phys Med Rehabil* 89:1594–1599, 2008.

39. Hakkinen K, Kraemer WJ, Kallinen M, et al: Bilateral and unilateral neuromuscular function and muscle cross-sectional area in middle-aged and elderly men and women, *J Gerontol A Biol Sci Med Sci* 51A:B21–B29, 1996.

40. Rogers MA, Evans WJ: Changes in skeletal muscle with aging: effects of exercise training, *Exerc Sport Sci Rev* 21:65–102, 1993.

41. Katula JA, Marsh A, Rejeski WJ: Strength training and quality of life in older adults: The POWER Study, *Health Qual Life Outcomes* 6:45, 2008.

42. Cancela JM, Varela S, Ayan C: Effects of high intensity training on elderly women: a pilot study, *Phys Occup Ther Geriatr* 27(2):160–169, 2008.

43. Tanaka H, Seals DR: Endurance exercise performance in masters athletes: age-associated changes and underlying physiological mechanisms, *J Physiol* 586(1):55–63, 2008.

44. Leyk D, Erley O, Ridder D, et al: Age-related changes in marathon and half-marathon performances, *Int J Sports Med* 28(6):513–517, 2007.

SUGGESTED READING

Guccione AA: Physical therapy diagnosis and the relationship between impairments and function, *Phys Ther* 71:499–504, 1991.

Purath J, Buchholz SW, Kark DL: Physical fitness assessment of older adults in the primary care setting, *J Am Acad Nurse Pract* 21(2):101–107, 2009.

Singh AS, Chin A Paw MJM, Bosscher RJ, et al: Cross sectional relationship between physical fitness components and functional performance in older persons living in long-term care facilities, *BMC Geriatr* 6:4, 2006.

CHAPTER 2

Theories Affecting Development

OBJECTIVES

After studying this chapter, the reader will be able to:

1. Define domains, periods, and concepts of development.
2. Discuss concepts of growth, maturation, adaptation, and learning in all developmental domains.

3. Identify theories of life span development.
4. Discuss how specific biophysical, psychological, and sociocultural theories are related to function at various ages.

Development is a topic covered in many professional education curricula, including biology, education, psychology, sociology, and health sciences programs. Each discipline focuses on aspects of development unique to its profession, and significant amounts of information exist within these specialized areas. Our collective knowledge substantiates that an individual develops across the broad continuum of the life span, strongly influenced by three interrelated domains. Thus normal human development is shaped by interaction between the biophysical, psychological, and sociocultural domains.

A general introduction to biophysical, psychological, and sociocultural theories of development describes how the different domains and disciplines are basic to our lives and the study of human behavior. For example, a child in the United States learns to eat with a fork within the first year of life. This social skill cannot develop until physical coordination is sufficiently advanced to allow fine controlled movements of the arm and hand. The child must cognitively understand the relationship between food, the fork, hunger, and the action taken to satisfy that hunger. Social customs shape how the child performs the skill. In fact, an Asian child will be meeting the same functional need at about the same age but will be using chopsticks.

HUMAN DEVELOPMENT

Human development refers to changes that occur in our lives from conception to death. Change can occur on many levels: the cell, tissue, organ, body systems, and in physical, psychological, and social domains. Change can be progressive, reorganizational, or regressive. In muscle, for example, where tissue increases during growth,

fiber types differentiate or atrophy because of use, loss of innervation, and nutrition. Form and function change during the process of development, as occurs when a sapling grows into an oak tree or a caterpillar turns into a butterfly. The form a movement takes is shaped by its intended function. Because functional demands vary with age, the movement forms that emerge during development change. Function or the way in which the body and its parts are used can change over time and can result in structural changes. Human behavior is the outward manifestation of development and changes through four processes: growth, maturation, adaptation, and learning. These processes occur simultaneously and concurrently in all domains of human development.

Domains of Development

The process of growth, maturation, adaptation, and learning operate at the same time in three different domains: biophysical, psychological, and sociocultural. Physical growth and development are accompanied by the acquisition of motor skills, intellectual development, and socioemotional development. For example, intellectually an infant may be unable to communicate verbally or even understand her own physical actions. The parent supplies meaning to the gestures, looks, or early sound production. This shapes the infant's actions to her parents' expectations for motor performance or communication. Thus, we, as parents, may interpret a random swipe as a reach or the sound "ma" as recognition of mother.

We see the interrelationships of development in multiple domains when the infant develops perceptual awareness concurrently with motor control, beginning cognition, and attachment. A social smile is evident in most 2-month-old infants, although it usually takes 2 additional months before the infant demonstrates sufficient head control to focus attention on caregivers or objects and to be able to direct reaching. This process of human development is interactive, and each domain exerts a positive or negative impact on the other domains. The temperament of a baby can affect the quality of interaction with the caregiver or therapist and thereby affect the attachment process. The biophysical, psychological, and sociocultural selves interact to produce a unique individual. Therefore, no two people are exactly alike.

Each domain contributes to our understanding of motor behavior. We are biological organisms that develop within a psychological and sociocultural environment. This relationship is schematically represented in Figure 1-4 Even though our primary therapeutic emphasis is on our client's ability to move, as therapists we must consider cognitive and psychosocial status, as well as the familial, cultural, and societal movement and life expectations. Indeed, motor behavior will reflect age, ability, level of maturation, experience, and cultural bias.

Periods of Development

The life span is most often divided into age-related segments or periods (Table 2-1). The prenatal period averages 38 weeks in length, beginning with conception

and culminating in birth. It is divided into three stages: the *germinal* period, the first 2 weeks of gestation; the *embryonic* period, when all major organ systems form (weeks 2 to 8); and the *fetal* period, when organ systems differentiate and rapid body growth occurs (weeks 9 to 38).

The lengthy postnatal period is usually divided into the categories of infancy, childhood, adolescence, and adulthood. *Infancy* spans the first 2 years of life, from birth to the second birthday. *Childhood* begins at 2 years of age for both girls and boys but ends at different ages because of the time difference in the onset of puberty. Classically, *adolescence* lasts 8 years, beginning at approximately age 10 for girls and age 12 for boys. It is divided into three stages: *prepubescence,* the 2 years before the onset of puberty; *pubescence,* the 4 years in which hormones produce secondary sexual characteristics; and *postpubescence*, the final 2 years of adolescence in which the final maturity of adulthood is reached.

Adulthood is concerned less with age than with role transition. Most of us are considered adult when we reach our 20s. Going to college, getting a job, and being able to vote have all been used as markers of adulthood, but no one task or age clearly defines this period. In fact, Jeffrey Arnett[1] has made a strong case that the transition from adolescence to adulthood is protracted and has introduced a new developmental stage he calls emerging adulthood. His theory of adult development will be discussed further in that section. For now adulthood can be divided loosely into young, middle, and older adulthood. Although transitions have been identified among the various divisions of adulthood, none appear to be as easily defined as the periods of child development.

Geriatrics and gerontology were established as fields of human service and research in the 1950s. Since that time, the field of gerontology has fostered an explosion of information on aging. Demographics document that the population continues to age. There were almost 37 million people age 65 and over living in the United States in 2006. This accounted for just over 12% of the total population.[2] By 2050, there are projected to be 21 million people over 85 years of age (Figure 2-1). The population of the oldest-old, those 85 years or older, went from 100,000 in 1990 to 5.3 million in 2006. The older Hispanic population is postulated to grow the fastest over the next decades. As research continues to focus on the oldest citizens, older adulthood has been divided into young-old, middle-old, and oldest-old. Many studies are only focusing on centenarians or those over age 100.

Table 2-1

Periods of Development

Period	Time Span
Prenatal	Conception to birth
• Germinal	• 1-2 weeks' gestation
• Embryonic	• 2-8 weeks' gestation
• Fetal	• 9-38 weeks' gestation
Infancy	Birth to 2 yr
Childhood	2-10 yr (female)
	2-12 yr (male)
Adolescence	10-18 yr (female)
	12-20 yr (male)
Young adulthood	18-40 yr
Middle adulthood	40-65 yr
Older adulthood	65 yr to death
• Young-old	• 65-74 yr
• Middle-old	• 75-84 yr
• Oldest-old	• 85 yr to death

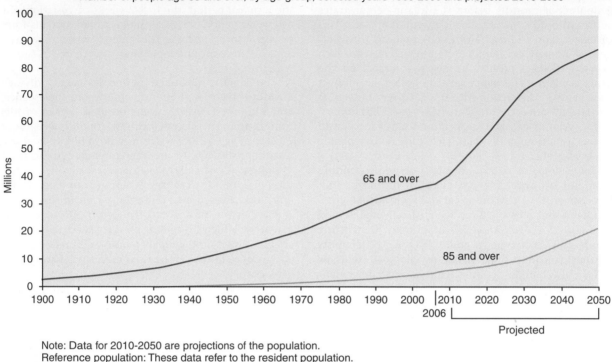

Number of people age 65 and over, by age group, selected years 1900-2006 and projected 2010-2050

Note: Data for 2010-2050 are projections of the population.
Reference population: These data refer to the resident population.
Source: U.S. Census Bureau, Decennial Census, Population Estimates and Projections.

Figure 2-1 Number of older Americans. (From Federal Interagency Forum on Aging-Related Statistics: *Older Americans 2008: key indicators of well-being* (website): www.agingstats.gov/. Accessed March 3, 2009.)

Concepts of Development

Maturity

Development from birth to the attainment of biophysical, psychological, and sociocultural maturity constitutes the first part of the life span. *Maturation* is the process whereby an organism continues to grow, differentiate, and change from conception until achieving the mature state. Maturity is usually attained during adulthood between 25 and 30 years of age. Biological maturation is typically attributed to an individual's genetic makeup, whereas psychological and social-emotional maturity results from a combination of maturation and learning. Maturation is not considered the only determinant of development.

Senescence

Development continues throughout adulthood with structural and functional changes seen as a normal part of healthy aging. Therefore, aging can be viewed as a continuation of the developmental process. The term *senescence*, however, is appropriately used to describe later life because aging can refer to any time-related process. *Senescence* is the progressive physiological decline that results in our increasing vulnerability to stress and the progressing likelihood of death. Just like other phases of development, senescence is not a single process but rather many processes. Age-related changes produced in our organ systems and personal identity result from a lifetime of interactions between our internal environment, culture, and society.

Life Span

The concept of life span development is not new. Baltes[3] originally identified five characteristics to use when assessing a theory for its life span perspective. The following list reflects the original four criteria and a new fifth one used to view development from a lifelong perspective:
- Lifelong
- Multidimensional
- Plastic
- Embedded in history
- Multicausal

Recently Baltes, Lindenberger, and Staudinger[4] revisited the theoretical underpinnings of life span theory. They reinforced the idea that development is *not* complete at maturity. The multidimensional quality of life span theory provides a complete framework for ontogenesis (development). Culture and the knowledge gained from all domains make a significant impact on a person's life course. Biological plasticity is accompanied by cultural competence, so there is a gain/loss dynamic that occurs during development. There are no gains without losses and no losses without gains. In essence this is the adaptive capacity of the person. Context, the original fifth criteria, has been replaced by the multicausal meaning that one can arrive at the same destination by different means or by a combination of means. Life span development is not constrained to travel a single course or developmental trajectory.

No one period of life can be understood without looking at its relationship to what came before and what lies ahead. History affects development in three ways as seen in Figure 2-2. The normative age-graded influence is seen in those developmental tasks described by Havighurst[5] for each period of development. Age-graded physical, psychological, and social milestones would fall into this category. Walking at 12 months and obtaining a driver's license at 16 years of age are examples of a physical age-graded task. Understanding simple concepts, such as all round objects bounce and getting along with same age peers in adolescence, are examples from the psychological and social domains. Secondly, normative history-graded influences come from the effect of when a person is born. Each of us is part of a birth cohort or group. Some of us are baby boomers and others are millennials. All people in an age cohort share the same history of events such as World War II, the Challenger disaster, or the terrorist attack of 9/11. When you were born makes a difference in expectations and behaviors; these historical events shape the life of the cohort. The last history-related influence

comes from things that happen to a person that have no norms or no expectations such as winning the lottery, losing a parent, or having a developmental disability. These are part of your own unique personal history. Life span development provides a holistic framework in which aging is a lifelong process of growing up and growing old. Development within the biophysical, psychological, and sociocultural domains is enriched when viewed through a life span perspective.

Life span is also defined as the maximum survival potential for a particular species. Most gerontologists agree that our life span is species specific and therefore intrinsically regulated. Theoretically, the maximum length of life biologically possible for a human is 120 years, although documentation exists for one individual who lived to be 122. Numerous social and environmental factors, such as war, famine, radiation, and toxic chemicals, can negatively affect this figure. Although catastrophic disease is often thought to dramatically shorten our life spans, statistics reveal that if all major causes of death were eradicated, only 15 years would be added to our life expectancy.[6]

Individual Differences

The development of human behavior is strongly influenced by both maturation and experience. Genetically, we are provided the physical base of our body that continually matures during our life span. The complete set of genes that are inherited is one's *genotype*. Each of us builds a sense of identity and psychological wholeness within our mind, influenced by experiences within the social environment of our family, culture, and society. The genetic instructions along with these environmental influences produce a *phenotype,* a person's physical, psychological, and behavioral features. The interplay of maturation and experience is unique for each individual (Figure 2-3).

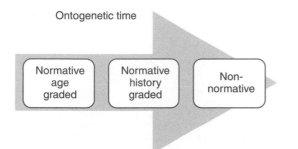

Figure 2-2 Three major biocultural influences on life span development.

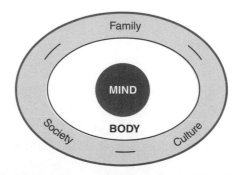

Figure 2-3 Depiction of the relationship of an individual's psychological (mind) and physical (body) self within the sociocultural environment.

Intelligence and personality can be influenced by the environment and heredity. Children exposed to enriched environments often improve their native intelligence. Conversely, environmental deprivation may contribute to a decrease in intellectual performance. Heredity can also influence the type of experiences an individual seeks, such as finding our niche in the world.[7] Picking a place for one's self in society by seeking social environments that fit with the person's heredity is called niche-picking.[7] Sociability has a genetic component that affects whether a child enjoys social interaction or prefers to observe the world from a distance. Shy children will tend to seek situations that allow peace and quiet, whereas extroverted children seek social contact. Researchers have found that environmental influences are what make siblings different within the same family. Despite the same parenting, siblings' social and cognitive development differ.[8]

Longevity is affected by genetics, environment, race, gender, and ethnicity. Heredity accounts for about 35% of our longevity.[9] In other words, one predictor of a longer life is to come from a family of long-lived people. The remaining 65% of our longevity is attributed to environmental influences: lifestyle as well as physical and social surroundings. Lifestyle factors considered to affect longevity include smoking, diet, stress, alcohol consumption, and exercise. Living in a hostile physical or social environment also can be counterproductive to a long life. African Americans have a shorter life expectancy than European Americans by about 5 years.[10] "Hispanic Americans' life expectancy exceeds European Americans at all ages, despite access problems to health care for many.[7]" Women in general live longer than men. However, when studying centenarians, Perls and Terry[11] found that despite the fact that men make up only 15 % of the over 100 population, they performed better in terms of cognitive and physical function. So women may be better off than men between the ages of 65 and 89 but do not do as well as men when they survive beyond 90 years of age.

Processes of Development

Growth refers to the changes in physical dimensions of the body. Growth rates vary for specific body systems and tissues. Figure 2-4 provides a comparison of the general growth curve with that of specific systems and tissues. The general growth curve reflects rapid growth in infancy, slower growth in childhood, and again rapid growth in adolescence. Head circumference, height, and weight are all examples of dimensions that can be used to assess growth and can be plotted on growth charts. Changes in growth can be used to assess development by comparing the percentile growth achieved in these anthropometrical measures. Growth that falls between the 10th and 90th percentiles is considered normal. Large variations among these measurements, such as when height and weight are at radically different percentiles, may signal a growth problem. Healthy children exhibit stable trends in growth through the developmental stages of life, although different body sections grow at proportionately different rates (Figure 2-5).

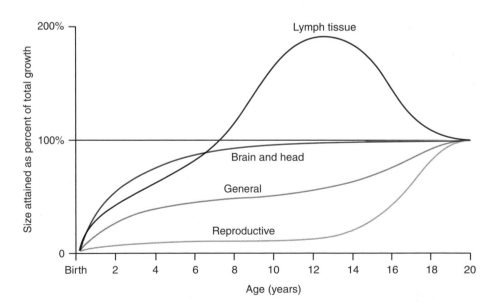

Figure 2-4 Differential rates of growth in three organ systems and tissues with the body's general growth curve.

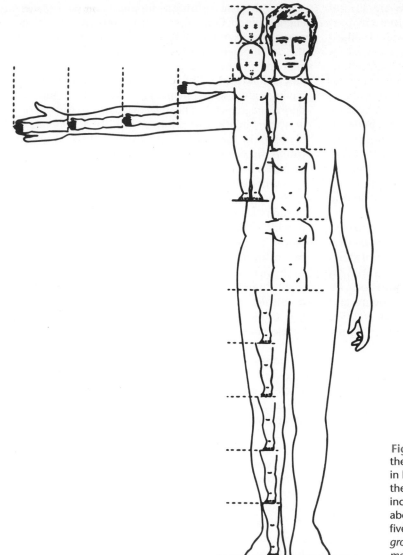

Figure 2-5 Proportional growth changes across the life span. While the whole body increases in length from birth to maturity, the length of the head increases about two times, the trunk increases about three times, the arms increase about four times, and legs increase about five times. (From Valadian I, Porter D: *Physical growth and development: from conception to maturity*, Boston, 1977, Little, Brown.)

Maturation contributes to development by producing physical changes that cause organs and body systems to reach their adult form and function. Changes that occur on a genetically controlled timetable can usually be attributed to the process of physical maturation. Maturation occurs in all body systems. One example from the skeletal system is the appearance of primary and secondary ossification centers in the bones (see Chapter 6). Reflexes and reactions emerge sequentially in response to maturation of the nervous system; myelination is one hallmark of nervous system maturation. Structures that function first are myelinated first,

thus paralleling the development of function of those neuroanatomical structures (see Chapter 9). The integrity of nervous system development can be assessed by evaluating the presence of developmentally appropriate reflexes and reactions. The genetic substrate of behavior does not simply imprint its code on the environment; rather, the genetic base allows us to adapt to our environment. The environment can also influence maturation through adaptation and learning.

Adaptation and learning are sometimes difficult to separate from maturation. *Adaptation* is the body's accommodation to the immediate environment. Some structures and functions of organ systems are adaptations to exposure to the internal or external environment. Adaptation, like development, can produce positive or negative change. A positive change is exhibited by the production of antibodies after exposure to chicken pox. An example of negative environmental effect has been seen in the delayed motor behavior of understimulated, institutionalized infants.[12] Exposure to some type of stimulus induces change, such as development of joints in the embryo, which requires primitive muscles to pull on bone to produce a joint cavity. If the muscles fail to produce movement, joint deformities occur in utero and result in *arthrogryposis*. Although each of us adapts differently, we all mature at varying rates in a similar manner.

Learning is a relatively permanent change in behavior resulting from practice and, as such, may be considered a form of adaptation. For example, rollerblading, or in-line skating, is an adaptation to having wheels on our shoes. To adapt to having wheels on our shoes, we must learn different ways to balance, start moving, and stop. To rollerblade takes practice. Many motor abilities, such as riding a bike, playing soccer, reading, writing, and speaking a foreign languages are learned. We do not know if there is an optimal time for learning these tasks. We do know that experience plays a crucial role in mastering abilities that are not innate.

Factors Affecting Development

The process of development is strongly influenced by four factors: genetics, maturation, environment, and culture. None of these influences alone can account for the many changes that occur throughout our life span. The interaction between maturation and experience within specific biophysical, psychological, and sociocultural domains may account for individual differences. Two children grow up in the same neighborhood; one becomes a CEO for a Fortune 500 companys and the other becomes a homeless drifter. What makes the difference? The values and life goals inherited from our family, society, and culture are just as real as our biological heritage.

Genetics and maturation contribute to and control our body's internal environment or milieu. The body's internal chemistry must be balanced to support growth, development, and functional activities such as movement. Hormones play a major role in controlling physical growth and initiating puberty, and they regulate the body's metabolism and ability to use chemical sources of energy for growth, maturation, adaptation, and learning.

Nutrition is part of the internal and external environment and contributes to the production of a healthy body. Adequate nutrition supplies fuel for efficient energy production, tissue development, and tissue repair. For example, adequate nutrition is critical for the development and function of the nervous system, enabling the execution and control of movement. A lack of folic acid is linked to an increased likelihood of having a child with a neural tube defect. Poor nutrition during pregnancy has been associated with intrauterine growth retardation, a significant cause of developmental disability in low-birth-weight infants. Prenatal malnutrition can cause permanent stunting of brain development. Fat must be present in the diet to produce myelin. Effects of nutritional deprivation on brain development have been so thoroughly established that U.S. manufacturers have added supplements to baby formula to provide sufficient fatty acids for nervous system maturation. Postnatal growth is supported by the secretion of growth hormones (see Chapter 11). Infants who fail to thrive (i.e., do not gain sufficient weight at an appropriate rate) have poorer motor skills than do adequately nourished peers. Inadequate nutrition especially during periods of rapid growth can have long-lasting effects on development. Appropriate nutrition supports prenatal and postnatal development.

Our external environment or surroundings and culture contribute to the definition of personal nutrition. There is a vast nutritional difference between having rice and fish as dietary mainstays and having red meat and potatoes. These two different diets have been associated with Asian and Western cultures, respectively, and have been linked to differing incidences of illness. Asian eating habits contribute to lower mortality from heart disease.[13] "In developed countries, almost as many cancer cases are attributable to an unhealthy diet and an inactive lifestyle as to smoking.[14]" Studies of the age at onset of puberty highlight the effect of adequate nutrition and health. In countries where health and nutrition are adequate, menarche occurs earlier than in countries with poorer health care and nutrition.[15] The effects of inadequate nutrition are painfully obvious in areas of the world that experience food shortages.

Culture helps us identify values and determine the task demands and roles that we play. There are similarities between cultural expectations as well as differences. Cultural expectations affect child-rearing practices and the attainment of adult status especially in selecting activities/actions that represent role transitions. Cultures vary in their focus on an individual or the group. Western cultures tend to focus on the individual, whereas Eastern cultures are collectivistic systems where the group is more important than the individual.

THEORETICAL ASSUMPTIONS

The theoretical approach used to describe human development provides a framework for a discussion of the reasons for change and allows us to test our hypotheses regarding the ability of a theory to predict future development. The major assumptions about development center on the role of maturation and learning and on the nature of developmental change over time. Theories and theorists differ in the way in which the origin of behavior is viewed. Is behavior innate, or is it a product of our experiences? Maturationists argue that our genetic blueprint produces commonalities in our growth and development. Behaviorists take the stand that experience plays a strong role in our personal and social development.

The theorists discussed here have tried to explain the nature of developmental change over time (Table 2-2).

All agree that orderly, sequential changes from simple to complex behavior occur in all domains of function. They differ on whether these changes occur in a smooth, continuous manner (continuity, or nonstage development) or with abrupt stops and starts (discontinuity, or stage development).

Continuity of development implies that later development is dependent on what came before. If development is viewed as continuous, earlier skills lead to the development of later skills. Continuity can be observed in psychological development.[16] In Erikson's theory,[17] successful resolution of each psychological dilemma is required to proceed to the next level. Development of cognition can be thought of as a continuous line from start to finish.

Stage theory provides another approach and can be thought of quantitatively: a stair-step arrangement specifies different motor skills, such as head control or

Table 2-2

Theories of Human Development

Domain	Life Span	Child Development	Adulthood	Senescence

Biophysical	Dynamic Systems
	• Thelen and Smith
	• Shroots and Yates
		Maturation
		• Gesell
				Programmed Aging
				• Hayflick
				• Free Radical/
				  Oxidative Damage
				• Harman Immune/
				  Neuroendocrine

Psychological	Stages of Psychosocial Development • Erikson	Stages of Intelligence • Piaget	Career Consolidation • Valliant	Cognitive Processing Speed • Salthouse
		Perceptual-Cognitive • Gibson	Emerging Adulthood • Arnett	Cognitive Reserve • Stern
		Information Processing	Seasons of Life • Levinson	
		Memory and Learning		
Sociocultural	Social Learning • Bandura	Behaviorist • Skinner Temperament • Thomas and Chess Attachment • Bowlby	Keeper of Meaning • Valliant	Selective Optimization with Compensation • Baltes
	Motivation • Maslow	Social Learning • Sears	Family Systems	Disengagement Activity
	Environmental • Bronfenbrenner	Zone of Proximal Development • Vygotsky Play	Leisure	Continuity

sitting on each step. Stage theory also postulates that there are qualitative changes that occur throughout development. At each successively higher level of development, or next step, a new characteristic appears that was not previously present. In stage development, discontinuity is more prevalent than continuity in motor development. For example, sitting and standing are sufficiently different to be considered stages in motor development, not continuous events.

A third viewpoint related to development is that of thinking that a child is a miniature adult. In some parts of the skeletal system, where miniature models of bones are first formed out of cartilage and then replaced by bone, it might appear that the theory is correct. Differential growth, however, occurs in the bones of the face during puberty, so that the adolescent looks much different from the child. Many body systems do not function on an adult level in the child. Because there are more instances in which this theory does not hold true, it is typically not accepted.

It is important to understand that theories provide a starting point from which to assess the complex process of human development. Regardless of the domain considered, theories attempt to explain why changes can and do occur over time. The time span covered by each developmental theory varies greatly. For example, Piaget's theory of intelligence begins at birth and ends in adolescence. Levinson's theory deals exclusively with adult development, a less well understood phenomenon than either early or later development. Erikson's theory of personality development is the most easily recognized life span approach because his theory accounts for changes that occur from birth to senescence.

LIFE SPAN THEORIES OF DEVELOPMENT

Biophysical Development

Most theories of biophysical development focus on one age group. The only theoretical approach that remotely approximates a life span perspective is the *dynamic systems theory*. Researchers from developmental psychology and gerontology have applied dynamic systems theory to early development and aging.[18,19] Lockman and Thelen[18] introduced the term *development biodynamics* to explain the organization of motor behavior based on interaction between perception and action. According to this theory, motor behavior emerges from that interaction rather than from nervous system maturation, as previously theorized. The relationship of dynamic systems theory to motor development is discussed in Chapter 3.

Dynamic systems theory grew out of *chaos theory*, which originated in mathematics and physical science to explain change over time in nonlinear systems. As a biological system, the human organism is an open system. Open systems are more complex. The human organism interacts with the internal and external environment. Open systems self-organize. "Dynamic systems theory hypothesizes that internal or external fluctuations of nonequilibrium systems can pass a critical point (transformation point) and create order out of disorder through a process of self-organization.[19]" Energy is used in the development of a single cell into interacting organ systems. Living systems exhibit periods of stability or equilibrium and periods of disequilibrium. During the period of disequilibrium, significant change may occur. Energy is also used to keep the body going, make repairs, and preserve capacities in all systems. Living systems fluctuate and behave in complex ways.

Schroots and Yates[19] applied dynamic systems theory to development and aging because they saw development and senescence as having similar features. These common features are (1) change over time, with gradients; (2) tapping of energy resources; and (3) the production of new structures and functions. Each new structure and function adds new dynamic constraints and information to the body through feedback to the genetic blueprint. Differences between early development and senescence are the degree and rate of change that take place. During early development, the system is highly changeable; when maturity is reached, the system is more stable. The rate of change is faster during early development and slower during senescence. The first processes are negentropic or anabolic and initially obscure the ongoing entropic or catabolic process of senescence. Homeodynamics is the process whereby complex systems maintain stability. The concept goes beyond homeostasis, which implies a static condition. In homeodynamics, the body's systems are working dynamically to cope with an ever-changing internal metabolism.

However, after maturity around the age of 30, the entropic processes dominate and lead to disorder.[20] The more disordered the system, the more vulnerable it is to disease and degradation, and eventual cessation of activity.

Psychological Development

Erikson[17] transformed Freud's psychoanalytical theory into a psychosocial view of human development. Erikson's view combined biological needs with cultural expectations, producing the most broadly applicable theory of human psychological development for

Table 2-3

Erikson's Eight Stages of Development

Life Span Period	Stage	Characteristics
Infancy	Trust vs. mistrust	Self-trust, attachment
Late infancy	Autonomy vs. shame or doubt	Independence, self-control
Childhood (preschool)	Initiative vs. guilt	Initiates own activity
School age	Industry vs. inferiority	Works on projects for recognition
Adolescence	Identity vs. role confusion	Sense of self: physically, socially, sexually
Early adulthood	Intimacy vs. isolation	Relationship with significant other
Middle adulthood	Generativity vs. stagnation	Guiding the next generation
Late adulthood	Ego integrity vs. despair	Sense of wholeness, vitality, and wisdom

From Erikson EH: *Identity, youth, and crisis*, New York, 1986, WW Norton.

present-day society by replacing Freud's sexual focus with traits of social interaction. Erikson also addressed the entire life span in his eight stages of psychosocial development, as outlined in Table 2-3 and discussed in detail later. These stages incorporate more than one domain of function and are identified as necessary for an individual's growth. Each revolves around a psychosocial conflict that must be resolved to advance in the developmental process. Interestingly, as Erikson aged, his work increasingly dealt with adult stages and aging. He and his colleagues[21] looked at generational differences and the role of expectations in aging.

Stage 1

The infant's first psychosocial conflict is whether to trust or mistrust the people within the world. Through physical contact and caregiving, the infant forms positive attachments that are mutually reinforcing. If a positive attachment does not occur, negative attachments or mistrust of others, of the environment, and even of self result. The basis of trust is seen in the establishment of positive contact with the environment and the people in it, including touch and the meeting of the infant's needs.

Stage 2

In toddlers, the basic trust learned in infancy is enhanced by resolving the next psychosocial conflict. The toddler expresses newfound independence using both motor and social skills, with the ever-popular statement, "Me do it." It is important during this stage that the toddler be permitted to be as independent as possible to prevent feelings of doubt concerning emerging abilities.

Learning to control one's movements and those of people and objects within the environment is very important in early development. However, with the assertion of this newfound independence can come conflict between the child's wants and parental boundaries, as seen in the so-called terrible twos.

Stage 3

Self-regulation develops slowly in the third stage as the child learns the boundaries of appropriate social behavior. Just as an infant learns the rules of moving by experimenting with movement, the child experiments with learning how to behave socially. A growing sense of identity plus parental guidance allow for the development of self-regulation, whether that means becoming toilet trained, learning to share, or learning to take turns. Between 3 and 5 years, the preschooler has learned to master many tasks and feels free to initiate her own activities. By teaching the child which behaviors are acceptable under what circumstances, the parents encourage the child's confidence in her own planning without fear of a negative result or the burden of guilt. During this time, the parents' most important task is to encourage self-regulation of behavior. When a child begins to regulate her own behavior, she begins to rely on internalized value and reward systems.

Stage 4

The school-age child deals with the conflict between industry and inferiority. The initiative developed in the previous stage is applied to learning how to work hard on a project and to enjoy the satisfaction of a job done well. A positive self-image grows out of achievement. Without success, the child may learn to be helpless, which in turn can produce a negative self-image. The initial self-image formed between 2 and 3 years of age is expanded during middle childhood in the struggle with success or failure in school. As the student increases awareness of her values, goals, and strategies, she becomes more sensitive to the needs and expectations of others. It is during this time that tasks are often undertaken to gain the approval of a favorite teacher.

Stage 5

Adolescence produces one of the most trying psychosocial dilemmas: identity versus role confusion. An adolescent's identity is a unique blend of what she was in childhood and what she will become in adulthood. Identity formation is affected by social and sexual experiences, cognitive abilities, and self-knowledge. An adolescent must be capable of the highest level of cognition to ponder the philosophical question of "Who am I?" Anticipation of what she will do in a variety of situations causes her to enact every possible life scenario before it actually transpires. Self-knowledge is gleaned from past life experiences. This knowledge includes physical information gained from the five senses as well as knowledge of bodily functions. Emotionally, self-knowledge includes self-esteem and self-image.

The self is very important to the adolescent, so much so that self-centeredness or egocentrism engenders a feeling of performing on stage. Although emotions are part of adolescent development, they play only one role in the development of a stable identity: achievement of emotional independence from parents and other adults. Socially, the adolescent is expected to develop appropriate behavior toward her own and the opposite sex. Sexual identity is established along with a moral ideology to guide socially responsible behavior. The successful end result is a unique and stable view of self, a life philosophy, and a career path. The pursuit of a career or vocation allows the adolescent to move away from her previous egocentrism.[17]

The term *role confusion* describes the failure to form an identity during adolescence. Role confusion may result if adequate support systems are not available. The inability to form an identity leaves an adolescent confused about her role in society and makes it difficult to formulate a life philosophy, forge a career, or start a family.

Stage 6

Once an identity has been established, the young adult must deal with the conflict of intimacy versus isolation. Forming an intimate relationship with a significant other involves sharing the values, hopes, goals, and fears found during the search for identity. A person learns to share love in many different forms: parental love, spousal love, child love, friend love, and spiritual love. The negative result from losing the battle for intimacy is to become self-absorbed and unable to relate openly with other people. Social and emotional isolation may lead to an overly developed sense of righteousness and outward prejudice toward those with whom we disagree.

Stage 7

Generativity is an unconscious desire to guide and assist the next generation. The traditional way that this assistance is given is through parenting, but it can also be expressed through an occupation such as teaching or an avocation such as Big Brother or Big Sisters. At the age of 80, Erikson[21] wrote that making creative contributions to the world and caring for other people's children could substitute for having our own children. The common denominator in this stage is fostering another's well-being. To help others, we must be productive and creative. Stagnation and cynicism are alternatives to generativity—the "Is that all there is?" attitude toward life.

Stage 8

The last hurdle of development is the conflict between integrity and despair—not ethical integrity, but ego integrity; a sense of wholeness of self related to the life already lived and life yet to be experienced. There is a sense of vitality, expectation, and wisdom that comes from the life cycle being reflected back on itself.[21] If the older adult does not achieve ego integrity because inner resources from successful handling of previous psychosocial dilemmas have not been built up, despair replaces vitality.

Realistically, we understand that all determinants of late life satisfaction are not under our control. The body ages physically as well as psychologically. The physical self and the life situation, including socioeconomic status, activity level, and availability of transportation, have an impact on successful aging. There is a complex relationship between internal and external factors that shape the end result of a process that includes our past achievements and how we reacted to them. The task of coming to terms with how we led our life, the choices made, and the paths not taken is not easy. The challenge is best met with a strong sense of self-respect and good sense of humor, remembering that "No one gets through this life alive."

Sociocultural Development

Social Learning

Bandura's social learning theory explains observational learning.[22] As such, it may be more relevant to understanding the abstract learning that occurs from adolescence through adulthood. However, an essential process in Bandura's cognitive social learning theory is that of *modeling*. Modeling is described as a type of cognitive patterning. Some skills are taught directly by modeling the behavior being taught, such as having a child watch an adult sweep the floor. More complicated behaviors, such as learning values and developing problem-solving approaches are transmitted more subtly. Adults are always amazed at what behaviors children pick up.

Social theory teaches us that experience is invaluable. We register personal experience with reference to our own level of biological and psychological maturity. A parent's raising her voice to a toddler may stop the child from an unwanted activity, but verbal warnings often go unnoticed by a teenager. Experience by itself is only an occurrence in time; experience paired with memory connotes learning. The pairing is possible because of the interaction between behavior, cognition, and the environment. Each area influences another; cognition can influence the environment, and the environment can influence behavior. For example, teaching children not to play with matches does not preclude them from learning how to safely light a campfire.

Observational learning is used in the socialization process of becoming a professional. Expectations play a large role in structuring or motivating performance. The clinical instructor expects a certain level of performance from a student therapist, and that expectation motivates the student to perform. Thus the reality that is observed in the clinic is more highly valued than a laboratory simulation. Learning is not the result of a single event but of many events within a context of interpersonal relationships.

Motivation

Maslow[23] generated a theory to counteract the seemingly nonhumanistic approach of the psychoanalysts and the behaviorists. His theory of motivation is based on his perceived human needs hierarchy (Figure 2-6) in which each life stage is seen from the perspective of fulfilling a specific need. We all have an innate drive to survive, grow, and find meaning to life. The sequence of needs progresses from the physiological needs related to survival and safety to the needs for love, self-esteem, and ultimately, self-actualization. The last stage occurs when we have become all that is possible for us to be, and it cannot be achieved unless all other needs have been met.

Ecology

Bronfenbrenner's ecological systems approach is the application of the biological concept of studying organisms in their natural habitat or ecosystem to human

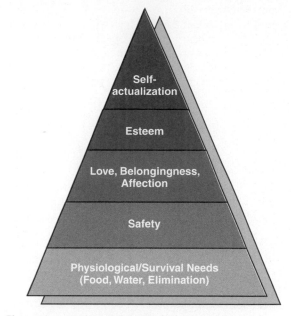

Figure 2-6 Maslow's hierarchy of needs.

development.[24] For example, a biologist studies trout in a trout stream, not in a saltwater marsh. The model in Figure 2-7 represents Bronfenbrenner's perception of the family, community, and culture as interacting systems of society. Each system is named for its relationship to the child and encompasses an ever-widening sphere of influence. The child interacts with the members of the family, community, and culture, and they in turn act on the child. The mesosystem connects the various microsystems as they are likely to influence one another. The exosystem does not affect the child directly but indirectly as it represents social settings. All three of these systems are embedded in the macrosystem. Research has focused on the effects of the varying levels of the system on developmental competence, child-rearing practices and developmental outcome, and parental attitudes within neighborhoods.[25]

THEORIES OF CHILD DEVELOPMENT

Biophysical Development

Maturationists

The maturationist's view of motor development correlates all movement acquisition with the onset of changes in the nervous system relative to the onset and integration of reflexes/reactions, hierarchy of control, and a timetable of myelination. As biologists, maturationists

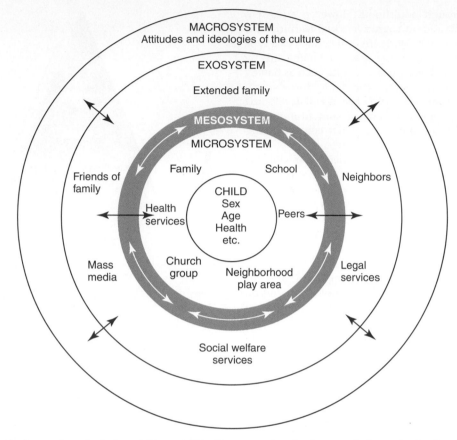

Figure 2-7 Bronfenbrenner's ecological model is one of the few comprehensive frameworks for understanding the role of the environment in the child's development. (From Kopp CB, Krakow JB: *The child: development in a social context*, 1982. Reprinted by permission of Pearson Education, Inc.)

might have considered the possibility that the maturation of other tissues, such as muscle or bone, could contribute to movement production. However, the theory was based on the idea that central nervous system maturation was the primary determinant of motor behavior. Gesell and McGraw are the primary proponents of a biological maturation theory of development. Our discussion will be confined to Gesell's contributions.

Gesell[26] coined the term *reciprocal interweaving* to describe the spiral-like development that alternates between periods of equilibrium and disequilibrium (Figure 2-8). Periods of equilibrium are marked by stable behavior, whereas periods of disequilibrium are marked by instability. The cycles occur frequently in the first year of life and decrease in frequency with increasing maturity. For example, head control in a newborn is relatively good. The newborn is able to hold the head in the midline if she is held upright and is able to lift

the head when held at one's shoulder or in the prone position. At 2 months, the head appears to be more wobbly; but at 4 months, control is again excellent in upright and in the prone position. The cycle of stability, instability, and regained stability is evident in the development of head control and the pattern of prone progression.

The maturationists attributed developmental change to genetics and tended to ignore the role of experience. Gesell and associates[26] studied motor development as a means to understand mental development. They applied the concept of reciprocal interweaving to all types of behavior: motor adaptive, linguistic, and personal-social. In the process, Gesell became known as the "father of developmental testing." Gesell viewed motor development as the physical entity that allowed functional behavior. A believer in structure, he defined stages of motor development that he thought

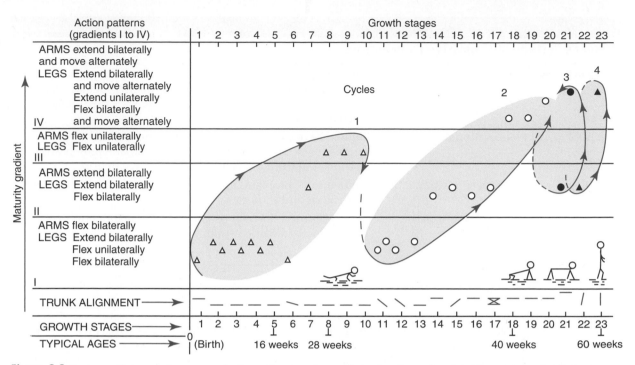

Figure 2-8 Reciprocal interweaving as seen in the patterning of prone behavior. (From Gesell A: The ontogenesis of infant behavior. In Carmichael L, editor: *Manual of child psychology*, ed 2, New York, 1954, John Wiley & Sons, pp 335-373.)

governed behavior during each age period. Gesell also recognized the role of individual differences in temperament as a variable during the development of stability and change in motor patterns.

Psychological Development

Intelligence

Piaget, a well-known developmental psychologist, identified four periods of cognitive development in children: sensorimotor, preoperational, concrete operational, and formal operational.[27] Each period is characterized by different ways of interacting with the environment, as identified in Table 2-4 and described in detail later. His theory explained how humans acquire and process information about the world. His theory of how children learn to think is predicated on an active construction of cognitive ability. Some researchers have questioned the exact ages that children demonstrate these abilities. Even Piaget recognized that children move through the periods and stages at their own rate, but he thought that the sequence was invariant.

Piaget[27] identified two basic functions of all organisms that make this mastery possible. The first function

is the individual's ability to *organize,* which is to make a coherent whole out of the parts. It involves integration at some level. The second basic function is *adaptation,* which is further divided into two processes of *assimilation* and *accommodation.* When a new way of acting becomes completely your own, you have assimilated it, taken it in, and made it a part of your own way of acting. Some objects or actions do not fit into existing structures or actions and require modification. The process of modification of the environment is accommodation. If an infant cannot grasp a block because something is covering it, the obstacle must be removed. The inborn strategies of adaptation—assimilation and accommodation—provide a basis for development of schemas.

Sensorimotor Period   Schemas are the basic unit of Piaget's cognitive structure. The infant begins to form these schemas by combining sensory and motor actions. Because the first two years of life are so critical to intellectual development, the sensorimotor period is divided into six stages. Each stage has its own hallmarks.[28]

Stage 1   Stage 1 is *reflexive* and lasts for only the first month of life when the infant's interactions with the world are largely based on reflexes such as rooting, sucking, and kicking. Sucking is not confined to

Table 2-4

Piaget's Periods of Cognitive Development

Life Span Period	Piaget's Period	Characteristics
Infancy	Sensorimotor six stages	Babies pair sensory and motor action schemes, such as sucking, hitting, and grasping, as a means to deal with the immediate surroundings in their world.
Preschool	Preoperational	Children have a one-dimensional awareness of the environment. They use symbols and internal representations to think, but thinking is illogical and unsystematic.
School age	Concrete Operational	Children solve problems and think systematically, but only with real objects and activities.
Pubescence	Formal Operational	Adolescents solve abstract problems by using induction and deduction. Systematic thinking is applied on a purely abstract level.

ingesting food. The infant sucks on its fingers, the blanket, and clothes. All kinds of objects are assimilated into the sucking scheme. Accommodation begins as the infant makes subtle adjustments of lips and head while feeding.

Stage 2   Stage 2 occurs from 1 to 4 months and is characterized by *primary circular reactions*. When an infant repeats a volitional act over again, it is considered a circular reaction. The initial action may be purely by chance. The reactions are considered primary because these activities are focused primarily on the infant's body. Examples would include thumb sucking or repetitive grasping of body parts or clothing.

Stage 3   Stage 3 brings about *secondary circular reactions*. Now the infant is broadening her horizons to events and objects in the external world. Grasping, shaking, and banging objects are all examples of such actions. Even vocalizations become greater as infants recognize that their noise-making prompts those around them to make noises back to them. This stage occurs from 4 to 8 months.

Stage 4   Stage 4 (8 to 12 months) brings big changes when there is *coordination of secondary schemes*. Now the infant can put two schemes together to accomplish a goal. Behavior becomes goal directed, and infants become capable of intentionality. When faced with an obstacle, the infant can begin to figure out how to remove it to get what is wanted. For example, an infant will push one toy out of the way to get to the toy that is partially exposed under it or use a stick to get to another object. *Object permanence* emerges during this stage. The ability to know that an object or person still exists even

if not in view is a profound realization. However, the concept is only emerging at this stage and will continue to mature over the next several months as evidenced by the following response to a hidden object. Infants at this stage may still be fooled if a toy is first hidden under one blanket then another. They will search only the first hiding place.

Stage 5   During the second year of life, 12-month olds begin to seek new, unexpected results by varying their actions. For example, the toddler may experiment with dropping various objects off the highchair tray to see the consequences. Another child might put her hand under the faucet while in the bathtub and observe the different results depending on how close the hand was to the faucet. Trial and error experimentation is an obvious primary activity for this stage, which is termed *tertiary circular reactions*. The child deliberately varies actions within schemes to observe the consequences. When playing with toy cars on a ramp, the toddler can comprehend that if the car is let go at the top of the ramp, it should be looked for at the bottom of the ramp. Before this time, the infant would still look for the toy car at the top of the ramp.

Stage 6   Stage 6, the last stage of the sensorimotor period, is the *beginning of thought* (18 to 24 months). The title for stage 6 is quite profound because it connotes the child's ability to exhibit mental representation. A person must be able to mentally represent objects or persons not in plain view in order to think symbolically. Once mental representation is possible, understanding causality becomes more sophisticated. Mentally being able to represent past events or actions allows for the ability to pretend. Deferred imitation is the ability to imitate in the absence of a model.

Preoperational Period The next few years of life are dedicated to acquiring verbal expression as well as to using symbols, words, or objects to represent things that are not present. Preschoolers exemplify the child in preoperational thought. The child labels all forms of transportation as "ride" or all four-footed animals as "dog" or "cat" depending on the frame of reference. Children in this period demonstrate egocentric behavior in that their reasoning is always in relation to themselves. They are unable to take another's viewpoint. Centration is exhibited when the child centers on only one characteristic of an object to the exclusion of other salient features. In deciding which beaker has more liquid, a typical 4-year-old may focus on the height of the liquid in a beaker and ignore the diameter (Figure 2-9). The last characteristic of the preoperational period is that of appearance as reality. Scary masks or costumes transform a known person into someone scary. Toward the end of this period, most children begin to have some understanding of time, which eventually allows them to learn how to wait.

Concrete Operational Period During this period, the school-age child develops the ability to classify objects according to their characteristics. The child can solve concrete problems, that is, those in which the actual objects are physically present, as in "Which cup is bigger?" or "Which string is longer?" Most of Piaget's famous conservation experiments were carried out to demonstrate a child's ability to transform objects from one set of circumstances to another while preserving the idea that the objects were unchanged. When a child in concrete operations is asked about which beaker has more liquid, as seen in Figure 2-9, all aspects of the container will be considered. Conservation of liquid is generally achieved by 7 years of age.[28] The school-age child demonstrates symbolic thinking and has acquired the ability to mentally reverse thoughts.

Formal Operational Period Piaget and Inhelder[29] described the highest level of cognitive development as formal operations in which early adolescents are able to think about and thus deal with hypothetical as well as real situations. Now instead of engaging in trial and error experimentation, the formal operations thinker formulates a hypothesis and plans a way to study a problem. For example, in the problem if Sally is shorter than Terry, and Terry is taller than Steve, the adolescent can figure out who is the tallest without having to line her classmates up and compare their heights. Being able to generate a hypothesis, engage in deductive reasoning, and check solutions are all characteristics of logical decision making. Not all adolescents and adults apply this type of thinking to all aspects of life. They may tend to selectively use the ability only in particular personal or professional situations.

Perceptual-Cognitive Theory

Perception has been linked to cognition from the beginning of the field of psychology. While Piaget linked sensation to movement as an initial step in the development of intelligence, it is Eleanor Gibson who is the champion of the perceptual-cognitive theory of cognition. She pioneered the view that perception has the ability to detect order and structure not just to organize sensory information. Gibsonian research focuses on how perception guides action.[30]

The goal of perception is action.[31] Perception of the surrounding environment, which includes objects and people, serves the functional purpose of bringing about contact and interaction. The objects afford the opportunity to act, and in acting, the object and action are changed. This is the concept of *affordance*.[32] Affordance goes beyond adaptation and integration because both the object and perceiver are changed in the encounter. A jungle gym may afford a seat for one child or a place to hang upside down for another child. Perception is the means by which the child comes in contact with the world and adapts to it. The ecological view of perceptual development does not require the child to construct actions with objects as did Piaget's model. Gibson's concept of environmental affordance highlights the ecological perspective of cognition. The quality of the learning environment and the affordances that are available to the learner can impact development of cognitive abilities. Perceptual development is further explored in Chapter 10.

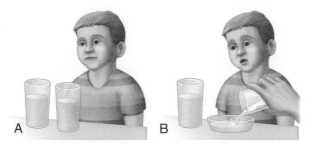

A   B

Figure 2-9 Conservation of liquids.

Information Processing With the advent of computers, information processing came into vogue as an explanation for the relationship between perception and cognition. The mind was viewed as a machine. Information processing theories are all based on the belief that thinking is information processing. The mind is described as working like a computer. When sensory information comes into the nervous system and is processed, that process is cognition. An information processing approach to development spans the biological and psychological domains and is concerned with memory, concept formation, and problem solving.[33] Neural structures and pathways are compared to hardware and software with speed of processing being the major change that occurs during development. Information processing on a physiological level is an integral part of motor control and is discussed in more depth in Chapter 4.

Memory Memory is necessary for learning and plays a pivotal role in information processing as a theory of cognition. Memories can be categorized by what is remembered. Table 2-5 compares the two largest types of memory. The memory for skills and information about doing a task is termed *implicit* memory. It is also known as *nondeclarative memory* or *procedural memory* and typically involves reflexive motor or perceptual skills. It is memory for doing and is recalled unconsciously. An example of procedural memory is that despite the fact that you may not have ridden a bike for many years, you have not forgotten how to ride. Procedural memory

is motor memory. *Priming,* another example of implicit memory, is the ability to identify or recognize an item due to a prior encounter. Implicit memory is stored in perceptual, motor, and emotional circuits of the brain.

The other type of memory is termed *explicit memory*, the memory of facts and events. This is also known as *declarative memory* and requires a conscious effort to be recalled. Explicit memory can be classified further into semantic or episodic. *Semantic memory* is memory for facts—how many inches are there in a foot? *Episodic memory* refers to being able to recall what you did on spring break last year. Explicit memory is stored in association cortices such that factual or semantic information is distributed in the cortex depending on the properties of the object to be identified.[34] The association areas in the prefrontal cortex appear to be involved in episodic information regarding where and when certain actions occurred. Developmental changes in memory are discussed in Chapter 9.

How are memories formed? It depends on whether one is talking about implicit or explicit memory. The process depicted in Figure 2-10 can be applied to either type of memory. Implicit memories build up slowly with repetition. In order to learn, one has to encode, store, and retrieve information as depicted in the flow diagram in Figure 2-10. Memories can be considered *immediate*, *short term*, or *long term* depending on their duration. Immediate memories last for only a few seconds or a few minutes. Short-term memories can last for days or weeks but will eventually be lost if they are not converted to long-term memory. Long-term memory

---

Table 2-5

Comparison of Types of Memory

Types	Implicit Memory	Explicit Memory
Alternate names	Nondeclarative memory Procedural memory	Declarative memory Recall memory Recognition memory
Level of awareness	Unconscious	Conscious
Neural substrate	Cortical-striatal-cerebellar system	Medial temporal-diencephalic system Prefrontal cortex
Examples	Priming Skills and habits Associative learning • Classic conditioning • Operant conditioning • Nonassociative learning • Habituation • Sensitization	Facts and general knowledge = semantic memory Memory of specific events = episodic memory

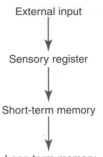

External input

↓

Sensory register

↓

Short-term memory

↓

Long-term memory

Figure 2-10 The process of memory formation.

can be recalled years later and is the result of structural changes at the level of the synapses that influence signal conduction. Memory encoding is the physiological process that occurs when a stimulus is attended to and processed. The longer the stimulus is attended to, the more likely it is to register and be processed into short-term memory. Memories can be stored for varying amounts of time. Short-term memory stores appear to be limited, while long-term stores seem almost limitless. Retrieval of information is the ability to use the information that is stored.

Working memory is a form of short-term memory. Encoding and retrieval both depend on the ability of the mind to use this form of short-term memory. If you have ever repeated a phone number to yourself several times or rehearsed what you are going to say to a person you are about to meet, you have engaged working memory. Working memory takes information from different sources and allows the person to create a response from the integrated information. If you become distracted, it is likely that you will lose the information. Thinking and reasoning depend on how well a person uses working memory. Short-term memory is also called *primary memory*. Information processed in short-term memory has the possibility of entering long-term memory. When short-term memory is converted to long-term memory, consolidation has occurred. Memory is not a unitary phenomenon. It consists of two major types and many subtypes and is dependent on many different areas of the central nervous system to function appropriately.

Sociocutural Development

Behaviorist

Probably the most famous behaviorist is B. F. Skinner,[35] the father of stimulus-response (S-R) psychology, whose experiments with rats and mazes clearly showed that certain behavior can be conditioned. He applied the principles of operant conditioning to the development of human behavior and believed that the environment was the most influential factor in determining behavioral outcomes. Skinner was even able to condition a fear response in a child. Although the value of reinforcement is universally accepted and behavioral modification is a legitimate form of therapeutic intervention, classic conditioning is not discussed as a formative aspect of development. Behaviorists do not represent a life span view of human development because they focus on development in childhood and adolescence, but they do represent the opposing side of the nature-nurture debate. According to behaviorists, all behavior is learned by observation and imitation and can be conditioned or shaped through reinforcement.

Temperament

Temperament is a person's characteristic way of responding. Temperament includes components of self-regulation and emotion.[36] It encompasses several dimensions such as activity level, affect (both positive and negative), persistence, and inhibition.[37] These dimensions have been distilled down from the original nine dimensions described in Thomas, Chess, and Birch's[38] original work. Three general types or clusters of temperament characteristics were identified based on their longitudinal study. These types and their characteristics are found in Table 2-6. Temperament is innate and relatively stable during infancy and the toddler years. Temperament can be influenced by the environment,

Table 2-6	
Temperament in Babies	
Temperament	**Characteristics**
Easy	Infants are easy going, have a positive disposition, are adaptable, and have regular body functions.
Difficult	Infants have negative moods, withdraw in a new situation, adapt slowly or not at all, or have irregular body functions.
Slow to Warm Up	Infants are relatively inactive, demonstrate calm reactions to their environment, are slow to adapt to new situations, and withdraw initially but later come around.

which includes child-rearing practices. Thomas, Chess, and Birch[38] introduced the concept of goodness of fit. This concept considered the infant's temperament and the parents' ability to match the environmental demands to foster mentally healthy and well-adjusted children. For example, a good fit would occur between an *easy* baby and a parent that would allow the infant to explore the environment pretty much self-directed. The majority of babies, about 40%, are categorized as *easy*. A poor fit would occur when a *difficult* baby was not directed to channel her negative energy into acceptable activities. *Difficult* babies make up about 10%, and the *slow to warm up* babies make up another 15%. The remaining infants are not able to be consistently categorized because they demonstrate a combination of characteristics. There are cultural differences in temperament. Chinese infants at 4 months are less vocal, less active, and less irritable than either their American or Irish counterparts.[39] Temperament can indirectly contribute to attachment. It may be more challenging for a mother to form an attachment to a difficult baby than to an easy baby.

Attachment

Once homeostasis is achieved in the first several months of life, the second stage of emotional development attachment begins to develop.[40] Infants who form attachments with adults are more likely to survive.[41] Figure 2-11 depicts the attachment system. Ainsworth[42] described four primary types of attachment. The ideal type of attachment is called *secure* attachment. The other three types are insecure attachments and include *anxious avoidant*, *resistant,* and *disorganized*. These categorizations are based on how the infant responds when separated from the mother. The infant who is securely attached may or may not cry when mom leaves, is happy

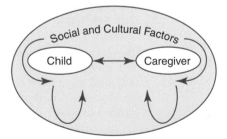

Figure 2-11 The attachment system depicting the bidirectional nature between the caregiver and the child as they are embedded in a sociocultural context. (From Barnekow KA, Kraemer GW: The psychobiological theory of attachment: a viable frame of reference for early intervention providers, *Phys Occup Ther Pediatr* 25[1/2]:3-15, 2005.)

to see mom when she returns, and stops crying on her return. The majority (60% to 65%) of babies are securely attached. The anxious avoidant attached infant is not upset when mom leaves but gives her the cold shoulder when she returns. Approximately 20% of infants demonstrate this type of insecure attachment. The resistant attached infant gets upset and remains upset and angry even after mom returns and is difficult to console. These infants make up about 10% to 15% of the population. Lastly, the disorganized or disoriented attached infants seem confused when mom leaves and when she returns, not appearing to understand what happened. These insecurely attached infants make up 5% to 10% of the group. Attachment is the primary basis for interpersonal relationships.[40] Parent-child relationships are expanded to include peer relationships. Children with secure attachments develop better peer relationships.[43]

Social Learning

Sears and colleagues[44] attempted to explain the early behavior of the child according to observable social interactions; that is, overt behavior. Although Sears used Skinner's S-R cycle, his theory became known as *social learning theory* and is predicated on identifying the common reinforcers used to produce social behavior. The theory states that behavioral development is learned with the parents as the first teachers, followed by the extended family and then the social group (Table 2-7).

Zone of Proximal Development

The person who really embraced the effect of cultural and society on cognitive development was Lev Vygotsky,[45] a Russian psychologist. He thought that cognitive development could take place only as a result of social interaction. The child partners with an adult who assists the child's learning. The adult provides the tools of the particular culture such as alphabetical and numbering schemes and its concepts about distance and time. He called the support given by the other person as *scaffolding*. Anyone who has watched a building being erected can grasp this concept. In this instance, the support is given for learning and problem solving. Unlike Piaget, who thought children became little scientists on their own, Vygotsky thought the nature of cognitive development could only be understood within a cultural and social context.[46] The *zone of proximal development* is the area of performance or level of performance that a child can demonstrate when assisted that is not possible when left to work on her own. This zone is the potential for growth in cognitive abilities that is made possible by the assistance of a skilled adult or peer. Vygotsky thought that children could not make significant progression alone.

Table 2-7

Sears' Phases of Social Learning

Life Span Period	Phase	Description
Infancy	I. Rudimentary behavior: initial behavioral learning	Basic need requirements met within intimate parental environment Positive reinforcement as primary socializing agent
Toddlerhood/preschool	II. Secondary motivational systems: family-centered learning	Socialization within larger family environment Negative reinforcement introduced as socializing agent
School age/adulthood	III. Secondary motivational systems: extrafamilial learning	Social penetration into neighborhood and beyond Controls universally defined and strictly enforced

From Sahler OJZ, McAnarney ER: *The child from three to eighteen*, St Louis, 1981, CV Mosby.

Play

Piaget[47] and Vygotsky[48] both appreciated the role of play in cognitive development. Play is a child's occupation.[49] Play promotes creativity and adaptation. Play is important for many reasons besides cognitive development, such as emotional development, socialization, and communication. Freud[50] and Erikson[51] used play to address wish fulfillment and coping. Modern day play therapy evolved from this perspective. Culture is embodied in play. Play mirrors the socialization process of society. Mead[52] thought that children learned rules and norms through play while Bateson[53] thought that play was important in communication but not socialization. The fact that children signal each other that they are playing is seen as a form of metacommunication. Play is not separate from reality; children know which is which, and this allows them to reflect and interpret culture. Why play is important is summarized in Table 2-8.

Children engage in different types of play.[54] A list of types of play and their characteristics can be found in Table 2-9. The first five types were originally described by Parten[55] to identify the various levels of social interaction. Play is important in a child's life because it is a major way of learning about the world. Play provides a rich opportunity for physical, cognitive, and language development. The quality of play changes dramatically and quickly early in life. *Solitary* play occurs alone. Peer interaction may be seen as early as 6 months of age when one infant may smile or point at another infant. *Parallel* play begins soon after the first birthday and is the most prevalent form of play observed in 1- and 2-year-olds. Simple social play in which there is some interaction between the toddlers is seen between 15 and 18 months. Toys may be offered one to the other. By age 2, young children may engage in several forms of play such as solitary, onlooker, or parallel play. *Associative* play is an example of simple social play that occurs in childhood. *Cooperative* play also begins as toddlers approach their second birthday and become children. Cooperative play involves rules and taking turns being "it" or being the leader or being the seeker in hide and seek. Game playing is social play as well. This type of play becomes the norm among 3- and 4-year-olds when parallel play is seen less frequently. Howes and Matheson[56] see the transition from parallel play to cooperative play as representative of a qualitative change, from less to more involved play.

Symbolic play, also called social pretend play, requires that a child be able to substitute another object for an absent object, such as when a ruler becomes a magic wand or a colander becomes a helmet. Michael Casby[57,58] notes that children exhibit beginning symbolic functioning in play during their second year of life (12 to 18 months). Symbolic play can be engaged in alone or in association or cooperation with others. For example, a child might put a bottle to a doll's mouth while playing alone. Between 18 and 24 months, multiple schemes may be observed such as the child pretending to comb her own hair and then the hair of another. Cooperative symbolic play is achieved by 30 months when the child puts out dishes and dolls for a pretend snack time. By age 4, the children exhibit complex social pretend play by being able to share fantasies and use verbal strategies based on agreed-upon rules. Play contributes unique developmental experiences that enrich the child's learning.

Other ways of describing play include the purpose of play: sensory/exploration, manipulation, imaginative/dramatic, or motor/physical play. The latter type is

Table 2-8

Why Play is Important

Type of Theory	Theorists	Summary of Tenets
Psychological (Cognitive)	Piaget and Vygotsky	Play is a cognitive process. Play is a voluntary act. Play contributes to cognitive development, problem solving, and creative thought. Play develops innovation, flexibility, enhanced problem solving, and adaptation.
Psychosocial	Freud and Erikson	These theories explain the role of play in the emotional development of children. Through play, children can play out wish fulfillment and master traumatic events in their lives.
Sociocultural		
Play as socialization	Mead	Through play with other children, children learn social rules and norms. Social roles are practiced through play.
Metacommunicative theory	Bateson	Play itself is the skill required to function within the real work of daily life. Children frame and reframe roles themselves. Play is learning about learning. Play is affected by the context in which it is played. Children signal that they are playing, and play is not an agent of socialization that develops skills for adulthood.

From Stagnitti K: Understanding play: the implications for play assessment, *Aust Occup Ther J* 51:3-12, 2004. Adaptation of part of Table 1 p 4. Mellou E: Play theories: a contemporary review, *Early Child Dev Care* 102:91-100, 1994.

Table 2-9

Types of Play

Type of Play	Characteristics
Solitary	Play is self-contained; examining and manipulating objects, toys, or people without reference to other(s) in the vicinity.
Onlooker	Observation of play of others with no actual participation beyond some communication, such as question/answer.
Parallel	Play with one or more child; each child is playing independently but aware of what the other is doing. There is no exchange of materials.
Associative	Play with one or more child with some shared material, activity, and communication. There is not a great deal of social exchange.
Cooperative	Play of longer duration in which there are rules or goals.
Symbolic	Play in which the child makes something stand for something else; also known as pretend play.

From Freiberg KL: *Human development: a life-span approach*, ed 3, Boston, 1987, Jones and Bartlett. Adaptation of Table 5-6, p 230.

thought to improve the child's awareness of the body in space. Imaginative/dramatic play is symbolic play when the child can act out conflicts or become the superhero. Piaget thought that symbolic play was very important not only for the child's development of cognition but also for emotional development. To play symbolically, the child has to be able to dually represent an object. In other words, the ruler she is holding has to be thought of as a wand capable of turning the stuffed frog into a handsome prince.

Regardless of how one categorizes play, it is an integral part of cognitive, social, and linguistic development.

THEORIES OF ADULT DEVELOPMENT

Adult development as a concept is a twentieth century phenomenon. Before this time, very little attention was paid to the longest period of human life, adulthood. Biological development is considered complete by the time a person is considered to be an adult. However, psychological and sociocultural development continues.

Career Consolidation

George Valliant, a psychiatrist and director of the Harvard study of adult development, inserted two new stages into Erikson's original eight stages: career consolidation and keeping the meaning. Career consolidation comes between intimacy and generativity. During this stage, a person chooses a career. It begins between 20 and 40 years of age, when young adults become focused on assuming a social identity within the work world. This is an extension of the person's personal identity forged in earlier stages. Valliant[59] identified four criteria that transform a "job" or "hobby" into a "career." They are competence, commitment, contentment, and compensation. The other stage will be discussed later in this section.

Emerging Adulthood

Jeffrey J. Arnett[1,60] espouses a new theory of emerging adulthood. He believes that there is a period of development between the end of adolescence and the beginning of adulthood. The period of emerging adulthood begins at 18 and ends at 25. Emerging adulthood is characterized by being the age of (1) identity exploration, (2) instability, (3) feeling in-between, (4) self-focus, and (5) possibility. Unlike Erikson, who thinks that identity is forged in adolescence, Arnett[1] believes that the transition to knowing who you are occurs later in time due to globalization and technological changes. Indeed Smith[61] and others[62] have discussed the prolongation of adolescence and the delay in taking on adult roles. Emerging adults face distinct challenges. They are on the one hand self-focused, highly content with their lives, and looking forward to the future, but at the same time are ambivalent about taking on adult roles. They see adulthood as a mixed blessing; there are rewards but there are constraints and limitations. During emerging adulthood there is relative independence from social roles and normative expectations.

Seasons of a Man's Life

Arnett is not the first to recognize the role of transitions in becoming an adult. Levinson[63] in his work on the Seasons of Life designated a 5-year period of time that bridged two developmental periods as a time of transition. The developmental periods are termed eras. There are four eras in life: preadulthood, up to 22; early adulthood, from 17 to 45; middle adulthood, from 40 to 65; and late adulthood, from 60 to ?. The transitions are the 5-year intervals between the eras: 17 to 22 for the early adult, 40 to 45 for midlife, and 60 to 65 for late adult.

What makes a person an adult? Is there a magic age or task to be attained that indicates when a person is an adult? Legally, you are an adult at 18. However, there are many 18-year-olds who would more than likely consider themselves as emerging adults. Regardless of the socioeconomic group a person belongs to, four criteria for adulthood continue to resound in the literature.[60] To be an adult, one must accept responsibility for actions, make independent decisions, be more considerate of others, and be financially independent. "Maturity requires the acceptance of responsibility and empathy for others.[64]"

Keeper of meaning is the additional stage Valliant[59] interjected between Erikson's generativity and integrity stages. It comes near the end of generativity, so the person is in late middle adulthood. The role of the keeper of meaning is to preserve one's culture rather than care for successive generations. The focus is on conservation and preservation of society's institutions. The keeper of meaning guides groups and preserves traditions.

Family Systems

The concept of family is very broad, with families having many different structures and life styles. Single-parent families have increased tremendously over the past decades. Regardless of structure, family function is affected by each member of the family. This can be thought of as family dynamics or in Bronfenbrenner's model as a system of interacting elements. Each parent affects the other, the child, or children, and in turn the child or children affect the parent. The family as a system is embedded in larger social systems, such as the extended family, neighborhood, school, and religious organizations. All of these systems can influence the family. Recognizing the family dynamics is very important when establishing a therapeutic relationship. Family-centered intervention is a life span approach.[65] Families have a life cycle in which stages and transitions have been identified.[66] However, the reader is referred to Carter and McGoldrick[67] for an expanded and updated discussion of family.

Leisure

Leisure is defined as "discretionary activity that includes simple relaxation, activities for enjoyment, and creative pursuits.[7]" Adolescents have been reported to spend up to 40% of their time in leisure activities.[68] However, in these days of organized sports and working for pay, that percentage appears high. The range of leisure activities engaged in by adults shows a trend with greater diversity in young adulthood and less in middle adulthood. In later adulthood, leisure time is spent engaging in less strenuous activities such as reading.

One of the big benefits from leisure is as a buffer against negative life events because the activity can serve as a distracter. The activities can generate optimism, help connect us with our past, and give a person a sense of well-being.[69]

Leisure may include play. The concept that adults play may seem foreign to most of the population, but play may be viewed as a form of leisure.[70] Focusing on the self often involves participating in fun activities purely for the pleasure it brings to the individual. Blanche[71] studied play in adults. Some activities involved novelty while others involved creativity or a sense or adventure. Many activities cited brought the individual a heightened self-awareness. Two final characteristics seen in adult play are mastery, such as becoming better at bridge or sudoku, and restoration, deriving pleasure from relaxation. Adults can engage in play at anytime. The time taken to grab a cup of coffee or a walk to the next meeting can be perceived as play. Play is not restricted to leisure time; it can be embedded in the daily routine. In summary, focusing on the self in play can promote a state of mind that can lead to self-actualization.[72]

THEORIES OF AGING

Development in the Older Adult

In contrast to adulthood where there are few theories, there are a multitude of theories on aging. Aging is a lifelong process, so in reality any life span theory could contribute to this discussion. Theorists observing the later aspect of the life span hypothesize that aging occurs because of biological or physical changes in the human body. A person is aging from the moment of birth; in fact, we celebrate birthdays as a social marker of the passage of time. Aging is seen by others as the number one health problem in the United States and developing countries.[73] Approximately 85% of all deaths were caused by age-related disease in 2003.[74] Aging transforms healthy individuals into people who are more susceptible to disease. These are the *frail elderly*. Homeostasis is unable to be maintained because of relentless physiological deterioration.[75] The physiological basis of frailty is depicted in Figure 2-12. Biological aging diminishes reserves in most physiological systems, eventually resulting in an irreparable breakdown and ultimately death. The aging process is modified by both genetic and environmental factors.[73]

Biophysical Theories

"A unified theory of biological aging involving genes, milieu, and chance is emerging.[76]" Biological theories of aging are usually subdivided into genetic and nongenetic. Genetic theory is based on the premise that aging is programmed in the cell nucleus. This process of cellular aging is considered a *purposeful event*.[77] Harman[78] calls cellular aging an inborn aging process (IAP) such that the human average life expectancy is limited to about 85 years. Nongenetic theory is related to environmental factors outside the cell nucleus. Here aging is viewed as part of the same continuum as the process of development—genetically controlled and probably programmed but subject to environmental influence.

Genetic Theories

Programmed Aging These theories grew out of biological investigation in the 1960s. Hayflick and Moorehead[79] made a profound observation while studying human tumor viruses. When growing human cells in tissue culture, they observed a waxing and waning of cellular proliferation, followed by senescence and eventual death of the cultures. Before this time, tissue cultures had been thought to be immortal. Hayflick and Moorehead[79] interpreted their findings to mean that aging was a cellular as well as an organismic phenomenon and dramatically changed the way we viewed aging.

Hayflick[80] subsequently described, in the *Hayflick limit theory*, the number of possible life span cell replications (population-doubling potential) to be about 50. The replicative life span of specific tissue types was then linked to the age of their donor cells when cultured.

The Physiologic Basis of Frailty

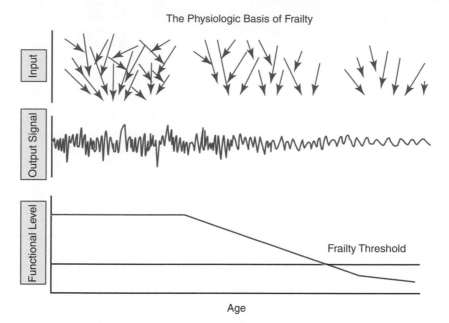

Figure 2-12 The physiological basis of frailty. (From Lipsitz LA: Dynamics of stability: the physiologic basis of functional health and frailty, *J Gerontol A Biol Sci Med Sci* 57A(3): B115-B125, 2002.)

The younger the donor cells, the greater was their life span. The replicative life span is also known as *replicative senescence*. In individuals with premature aging, called *progeria,* the donor cells show a lower Hayflick limit.[81] Chromosome dysfunction is the root cause of premature aging.[82]

Programmed cell death, called *apoptosis,* is apparent during early development when unwanted or unused cells are destroyed. Apoptosis can also occur in response to DNA damage that cannot be repaired. Deficits in DNA repair pathways can also lead to cancer-causing mutations. To prevent this, cellular senescence or apoptosis is induced and indirectly causes certain aspects of aging.[82] Prevention of the accumulation of damaged molecules in theory would slow the aging process.

Scientists have identified *longevity determinant genes* or *longevity assurance genes* (LAG).[82,83] Puca and associates[84] noted a linkage of a locus on chromosome 4 with exceptional longevity in humans. It is thought that at least one or more genes could exert a positive influence on a person's ability to reach old age. Many such genes have been found in mice and fruit flies. Originally these genes and their pathways were studied in mice as part of cancer research. The LAG ensure a healthy life span because they code for proteins that reduce cancer incidence. Hasty believes that "some aspects of normal aging are the consequence of anticancer mechanisms designed to deal with damaged DNA.[82]" Cutler and Mattson[73] state that most of the genes studied in lower organisms relate to developmental growth factors and oxidative stress.

Nongenetic Theories

Nongenetic theories assume that aging changes occur because of influences outside the cell nucleus and involve some maladaptive response to cell, tissue, or system damage. The damage may be from external, environmental sources or from internal sources. These events eventually reach a level that is no longer compatible with life. If the events occur randomly and represent environmental insults to the human body, they are called *stochastic changes*. The major stochastic theories include the free radical theory, cross-linkage theory, immune system theory, and the neuroendocrine system theory. In light of recent research, only one of these theories will be discussed in detail. The others will be mentioned tangentially.

The major biological theory of aging is the *free radical theory* first postulated by Harman.[85] It is also known as the *oxidative damage hypothesis*. The theory states that aging is due to the accumulation of oxidative damage to macromolecules. Macromolecules are considered DNA (nuclear and mitochondrial), RNA, protein, carbohydrates, lipids, and molecular conjugates. Reactive oxygen species (ROS) and free radicals (FR) are formed as by-products of cellular metabolism using oxygen. Mitochondria are the main generators of ROS. During electron transport in oxidative phosphorylation, electrons are leaked to oxygen. This mechanism is a major way lipids, proteins, and DNA are damaged. Both muscle and nervous system tissue are prone to oxidative damage because of their high metabolic rate and, therefore, high rate of ROS generation.[86] Mitochondria play a crucial role in the aging process because of their role in not only producing ROS but being a target of ROS attack.[87]

Free radicals are highly charged ions with an orbiting unpaired electron. The separated electron with its high energy level attacks neighboring molecules. Free radicals have an affinity for lipid molecules, which are found in abundance in mitochondrial and microsomal membranes. These membranes are damaged by a chemical process called lipid peroxidation, which leads to structural changes and malfunctions in the cell. One of the results of the oxidative reactions within the cells is the deposition of lipofuscin, an aging pigment. Lipofuscin consists of lipid and protein, most of which has been oxidized.

Lipofuscin accumulates in many organs with aging, particularly in postmitotic organs, such as the heart, skeletal muscle, and central nervous system, that are no longer dividing. Its formation has been postulated to be advantageous early on in the aging process, but once a critical amount of lipofuscin is formed, cell viability is threatened.[88]

In addition to forming age pigments, free radicals produce cross-linkages in some cells that can damage DNA. If a cross-link attaches to only one strand of DNA, it can be repaired. However, if two strands of DNA are cross-linked, the strands are unable to part normally. With aging, the body's ability to repair cross-linkages declines, causing an increase in cell death related to incomplete division. Cross-links also occur in the skin with age. Cross-linkages between collagen and elastin lead to a loss of tissue elasticity and the production of wrinkles. Sun exposure can hasten this process. Loss of flexibility due to these age-related changes in collagen can be partially compensated for by diet and exercise.[89]

Oxidative stress has been implicated to have a role in several neurodegenerative disorders from Alzheimer to Parkinson disease. The brain is highly susceptible to damage from free radicals. Free radicals play a role in formation of neuritic plaques, a structural hallmark of Alzheimer disease. Plaques are derived from beta amyloid. The amyloid is neurotoxic and leads to production of ROS that promote more aggregation of amyloid. Free radical production eventually destroys the neurons. The other structural hallmark of Alzheimer disease is the neurofibrillary tangle that contains a tau protein. This protein is also neurotoxic and causes neuron death by the accumulation of free radicals. The accumulation of ROS in the form of free radicals increases with age,

regardless of the presence of pathology. The body's ability to produce antioxidants to counteract the effects of ROS declines with age. Oxidative stress is definitely involved in aging and in age-related diseases.[73,87] See Chapter 9 for more age-related changes in the brain and the clinical implications of Alzheimer disease.

Immune   The immune system consists of the bone marrow, thymus gland, spleen, and lymph nodes. The first two are primary organs of immunity; the latter two are considered peripherally or secondarily responsible for developing immunity. The bone marrow and thymus are the two organs most affected by the aging process. The thymus involutes with age. By age 50, it is 5% to 10% of its peak mass.[90] After young adulthood, the thymus loses its ability to produce the differentiated T cells needed for cell-mediated immune responses. As the bone marrow becomes less efficient, the rate of infections, autoimmune disorders, and cancer rises. The term *immunosenescence* is used to describe the dysfunctional immunity seen in older adults.[91] Oxidative damage has been implicated in producing the immune function decline seen with increasing age. The central nervous system and the immune system are in constant communication; what affects one, affects the other. Specific cytokines, synthesized by lymphocytes, have been linked to the aging process.[92] The cytokine response to nonspecific inflammation has also been linked to functional decline, frailty, and even death in older adults.[93,94]

Neuroendocrine   The nervous system and endocrine systems work together with the immune system to maintain homeostasis. The autonomic nervous system, especially the sympathetic division, and the hormones produced by the neuroendocrine system via the pituitary affect the brain and the immune system. Neural and endocrine function can be changed by immune system responses, and in turn, endocrine and neural activity can modify immune functions. As we age, the hormones produced by the endocrine system appear to be intact and potent, although their effective interaction with target body cells is decreased. Put another way, the body's tissues are less responsive. The hypothalamic-pituitary-adrenal (HPA) interconnections act as a system to control the body functions of growth, reproduction, and metabolism. The pituitary gland controls the thyroid gland that manages the metabolic rate of the body through the secretion of thyroxine. As physiological reserve is lowered with advanced age and threatened by accumulated stress, the neuroendocrine system's initial response is adequate, but the response may persist and may be harmful. Moderate exercise and endurance training have been shown to improve immune function and to protect against the deleterious effects of stress.[95]

Psychological Theories

Intelligence

After peaking in early adulthood, intelligence declines through late adulthood. Horn and Cattel[96] described two dimensions of intelligence: fluid and crystallized. *Fluid intelligence* refers to learning reflective of induction, deduction, and abstract thinking, whereas *crystallized intelligence* is related to knowledge of life experiences and education or cultural knowledge. Fluid intelligence declines at some point in adulthood, whereas crystallized intelligence is maintained or may even increase during the adult years (Figure 2-13). Fluid intelligence is more dependent on physiological functioning, especially the neurological system, both of which decline with advancing age.

Cognition is a complex phenomenon and is a composite of the interactions between multiple domains, including memory, information processing, and perception. Humans demonstrate age-related decline in memory, mental speed, fluid reasoning, and spatial ability.[97] These interactions are referred to as a general cognitive factor.[88] There appears to be more of a decline in the general factor with certain domains being selectively affected. Salthouse[98] and colleagues[99] reported that executive function (problem solving) and mental speed are more vulnerable to aging effects than other domains of cognition. During advanced aging, the majority of elderly develop diffuse plaques and neurofibrillary tangles, which may be linked to cognitive decline. Diffuse plaques are different from the neuritic plaques indicative of Alzheimer. Neurofibrillary tangles are also a hallmark of Alzheimer disease. However, they may also be found in dementia-free elderly. There can be a great deal of difference between pathology and cognitive impairment in older individuals. There is no one-to-one relationship between the degree of pathology and degree of functional decline.

Cognitive Processing Speed

Information-processing theories of cognition have been used to assess the age-related differences seen in attention, reaction time, and working memory. The *processing-speed theory* states that a decrease in the speed of processing operations leads to impairment in cognitive functioning.[98] Older adults are slower to respond, with increased reaction time being well documented.[100] The degree to which the response time slows depends on the difficulty of the task being performed. Attending to tasks of increasing complexity is more difficult for older than younger adults.[101,102]

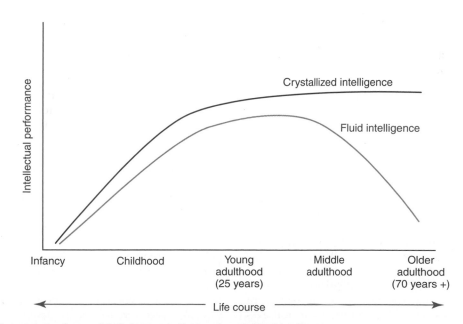

Figure 2-13 Comparison of age-related changes in fluid and crystallized intelligence.

Cognitive Reserve Theory

The theoretical construct of holding something in reserve has been applied to cognitive abilities in late adulthood. Just as Schroots and Yates[19] devised resiliency curves that mirrored the body's ability to bounce back from a stressor, Whalley and colleagues[103] have articulated the neurobiology of cognitive aging. The cognitive reserve hypothesis proposes that people with more cognitive reserve can successfully sustain neuropathology that would cause clinical dementia in those individuals with a lower cognitive ability.[88]

Education, intelligence, and occupation are often listed as components of the cognitive reserve. Educational experiences can be thought of as enrichment. When formal education is studied as a predictor of cognitive vitality, it is usually found to have a protective effect.[104,105] Intelligence in childhood is highly correlated to intelligence in adulthood. Childhood intelligence is also strongly associated with the level of education attained and occupational complexity. Shimamura and colleagues[106] studied university professors and found a lower effect of aging on cognitive function. Low education level and low occupational status are risk factors for Alzheimer disease.[103] Kramer and associates[105] also identified lifestyle and fitness as modifiers of the developmental trajectory of cognition from young to older adulthood. Dementia is not inevitable if you live to be 100; about 15% to 25% of centenarians are functionally cognitively intact.[107] These findings support the premise of a cognitive reserve. In fact, of those over 100 who did have some form of cognitive impairment, more than 90% of them did not demonstrate problems until well into their 90s.[108]

Sociocultural Theories

Aging may be the only thing a group of older adults have in common. Life histories and experiences are only a few of the variables present in our life course. Older adults may work for a longer period of time out of necessity. Other older adults take up volunteerism with great gusto and fervor. For those retirees who are healthy, there are many more years of leisure than ever before. Previously, selective optimization with compensation had been discussed under the psychological theories of aging but it is really a social theory of adaptation. So we will begin with it and then revisit disengagement, activity, and continuity theories as well.

Selective Optimization with Compensation

This theory was originally postulated by Baltes[4] to explain why some individuals compensate for age-related declines in function. He has recently expanded this theory to encompass the life span as a way of explaining the adaptation that occurs over the entire life course. Successful aging is viewed as optimizing gains while minimizing losses. Selection involves deciding what direction to take, making goals, and specifying outcomes. Compensation involves making a functional response in the face of a loss of a previously available means of attaining a goal.[4] For example, the pianist Arthur Rubinstein, at age 80 practiced fewer pieces (selection) more frequently (optimization), compensating for his slower speed by purposefully slowing down before rapid sequences to increase the contrast in movement speed.[109] Selective optimization with compensation (SOC) is a general model of successful aging. As both physical and sociocultural resources become limited with advanced age, focus is shifted to optimizing achievements and compensating for limitations. Reallocation of resources provides the best possible outcome, leading to an effective life.

Disengagement

Cumming and Henry[110] proposed the *disengagement theory*, suggesting that aging adults turned inward as a means of withdrawal from family and society. This served to ease the eventual loss of the older adult on the family. It has been suggested that mandatory retirement, which compels the older adult to withdraw from work-related roles, hastens the disengagement process.[46] Socially, the older adult may engage in less day-to-day and face-to-face encounters. Society in some ways begins to disengage from the older adult. The theory suggests that disengagement is a mutual process.[46]

While disengagement has a negative connotation, in actuality it may be beneficial to the older adult. Withdrawing from some social relationships may provide more time for those that are more beneficial. Investing less emotionally may make dealing with the increasing frequency of illness and death among their peer group easier. The initial research found some support for disengagement, but later research found that complete disengagement was neither normal nor natural.[111] Disengagement occurs after the loss of spouse and retirement, but many older adults return to being more actively engaged after a period of time. Disengagement is not universal for everyone in late adulthood.

Activity

In sharp contrast to the disengagement theory, the *activity theory*, postulated by Neugarten and associates,[112] suggested that staying actively involved with friends, family, and society was necessary for successful aging. Activity was positively correlated with happiness in old age. Being active allowed for adaptation, which has always been part of life and becomes an even more important part of aging. Critics of this theory point out that not every older adult wants to be active; many look forward to slowing down and for some "less is more." The theory does not clearly delineate which activities are important to continue. Depending on life circumstances, the older adult may need to adjust to less income, increased dependency, loss or change of job role, or an inability to participate in leisure activities. Neither the disengagement theory nor the activity theory completely addresses the picture of successful aging.

Continuity

Continuity theory has replaced the need for debating the merits of the activity and disengagement theories. Atchley[113] described this widely accepted theory as one in which the individual seeks continuity by linking things in the past with changes in the future. For example, applying a study strategy used in college to taking on a new task at work is combining prior knowledge for future change. There are three degrees of continuity; too little, too much, and optimal.[113] Too little continuity produces an unsettled feeling that one's life is too unpredictable. Too much continuity is boring and totally predictable. The optimal amount of continuity provides sufficient challenge for change but not so much challenge that the person is overwhelmed.

Continuity can be internal or external. Internal continuity comes from those aspects of a person's personality such as temperament, emotions, and experiences unique to the individual. Internal continuity connects you to your past. External continuity comes from the environment, physical and social, and includes the roles each of us is involved in and the jobs we perform. Friendships and phasing out of employment are examples of maintaining external continuity in older adulthood. Phasing out of employment means that there will be more time for family and friends and volunteer pursuits. Internal continuity is lost in a patient with Alzheimer who loses awareness of herself, but external continuity allows adaptation to changing environmental demands.

The range of sociocultural theories is vast and mutilayered. Aging is viewed within the context of our relationship with the larger society and culture. Our relationships can be defined in terms of sociocultural roles, as in SOC and continuity theory, or as a linkage to the larger group, as seen in the activity or disengagement theories.

Successful Aging

Rowe and Kahn[114] identified three components of successful aging based on longitudinal studies by the MacArthur Foundation. The number one component is avoiding disease and disability, number two is having a high cognitive and physical functional capacity, and number three is active engagement with life. Unlike the activity theorist, Rowe and Kahn[114] defined activity as something that holds societal value. The activity does not have to be remunerated for it to be considered productive.

SUMMARY

Development, as a process of change, reflects the transactional nature of our interaction with the environment and encompasses our need to survive, organize, and adapt to our surroundings. As a child changes during the course of her development, the people and things with which that child interacts also change. Each person's experience is different. The variables within the physical, psychological, and sociocultural environments encountered by a person need to be considered in the development of that person's functional skills. We should not envision this interaction as a robotlike series of actions but as actions with endless possible variations to produce a unique adaptive response. The environment includes people, places, and things. We develop a sense of identity through psychological interaction with all components of our environment. Motor learning occurs as a function of the interactions between our physical body and environmental task demands. Although it may be true that "just because your father was concert pianist, it doesn't mean that you will inherit his musical talent," our genetic makeup will predispose us to certain traits. The physical, psychological, and sociocultural environment in which we develop, however, can have an equally potent effect.

Theories of development have evolved over time and been modified to reflect what we currently know about development and to provide a basis for our clinical decision making. We no longer believe that development of functional movement is solely based on neuromaturation. We believe that the environment and the task goal shape the form of the functional movement that emerges. Motor learning is necessary for motor development; therefore, therapeutic intervention must incorporate knowledge of results and practice at solving movement problems. We must remember that theories are changeable; none are totally correct. As theorists of human development and clinicians seek to integrate the changes in all domains of function across the life span, the process of development of functional movement will become clearer.

REFERENCES

1. Arnett JJ: Emerging adulthood: a theory of development from the late teens through the twenties, *Am Psychol* 55:469–480, 2000.
2. Federal Interagency Forum on Aging-Related Statistics: *Older Americans 2008: key indicators of well-being*, (website): www.agingstats.gov/. Accessed March 3, 2009.
3. Baltes PB: Theoretical propositions of life-span developmental psychology: on the dynamics between growth and decline, *Dev Psychol* 23:611–626, 1987.
4. Baltes PB, Lindenberger U, Staudinger UM: Life span theory in developmental psychology. In Damon W, Lerner RM, editors: *Handbook of child psychology*, ed 6, New York, 2006, John Wiley & Sons, pp 569–664.
5. Havighurst RJ: *Developmental tasks and education*, ed 3, New York, 1972, David McKay Co, Inc.
6. Hayflick L: New approaches to old age, *Nature* 403:365, 2000.
7. Kail RV, Cavanaugh JC: *Human development: a life-span view*, ed 4, Belmont, Calif, 2007, Thompson Wadsworth.
8. Plomin R, Spinath F: Intelligence: genes, genetics, and genomics, *J Pers Soc Psychol* 86:112–129, 2004.
9. Finch CE, Tanzi RE: Genetics of aging, *Science* 278:407–411, 1997.
10. National Center for Health Statistics: *Older Americans 2004: key indicators of well-being*, (website): http://www.agingstats.gov/chartbook2004/tables-population.html. Accessed March 16, 2007.
11. Perls T, Terry D: Genetics of exceptional longevity, *Exp Gerontol* 38:725–730, 2003.
12. Gunnar MR, Bruce M, Grotevant HD: International adoption of institutionally reared children: research and policy, *Dev Psychopathol* 12:677–692, 2000.
13. Yamori Y: Food factors for atherosclerosis prevention: Asian perspective derived from analyses of worldwide dietary biomarkers, *Exp Clin Cardiol* 11(2):94–98, 2006.
14. World Health Organization: *Global action against cancer, updated edition 2005*, (website): http://www.who.int/cancer/media/GlobalActionCancerEnglfull.pdf. Accessed March 28, 2007.
15. Leenstra T, Peterson LT, Kariuki SK, et al: Prevalence and severity of malnutrition and age at menarche: cross-sectional studies in adolescent schoolgirls in western Kenya, *Eur J Clin Nutr* 59(1):41–48, 2005.
16. Gottlieb G, Wahlsten D, Lickliter R: The significance of biology for human development: a developmental psychobiological systems view. In Damon W, Eisenberg N, editors: *Handbook of child psychology*, ed 5, New York, 1998, John Wiley & Sons, pp 233–273.
17. Erikson EH: *Identity, youth, and crisis*, New York, 1968, WW Norton.
18. Lockman JJ, Thelen E: Developmental biodynamics: brain, body, behavioral connections, *Child Dev* 64:953–1050, 1993.
19. Schroots JJ, Yates RE: On the dynamics of development and aging. In Bengtson VL, Schaie KW, editors: *Handbook of theories of aging*, New York, 1999, Springer, pp 417–433.
20. Yates FE, Benton LA: Rejoinder to Rosen's comments on biological senescence: loss of integration and resilience, *Can J Aging* 14:125–130, 1995.
21. Erikson EH, Erikson JM, Kivnick HQ: *Vital involvement in old age*, New York, 1986, WW Norton.
22. Bandura A: *Social foundation of thought and action: a social cognitive theory*, Englewood Cliffs, NJ, 1986, Prentice-Hall.
23. Maslow A: *Motivation and personality*, New York, 1954, Harper & Row.
24. Bronfenbrenner U: *The ecology of human development. Experiments by nature and design*, Cambridge, Mass, 1979, Harvard University Press.
25. Bronfenbrenner U, Morris PA: The ecology of developmental processes. In Damon W, Lerner RM, editors: *Handbook of child psychology*, ed 6, New York, 2006, John Wiley & Sons, pp 793–828.
26. Gesell A, Ilg FL, Ames LB, et al: *Infant and child in the culture of today*, revised. New York, 1974, Harper & Row.
27. Piaget J: *Origins of intelligence*, New York, 1952, International Universities Press.
28. Crain WC: *Theories of development: concepts and applications*, ed 6, Upper Saddle River, NJ, 2005, Pearson Prentice Hall.
29. Piaget J, Inhelder B: *The child's concept of space*, New York, 1967, WW Norton.
30. Pick HL, Gibson EJ: Learning to perceive and perceiving to learn, *Dev Psychol* 28:787–794, 1992.
31. Gibson EJ: *The ecological approach to visual perception*, Boston, 1979, Houghton Mifflin.
32. Gibson EJ: The concept of affordance in development: the renaissance of functionalism. In Collins WA, editor: *Minnesota symposium on child psychology*, vol 15, Hillsdale, NJ, 1982, Erlbaum.
33. Klar D, MacWhinney B: Information processing. In Damon W, Kuhn D, Siegler RS, editors: *Handbook of child psychology*, ed 5, New York, 1998, John Wiley & Sons, pp 631–678.
34. Kandel ER, Kupfermann I, Iversen S: Learning and memory. In Kandel ER, Schwartz JH, Jessell TM, editors: *Principles of neural science*, New York, 2000, McGraw-Hill, pp 1227–1246.
35. Skinner BF: *The behavior of organisms: an experimental analysis*, New York, 1938, Appleton-Century-Crofts.
36. Rothbart MK, Derryberry D: Temperament in children. In vonHofsten C, Blackman L, editors: *Psychology at the turn of the millennium: vol 2. Social, developmental, and clinical perspectives*, New York, 2002, Taylor & Francis, pp 17–35.
37. Caspi A, Shiner RL: Personality development. In Damon W, Lerner RM, editors: *Handbook of child psychology*, ed 6, New York, 2006, John Wiley & Sons, pp 300–428.
38. Thomas A, Chess S, Birch HG: *Temperament and behavior disorders in children*, New York, 1968, University Press.
39. Kagan J, Arcus D, Snidman N, et al: Reactivity in infants: a cross-national comparison, *Dev Psychol* 30:342–345, 1994.
40. Greenspan SI: *Infancy and early childhood: the practice of clinical assessment and intervention with emotional and developmental challenges*, Madison, Wis, 1992, International Universities Press.

41. Bowlby J: *Attachment and loss*, vol 1. New York, 1969, Basic Books.
42. Ainsworth MS: Attachment as related to mother-infant interaction, *Adv Infancy Res* 8:1–50, 1993.
43. Schneider BA, Atkinson L, Tardif C: Child-parent attachment and children's peer relations: a quantitative review, *Dev Psychol* 37:86–100, 2001.
44. Sears RR, Rau L, Alpert R: *Identification and child rearing*, Stanford, Calif, 1965, Stanford University Press.
45. Vgotsky L: *Thought and language*, MIT Press (Kozulin A, translator), Cambridge, Mass, 1986.
46. Feldman RS: *Development across the life span*, ed 3, Upper Saddle River, NJ, 2003, Prentice Hall.
47. Piaget J: *Play, dreams, and imitation in childhood*, London, 1951, Heinemann.
48. Vygotsky L: Play and its role in the mental development of the child, *Sov Psychol* 12:62–76, 1966.
49. Parham LD: Play and occupational therapy. In Parham LD, Fazio LS, editors: *Play in occupational therapy*, ed 2, St Louis, 2007, Mosby, pp 3–39.
50. Freud S: *Beyond the pleasure principle*, New York, 1961, Norton.
51. Erikson EH: Play and actuality. In Bruner JS, Jolly A, Sylva K, editors: *Play: its role in development and evolution*, New York, 1985, Penguin Books, pp 688–704.
52. Mead GH: *Mind, self, and society*, Chicago, 1934, University of Chicago Press.
53. Bateson G: *Steps to an ecology of mind*, New York, 1972, Ballantine Books.
54. Freiberg KL: *Human development: a life-span approach*, ed 3, Boston, 1987, Jones and Bartlett.
55. Parten MB: Social participation among preschool children, *J Abnorm Psychol* 27:243–269, 1932.
56. Howes C, Matheson CC: Sequences in the development of competent play with peers: social and social pretend play, *Dev Psychol* 28(5):961–974, 1992.
57. Casby MW: The development of play in infants, toddlers, and young children, *Commun Disord Q* 24(4):163–174, 2003.
58. Casby MW: Developmental assessment of play: a model for early intervention, *Commun Disord Q* 24(4):175–183, 2003.
59. Valliant GE: *Aging well*, New York, 2002, Little, Brown.
60. Arnett JJ: Emerging adulthood in Europe: a response to Bynner, *J Youth Stud* 9(1):111–123, 2006.
61. Smith TW: *Coming of age in 21st century America: public attitudes towards the importance and timing of transitions to adulthood*, GSS Topical Report No. 35, Chicago, 2004, University of Chicago, National Opinion Research Center.
62. Arnett JJ, Tanner JL, editors: *Emerging adults in America: coming of age in the 21st century*, Washington, D.C., 2006, American Psychological Association.
63. Levinson DF: A conception of adult development, *Am Psychol* 41:3–13, 1986.
64. Purtillo R, Haddad A: *Health professional and patient interaction*, ed 6, Philadelphia, 2002, Saunders.
65. Chiarello LA: Family-centered intervention. In Effgen SK, editor: *Meeting the physical therapy needs of children*, Philadelphia, 2005, FA Davis, pp 108–127.
66. Duvall EM: *Family development*, ed 4, Philadelphia, 1971, Lippincott.
67. Carter B, McGoldrick M: *Expanded family life cycle: individual, family, and social perspectives*, ed 3, Boston, 2005, Allyn and Bacon.
68. Csikszentmihalyi M, Larson R: *Being adolescent*, New York, 1984, Basic Books.
69. Kleiber DA, Hutchinson SL, Williams R: Leisure as a resource in transcending negative life events: self-protection, self-restoration, and personal transformation, *Leisure Sci* 24:219–235, 2002.
70. Huizina J: *Homo ludens*, Boston, 1955, Beacon Press.
71. Blanche EI: Play and process: adult play embedded in the daily routine. In Reifel S, Roopnarine JL, editors: *Play and culture studies: vol 4. Conceptual, social-cognitive, and contextual issues in the field of play*, Westport, Conn, 2002, Ablex, pp 249–278.
72. Sutton-Smith B: *The ambiguity of play*, Cambridge, Mass, 1997, Harvard Press.
73. Cutler RG, Mattson MP: Introduction: the adversities of aging, *Ageing Res Rev* 5:221–238, 2006.
74. CDC, National Center for Health Statistics: *National vital statistic report vol 54, no 13; final mortality for 2003*, (website): http://www.cdc.gov/nchs/data/nvsr/nvsr54/nsvr54_13.pdf. Accessed April 5, 2007.
75. Harman D: Aging: overview, *Ann N Y Acad Sci* 928:1–21, 2001.
76. Rattan SI: Theories of biological aging: genes, proteins, and free radicals, *Free Radic Res* 40(123):1230–1238, 2006.
77. Cavanaugh JC: Theories of aging in the biological, behavioral, and social sciences. In Cavanaugh JC, Whitbourne SK, editors: *Gerontology: an interdisciplinary perspective*, New York, 1999, Oxford University Press, pp 1–32.
78. Harman D: Free radical theory of aging: an update, *Ann N Y Acad Sci* 10067:10–21, 2006.
79. Hayflick L, Moorehead PS: The serial cultivation of human diploid cell strains, *Exp Cell Res* 24:585–621, 1961.
80. Hayflick L: The limited in vitro lifetime of human diploid cell strains, *Exp Cell Res* 25:614–636, 1965.
81. Freis I, Crapo L: *Vitality and aging*, San Francisco, 1981, WH Freeman.
82. Hasty P: The impact of DNA damage, genetic mutation and cellular responses on cancer prevention, longevity and aging: observations in humans and mice, *Mech Ageing Dev* 126:71–77, 2005.
83. Cutler RG, Guarante LP, Kensler TW, et al: Longevity determinant genes: What is the evidence? What is the importance? Panel discussion, *Ann N Y Acad Sci* 1055:58–63, 2005.
84. Puca AA, Daly MJ, Brewster SJ, et al: A genome-wide scan for linkage to human exceptional longevity identifies a locus on chromosome 4, *Proc Natl Acad Sci U S A* 98:10505–10508, 2001.
85. Harman D: A theory based on free radical and radiation chemistry, *J Gerontol* 11:298–300, 1956.
86. Halliwell B, Gutteridge JM: *Free radicals in biology and medicine*, ed 3, Oxford, UK, 1999, Oxford University Press.

87. Mariani E, Polidori MC, Cherubini A, et al: Oxidative stress in brain aging, neurodegenerative and vascular diseases: an overview, *J Chromatogr B Analyt Technol Biomed Life Sci* 827:65–75, 2005.

88. Keller JN: Age-related neuropathology, cognitive decline, and Alzheimer's disease, *Ageing Res Rev* 5:1–13, 2006.

89. Lee IM, Paffenbarger RS Jr: Association of light, moderate, and vigorous intensity physical activity with longevity. The Harvard alumni health study, *Am J Epidemiol* 151:293–299, 2000.

90. Whitbourne SK: Physical changes. In Cavanaugh JC, Whitbourne SK, editors: *Gerontology: an interdisciplinary perspective*, Baltimore, 1999, Williams & Wilkins, pp 91–122.

91. Pawelec G, Koch S, Franceschi C, et al: Human immunosenescence. Does it have an infectious component? *Ann N Y Acad Sci* 1067:56–65, 2006.

92. Morley JE, Baumgartner RN: Cytokine-related aging process, *J Gerontol A Biol Sci Med Sci* 59(9):M924–M929, 2004.

93. Fried LP, Ferrucci L, Darer J, et al: Untangling the concepts of disability, frailty, and comorbidity: implications for improved targeting and care, *J Gerontol A Biol Sci Med Sci* 59:255–263, 2004.

94. Morley JE, Perry HM, Miller DK: Something about frailty, *J Gerontol A Biol Sci Med Sci* 57A:798–808, 2002.

95. Fleshner M: Exercise and neuroendocrine regulation of antibody production: protective effect of physical activity on stress-induced suppression of the specific antibody response, *Int J Sports Med* 21(Suppl 1):S14–S19, 2000.

96. Horn JL, Cattell RB: Refinement and test of a theory of fluid and crystallized intelligence, *J Educ Psychol* 57:253–270, 1966.

97. Dreary IJ: *Looking down on human intelligence*, Oxford, UK, 2000, Oxford University Press.

98. Salthouse TA: The processing-speed theory of adult age differences in cognition, *Psychol Rev* 103:403–428, 1996.

99. Salthouse TA, Atkinson TM, Berish DE: Executive function as a potential mediator of age-related cognitive decline in normal adults, *J Exp Psychol* 132:566–594, 2003.

100. Kail KM, Salthouse TA: Processing speed as a mental capacity, *Acta Psychol (Amst)* 86:199–225, 1994.

101. Stine-Morrow EAL, Soederberg Miller LM: Basic cognitive processes. In Cavanaugh JC, Whitbourne SK, editors: *Gerontology: an interdisciplinary perspective*, New York, 1999, Oxford University Press, pp 186–212.

102. Gorus E, De Raedt R, Mets T: Diversity, dispersion and inconsistency of reaction time measures: effects of age and task complexity, *Aging Clin Exp Res* 18(5):407–417, 2006.

103. Whalley LJ, Deary IJ, Appleton CL, et al: Cognitive reserve and neurobiology of cognitive aging, *Ageing Res Rev* 3:369–382, 2004.

104. LeCarret N, Lafont S, Mayo W, et al: The effect of education on cognitive performances and its implication for the constitution of the cognitive reserve, *Dev Neuropsychol* 23:317–337, 2003.

105. Kramer AF, Bherer L, Colcombe SJ, et al: Environmental influences on cognitive and brain plasticity during aging, *J Gerontol A Biol Sci Med Sci* 59(9):M940–M957, 2004.

106. Shimamura AP, Berry HJM, Mangels JA, et al: Memory and cognitive abilities in university professors: evidence for successful aging, *Psychol Sci* 6:271–277, 1996.

107. Perls T: Centenarians who avoid dementia, *Trends Neurosci* 27(10):633–636, 2004.

108. Hitt R, Young-Xu Y, Perls T: Centenarians: the older you get, the healthier you've been, *Lancet* 354(9179):652, 1999.

109. Baltes PB, Lindenberger U, Staudinger UM: Life span theory in developmental psychology. In Damon W, Eisenberg N, editors: *Handbook of child psychology*, ed 5, New York, 1998, John Wiley & Sons, pp 1029–1144.

110. Cumming E, Henry WE: *Growing old: the process of disengagement*, New York, 1961, Basic Books.

111. Atchley RC, Barusch AS: *Social forces and aging*, ed 10, Belmont, Calif, 2004, Wadsworth.

112. Neugarten BL, Havinghurst RJ, Tobin SS: Personality and patterns of aging. In Neurgarten BL, editor: *Middle age and aging*, Chicago, 1968, University of Chicago Press, pp 173–177.

113. Atchley RC: A continuity theory of normal aging, *Gerontologist* 29:183–190, 1989.

114. Rowe JW, Kahn RL: Successful aging, *Gerontologist* 37:433–440, 1997.

3

Motor Development

OBJECTIVES

After studying this chapter, the reader will be able to:

1. Define motor development.
2. Understand the relationship between motor development and dynamic systems theory.

3. Identify variables that influence motor development.
4. Describe motor skill development across the life span.

Development results from the interrelated processes of maturation, physical growth, and learning and may be observed in genetic and environmental adaptation. *Maturation* guides development genetically in the physical changes that occur during organ differentiation in the embryo, myelination of nerve fibers, and the appearance of primary and secondary ossification centers. *Growth* is the process whereby changes in physical size and shape take place, as witnessed during adolescence when dramatic changes in facial and body growth occur. *Adaptation,* on the other hand, is the body's response to environmental stimuli. A muscle increases bulk with strength training, the immune system produces antibodies when exposed to a pathogen, bones heal after a fracture. All of these processes illustrate adaptation.

MOTOR DEVELOPMENT

Motor development is the change in motor behavior experienced over the life span. The process and the product of motor development are related to age, and motor development's study has roots in biology and psychology. Typically, researchers in motor development study individuals of different ages performing the same task, describe age differences in terms of performance, and suggest age-appropriate standards for judging the motor performance of infants, children, teenagers, adults, and older adults. Motor development studies are less likely to be concerned with changing one's performance than with documenting naturally occurring age-related change.

Motor behavior changes occur to meet our needs across the life span. Observable changes are the result of the interaction between biological and environmental factors. Biological factors are not stable over time and are evidenced by differences in rate of growth, magnitude of growth, sensory processing, flexibility, strength, and speed of response. Maturation and learning depend on each other because learning does not occur unless the system is ready to learn. The rate of maturation is affected by the amount and type of learning experiences, and the type of learning experiences is affected by the sociocultural environment. Environmentally, the variables are infinite and include physical surroundings, family structure, access to motor learning experiences, and culture. Needs are related to survival, safety, motivation, psychological development, and sociocultural expectations. Together, all of these factors produce change or adaptation in the motor behaviors of the individual.

Changes in growth are used as markers for development. Growth charts are familiar ways in which a child's height, weight, and head circumference are monitored during the course of development. Children can be classified as an early, an average, or a late maturer according to the relationship between physiological growth parameters and chronological age. Despite the smooth trajectories seen on standard growth curves, a child's growth is not continuous but episodic. Growth is episodic at all ages with more growth occurring at night than during the day.[1,2] The effects of physical size and body proportion on motor skill acquisition or movement proficiency have been examined in adolescence but are only now being explored in younger age groups.[3] Does the changing weight and proportion of the limb segments constrain the production of movement? Thelen and Fisher's[4] research supports the real possibility that infants cease reflex stepping because the limbs get too heavy, not because of any change in the nervous system.

Other factors that affect how a person develops movement are genetic coding and culture. Genes code for growth and maturation. Various sets of genes are associated with newborn length and weight, adult height and weight, and rate of growth in body size.[5] Genetics can contribute to motor performance and learning although the effect varies from task to task. The reader is referred to a review by Bouchard and colleagues[6] for more information. Children born with genetic disorders will usually exhibit delays in motor development. Group differences are reflected in gender and in the culture in which children are raised. Males have an innate ability to develop more muscle and greater strength.[5] Why does one person become a triathlete and another a prima ballerina, whereas others have difficulty riding a bike, water-skiing, or hitting a ball? Genes and the environment contribute in a complex way to human athletic performance. (See Brutsaert and Para[7] for a review of the evidence in support of a genetic basis to and environmental influences on athletic performance.) A child's experience gleaned from various child-rearing practices (including physical handling), sensory and motor feedback, and sensorimotor integration combines with a genetic predisposition to produce movement skills. As a result of the Back to Sleep campaign to decrease the incidence of sudden infant death syndrome, infants spend less time on their tummy. The lack of tummy time has been associated with delays in motor development.[8,9] Culture and child rearing practices influence movement skill acquisition by rewarding some motor behaviors and avoiding others.

Motor Development Goals

Motor development is both a process and a product. The process of motor development requires motor control and motor learning. Movement is guided by sensation and changed by sensory feedback. The goals of motor development are to acquire functional synergies that can be used to the mover's advantage, to become a competent mover, to become an efficient mover, to adapt movement to intrinsic and extrinsic demands, and lastly to achieve task goals. Movement allows for exploration, affording perception, making choices, and acquiring skills.

Motor Development Concepts

Many conceptual themes have been used to describe the acquisition and production of movement across the life span. One major concept related to movement skill acquisition is that it is sequential. Another framework that appears to influence movement outcomes seen across the life span is the direction in which growth and development, and hence change, occur. Movement, by its nature, also requires a point of mobility and a point of stability. Last, sensation plays a very important role in the acquisition and refinement of movement skill acquisition.

Developmental Sequence

One of the most important concepts about movement, and possibly the most universal concept, is that movement skill development is sequential. Movement development in the broadest sense is based on what came before. Each movement learned is used again in a slightly different way to achieve something else. Although the rate of development may vary normally from individual to individual and is referred to by the term *individual differences,* the sequence is the same for similar populations and cultures. In Western cultures, infants master sitting before creeping, standing, or walking. The typical sequence of motor skill acquisition will be presented at the end of this chapter.

Directional Concepts

Cephalocaudal Traditionally, development is said to progress *cephalocaudally,* that is, from the head to the foot. Head control develops before trunk control. Control of arm movements for reaching develops before control of leg movements for creeping. The first part of the body to develop is the neck. In utero, the neural tube closes first at the level of the fourth cervical vertebra and continues to close in two directions: toward the head (cephalo) and toward the feet (caudal). From this perspective, development is said to proceed from the neck cervicocephalocaudally.

Proximal-Distal The second concept of directional development is that development occurs from proximal to distal. In this case, *proximal* refers not only to the proximal parts of the extremities, such as the shoulder or pelvic girdles, but also to the midline of the neck and the midline of the trunk. The infant controls the midline of the neck, the midline of the trunk, the shoulders, and the pelvis before controlling the arms, legs, hands, and feet.

Proximal and distal structures are inseparable because the body is a system of linked structures. Movement in one area affects the relationship of the structures not only in the moving part but also in the other parts. Although the infant has not developed sufficient trunk control to sit alone, the infant can reach for and hold objects. Control of the midline of the trunk occurs before shoulder and pelvic girdle control is established.

Mobility and Stability

Controlled movement occurs within the framework of mobility and stability, or movement and posture. The relationship between *stability* (holding a posture) and *mobility* (moving) is called *postural control*. Mobility is present before stability. Once a stable posture is established, movement control within that posture develops.

Infants are very mobile and initially demonstrate random movements such as kicking in the supine position. These random leg movements occur within the available range of motion. Some postures are assumed briefly, such as head lifting in the prone position. Next, the infant learns to hold postures such as propping on elbows in prone (prone on elbows). Stable postures provide a base from which movement can occur. Infants and children are able to maintain a posture such as sitting before they are able to attain the posture independently, move in and out of the posture, or demonstrate the ability to preserve the posture if balance is disturbed.

Some postures are inherently stable and require little or no muscular effort. A prime example is W-sitting (Figure 3-1), in which the legs are internally rotated, the pelvis in anteriorly tilted, and the knees are flexed.

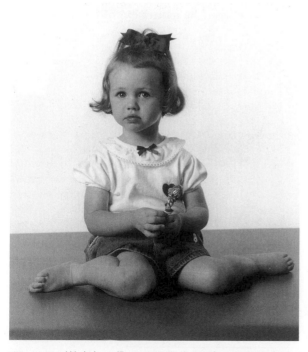

Figure 3-1 W-sitting. (From Martin S, Kessler M: *Neurologic interventions for physical therapy*, ed 2, St Louis, 2007, Saunders.)

It is as if a peg (the trunk) has been placed in a puzzle hole (the pelvis). Biomechanically, the child is locked in place with no need for active trunk control and is free to use the hands for play rather than support. The child is exhibiting *positional stability*, the stability that comes from the mechanics of the position, not from muscular control of the trunk. W-sitting is not an ideal position because it is a compensation for weakness or poor motor control. *Dynamic stability* is the use of muscular control to maintain a position. Frequently, infants use mechanical stability before sufficient muscular control has developed. For example, an infant elevates the shoulders to assist in maintaining the head in a midline position when first supported in an unstable sitting position. Once dynamic stability is established, the infant no longer needs the shoulders, the head can be turned easily, and there is separation of head and arm movement.

Dynamic stability is necessary for the child to develop skilled movements such as walking, running, and climbing. A child must be able to move into and out of postures, make subtle corrections to maintain balance, and control movement over a stable base for these functional movement patterns to emerge. Dynamic postural control is necessary to move safely from one posture to another and involves both dynamic stability and controlled mobility.

Sensation

Sensory information plays an important role in movement skill acquisition. The first movements experienced by the newborn are reflexively cued by sensation. Before vision, touch cues help the newborn find food. "Sensation is an ever-present cue for motor behavior in the seemingly reflex-dominated infant.[10]" Voluntary movement emerges as the nervous system and body mature. Sensory information from visual, somatosensory, and vestibular systems cues automatic postural responses in a reactive manner as postural control is acquired. Sensation from weight bearing reinforces postures such as quadruped, kneeling, and standing. Sensory information is used by the infant, toddler, or child to entice, direct, or guide interaction with objects and navigate the environment. Later, sensory information is used to cue postural readiness, such as when a person sees a bulging grocery sack and she needs to recruit a few more muscles before lifting it.

Comparison of Motor Development, Motor Control, and Motor Learning

The studies of motor development, motor control, and motor learning all uniquely contribute to our understanding of functional motor behavior. It is important to appreciate the similarities and differences in these three areas to have a full understanding of how functional movement is produced and controlled.

Motor control theory was influenced by a developmental model of neural function, one that grew from a view of how the nervous system evolved. This developmental model was championed by maturationists such as Gesell and McGraw, who based their model on observation of behavior. Similarly, motor development scholars were strongly influenced by studies of reflexes,[11] which have long been considered a fundamental unit of motor control. Motor learning and motor control theory share common themes such as the use of feedback, and researchers in these areas share ideas that mutually influence each other's work.[12] An understanding of the differences between these areas helps one to appreciate the unique contributions of each to our knowledge of motor behavior.

Time Frames

One way to distinguish between motor development, motor control, and motor learning is to focus on the time base that is used to study motor behavior within each area (Figure 3-2).[13] Motor development processes transpire across intervals typically referred to as "age." Commonly, age is measured in years. Motor control processes occur within very small intervals, typically,

fractions of seconds. Motor learning is a process that occurs across hours, days, and weeks and is discussed in Chapter 4.

Maturation of Systems

The development of motor control begins with the control of self-movements and proceeds to the control of movements in relationship to changing conditions. Control of self-movement is largely due to the development of the neuromotor systems. As the nervous and muscular systems mature, movement emerges. Motor control allows the nervous system to direct which muscles should be used and in what order and how quickly to solve a movement problem. The infant's first movement problem relates to overcoming the effect of gravity. A second but related problem is how to move a proportionately larger head in relation to a smaller body to establish head control. Later, movement problems are related to controlling the interaction between stability and mobility of the head, trunk, and limbs. Control of task-specific movements such as stringing beads or riding a tricycle is dependent on cognitive and perceptual abilities. The task to be carried out by the person within the environment dictates the type of movement solution that is going to be needed.

Because the motor abilities of a person change over time, the motor solutions to a given motor problem also may change. The motivation of the individual to

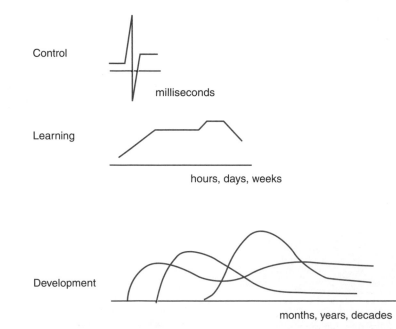

Control   milliseconds

Learning

hours, days, weeks

Development

months, years, decades

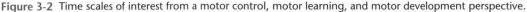

Figure 3-2 Time scales of interest from a motor control, motor learning, and motor development perspective.

move may also change over time and affect the intricacy of the movement solution. An infant encountering a set of stairs sees a toy on the top stair. She creeps up the stairs but then has to figure out how to get down. She can cry for help, bump down on her buttocks, creep down backwards, or even attempt to creep down forward. A toddler faced with the same dilemma may walk up the same set of stairs one step at a time holding onto a railing and descend sitting, holding the toy, or she may be able to hold the toy with one hand and the railing with the other and descend the same way she came up. The child will go up and down stairs without holding on, and an even older child may run up those same stairs. An older adult may go up and down stairs marking time when balance is impaired. The relationship between the task, the individual, and the environment is depicted graphically in Figure 3-3. All three components must be considered when thinking about motor development, motor control, and motor learning.

Motor Control Dependency on Maturation

The degree of maturation of the body's systems affects motor control because motor control occurs on a physiological level. Physiological maturation occurs in all body systems involved in movement production: muscular, skeletal, nervous, cardiovascular, and pulmonary. For example, if maturation of the contractile properties of muscle is incomplete, certain types of movements may not be possible. Weakness can impair movement. If synaptic connections are not complete, movement quality could be affected. Inability to perceive a threat visually will prevent a person from making a protective

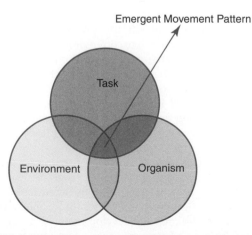

Figure 3-3 Systems model indicating the emergent pattern of movement arising from the interaction of system elements. (From Holt KG: Biomechanical models, motor control theory, and development, *Inf Child Dev* 14:524-527, 2005.)

movement. Muscle strength, posture, and perceptual abilities exhibit maturation and can affect the rate of motor development by affecting the process of motor control.

Motor Development Theories

Motor development scholars describe changes in motor behavior that are related to age. The three most prevalent theories of motor skill acquisition are the maturation perspective, the perceptual-cognitive perspective, and the dynamic systems perspective. The first two of these theories and theorists were discussed in Chapter 2. The maturationists predicated motor development and emerging motor behaviors on the neuromaturation of the cerebral cortex. The perceptual-cognitivists viewed information processing/perceptual development as a foundation for movement. In the dynamic systems theory, multiple systems of the body interact, and in that interaction, movement emerges.[14] Dynamic systems theory (DST) is highlighted because it is has been described in the literature as the grand theory of development (Spencer et al, 2006) and therefore most appropriate to be used to explain motor development.

Dynamic Systems Theory

Thelen and Smith[14,16,17] proposed a functional view of the process of motor development. In this perspective, movement is described as emerging from the interaction of multiple body systems. DST incorporates developmental biomechanical aspects of the mover, along with the developmental status of the mover's nervous system and the environmental context in which the movement occurs. Movement abilities associated with the developmental sequence are the result of motor control, which organizes movements into efficient patterns. DST is both a theory of motor control and of motor development.

Themes Relative to Dynamic Systems Theory A dynamic system is any system that demonstrates change over time.[18] Behavior emerges over a period of time. Motor development occurs over a period of months and years and because movement takes time to emerge, every movement made is potentially modifiable. Two main themes relative to DST have been identified:
1. "Development can only be understood as the multiple, mutual, and continuous interaction of all the levels of the developing system, from the molecular to the cultural.
2. Development can only be understood as nested processes that unfold over many time scales, from milliseconds to years.[14]" Development is depicted as a

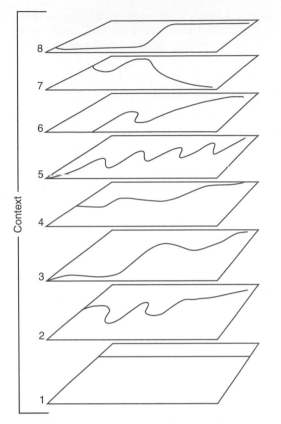

Figure 3-4 Development as a layered system where many, parallel developing components exhibit asynchronous trajectories. (From Thelen E: Motor development: a new synthesis, *Am Psychol* 50(2):79-95, 1995.)

layered system in Figure 3-4. The bottom layer could be the molecular layer, followed by the tissue layer, followed by a system layer or each layer could represent one or more body systems or developmental behaviors, such as the musculoskeletal, neurological, cognitive, perceptual, or socioemotional. Regardless of the components, each interacts with the other. Change is happening in all the layers but not at the same time as development unfolds over time.

The four processes that support development—growth, maturation, adaptation, and learning—overlap or are nested within one another as in a child's set of stacking cups. The themes espoused by Thelen and Smith[14] encompass four assumptions:

1. Every action, such as walking, requires the cooperation of numerous systems, including neuromuscular, sensory, perceptual, cardiovascular, and pulmonary.
2. There are "self-organizing properties" inherent in developing systems. Movement patterns arise from an interaction of these component parts.

3. Component structures and skill processes develop in an asynchronous, nonlinear manner.
4. Shifts from one behavioral mode to another are discontinuous.

Components such as posture, strength, flexibility, muscular maturation, and nervous system maturation can limit emergence of movement.

Lewis[19] viewed *self-organization* as the unifying theme that could establish DST as the single theory of development because this concept integrates diverse viewpoints and multiple facets of development. Self-organizing systems permit true novelty, so the structure of movement is emergent. For example, the stages seen in the developmental sequence represent periods of stability that emerge from the self-organization of multiple body systems. Self-organizing systems have the possibility of becoming more complex. The complexity serves the purpose of adapting to varying functional needs. A self-organizing system is able to reorganize and transition to new patterns of movement after or during a period of instability. Phase transitions are points of instability that occur when old patterns break down and new ones appear. For example, stereotypical rhythmic movements described by Thelen[20] (Figure 3-5) appear to represent transitional behaviors that emerge as the child is gaining control over a new posture. Lastly, self-organizing systems are both sensitive to change and inherently stable. The self-organizing system recognizes aspects of the environment via feedback. However, the repetition of a pattern of movement such as walking increases the likelihood that the preferred pattern of coordinative movement continues.

In the latest review of DST,[15] four central concepts were identified as being central to the theory as it has evolved over the last two decades. These central concepts do not diminish the previously discussed assumptions or themes but do represent extensions of our knowledge that motor development is constantly changing. The first concept is that dynamic system theory promotes a new look at *time*. The second concept of DST is that motor behavior is *multiply determined* and *soft assembled*. Many factors determine the form a movement takes: the mover's body, maturation of the mover's musculoskeletal and nervous systems, and the mover's motivation to name a few. Movement is initially loosely put together or soft assembled, the final product yet to be determined. The final form of the movement may require many revisions. Figure 3-4 depicts development as a layered system where each layer represents a component developing in parallel, all having asynchronous trajectories. At any given time, the movement outcome is a product of the components within a context. Some examples

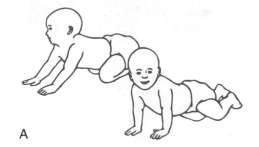

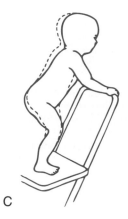

Figure 3-5 Stereotypical rhythmic movements. **A,** Hands and knees rocking. **B,** Arm banging against a surface. **C,** Stand-bouncing. (Modified from Thelen E: Rhythmical stereotypies in infants, *Anim Behav* 27(3):699-715, 1979.)

of components are strength, posture, and flexibility. Longitudinal studies show many influences over different time scales.[21,22] Behavior emerges in a moment and is subject to change based on the results of the movement or a change in the motivation of the mover or the environment in which the movement takes place. The concept of soft assembly allows for adaptability. Soft assembly provides a foundation for exploration and selection. The infant mover adapts to the changing world. Each infant learns a new movement in a different way; solutions are unique and within the context of the mover.

The third concept is *embodiment.* Embodiment includes the sensory information that occurs before, during, and after a movement, as well as the perception of the mover about what is happening. Sensation and perception are crucial to the integration of perception, action, and cognition. Movement happens in the context of the surrounding environment. Action or moving is a form of perception. Infants generate motor behaviors to gain perceptual information that they in turn use to learn how to make other actions possible. How will it feel if I wave my arm? Is it different if I

have something in my hand? Many forms of sensory information are dependent on movement such as vestibular, touch, vision, and proprioception/kinesthesia. Feedback from movement affords the possibility for sensation to be used as an anticipatory cue for movement. "Movement is ... the vehicle that drives spatial and temporal correlation and thus learning and skill performance.[23]" Sensation and movement are inextricably linked throughout motor development.

Nested actions such as looking and reaching are embedded in posture. These actions require a postural base. Maintaining a posture allows the sensory receptors to function in acquiring perceptions. Posture affords the infant the possibility for interaction such as looking, reaching for objects, holding objects, or moving somewhere. In Figure 3-6, each image of the infant is a moment in time with time moving from left to right. The infant must shift among stable solutions to reach for the ball or the box.

The fourth concept is a new respect for *individuality.* Each mover is an individual with unique needs. Novice movers show incredible variability. In fact, variability has always been considered a hallmark of typical

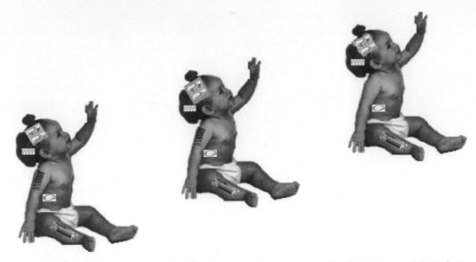

Figure 3-6 A view of learning and development from a dynamic systems perspective. Each image of the infant captures one time point, with time moving from left to right. (From Spencer JP, Clearfield M, Corbetta D et al: Moving toward a grand theory of development: in memory of Esther Thelen, *Child Dev* 77(6):1521-1538, 2006.)

development. DST encourages researchers and clinicians to embrace variability as a possible causal agent of change rather than just a marker of normalcy. If an infant is going to change the way she moves, the movement must be less stable or more variable.

Theory of Neuronal Group Selection Neuronal group selection[23] proposes that motor skills result from the interaction of developing body dynamics and the structure/functions of the brain. The brain's structures are changed by how the body is used (moved). The brain's growing neural networks are sculpted to match

efficient movement solutions. Three requirements must be met for neuronal selection to be effective in a motor system. First, a basic repertoire of movement must be present. Second, sensory information has to be available to identify and select adaptive forms of movement, and third, there must be a way to strengthen the preferred movement responses.

The infant is genetically endowed with spontaneously generated motor behaviors. Figure 3-7 illustrates rudimentary neural networks that subserve initial motor behaviors. This example involves activation of postural muscles in sitting infants. As the infant's multiple

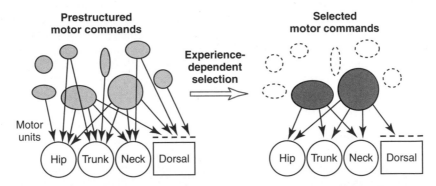

Figure 3-7 A developmental process according to the neuronal group selection theory is exemplified by the development of postural muscle activation patterns in sitting infants. Before independent sitting, the infant exhibits a large variation of muscle activation patterns in response to external perturbations, including a backward body sway. Various postural muscles on the ventral side of the body are contracted in different combinations, sometimes together with inhibition of the dorsal muscles. Among the large repertoire of response patterns are the patterns later used by adults. With increasing age, the variability decreases and fewer patterns are elicited. Finally, only the complete adult muscle activation patterns remain. If balance is trained during the process, the selection is accelerated. (Redrawn from Forssberg H: Neural control of human motor development, *Curr Opin Neurobiol* 9:676-682, 1999.)

sensory systems provide perception, the strength of synaptic connections between brain circuits is varied with selection of some networks that predispose one action over another. Environmental and task demands become part of the neural ensemble for producing movements. Spatial maps are formed and mature neural networks emerge as a product of use and sensory feedback. The maps that develop via the process of neuronal selection are preferred pathways. They become preferred because they are the ones that are used more often. These pathways connect large amounts of the nervous system and provide an interconnected organization of perception, cognition, emotion, and movement.[24]

The theory of neuronal group selection supports a dynamic systems theory of motor control/motor development. According to neuronal group selection, the brain and nervous system are guided during development by a genetic blueprint and initial activity, which establishes rudimentary neuronal circuits. This soft assembly is an example of self-organization. The use of certain circuits over others reinforces synaptic efficacy and strengthens those circuits. This is the selectivity that comes from exploring different ways of moving. Last, maps are developed that provide the organization of patterns of spontaneous movement in response to mover and task demands. The linking of these early perception-action categories is the cornerstone of development.[25] Other body systems, such as the skeletal, muscular, cardiovascular, and pulmonary systems, develop and interact with the nervous system so the most efficient movement pattern is chosen for the mover. There are no motor programs, and the brain should not be thought of as a computer or as hard wired. This theory supports the idea that neural plasticity may be a constant feature across the life span.

Order parameters are expressions of complex relationships within a motor behavior. They represent observable collective variables involved in temporal and spatial phasing between limbs. According to neuronal selection theory of motor control, the most appropriate neuronal group would be selected based on the task requirements, the environmental conditions, and the state of the body systems. Movement variability has always been considered a hallmark of normal movement. This integration of multiple systems allows for a variety of movement strategies to be available to perform a functional task; think of how many different ways it is possible to move across a room.

Theory Summary The DST has advanced our understanding of the changing form of movements that we observe in typically developing infants and children. By manipulating the subsystems involved in stepping behavior, Ulrich and colleagues[26] demonstrated that infants with Down syndrome can achieve walking earlier than expected. Down syndrome is a genetic disorder in which the child exhibits mental retardation and delayed motor skill acquisition. Infants with Down syndrome were trained to walk on a treadmill while supported by a parent. The children continued to receive physical therapy weekly in addition to stepping practice on the treadmill. In this case, the rate of acquisition of a motor skill was significantly impacted.

The DST is both a theory of motor development and motor control. Motor development can be seen as a model of general development. The nervous system is going to take advantage of the inherent properties of the musculoskeletal system and produce the most efficient movement possible in light of the demands of the task and the environment in which the movement takes place. Movement takes place in real time and each time a movement occurs the mover and the movement have the potential for change. A new solution to the movement problem may emerge. Some components limit the rate at which motor development changes. Some of these are strength, posture, muscular maturation, and nervous system maturation. "At any given point in development, the critical, rate-limiting factor that triggers the system to reorganize into a new configuration might be a psychological function governed by the CNS (e.g., motivation, balance control), or it might be a more peripheral factor such as gravity or leg fat.[27]"

FUNCTIONAL IMPLICATIONS

The functional implication of motor development is that movement abilities change over time or across the life span. Each individual develops functional movement in a similar sequence, but the rate of acquisition shows variation. The ages noted in the following discussion of typical motor development are approximations. There is a great deal of individual variation in the rate of change.

Life Span Changes in Motor Development and Function

Infancy

An infant's movements are intimately associated with reflexes for the first 3 months of life. Although a typically developing infant is not limited to reflex motor behavior, reflexes do play a role in pairing sensory and motor action. Reflexes are stereotypical responses to sensory stimuli. Reflexes occur early in developmental time, with some appearing during gestation or shortly

Table 3-1

Primitive Reflexes

Reflex	Age at Onset	Age at Integration
Suck-swallow	28 weeks' gestation	2-5 mo
Rooting	28 weeks' gestation	3 mo
Flexor withdrawal	28 weeks' gestation	1-2 mo
Crossed extension	28 weeks' gestation	1-2 mo
Moro	28 weeks' gestation	4-6 mo
Plantar grasp	28 weeks' gestation	9 mo
Positive support	35 weeks' gestation	1-2 mo
Asymmetrical tonic neck	Birth	4-6 mo
Palmar grasp	Birth	9 mo
Symmetrical tonic neck	4-6 mo	8-12 mo

Data from Barnes MR, Crutchfield CA, Heriza CB: *The neurophysiological basis of patient treatment*, vol 2, Atlanta, Stokesville, 1982.

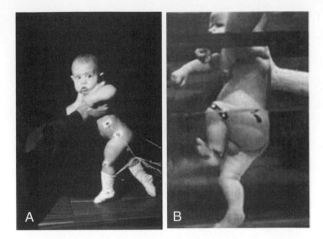

Figure 3-8 **A,** A newborn stepping. **B,** The reemergence of stepping when the infant is placed in water. (From Spencer JP, Clearfield M, Corbetta D et al: Moving toward a grand theory of development: in memory of Esther Thelen, *Child Dev* 77(6):1521-1538, 2006.)

Table 3-2

Gross Motor Milestones

Milestone	Age
Head control	4 mo
Rolling	6-8 mo
Sitting	8 mo
Creeping	9 mo
Cruising	10 mo
Walking	12 mo

From Martin ST, Kessler M: *Neurologic intervention for physical therapist assistants*, Philadelphia, 2000, WB Saunders, p 57.

Table 3-3

Fine Motor Milestones

Milestone	Age
Palmar grasp reflex	Birth
Raking	5 mo
Voluntary palmar grasp	6 mo
Radial palmar grasp	7 mo
Radial digital grasp	9 mo
Inferior pincer grasp	9-12 mo
Superior pincer grasp	12 mo
Three-jaw chuck	12 mo

From Martin ST, Kessler M: *Neurologic intervention for physical therapist assistants*, Philadelphia, 2000, WB Saunders, p 57.

after birth, and are integrated by 4 to 6 months of age. A list of primitive, or early occurring, reflexes is found in Table 3-1. Reflexes are often thought to be invariant but in many cases, the responses are modified by the alertness or satiation of the infant. Some reflex behavior can also be influenced by the environment. A stepping reflex can be elicited in a newborn but by several months of age the reflex "disappears." The case of the disappearing reflex was studied by Thelen and colleagues (Figure 3-8).[28,29] The usual explanation for the loss of stepping was that the nervous system matured and the reflex was integrated into the system. Thelen proved that the reason infants no longer exhibit a stepping reflex was that their legs got too heavy to perform the movement. When weight was not an issue, as when the infants were placed in water up to their chest, they once again exhibited the ability to step.

Motor skill development progresses sequentially over the first year of life, with the infant able to roll, sit, creep, pull to stand, and walk by 1 year. Reaching and prehension change from swiping at objects at 5 months to discrete movement of the thumb and index finger by 10 months. Reaching and prehension are discussed at length in Chapter 14. The motor milestones and the ages at which these skills can be expected to occur can be found in Tables 3-2 and 3-3. Action requires a stable postural base.

Birth to 3 Months

Newborns assume a flexed posture regardless of their position because physiological flexion dominates at birth. Initially, the newborn is unable to lift the head from a prone position. The newborn's legs are flexed under the pelvis and prevent the pelvis from coming into contact with the supporting surface. If you put yourself into that position and try to lift your head, even as an adult, you will immediately recognize that the biomechanics of the situation are against you. With your hips in the air, your weight is shifted forward, thus making it more difficult to lift your head even though you have more muscular strength and control than a newborn. Although you are strong enough to overcome this mechanical disadvantage, the infant is not. The infant must wait for gravity to help lower the pelvis to the support surface and for the neck muscles to strengthen to be able to lift the head when in the prone position. The infant will be able to lift the head first unilaterally (Figure 3-9, *A*), then bilaterally.

Over the next several months, neck and spinal extension develop and allow the infant to lift the head to one side, to lift and turn the head, and then to lift and hold the head in the midline. As the pelvis lowers to the support surface, neck and trunk extensors become stronger. Extension proceeds from the neck down the back in a cephalocaudal direction, so the infant is able to raise the head up higher and higher in the prone position. By 3 months of age, the infant can lift the head to 45 degrees from the supporting surface. Spinal extension also allows the infant to bring the arms from under the body into a position to support herself on the forearms (Figure 3-9, *B*). This position also makes it easier to extend the trunk. Weight bearing through the arms and shoulders provides greater sensory awareness to those structures and allows the infant to view the hands while in a prone position.

When in the supine position, the infant exhibits random arm and leg movements. The limbs remain flexed, and they never extend completely. In supine, the head is kept to one side or the other because the neck muscles are not yet strong enough to maintain a midline position. If you wish to make eye contact, approach the infant from the side because asymmetry is present. An asymmetrical tonic neck reflex may be seen when the baby turns the head to one side (Figure 3-10). The arm on the side to which the head is turned may extend and may allow the infant to see the hand while the other arm, closer to the skull, is flexed. This "fencing" position does not dominate the infant's posture, but it may provide the beginning of the functional connection between the eyes and the hand that is necessary for visually guided reaching. Initially the baby's hands are normally fisted, but in the first month they open. By 2 to 3 months, eyes and hands are sufficiently linked to allow for reaching, grasping, and shaking a rattle. As the eyes begin to track ever-widening distances, the infant will watch the hands and explore the body.

When an infant is pulled to sit from a supine position before the age of 4 months, the head lags behind the body. Postural control of the head has not been

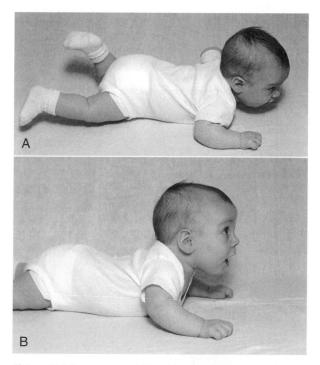

Figure 3-9 Prone progression of head control. **A,** Head lifting in prone. Infant momentarily lifts head at 1 month. **B,** Prone on elbows. A 4-month-old infant lifts and maintains head past 90 degrees. (From Wong DL, Perry SE: *Maternal child nursing care,* ed 3, St Louis, 2005, CV Mosby, p 1031.)

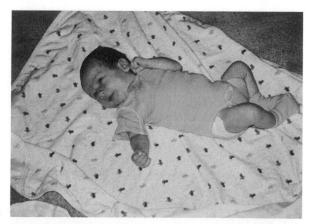

Figure 3-10 Asymmetrical tonic neck reflex in an infant.

established. The baby lacks sufficient strength in the neck muscles to overcome the force of gravity. Primitive rolling may be seen as the infant turns the head strongly to one side. The body may rotate as a unit in the same direction as the head moves. The baby can turn to the side or may turn all the way over from supine to prone or from prone to supine. This turning as a unit is the result of a primitive neck righting reflex. More discussion of postural reflexes and reactions is presented in Chapter 12. In this stage of primitive rolling, separation of upper and lower trunk segments around the long axis of the body is missing.

Four Months

Four months is a critical time in motor development because posture and movement change from asymmetric to more symmetric. When the infant is pulled to sit from a supine position, the head is in line with the body. Midline orientation of the head is present when the infant is at rest in the supine position. The infant is able to bring her hands together in the midline and to watch them. In fact, the first time the baby gets both hands to the midline and realizes that her hands, to this point only viewed wiggling in the periphery, are part of her body, a real "aha" occurs. Initially, this discovery may result in hours of midline hand play. The infant can now bring objects to the mouth with both hands. Bimanual hand play is seen in all possible developmental positions. The hallmark motor behaviors of the 4-month-old infant are head control and midline orientation.

Head control in the 4-month-old infant is characterized by being able to lift the head past 90 degrees in the prone position (see Figure 3-9), to keep the head in line with the body when the infant is pulled to sit, and to maintain the head in midline with the trunk when the infant is held upright in the vertical position and is tilted in any direction. Midline orientation refers to the infant's ability to bring the limbs to the midline of the body, as well as to maintain a symmetric posture regardless of position. When held in supported sitting, the infant attempts to assist in trunk control. The positions in which the infant can independently move are still limited to supine and prone at this age. Lower extremity movements begin to produce pelvic movements. Pelvic mobility begins in the supine position when, from a hooklying position, the infant produces anterior pelvic tilts by pushing on her legs and increasing hip extension, as in bridging.[30] Active hip flexion, adduction, and abdominals in supine produce posterior tilting. Random pushing of the lower extremities against the support surface provides further practice of pelvic mobility that will be used later in development, especially in gait.

Five Months

Even though head control as defined earlier is considered to be achieved by 4 months of age, control of the head against gravity in a supine position is not achieved until 5 months of age. At 5 months, the infant exhibits the ability to lift the head off the support surface (*antigravity neck flexion*). Antigravity neck flexion may first be noted by the caregiver when putting the child down in the crib for a nap. The infant works to keep the head from falling backward as she is lowered toward the supporting surface. This is also the time when infants look as though they are trying to climb out of their car or infant seat by straining to bring the head forward. When the infant is pulled to sit from a supine position, the head now leads the movement with a chin tuck. The head is in front of the body. In fact, the infant often uses forward trunk flexion to reinforce neck flexion and to lift the legs to counterbalance the pulling force.

As extension develops in the prone position, the infant may occasionally demonstrate a "swimming" posture (Figure 3-11). In this position, most of the weight is on the tummy, and the arms and legs are able to be stretched out and held up off the floor or mattress. This posture is a further manifestation of extensor control against gravity. The infant plays between this swimming posture and a prone-on-elbows or prone-on-extended-arms posture. The infant makes subtle weight shifts while in the prone-on-elbows position and may attempt reaching. Movements at this stage show *dissociation* of head and limbs, as exemplified by the following movement sequences:

1. Bilateral arm and leg movements are present as compared with previous unilateral movements. The proximal joints, such as the shoulder and pelvic girdles,

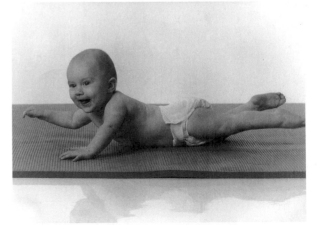

Figure 3-11 "Swimming" posture, antigravity extension of the body. (From Martin S, Kessler M: *Neurologic interventions for physical therapy*, ed 2, St Louis, 2007, Saunders.)

direct reaching and kicking movements. Just as the pattern of reaching is influenced by shoulder position, kicking can be changed by the position of the pelvis before and during the movement.

2. Pedaling is seen in the lower extremities. Starting with both hips flexed, the infant extends one leg, then the other, and then returns both legs to the original starting position. This leads to reciprocal kicking in which both legs continue to perform reciprocal alternating movements.

3. From a froglike position, the infant is able to lift her bottom off the support surface and to bring her feet into her visual field. This "bottom lifting" allows her to play with her feet and even to put them into her mouth for sensory awareness. This play provides lengthening for the hamstrings and prepares the baby for long sitting. The lower abdominals also have a chance to work while the trunk is supported.[31]

Six Months

A 6-month-old infant becomes mobile in the prone position by pivoting in a circle (Figure 3-12). The infant is also able to shift weight onto one extended arm and to reach forward with the other hand to grasp an object. The reaching movement is counterbalanced by a lateral weight shift of the trunk that produces lateral head and trunk bending away from the side of the weight shift (Figure 3-13). This lateral bending in response to a weight shift is called a *righting reaction*. Righting reactions of the head and trunk are discussed in Chapter 9. Maximum extension of the head and trunk is possible in the prone position along with extension and abduction of the limbs away from the body. This extended posture

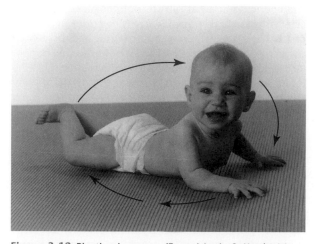

Figure 3-12 Pivoting in prone. (From Martin S, Kessler M: *Neurologic interventions for physical therapy*, ed 2, St Louis, 2007, Saunders.)

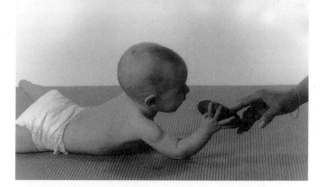

Figure 3-13 Lateral righting reaction. (From Martin S, Kessler M: *Neurologic interventions for physical therapy*, ed 2, St Louis, 2007, Saunders.)

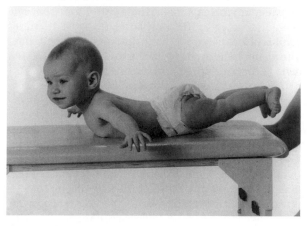

Figure 3-14 Spontaneous Landau reflex. (From Martin S, Kessler M: *Neurologic interventions for physical therapy*, ed 2, St Louis, 2007, Saunders.)

is called the *Landau reflex* and represents total body righting against gravity. It is mature when the infant can demonstrate hip extension when held away from the support surface, supported only under the tummy. The infant appears to be flying (Figure 3-14). This final stage in the development of extension can occur only if the hips are relatively adducted. Too much hip abduction puts the gluteus maximus at a biomechanical disadvantage and makes it more difficult to execute hip extension. Excessive abduction is often seen in children with low muscle tone and increased range of motion such as in Down syndrome. These children have difficulty performing antigravity hip extension.

Segmental rolling is now present and becomes the preferred mobility pattern when rolling, first from prone to supine, which is less challenging, and then from supine to prone. Antigravity flexion control is needed to roll from supine to prone. The movement usually begins with flexion of some body part, depending on the infant and the circumstances. If enticed with a toy, the infant may reach up and over the body for the toy with the upper extremity. Another infant may lift one leg up and over the body, and may allow the weight of the pelvis to initiate trunk rotation. Still another infant may begin the roll with head and neck flexion. Regardless of the body part used, segmental rotation is essential for developing transitional control. *Transitional movements* are those that allow a change of position, such as moving from prone to sitting, from the four-point position to kneeling, and from sitting to standing. Only a few movement transitions take place without segmental trunk rotation, such as moving from the four-point position to kneeling and from sitting to standing. Individuals with movement dysfunction often have problems making the transition from one position to another smoothly and efficiently. This difficulty is often due to a lack of segmental trunk rotation. The quality of movement affects the individual's ability to perform transitional movements.

The 6-month-old infant can sit up if placed and supported at the low back or pelvis. The typically developing infant can sit in the corner of a couch or on the floor if propped on extended arms. A 6-month-old cannot purposefully move into sitting from a prone position but may incidentally push herself backward along the floor. Coincidentally, while pushing, her abdomen may be lifted off the support surface, allowing the pelvis to move over the hips, with the end result of sitting between the feet. Sitting between the feet is called *W-sitting* and should be avoided in infants with developmental movement problems because it can make it difficult to learn to use trunk muscles for balance. The posture provides positional stability, but it does not require active use of the trunk muscles. Concern also exists about the abnormal stress this position places on growing joints. Concern about this sitting posture in typically developing children is less because these children move in and out of the position more easily, rather than remaining in it for long periods of time.

Having developed trunk extension in the prone position, the infant can sit with a relatively straight back with the exception of the lumbar spine (Figure 3-15). The upper and middle back are not rounded as in previous months, but the lumbar area may still demonstrate forward flexion. Although the infant's arms are needed for support initially, with improving trunk control, first one hand and then both hands will be freed from providing postural support to explore objects and to engage in more sophisticated play. When balance is lost during sitting, the infant extends the arms for protection while

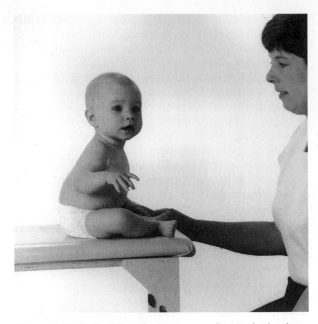

Figure 3-15 Early sitting showing a rounding in the lumbar area. (From Martin S, Kessler M: *Neurologic interventions for physical therapy*, ed 2, St Louis, 2007, Saunders.)

falling forward. In successive months, this same upper extremity protective response will be seen in additional directions such as laterally and backward.

The pull-to-sit maneuver with a 6-month-old often causes the infant to pull all the way up to standing (Figure 3-16). The infant will most likely reach forward for the caregiver's hands as part of the task. A 6-month-old likes to bear weight on the feet and will bounce in this position if she is held. Back and forth rocking and bouncing in a position seem to be prerequisites for achieving postural control in a new posture.[20] Repetition of rhythmic upper extremity activities is also seen in the banging and shaking of objects during this period. Reaching becomes less dependent on visual cues as the infant uses other senses to become more aware of body relationships. The infant may hear a noise and may reach unilaterally toward the toy that made the sound.[32]

Seven Months

Functional ability in sitting improves at this age. Trunk control improves in sitting and allows the infant to free one hand for playing with objects. The infant can narrow her base of support in sitting by adducting the lower extremities as the trunk begins to be able to compensate for small losses of balance. Dynamic stability develops from muscular work of the trunk. An active trunk supports dynamic balance and complements the positional stability derived from the configuration of the base of

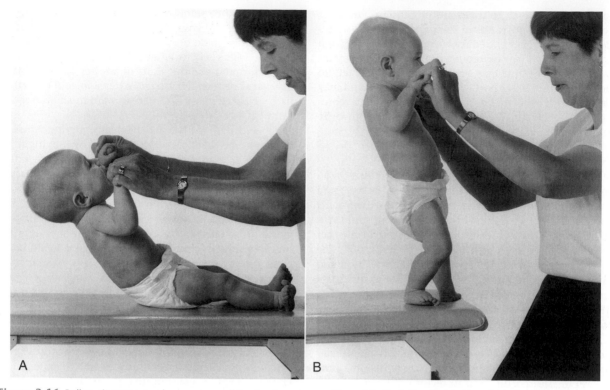

Figure 3-16 Pull-to-sit maneuver becomes a pull-to-stand maneuver. (From Martin S, Kessler M: *Neurologic interventions for physical therapy*, ed 2, St Louis, 2007, Saunders.)

support. The different types of sitting postures such as ring sitting, wide abducted sitting, and long sitting provide the infant with different amounts of support. Lateral protective reactions begin to emerge in sitting at this time. Unilateral reach is displayed by the 7-month-old infant, as is an ability to transfer objects from hand to hand.

Eight Months

Sitting is the most functional and favorite position of an 8-month-old infant. Because the infant's back is straight, the hands are free to play with objects or extend and abduct to catch the infant if a loss of balance occurs, as happens less frequently at this age. Upper trunk rotation is demonstrated during play in sitting as the child reaches in all directions for toys. If a toy is out of reach, the infant can prop on one arm and reach across the body to extend the reach using trunk rotation and reverse the rotation to return to an upright sitting position. With increased control of trunk rotation, the body moves more segmentally and less as a whole. This trend of dissociating upper trunk rotation from lower trunk movement began at 6 months with the beginning of

segmental rotation. Dissociation of the arms from the trunk is seen as the arms move across the midline of the body. More external rotation is evident at the shoulder (turning the entire arm from palm down, to neutral, to palm up) and allows supinated reaching to be achieved. By 8 to 10 months, the infant's two hands are able to perform different functions such as holding a bottle in one hand while reaching for a toy with the other.[32]

Now the infant can move into and out of sitting by deliberately pushing up from side lying. She may bear weight on her hands and feet and may attempt to "walk" in this position (*bear walking*) after pushing herself backward while belly crawling. Some type of prewalking progression, such as belly crawling, creeping on hands and knees, or sitting and hitching, is usually present by 8 months. Hitching in a sitting position is an alternative way for some children to move across the floor. The infant scoots on her bottom with or without hand support. We have already noted how pushing up on extended arms can be continued into pushing into sitting. Pushing can also be used for locomotion. Because pushing is easier than pulling, the first type of straight plane locomotion achieved by the infant in a prone position may be backward propulsion. Pulling is seen as strength increases in the upper back and shoulders. All this upper extremity work in a prone position is accompanied by random leg movements. These random leg movements may accidentally cause the legs to be pushed into extension with the toes flexed and may thus provide an extra boost forward. In trying to reproduce the accident, the infant begins to learn to belly crawl or creep forward.

Nine Months

A 9-month-old is constantly changing positions, moving in and out of sitting, including side sitting, and into the four-point position. As the infant experiments more and more with the four-point position, she rhythmically rocks back and forth and alternately puts her weight on her arms and legs. In this endeavor, the infant is aided by a new capacity for hip extension and flexion, which affords more opportunities to dissociate movements of the pelvis from movements of the trunk. The hands and knees position, or quadruped position, is a less supported position requiring greater balance and trunk control. As trunk stability increases, simultaneous movement of an opposite arm and leg is possible while the infant maintains weight on the remaining two extremities. This form of reciprocal locomotion is called *creeping*. Creeping is often the primary means of locomotion for several months, even after the infant starts pulling to stand and cruising around furniture. Creeping provides fast and stable travel for the infant and allows for exploration of the environment.

Reciprocal movements used in creeping require counterrotation of trunk segments; the shoulders rotate in one direction while the pelvis rotates in the opposite direction. Counterrotation is an important element of erect forward progression (walking), which comes later. Other major components needed for successful creeping are extension of the head, neck, back, and arms, and dissociation of arm and leg movements from the trunk. Extremity dissociation depends on the stability of the shoulder and pelvic girdles and on the infant's ability to control rotation in opposite directions.

When playing in the quadruped position, the infant may reach out to the crib rail or furniture and may pull up to a kneeling position. Balance is maintained by holding on with the arms rather than by fully bearing weight through the hips. The infant at this age does not have the control necessary to balance in a kneeling or half-kneeling (one foot forward) position. Even though kneeling and half-kneeling are used as transitions to pull to stand, only after learning to walk is such control possible for the toddler. Pulling to stand is a rapid movement transition with little time spent in

either true knee standing or half-kneeling. Early standing consists of leaning against a support surface, such as the coffee table or couch, so the hands can be free to play. Legs tend to be abducted for a wider base of support, much like the struts of a tower. Knee position may vary between flexion and extension, and toes alternately claw the floor and flare upward in an attempt to assist balance.

Once the infant has achieved an upright posture at furniture, she practices weight shifting by moving from side to side. While in upright standing and before cruising begins in earnest, the infant practices dissociating arm and leg movements from the trunk by reaching out or backward with an arm while the leg is swung in the opposite direction. When side-to-side weight shift progresses to actual movement sideways, the baby is cruising. Cruising is done around furniture and between close pieces of furniture. This sideways "walking" is done with arm support and may be a means of working the hip abductors to ensure a level pelvis when forward ambulation is attempted. These maneuvers always make us think of a ballet dancer warming up at the barre before dancing. In this case, the infant is warming up, practicing counterrotation in a newly acquired posture, upright, before attempting to walk (Figure 3-17). Over the next several months, the infant will develop better pelvic and hip control to perfect upright standing before attempting independent ambulation.

Toddler

Twelve Months The infant becomes a toddler at 1 year. Most infants attempt forward locomotion by this age. The caregiver has probably already been holding the infant's hands and encouraging walking, if not placing the infant in a walker. Use of walkers has raised some safety issues[33]; also use of walkers too early does not allow the infant to sufficiently develop upper body and trunk strength needed for the progression of skills seen in the prone position. Typical first attempts at walking are lateral weight shifts from one widely abducted leg to the other (Figure 3-18). Arms are held in *high guard* (arms held high with the scapula adducted, shoulders in external rotation and abducted, elbows flexed, and wrist and fingers extended). This position results in strong extension of the upper back that makes up for the lack of hip extension. As an upright trunk is more easily maintained against gravity, the arms are lowered to *midguard* (hands at waist level, shoulders still externally rotated), to *low guard* (shoulders more neutral, elbows extended), and finally to no guard.

The beginning walker keeps hips and knees slightly flexed to bring the center of mass closer to the ground. Weight shifts are from side to side as the toddler

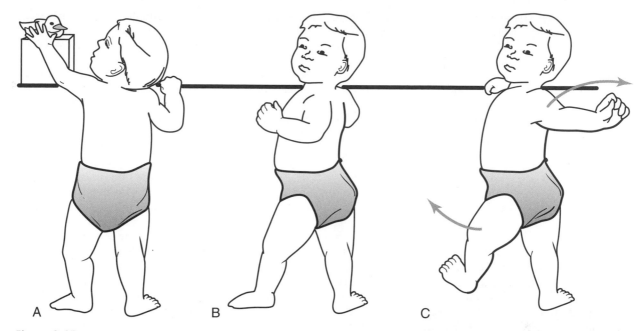

Figure 3-17 Cruising maneuvers. **A,** Cruising sideways, reaching out. **B,** Standing, rotating upper trunk backward. **C,** Standing, reaching out backward, elaborating with swinging movements of the same-side leg, thus producing counterrotation. (Redrawn by permission of the publisher from Conner FP, Williamson GG, Siepp JM: *Program guide for infants and toddlers with neuromotor and other developmental disabilities*, New York, 1978, Teacher's College Press, p 121.)

moves forward by total lower extremity flexion, with the hip joints remaining externally rotated during the gait cycle. Ankle movements are minimal, with the foot pronated as the whole foot contacts the ground. Toddlers take many small steps and walk slowly. The instability of their gait is seen in the short amount of time they spend in single-limb stance. As trunk stability improves, the legs come farther under the pelvis. As the hips and knees become more extended, the feet develop the plantar flexion needed for the push-off phase of the gait cycle. New walkers engage in massive walking practice, often taking more than 9000 steps a day, the equivalent of traversing more than 29 football fields.[34]

Sixteen to Eighteen Months By 16 to 17 months, the toddler is so much at ease with walking that a toy can be carried or pulled at the same time. With help, the toddler goes up and down stairs, one step at a time. Without help, the toddler creeps up the stairs and may creep or scoot down on her buttocks. Most children will be able to walk sideways and backward at this age if they started walking at 12 months or earlier. The typically developing toddler comes to stand from a supine position by rolling to prone, pushing up on hands and knees or hands and feet, assuming a squat, and rising to standing (Figure 3-19).

Most toddlers exhibit a reciprocal arm swing and heel strike by 18 months of age, with other adult gait characteristics manifested later. They walk well and demonstrate a "running-like" walk. Although the toddler may still occasionally fall or trip over objects in her path because eye-foot coordination is not completely developed, the decline in falls appears to be the result of improved balance reactions in standing and the ability to monitor trunk and lower extremity movements kinesthetically and visually. The first signs of jumping appear as a stepping off "jump" from a low object such as the bottom step of a set of stairs. Children are ready for this first step-down jump after being able to walk down a step while they hold the hand of an adult.[35] Momentary balance on one foot is also possible.

Childhood

A 2-year-old child can go up and down stairs one step at a time, jump off a step with a 2-foot takeoff, stand on one foot for 1 to 3 seconds, kick a large ball, and throw a small ball. Stair climbing and kicking are indicative of improved stability while shifting body weight from one leg to another.[31] The child can easily step over low objects encountered in the environment. True running emerges in the second year and is characterized by a flight phase when both feet are off the ground at the

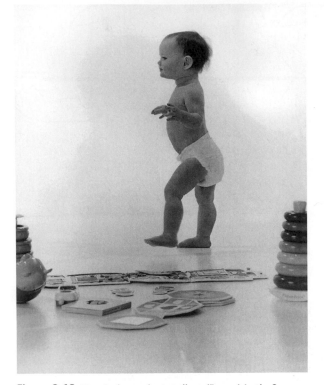

Figure 3-18 New independent walker. (From Martin S, Kessler M: *Neurologic interventions for physical therapy*, ed 2, St Louis, 2007, Saunders.)

same time. Despite the running, quick starts and stops remain difficult, with directional changes requiring a large area to make a turn. Jumping off the ground with both feet is eventually mastered. Beginning attempts result in only one foot leaving the ground, followed by the second foot as if the child were stepping in air.

Fundamental motor patterns such as hopping, galloping, and skipping develop from 3 to 6 years of age. Wickstrom[35] also includes running, jumping, throwing, catching, and striking in this category. Other reciprocal actions mastered by age 3 are pedaling a tricycle and climbing a jungle gym or ladder. Locomotion can be started and stopped based on the demands from the environment or from a task such as playing dodgeball on a crowded playground. A 3-year-old child can make sharp turns while running and can balance on toes and heels in standing. Standing with one foot in front of the other, known as tandem standing, is possible, as is standing on one foot for at least 3 seconds. A reciprocal gait is now used to ascend stairs with the child placing one foot on each step in alternating fashion but marking time (one step at a time) when descending.

Hopping on one foot is a special type of jump requiring balance on one foot and the ability to push off the loaded foot. It does not require a maximum effort. "Repeated vertical jumps from two feet can be done before true hopping can occur.[35]" Neither type of jump is seen at an early age. Hopping one or two times on the preferred foot may also be accomplished by age 3½ years when there is the ability to stand on one foot and balance long enough to push off on the loaded foot. A 4-year-old child should be able to hop on one foot four to six times. Improved hopping ability is seen when the child learns to use the nonstance leg to help propel the body forward. Before that time, all the work is done by pushing off with the support foot. A similar pattern is seen in arm use; at first, the arms are inactive, and later they are used opposite the action of the moving leg. Sexual differences for hopping are documented in the literature, with girls performing better than boys.[35] This may be related to the fact that girls appear to have better balance than do boys in childhood.

Rhythmic relaxed galloping is possible for a 4-year-old child. Galloping consists of a walk on the lead leg followed by a running step on the rear leg. Galloping is an asymmetrical gait. A good way to visualize galloping is to think of a child riding a stick horse. Toddlers have been documented to gallop as early as 20 months after learning to walk,[36] but the movement is stiff with arms held in high guard as in beginning walking.

At 5 years of age, a child can stand on either foot for 8 to 10 seconds, walk forward on a balance beam, hop 8 to 10 times on one foot, make a 2- to 3-foot standing broad jump, and skip on alternating feet. Skipping requires bilateral coordination. A 6-year-old child is well coordinated and can stand on one foot for more than 10 seconds, with eyes open or eyes closed. This ability is important to note because it indicates that vision can be ignored and balance maintained. The 6-year-old child can walk on a balance beam in all directions without stepping off. The child also uses alternate forms of locomotion, such as riding a bicycle or roller skating.

Fundamental game-playing skills are learned in early childhood (3 to 6 years). All children typically develop the ability to run, jump, throw, and catch. These patterns of movement form the basis for later sports skills. Between 6 and 10 years of age, a child masters the adult forms of running, throwing, and catching. Throughout the process of changing motor activities and skills, the nervous, muscular, and skeletal systems are maturing, and the body is growing in height and weight. Power develops slowly in children because strength and speed within a specific movement are required.[37]

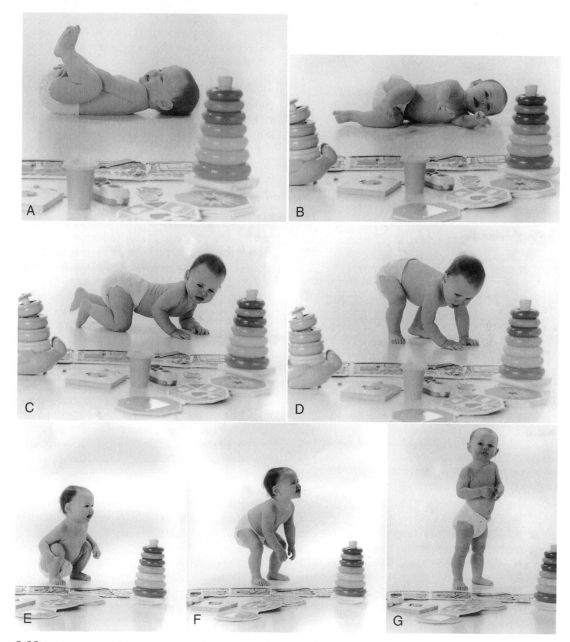

Figure 3-19 Progression of rising to standing from supine. **A,** Supine; **B,** rolling; **C,** four-point position; **D,** plantigrade; **E,** squat; **F,** semisquat; **G,** standing.

Fundamental motor skills demonstrate changes in form over time. Figure 3-20 depicts when 60% of children were able to demonstrate a certain developmental level for the listed fundamental motor skills. A marked gender difference is apparent in overhand throwing. It is not uncommon to see young children demonstrate a mature pattern of movement at one age and a less mature pattern at a later age. Regression of patterns is possible when the child is attempting to combine skills. For example, a child who can throw overhand while standing may revert to underhand throwing when running. Alterations between mature

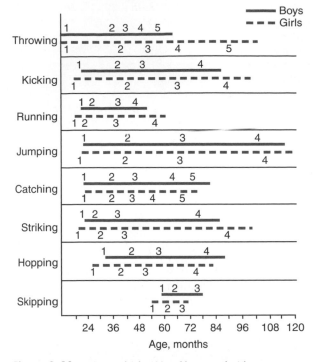

Figure 3-20 Ages at which 60% of boys and girls were able to perform at specific developmental levels for several fundamental motor skills. Stage 1 is immature; stage 4 or 5 is mature. (Reprinted by permission from Seefeldt V, Haubenstricker J: Patterns, phases, or stages: an analytical model for the study of developmental movement. In Kelso JAS, Clark JE, editors: *The development of movement control and coordination,* 1982, p 314.)

and immature movement is in line with Gesell's concept of reciprocal interweaving (see Chapter 2). Individual variation in motor development is considerable during childhood. Even though 60% of children have achieved the fundamental motor skills listed in Figure 3-20, 40% of the children have not achieved them by the ages given.

Assessment of motor development is clinically important in the context of screening, diagnosis, and intervention. Commonly used tools include the Bayley Scales of Infant Development, the Peabody Developmental Motor Scales, and the Bruininks-Oseretsky Test of Motor Proficiency. A thorough discussion of tools is beyond the scope of this chapter. The reader is referred to Campbell and colleagues[38] and Effgen[39] for a discussion of these and other tests and measures. Behavioral observation including an assessment of play is a useful adjunct to information obtained from a standardized tool of motor skill acquisition. Play assessment tools such as the Knox Preschool Play Scale and Bundy's Test of Playfulness are discussed in Parham and Fazio.[40]

Adolescence

The onset of puberty occurs 2 years earlier in girls than in boys. Static strength increases in females during adolescence, but the gains are not as great as in males. Although strength changes are related to skeletal maturity, such as peak height velocity (rate of fastest growth), motor performance is not.[5] Although females demonstrate an increase in motor performance to around 14 years of age,[41] performance on tasks is highly variable during the remainder of adolescence. The variability is probably due to a complex interaction of strength, peak height velocity, and the onset of menses. Motivation, interest, and attitudes toward physical activity may also be factors.

The onset of puberty can have a short-term positive effect on motor performance of boys, which is related to an increase in adrenergic hormones. Boys who mature early demonstrate greater strength and endurance than do boys who have not yet matured. The height growth spurt seen in adolescent males is marked by rapid gain in strength. The acceleration peaks around 14 years of age and stops at about 18 years of age. Motor performance peaks during late adolescence, which for males occurs around 17 to 18 years of age.

The adolescent may continue to gain prowess in motor skills with practice. Parameters of performance such as power, speed, accuracy, form, and endurance can be changed. The amount of change is highly variable and depends on practice and innate ability. The maximum degree of skill possible on most tasks is related to the individual's satisfaction with her performance within the limits of cognitive, structural (physical), or sociocultural factors.[42] In other words, working with the resources at hand, the movement is as efficient as possible given the raw materials of the individual within the environment. Some improvement in motor performance in most sports has been thought to occur relatively early.

Spirduso[43] examined the effect of age on sport-specific abilities. Generally, peak performance of sports requiring explosive bursts of power or speed over time occurs in the person's early 20s. However, because older athletes (30s) put in record-breaking performances in the 1990s, she thinks the concept of age at peak performance may need to be reevaluated. Years of training and a competitive edge may allow an over-30 athlete to triumph over a more physiologically robust 20-year-old in some sports. The physical demands of the task, such as power, speed, or endurance, must be taken into consideration.

Age-Related Differences in Movement Patterns Beyond Childhood

Many developmentalists have chosen to look only at the earliest ages of life when motor abilities and skills are being acquired. The belief that mature motor behavior is achieved by childhood led researchers to overlook the possibility that movement might change as a result of factors other than nervous system maturation. Although the nervous system is generally thought to mature by the age of 10, changes in movement patterns do occur in adolescence and adulthood.

VanSant[44,45] and Sabourin[46] studied the movement patterns used by people of different ages to accomplish a simple motor task. VanSant and others[44,45] studied the task of rising from supine to standing by describing the movement components for different regions of the body. Although an explanation of the method used in the many studies is beyond the scope of this text, a summary of the results is most appropriate.

Research shows a developmental order of movement patterns across childhood and adolescence with trends toward increasing symmetry with increasing age.[44] VanSant[45] identified three common ways in which adults move from supine to standing (Figure 3-21). The most common pattern was to use upper extremity reach; symmetrical push; forward head, neck, and trunk flexion; and a symmetrical squat. The second most common pattern was identical to the first pattern up to an asymmetrical squat. The third most common pattern involved an asymmetrical push and reach followed by a half-kneel. In a separate study of adults in their 20s through 40s, there was trend toward increasing asymmetry with age.[47] Adults in their 40s were more likely to demonstrate the asymmetrical patterns of movement seen in young children.[13] The asymmetry of movement in 40-year-old adults may reflect less trunk rotation due to stiffening of joints or lessening of muscle strength, making it more difficult to come straight forward to sitting from a supine position.

Thomas and colleagues[48] studied movement from a supine position to standing in older adults using VanSant's descriptive approach. In a group of community dwelling older adults with a mean age of 74.6 years, the 70- and 80-year-old adults were more likely to use asymmetrical patterns of movement in the upper extremity and trunk regions, whereas those younger than 70 demonstrated more symmetrical patterns in the same body regions. Furthermore, the researchers found a shorter time to rise was related to lower age, greater knee extension strength, and greater hip and ankle range of motion (flexion and dorsiflexion, respectively). However, older adults who maintain their strength and flexibility rise to standing faster and more symmetrically than do those who are less strong and flexible.[48]

Although the structures of the body are mature at the end of puberty, changes in movement patterns continue throughout a person's life. Mature movement patterns have always been associated with efficiency and symmetry. Early in motor development, patterns of movement appear to be more homogeneous and follow a fairly prescribed developmental sequence. As a person matures, movement patterns become more symmetrical. With aging, movement patterns again become more asymmetrical. In general, more mature patterns of movement are symmetrical. Because an older adult may exhibit different ways of moving from supine to standing than a younger person, treatment interventions should be taught that match the individual's usual patterns of movement.

SUMMARY

Motor development includes the change in motor behavior over the life span and the sequential, continuous, age-related process of change. It is determined by the merging of our genetic predisposition for movement and our experiences. The soft assembled movements allow exploration and skill refinement. The mover and the environment are both changed in the process. Movement emerges from the dynamic interaction of multiple components and systems to meet intrinsic or extrinsic demands. Motor control is the physiological process whereby motor development occurs, and motor learning allows motor development to occur systematically, resulting in a permanent change in motor behavior due to experience. In the following chapter, motor control and motor learning will be explored.

In 1989 Roberton[49] proposed that the dynamic systems theory be applied to life-span motor development research. Thelen and Smith[14,16,17] have done so with great effect. The DST, along with its underlying premise, neuronal selection theory, continues to be hailed as the unifying theme for understanding motor development.[15] If motor development is viewed as the study of change in motor behavior across a lifetime, age becomes a marker variable and may not be the cause of change. Altering the way in which we think about age may allow therapists

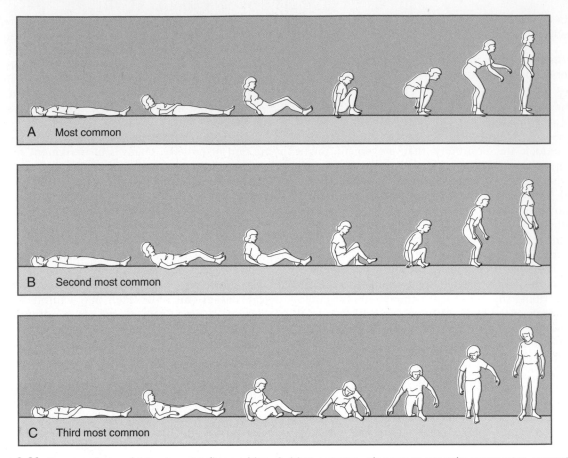

A Most common

B Second most common

C Third most common

Figure 3-21 Common forms of rising to a standing position. **A,** Most common using upper extremity component, symmetrical push; axial component, symmetrical; lower extremity component, symmetrical squat. **B,** Second most common using upper extremity component, symmetrical push; axial component, symmetrical; lower extremity component, asymmetrical squat. **C,** Third most common using upper extremity component, asymmetrical push and reach; axial component, partial rotation; lower extremity component, half-kneel. (Adapted and reprinted from VanSant AF: Rising from a supine position to erect stance: Description of adult movement and a developmental hypothesis, *Phys Ther* 68:185-192, 1988, with permission of the American Physical Therapy Association.)

and researchers to discover new information about why individuals move the way they do at different times in their lives. Knowledge of motor development across the life span is critical for therapists to ascertain the most appropriate therapeutic strategies for people to function optimally regardless of age, occupation, or disability.

REFERENCES

1. Lampl M, Johnson ML, Frongillo EA: Mixed distribution analysis identifies saltation and stasis growth, *Ann Hum Biol* 28:403–411, 2001.
2. Noonan KJ, Franum CE, Leiferman EM, et al: Growing pains: are they due to increased growth during recumbency as documented in a lamb model? *J Pediatr Orthop* 24:726–731, 2004.
3. Adolph KE, Avolio AM: Walking infants adapt locomotion to changing body dimensions, *J Exp Psychol* 26(3):1148–1166, 2000.
4. Thelen E, Fisher DM: Newborn stepping: an explanation for a disappearing reflex, *Dev Psychol* 18:760–775, 1982.
5. Malina RM, Bouchard C, Bar-Or O: *Growth, maturation and physical activity*, ed 2, Champaign, Ill, 2004, Human Kinetics.
6. Bouchard C, Malina RM, Perusse L: *Genetics of fitness and physical performance*, Champaign, Ill, 1997, Human Kinetics.
7. Brutsaert TD, Parra EJ: What makes a champion? Explaining variation in human athletic performance, *Respir Physiol Neurobiol* 151:109–123, 2006.
8. Liao PJ, Zawacki L, Campbell SK: Annotated bibliography: effects of sleep position and play position on motor development in early infancy, *Phys Occup Ther Pediatr* 25:149–160, 2005.

9. Pin T, Eldridge B, Galea MP: A review of the effects of sleep position, play position, and equipment use on motor development, *Dev Med Child Neurol* 49:858–867, 2007.

10. Martin S, Kessler M: *Neurologic interventions for physical therapy*, ed 2, St Louis, 2007, Saunders.

11. Wyke B: The neurological basis for movement: a developmental review, *Clin Dev Med* 55:19–33, 1975.

12. Schmidt RA, Lee TD: *Motor control and learning: a behavioral emphasis*, ed 3, Champaign, Ill, 1999, Human Kinetics.

13. VanSant AF: Life-span motor development. In Lister M, editor: *Contemporary management of motor control problems. Proceedings of the II step conference*, Alexandria, Va, 1991, Foundation for Physical Therapy, pp 77–83.

14. Thelen E, Smith LB: Dynamic systems. In Damon W, Lerner RM, editors: *Handbook of child psychology*, ed 6, New York, 2006, John Wiley & Sons, pp 258–312.

15. Spencer JP, Clearfield M, Corbetta D, et al: Moving toward a grand theory of development: in memory of Esther Thelen, *Child Dev* 77(6):1521–1538, 2006.

16. Thelen E, Smith LB: *A dynamic systems approach to the development of cognition and action*, Cambridge, Mass, 1994, MIT Press.

17. Thelen E, Smith LB: Dynamic systems. In Damon W, editor: *Handbook of child psychology*, ed 5, New York, 1998, John Wiley & Sons, pp 563–634.

18. Heriza C: Motor development: traditional and contemporary theories. In Lister M, editor: *Contemporary management of motor control problems. Proceedings of the II step conference*, Alexandria, Va, 1991, Foundation for Physical Therapy, pp 99–126.

19. Lewis MD: The promise of dynamic systems approaches for an integrated account of human development, *Child Dev* 71:36–43, 2000.

20. Thelen E: Rhythmical stereotypies in infants, *Anim Behav* 27(3):699–715, 1979.

21. Thelen E, Ulrich BD: Hidden skills: a dynamic systems analysis of treadmill stepping during the first year, *Monogr Soc Res Child Dev* 56(1, No. 223):1–104, 1991.

22. Thelen E, Corbetta D, Kamm K, et al: The transition to reaching: mapping intention and intrinsic dynamics, *Child Dev* 64:1058–1098, 1993.

23. Andreatta R: Power point, course notes RHB 710, *Neural Plast* Fall 2006.

24. Campbell SK: Revolution in progress: a conceptual framework for examination and intervention. Part II, *Neurol Rep* 24:42–46, 2000.

25. Edelman GM: *Neural Darwinism*, New York, 1987, Basic Books.

26. Ulrich DA, Ulrich BD, Angulo-Barroso RM, et al: Treadmill training of infants with Down syndrome: evidence-based developmental outcomes, *Pediatrics* 108:1–7, 2001.

27. Adolph KE, Berger SE: Motor development. In Damon W, Lerner RM, editors: *Handbook of child psychology*, ed 6, New York, 2006, John Wiley & Sons, pp 161–213.

28. Thelen E, Fisher DM, Ridley-Johnson R: The relationship between physical growth and a newborn reflex, *Infant Behav Dev* 7:479–493, 1984.

29. Thelen E: Motor development: a new synthesis, *Am Psychol* 50(2):79–95, 1995.

30. Bly L: *Motor skill acquisition in the first year of life*, San Antonio, Tex, 1994, Therapy Skill Builders.

31. Conner FP, Williamson GG, Siepp JM: *Program guide for infants and toddlers with neuromotor and other developmental disabilities*, New York, 1978, Teacher's College Press.

32. Duff SV: Prehension. In Cech D, Martin S, editors: *Functional movement development across the life span*, ed 2, Philadelphia, 2002, WB Saunders.

33. American Academy of Pediatrics, Committee on Injury and Poison Prevention: Injuries associated with infant walkers, *Pediatrics* 108(3):790–792, 2001.

34. Adolph KE, Vereijken B, Shrout PE: What changes in infant walking and why, *Child Dev* 74:474–497, 2003.

35. Wickstrom RL: *Fundamental movement patterns*, ed 3, Philadelphia, 1983, Lea & Febiger.

36. Whithall J: A developmental study of the inter-limb coordination in running and galloping, *J Mot Behav* 21:409–428, 1989.

37. Bernhardt-Bainbridge D: Sports injuries in children. In Campbell SK, Vander Linden DW, Palisano RJ, editors: *Physical therapy for children*, ed 3, St Louis, 2006, Saunders, pp 517–556.

38. Campbell SK, Vander Linden DW, Palisano RJ, editors: *Physical therapy for children*, ed 3, St Louis, 2006, Saunders.

39. Effgen SK: *Meeting the physical therapy needs of children*, Philadelphia, 2005, FA Davis.

40. Parham LD, Fazio LS, editors: *Play in occupational therapy for children*, ed 2, St Louis, 2008, Mosby.

41. Bailey DA, Malina RM, Mirwald RL: Physical activity and growth of the child. In Falkner FT, Tanner JM, editors: *Human growth: a comprehensive treatise*, vol 2, ed 2, New York, 1986, Plenum, pp 147–170.

42. Higgins S: Motor skill acquisition, *Phys Ther* 71:123–139, 1991.

43. Spirduso WW: *Physical dimensions of aging*, Champaign, Ill, 1995, Human Kinetics.

44. VanSant AF: Age differences in movement patterns used by children to rise from a supine position to erect stance, *Phys Ther* 68:1130–1138, 1988.

45. VanSant AF: Rising from a supine position to erect stance: description of adult movement and a developmental hypothesis, *Phys Ther* 68:185–192, 1988.

46. Sabourin P: *Rising from supine to standing: a study of adolescents*, 1989, Virginia Commonwealth University unpublished master's thesis.

47. Ford-Smith CD, VanSant AF: Age differences in movement patterns used to rise from a bed in the third through fifth decades of age, *Phys Ther* 73:300–307, 1993.

48. Thomas RL, Williams AK, Lundy-Ekman L: Supine to stand in elderly persons: relationship to age, activity level, strength, and range of motion, *Issues Aging* 21:9–18, 1998.

49. Roberton MA: Motor development: recognizing our roots, charting our future, *Quest* 41:213–223, 1989.

CHAPTER 4

Motor Control and Motor Learning

OBJECTIVES

After studying this chapter, the reader will be able to:

1. Define motor control and motor learning.
2. Discuss the basic theories of motor control and motor learning.

3. Understand the age-related changes in motor control and motor learning.

Motor control theories provide a framework for interpreting movement and behavior. Motor control is the ability to organize and control functional movement. The field of motor control grew primarily from the specialized study of neurophysiology in an attempt to explain how functional movement is produced and regulated in humans. From a historical perspective, several different theories and models have been proposed. Some models approach motor control from a physiological perspective, and others have a psychological perspective. Regardless, it is important to realize that these theories are ever-changing and evolving based on contemporary thought and the current research. When the explanations of an existing theory are no longer sufficient to interpret the research data, new theories are developed.

During the twentieth century, scholars attempted to explain the mechanisms of motor control. Initially, it was thought that the brain organized movement through reflexes alone or as a hierarchy. Later models were developed that described feedback and programming within the nervous system. A systems model is the most contemporary model of motor control at this time. Motor control is the ability to organize and control functional movement. Each of these models is discussed in turn.

MOTOR CONTROL THEORIES

Early perspectives of motor control date back to the late 1800s, when two similar views were proposed that pointed to a hierarchical organization. In separate research, the authors claimed that sensory input was necessary for the control of motor output. James[1] suggested that a successive chain of muscular contractions inherent in a habitual motor act were triggered in sequence by associated sensations, or *chaining*. By the turn of the century, Sherrington[2] proposed his *reflex model*, wherein a sequence of reflexes formed the building blocks of complex motor behavior. Unfortunately, these two related theories did not explain movement that occurs without a sensory stimulus, nor did they explain how actions are modified depending on the context in which they occur (e.g., varying speed, novel conditions).

Reflex Model

The original reflex model of Sherrington[2] was predicated on the reflex being the basic unit of movement. Reflexes are stereotypical responses to specific sensory stimuli. Sensory information triggers a motor response. There is no response without sensory input. A deep tendon reflex is an example of a monosynaptic reflex. Other reflexes are more complicated and involve more than one level of the nervous system such as an asymmetrical tonic neck reflex. Sherrington thought that voluntary movement was the product of chains of reflexes put together by the brain. Although this explanation of movement being based on reflexes persisted for quite some time, it is incorrect. Movement can occur without a sensory trigger. Reflexive movement tends to be very stereotypical with little or no variability. The nervous system does have local circuits at the spinal cord level that coordinate reflexes. Reflexive movement is only one category of movement.

Hierarchical Model

In the hierarchical model of motor control, specific reflexes or reactions are associated with a specific neuroanatomical level (Figure 4-1). Reflexes mediated in the spinal cord are deemed phasic because they are typically of short duration. The monosynaptic stretch reflex and the flexor withdrawal are examples of phasic reflexes. Spinal reflexes are characterized by patterns of reciprocal innervation. Reflexes mediated at the brain stem level are characterized as tonic because of their long duration. Tonic reflexes such as the asymmetrical tonic neck reflex and tonic labyrinthine reflex produce changes in tone and posture. Cocontraction of agonist and antagonist muscles enables primitive forms of posture. The positive support reflex, brought about by pressure on the ball of the foot, turns the lower limb into a pillar of support.

The midbrain or subcortical structures were associated with compensatory behaviors that align the body with respect to gravity. These righting reactions are brought about by complex sensory signals arising from a variety of sources, including the eyes, the labyrinths of the ears, and the cutaneous and proprioceptive receptors of the body. The movements produced are more variable than reflexes and as a result are termed reactions. See Chapter 12 for a description of various righting reactions as they relate to reactive postural control.

Each subsequent level of the neural axis exhibits control over the lower levels, resulting in a top-down model of control. The highest level of motor control in the hierarchical model is at the cortical level. The cortex in this model is considered the director of movement. The cortex is the site of the will, or volitional functions that inhibit and control reflexes and initiate purposeful action.

Neurologists have explained motor behavior exhibited by patients with brain injury using this traditional hierarchy.[3-5] According to classic theory, disease or damage to the brain causes "dissolution" of brain function. *Dissolution* means that neural function regresses to a primitive level characteristic of an earlier phase of nervous system development. After the therapist performs a clinical test of reflexes, the behavior of the patient is interpreted to represent a particular level of function. For example, if the patient's behavior is dominated by tonic reflex responses, the behavior is interpreted as representing brain stem-level function. Classic treatment and intervention strategies for individuals with brain damage were founded on this view of motor control.

In both the reflex and the hierarchical models, volitional movement is thought to replace reflexive movement. As stated earlier, when an individual is able to exert cortical control over her actions, she is displaying volitional control of movement. The ability of the cortex to use feedback related to the performance of motor tasks contributes to the volitional control of movement. Use of sensory information in the form of feedback is an important factor in both motor control and motor learning. Various motor control models further examines the concept of feedback.

FEEDBACK CONTROL

Feedback is a very crucial feature of motor control. *Feedback* is defined as sensory or perceptual information received as a result of movement. There is intrinsic feedback, or feedback produced by the movement. Sensory feedback can be used to detect errors in movement. Feedback and error signals are important for two reasons. First, feedback provides a means to understand

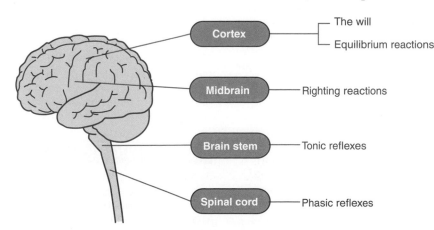

Figure 4-1 The classic reflex hierarchy with reflexes or reactions assigned to specific neuroanatomical levels.

the process of self-control. Reflexes are initiated and controlled by sensory stimuli from the environment surrounding the individual. Motor behavior generated from feedback is initiated as a result of an error signal produced by a process within the individual. The highest level of many motor hierarchies is a volitional, or self-control, function, but there has been very little explanation of how it operates.

Second, feedback also provides the fundamental process for learning new motor skills. Intrinsic feedback comes from any sensory source from inside the body such as from proprioceptors or outside the body when the person sees that the target was not hit or the ball was hit out of bounds.[6] Extrinsic feedback is extra or augmented sensory information given to the mover by some external source.[6] A therapist or coach may provide enhanced feedback of the person's motor performance. For this reason, feedback is a common element in motor control and motor learning theories.

Closed-Loop Control Model

Closed-loop control is the term used to designate the motor control process that is based on feedback. If one were to draw a model of a feedback or closed-loop control process, it would look like Figure 4-2. The information regarding a motor action is fed back into the nervous system to assist in planning the next action or modifying an ongoing action. A loop between sensory information and motor actions is created; this is a closed loop. By using feedback, errors can be detected and corrections made to maintain or improve performance. An example of a closed-loop action can be seen in many computer games that require guiding a figure or object across a screen. No one can learn without feedback. Whether one relies on a teacher or coach to provide the feedback or on one's capacity to gather information about performance, feedback is necessary to correct faulty actions. Closed-loop control is used to control deliberate movements carried out at relatively slow speeds and is necessary for motor learning.

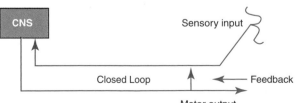

Figure 4-2 A model of closed loop control. *CNS,* central nervous system.

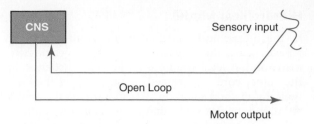

Figure 4-3 A model of open loop control. *CNS,* central nervous system.

Open-Loop Control Model

An open-loop control process is depicted in Figure 4-3. Movement is anticipated in this type of control and proceeds without waiting for feedback. Feedforward control or open-loop control is driven by either a centrally preprogrammed command[6] or sensory information from the peripheral environment. This is particularly true for very fast actions termed *ballistic movements.* For example, when a baseball pitcher fires off his favorite pitch, the movement occurs so fast that it is completed before feedback loops can provide information that would alter the action. The sensory cue in this instance is fed forward to trigger the action rather than fed back after the action. The blaring of a fire alarm immediately generates rapid movement in individuals to move to an exit. Open-loop control can occur after a movement is well learned and allows for increased speed of performance that would not be possible if the person waited to receive feedback.

Feedforward control requires experience and sensory information to work correctly. It has therefore more aptly been called *anticipatory control.* Feedforward control is imperative for a rapid response. Feedforward control requires that the nervous system be able to predict what is going to happen as a result of a sensory experience. For example, think of a batter hitting a ball that then comes straight to you. You must react quickly and rapidly to position your gloved hand to catch the ball on the fly. Feedforward control is one important aspect of control of posture and movement.[7] More aspects of control of posture will be discussed in Chapter 12.

MOTOR PROGRAM MODELS

As a result of a debate over the role of sensory information in motor actions, another concept of importance to current motor control and learning theories arose.[8] That concept is the motor program. A motor program is a memory structure that provides instructions for the control of actions. A program is a plan that has been stored for future use. The concept of a motor program is useful because it provides a means by which the nervous system can avoid having to create each action from scratch and thus can save time when initiating actions. There has been much debate over what is contained in a motor program. Different researchers have proposed a variety of programs.

During the 1900s, different perspectives emerged in an attempt to demonstrate that movement could be generated from within the nervous system, not just following a sensory stimulus, and that motor control may be distributed throughout the nervous system. *Motor program theory* was developed to directly challenge the notion that all movement was generated through chaining or reflexes because even slow movements occur too fast for sensory input to influence them.[9] The implication is that in order for efficient movement to occur in a timely manner, an internal representation of movement actions must be available to the mover. "Motor programs are associated with a set of muscle commands specified at the time of action production, which do not require sensory input.[10]" Schmidt[11] expanded motor program theory to include the notion of a generalized motor program or an abstract *neural representation* of an action, distributed among different systems. Being able to mentally represent an action is part of developing motor control.[12]

Systems Models

A systems model disputes the assumption that motor control is hierarchically organized and instead argues that it is distributed throughout the nervous system.[13] Although the CNS is organized in a hierarchical fashion to a certain degree, the direction of control is not simply from the top down.[9,14] For example, lower levels of the nervous system can assume control over higher levels depending on the goals and constraints of the task.

The brain undergoes anatomical growth during development, which includes cell proliferation, migration, and differentiation,[15] as well as functional and organizational changes in response to environmental and task demands. Because the nervous system has the ability to self-organize, it is feasible that several systems are engaged in resolving movement problems; therefore, solutions typically are unique to the context and goal of the task at hand.[16,17] The advantage of the systems model is that it can account for the flexibility and adaptability of motor behavior in a variety of environmental conditions. Functional goals, as well as environmental and task constraints, are thought to play a major role in determining movement.[14] This frame of reference provides a foundation for developing intervention strategies based on task goals that are aimed at improving motor skills.

Dynamic Systems Model

A dynamic system is any system that changes over time.[18] Development of control of the body systems involved in movement occurs asynchronously. However, all systems of the body interact with each other and with the environment in which the movement takes place on an ongoing basis. The interface of the mover, the task, and the environment is where the movement pattern emerges to best fit the needs at that time. Not only are the body systems involved in movement maturing over time, but so is the psychological understanding of the mind and body maturing to provide motivation, ideation, and an understanding of how things work. The common solutions to early movement dilemmas, such as gravity and changing body proportions that are the developmental sequence, support this view of motor control. A further discussion of dynamic systems theory as it relates to motor development is found in Chapter 3.

Motor control theories continue to be developed, and although the associated assumptions may differ, most current models have incorporated a systems view of distributed control of the nervous system. One assumption that remains controversial is whether a central neural representation of movement exists. Bernstein[19] suggested that the outcome of a movement is represented in a motor plan (e.g., aiming a ball toward a target) and distributed at different levels of the CNS. Many theorists have adopted this concept. *Early motor program theory* suggested that some form of neural storage of motor plans took place.[20] It is questionable whether the CNS has the capacity to store motor plans or whether the motor plan is a hypothetical concept.[21] Conversely, DST proposes that nothing is stored; instead, movement is an emergent property.[22] Although the specific organization of motor plans is not known, flexible neural representations of the dynamic and distributed processes through which the nervous system can solve motor problems seem to exist.[23,24] It is thought that motor learning evolves from an interaction and strengthening among multiple systems and that there may be strong neural connections between related systems that can be crudely viewed as representations.

ISSUES RELATED TO MOTOR CONTROL

Top-Down or Distributed Control

The issue of where the control of movement resides has always been at the heart of the discussion of motor control. Remember that motor control occurs in milliseconds as compared with the time it takes to learn a movement or to develop a new motor skill. The reflex hierarchical models are predicated on the cortex being the controller of movement. However, if there is no cortex, movement is still possible. The cortex can initiate movement, but it is not the only neural structure able to do so. From studying pathology involving the basal ganglia, it is known that movement initiation is slowed in people with Parkinson disease. Other neural structures that can initiate/control movement include the basal ganglia, the cerebellum, and the spinal cord. The spinal cord can produce rudimentary reciprocal movement from activation of central pattern generators. The reflexive withdrawal and extension of the limbs have been modified to produce cyclical patterns of movement that help locomotion be automatic but are modifiable by higher centers of the brain. Lastly, the cerebellum is involved in movement coordination and timing of movements. The fact that more than one structure within the nervous system can affect and control movement lends credence for a distributed control of movement.

There is no one seat of control in the systems view of movement; the movement emerges from the combined need of the mover, the task, and the environment. The structures, pathways, and processes needed to most efficiently produce the movement are discovered as in finding the best way to get the task done. The structures, pathways, or processes that are continually used get better at the task and become the preferred way of performing that particular task. Developmentally, only certain structures, pathways, or processes are available early in development so that movements become refined and control improves with age. Movement control improves not only because of the changes in the CNS but because of the maturation of the musculoskeletal system. Because the musculoskeletal system carries out the movement, its maturation can affect movement outcome.

Degrees of Freedom

How is the degrees of freedom problem inherent in movement solved? The mechanical definition of *degrees of freedom* is "the number of planes of motion possible at a single joint.[25]" The degrees of freedom of a system have been defined as all of the independent movement elements of a control system and the number of ways each element can act.[6] There are multiple levels of redundancy within the CNS. Bernstein[19] suggested that a key function of the CNS was to control this redundancy by minimizing the degrees of freedom or the number of independent movement elements that are used. For example, muscles can fire in different ways to control particular movement patterns or joint motions. In addition, many different kinematic or movement patterns

can be executed to accomplish one specific outcome or action. During the early stages of learning novel tasks, the body may produce very simple movements, often "linking together two or more degrees of freedom[9]" and limiting the amount of joint motion by holding some joints stiffly via muscle cocontraction. As an action or task is learned, we first hold our joints stiffly through muscle coactivation, and then, as we learn the task, we decrease coactivation and allow the joint to move freely. This increases the degrees of freedom around the joint.[26] This concept is further discussed later in the chapter.

Certainly, an increase in joint stiffness used to minimize degrees of freedom at the early stages of skill acquisition may not hold true for all types of tasks. In fact, different skills require different patterns of muscle activation. For example, Spencer and Thelen[27] reported that muscle coactivity increases with learning of a fast vertical reaching movement. They proposed that high velocity movements actually result in the need for muscle coactivity to counteract unwanted rotational forces. However, during the execution of complex multijoint tasks, such as walking and rising from sitting to standing, muscle coactivation is clearly undesirable and may in fact negatively affect the smoothness and efficiency of the movements. The resolution of the degrees of freedom problem varies depending on the characteristics of the learner as well as on the components of the task and environment. Despite the various interpretations of Bernstein's original hypothesis,[19] the resolution of the degrees of freedom problem continues to form the underlying basis for a systems theory of motor control.

Use of Sensory Information

Movement occurs within an environmental context. First, sensation is paired with movement reflexively, after which sensation can be used to learn movement as when feedback occurs. Finally, sensation can cue movement in a feedforward manner. Sensory information most pertinent to motor control comes from three key sources: somatosensory (proprioceptive and tactile), visual, and vestibular processes. Sensory processing improves through childhood and adolescence, as does the integration of sensory information for planning and executing movements. Vision is extremely important for postural control and balance early in life. The vestibular system provides information about the infant's relationship to gravity and head movements. Proprioception of the upper limb is particularly important in the development of accuracy of motor performance in children. Depending on the type of task employed, studies have shown that proprioceptive abilities are stable by age 8 or that proprioceptive ability continues to improve well into adolescence.[28,29] Loss of proprioceptive sensibility in older adults has functional consequences for movement.[30] The effects of these sensory systems relative to posture and balance are discussed in Chapter 12.

Optimization Principles

Optimization theory suggests that movements are specified to optimize a select cost function.[31-33] Cost functions are those kinematic (spatial) or dynamic (force) factors that influence movement at an expense to the system. Motor skill development or relearning is aimed at achieving select objectives while minimizing cost to the system. Reducing such cost while meeting task demands and accommodating to task constraints theoretically solves the degrees of freedom problem and enhances movement efficiency.

Flash and Hogan[34] theorized that the cost function being reduced during point-to-point reaching movements is *jerk* (rate of change in acceleration). This results in a straighter hand path, as exemplified in a 1997 study by Konczak and Dichgans (Figure 4-4).[35] These authors found that the distance the hand traveled

during reaching movements in young infants was initially prolonged with a noticeable curvature in the sagittal hand path or paths. However, with practice, the distance the hand traveled was reduced, the hand path became straighter, and the overall movement was smoother. Hypothetically, optimization principles drive the nervous system toward greater efficiency within the confines of task demands, environmental constraints, and performer limitations.

As children and adults struggle to achieve functional gains during development or during recovery from neural injury, they may appear to use inefficient movement strategies, at least from an outside view. In actuality, they may be expressing the most efficient movements available to them given their current resources. For example, a child with hemiplegic cerebral palsy may have the physical constraints of shoulder or wrist weakness and reduced finger fractionation (isolation). In an effort to reduce cost to the system while meeting tasks demands, she may use a "flexion synergy," in which elbow flexion is used in combination with shoulder elevation and lateral trunk flexion to reach for objects placed

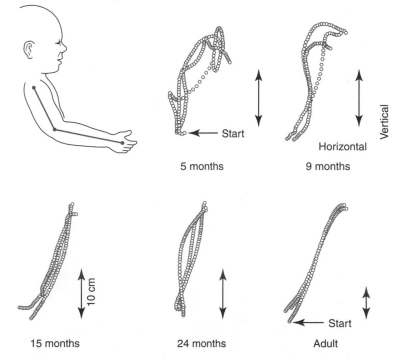

Figure 4-4 Progressive smoothing of sagittal hand paths during reaching, from infancy to adulthood. (Redrawn from Konczak J, Dichgans J: The development toward stereotypic arm kinematics during reaching in the first 3 years of life, *Exp Brain Res* 117:346-354, 1997.)

at shoulder height. This flexion synergy is a strategy that seems to reduce the number of movement elements yet allows for successful attainment of the target object. Although this strategy may be useful in a specific situation, it may become habitual and may not be effective in performing a wide range of tasks. Researchers have found that children with hemiplegic cerebral palsy as a result of right hemisphere damage have deficits in using proprioceptive feedback to recognize arm position.[30]

AGE-RELATED CHANGES IN MOTOR CONTROL

The development of motor control is thought to be linked to the development of the ability to form a mental representation of movement, which has been studied using a motor imagery paradigm. Motor imagery is an active cognitive process whereby representation of an action is internally reproduced in working memory.[36] This internal representation occurs without motor output. Motor imagery has frequently been used to study how adults plan and control movements,[37] but children have been less frequently studied.

Children

In a recent review article, Gabbard[12] presented current findings on motor imagery in children. A relationship exists between the ability to mentally represent an action by forming internal models and motor imagery. Using a water tilting task, Frick and colleagues[38] tried to determine if motor or visual information about movement of water in a glass that was tilted would make it easier to perform the task successfully. Movement of the glass provided information to the youngest children studied who were 5 years old. The experimental setups are shown in Figure 4-5. Funk and colleagues[39] also noted that motor processes guided 5- and 6-year-old children in performing a mental rotation task. Gabbard[12] concluded that by the age of 5, children appear to be able to use mental imagery to represent actions.

Feedforward control develops rapidly between 6 and 10 years of age.[40] The connection between motor imagery and motor action gets stronger with age and probably represents the maturation of neural networks. As children age, they improve in their ability to generate internal models of movement that are scaled

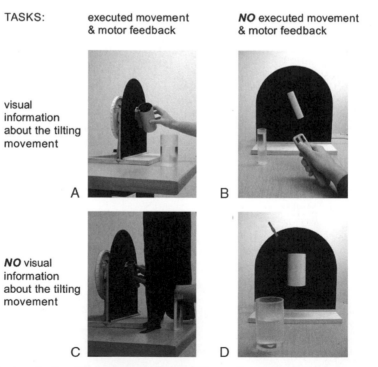

Figure 4-5 Experimental setups for the different tasks: **A,** Manual tilting task—experiment 1; **B,** remote control task—experiment 2; **C,** blind tilting task—experiment 3; **D,** judgment task—experiment 4. (From Frick A, Daum MM, Wilson M, et al. Effects of action on children's and adult's mental imagery. *J Exp Child Psych* 104:34-51, 2009.)

to their intrinsic biomechanics. Caeyenberghs and fellow researchers studied a cross section of children from 7 to 12 years of age to assess their development of motor imagery using a radial pointing task and a hand rotation task.[40] There was a strong relationship between motor imagery and motor skills with clear age differences.

Adolescents and Adults

The ability to generate accurate mental images of actions improves and is refined with age. Adolescents and adults show changes in motor imagery that could not be accounted for by general cognitive changes. Choudhury and associates[41] assessed movement execution time in adolescents and adults while performing two different hand movements and while imagining performing the same two different hand movements. There was a definite tight correlation between the time it took to perform the real and the imagined movements. The ability to form motor images was better in adults than adolescents. The researchers attributed this difference to the fact that the adolescent brain is experiencing ongoing maturation of the parietal cortex. The parietal cortex is thought to be involved with storage and modification of internal models of actions.[42]

Older Adults

In contrast to adults, older adults demonstrate a lack of ability to accurately simulate imagined movements. In other words, older adults show a decline in the ability to match the timing and spatial components of a mentally simulated movement compared with adults.[43-45] These researchers studied arm movements in a series of experiments that compared the performance of healthy older adults and healthy younger adults. Based on these experiments, they concluded mental representation of arm movements appears to weaken with age. Additionally, Skoura and associates[45] found more of a decline in the nondominant arm. Skoura and associates[46] also showed that young and old adults displayed similar timing for a walking and pointing task that was imagined or performed. However, the groups were dissimilar in the timing of a stand-sit-stand task. Both young and older adults demonstrated a shorter time for the imagined task than for the actual task. The authors thought that this was related to the fact that when actually performing the movement, the sit-to-stand part of the task was performed more quickly than the stand-to-sit portion of the task. They surmised that occurred because of a lack of visual information regarding movement into backward space.

MOTOR LEARNING

Across the life span, individuals are faced with new motor challenges and must learn to perform new motor skills. An infant must learn how to hold up her head, roll over, sit, crawl, and eventually walk. Each skill takes time to master and occurs only after the infant has practiced each skill in several different ways. The young child then masters running, climbing on furniture, walking up stairs, jumping, and playing ball. The school-age child takes these tasks further to specifically kick a soccer ball into a net, throw a ball into a basketball hoop, ride a bike, or skateboard. As teens and adults learn new sports, they refine their skills, becoming more efficient at turning while on snow skis or pitching a baseball into the strike zone with more force. Adults also learn to efficiently perform tasks related to their occupation. These tasks vary widely from one occupation to another and may include efficient computer keyboarding, climbing up a ladder, or lifting boxes. Older adults may need to modify their motor skill performance to accommodate for changes in strength and flexibility. For example, the older adult golfer may change her stance during a swing or learn to use a heavier golf club to maximize the distance of her drive. Often injury or illness requires an individual to relearn how to sit up, walk, put on a shirt, or get into or out of a car. The method each individual uses to learn new movements demonstrates the process of motor learning. Motor learning examines how an individual learns or modifies a motor task. As discussed in the section on motor control, characteristics of the task, the learner, and the environment will impact the performance and learning of the skill. With motor learning, general principles apply to individuals of any age, but variations also have been found between the motor learning methods used by children, adults, and older adults.

Motor Learning Defined

In its simplest terms, motor learning can be defined as a permanent change in motor performance that occurs as a result of practice. More formally, motor learning has been defined as: "Changes in internal processes that determine an individual's capability for producing a motor task. The level of an individual's motor learning improves with practice and is often inferred by observing relatively stable levels of the person's motor performance.[6]"

THEORIES OF MOTOR LEARNING

There are two theories of motor learning that have generated a great deal of study about how we control and acquire motor skills. Both theories use programs to explain how movements are controlled and learned; they are Adams' closed-loop theory of motor learning[47] and Schmidt's schema theory.[48] The two theories differ in the amount of emphasis placed on open-loop processes that can occur without the benefit of ongoing feedback.[49] Schmidt incorporated many of Adams' original ideas when formulating his schema theory in an attempt to explain the acquisition of both slow and fast movements. Intrinsic and extrinsic feedback, as defined earlier in this chapter, are both important factors in these two theories.

Adams' Closed-Loop Theory

The name of Adams' theory emphasizes the crucial role of feedback. The concept of a closed loop of motor control is one in which sensory information is funneled back to the central nervous system for processing and control of motor behavior. The sensory feedback is used to produce accurate movements.

The basic premise of Adams' theory is that movements are performed by comparing the ongoing movement with an internal reference of correctness that is developed during practice. This internal reference is termed a *perceptual trace*, which represents the feedback one would receive if the task were performed correctly. Through ongoing comparison of the feedback with the perceptual trace, a limb may be brought into the desired position. To learn the task, it would be necessary to practice the exact skill repeatedly, strengthening the correct perceptual trace. The quality of performance is directly related to the quality of the perceptual trace. A perceptual trace, formed as the learner repeatedly performs an action, is made up of a set of intrinsic feedback signals that arise from the learner. Intrinsic feedback here means the sensory information that is generated through performance, for example, the kinesthetic feel of the movement. As a new movement is learned, correct outcomes reinforce development of the most effective, correct perceptual trace, while perceptual traces leading to more incorrect outcomes are discarded. The perceptual trace becomes stronger with repetition and more accurately represents correct performance as a result of feedback.

Limitations of the closed-loop theory of motor learning have been identified, as motor control and learning have been studied in more detail. One limitation is that the theory does not explain how movements can be explained when sensory information is not available. The theory also does not explain how individuals can often perform novel tasks successfully, without the benefit of repeated practice and the perceptual trace. The ability of the brain to store individual perceptual traces for each possible movement has also been questioned, considering the memory storage capacity of the brain.[48]

Schmidt's Schema Theory

Schmidt's schema theory was developed in direct response to Adams' closed-loop theory and its limitations. Schema theory is concerned with how movements that can be carried out without feedback are learned, and it relies on an open-loop control element, the motor program, to foster learning. The *motor program* for a movement reflects the general rules to successfully complete the movement. These general rules, or schema, can then be used to produce the movement in a variety of conditions or settings. For example the general rules for walking can be applied to walking on tile, on grass, going up a hill, or on an icy sidewalk. The motor program provides the spatial and temporal information about muscle activation needed to complete the movement.[49] The motor program is the schema, or abstract memory, of rules related to skilled actions.

According to schema theory, when a person produces a movement, four kinds of information are stored in short-term memory.

1. The initial conditions under which the performance took place (e.g., the position of the body, the kind of surface on which the individual carried out the action, or the shapes and weights of any objects that were used to carry out the task)
2. The parameters assigned to the motor program (e.g., the force or speed that was specified at the time of initiation of the program)
3. The outcome of the performance
4. The sensory consequences of the movement (e.g., how it felt to perform the movement, the sounds that were made as a result of the action, or the visual effect of the performance)

These four kinds of information are analyzed to gain insight into the relationships between them and to form two types of schema: the recall schema and the recognition schema.

The *recall schema* is used to select a method to complete a motor task. It is an abstract representation of the relationship among the initial conditions surrounding performance, parameters that were specified within the motor program, and the outcome of the performance. The learner, through the analysis of parameters that were specified in the motor program and the outcome, begins to understand the relationship between these two factors. For example, the learner may come to understand how far a wheelchair travels when varying amounts of force are generated to push the chair on a gravel pathway. The learner stores this schema and uses it the next time the wheelchair is moved on a gravel path.

The *recognition schema* helps assess how well a motor behavior has been performed. It represents the relationship among the initial conditions, the outcome of the performance, and the sensory consequences that are perceived by the learner. Because it is formed in a manner similar to that of the recall schema, once it is established, the recognition schema is used to produce an estimate of the sensory consequences of the action that will be used to adjust and evaluate the motor performance of a given motor task.

In motor learning, the motor behavior is assessed through use of the recognition schema. If errors are identified, they are used to refine the recall schema. Recall and recognition schema are continually revised and updated as skilled movement is learned.

Limitations of the schema theory have also been identified. One limitation is that the formation of general motor programs is not explained. Another question has arisen from inconsistent results in studies of effectiveness of variable practice on learning new motor skills, especially with adult subjects.

STAGES OF MOTOR LEARNING

It is generally possible to tell when a person is learning a new skill. The person's performance lacks the graceful, efficient movement of someone who has perfected the skill. For example, when adults learn to snow ski, they generally hold their bodies stiffly, with knees straight and arms at their side. Over time, as they become more comfortable with skiing they will bend and straighten their knees as they turn. Finally, when watching the experienced skier, the body fluidly rotates and flexes/extends as she maneuvers down a steep slope or completes a slalom race. The stages associated with mastery of a skill have been described and clearly differentiate between the early stages of motor learning and the later stages of motor learning. Two models of motor learning stages are described below and in Table 4-1.

In the early stages of motor learning, individuals have to think about the skill they are performing and may even "talk" their way through the skill. For example, when learning how to turn when snow skiing, the novice skier may tell herself to bend the knees as initiating the turn, then straighten the knees through the turn, and then bend the knees again as the turn is completed. The skier might even be observed to say the words "bend, straighten, bend" or "down, up, down" as she turns. Early in the motor learning process, movements tend to be stiff and inefficient. The new learner may not always be able to successfully complete the skill or might hesitate, making the timing movements within the skill inaccurate.

In the later stages of motor learning, the individual may not need to think about the skill. For example, the skier will automatically go through the appropriate motions with the appropriate timing as she makes a turn down a steep slope. Likewise, the baseball player steps up to the plate and does not think too much about how she will hit the ball. The batter will swing at a ball that comes into the strike zone automatically. If either the experienced skier or batter makes an error, she will self-assess her performance and try to correct the error next time.

Table **4-1**

Stages of Motor Learning

Model	Stage 1	Stage 2	Stage 3
Fitts' stages of motor learning[50]	Cognitive Stage Actively think about goal Think about conditions	Associative Stage Refine performance Error correction	Autonomous Stage Automatic performance Consistent, efficient performance
"Neo-Bernsteinian" model of motor learning[26]	Novice Stage Decreased number of degrees of freedom	Advanced Stage Release some degrees of freedom	Expert Stage Uses all degrees of freedom for fluid, efficient movement
General characteristics	Stiff looking Inconsistent performance Errors Slow, nonfluid movement	More fluid movement Fewer errors Improved consistency Improved efficiency	Automatic Fluid Consistent Efficient Error correction

Fitts' Stages

In analyzing acquisition of new motor skills, Fitts[50] described three stages of motor learning. The first stage is the *cognitive phase* where the learner has to consciously consider the goal of the task to be completed and recognize the features of the environment to which the movement must conform.[51] In a task such as walking across a crowded room, the surface of the floor and the location and size of people within the room are considered regulatory features. If the floor is slippery, a person's walking pattern is different than if the floor is carpeted. Background features such as lighting or noise may also affect task performance. During this initial cognitive phase of learning, an individual tries a variety of strategies to achieve the movement goal. Through this trial and error approach, effective strategies are built upon and ineffective strategies are discarded.

At the next stage of learning, the *associative phase,* the learner has developed the general movement pattern necessary to perform the task and is ready to refine and improve the performance of the skill. The learner makes subtle adjustments to adjust errors and to adapt the skill to varying environmental demands of the task. For example, a young baseball player may learn that she can more efficiently and consistently hit the ball if she chokes up on the bat. During this phase, the focus of the learner switches from "what to do" to "how to do the movement.[11]"

In the final stage of learning, the *autonomous stage*, the skill becomes more "automatic" because the learner does not need to focus all of her attention on the motor skill. She is able to attend to other components of the task, such as scanning for subtle environmental obstacles. At this phase, the learner is better able to adapt to changes in features in the environment. The young baseball player will be relatively successful at hitting the ball when using different bats or if a cheering crowd is present.

"Neo-Bernsteinien" Model

This model of staging motor learning considers the learners' ability to master multiple degrees of freedom as they learn the new skill.[19,26] Within this model the initial stage of motor learning, the *novice stage*, is when the learner reduces the degrees of freedom that need to be controlled during the task. The learner will "fix" some joints so that motion does not take place and the degree of freedom is constrained at that joint. For example, think of the new snow skier who holds her knees stiffly extended while bending at the trunk to try to turn. The resultant movement is stiff looking and not always effective. For example, if the slope of the hill is too steep, or if the skier tries to turn on an icy patch, she may not be effective. The second stage in this model, the *advanced stage,* is seen when the learner allows more joints to participate in the task, in essence releasing some of the degrees of freedom. Coordination is improved as agonist and antagonist muscles around the joint can work together to produce the movement, rather than cocontracting as they did to "fix" the joint in earlier movement attempts. The third stage of this model, the *expert stage,* is when all degrees of freedom necessary to perform a task in an efficient, coordinated manner are released. Within this stage, the learner can begin to adjust performance to improve the efficiency of the movement by adjusting the speed of the movement. Considering the skier, the expert may appreciate that by increasing the speed of descent, a turn may be easier to initiate.

IMPORTANT ELEMENTS OF THE MOTOR LEARNING PROCESS

Practice

As defined earlier in this chapter, motor learning is a permanent change in motor behavior resulting from practice. Practice is therefore a key component of motor learning. Many factors need to be considered when designing the practice component for learning different tasks. The amount of practice and a practice schedule should be considered. The order in which tasks are practiced can also influence learning, as can whether a task is practiced as a whole skill or is broken down into its parts.

Massed Versus Distributed Practice

The difference between massed and distributed practice schedules is related to the proportion of rest time and practice time during the session. In *massed practice*, greater practice time than rest time occurs in the session. The amount of rest time between practice attempts is less than the amount of time spent practicing. In *distributed practice* conditions, the amount of rest time is longer than the time spent practicing. In some clinical settings, tasks may be more safely learned with a distributed practice schedule than massed practice, especially tasks in which a person might fatigue. If the learner becomes too fatigued and is at risk for injuring themselves or not being able to maintain correct form during an activity, it is better to give her a rest period. In contrast, some tasks such as picking up a coin or buttoning a button, do not take excessive energy and may be better learned with less rest between trials. One example of how

CLINICAL IMPLICATIONS Box 4-1

Constraint-induced Movement Therapy: Use of Massed Practice for Improvement of Upper Extremity Function in the Patient with Hemiplegia

Constraint-induced movement therapy (CIMT) is a treatment approach that has been used with individuals with hemiplegia. CIMT involves both constraint of the noninvolved upper extremity of an individual with hemiplegia and repetitive practice of skilled activities or functional tasks. The intense, repetitive practice in this therapeutic approach reflects the use of massed practice strategies in rehabilitation.

In CIMT, massed practice of tasks by the involved upper extremity of the patient with hemiplegia is completed while the noninvolved extremity is constrained. Practice refers to the repetitive performance of a functional skill, generally for 15 to 20 minutes. Shaping is also incorporated into the practice session. Shaping incorporates the motor learning concept of part practice as a task is learned in small steps, which are individually mastered. Successive approximation of the completed task is made until the individual is able to perform the whole task. Both repetitive practice and shaping approaches to functional task mastery are included in constraint-induced therapy.

Originally studied in adults with hemiplegia, evidence indicates that constraint-induced therapy is effective in improving use of the involved arm for functional tasks.[91–93] When first introduced, constraint of the upper extremity was maintained for 90% of waking hours and practice sessions of 6 hr/day were

recommended. Modified approaches have decreased the percent of time a person wears a constraint during the day and the hours of practice. Lin[93] has demonstrated improved motor control strategies during goal-directed reaching tasks, implying that the CIMT improved reaction time and use of feedforward motor control strategies.

CIMT has also been used with children with hemiplegia from infancy through adolescence. Modified CIMT approaches have been suggested to decrease the amount of time the constraint is worn and to use practice sessions as short as 1 to 3 hr/day.[94,95] Activities are also selected to reflect a child's interests and maintain attention, incorporating both games and functional activities. Within pediatric CIMT, the two basic components of CIMT (constraint of the noninvolved upper extremity and repetitive practice) are maintained. Pediatric CIMT studies have demonstrated improved functional use and efficiency of movement in the involved upper extremity of children with hemiplegia.[94–96]

In the case of CIMT, the massed practice of tasks is thought to contribute to cortical reorganization and mapping, which increases efficiency of task performance with the hemiplegic upper extremity.[96–98] These findings reflect the influence of CIMT on activity-dependent neural plasticity.

---

massed practice is used in rehabilitation is the use of constraint-induced movement therapy (Clinical Implications Box 4-1). Constraint-induced therapy can be considered a modified form of massed practice in which learned nonuse is overcome by shaping or reinforcement.[52] In an individual with hemiplegia, the uninvolved arm or hand is constrained, thereby necessitating use of the involved (hemiplegic) upper extremity in functional tasks.

Random Versus Blocked Practice

Another consideration in structuring a practice session is the order in which tasks are practiced. *Blocked practice* occurs when the same task is repeated several times in a row. One task is practiced several times before a second task is practiced. *Random practice* occurs when a variety of tasks are practiced in a random order, with any one skill rarely practiced two times in a row. Figure 4-6

shows the difference between blocked and random practice. *Mixed practice* sessions may also be useful in some situations, where episodes of both random and blocked practice are incorporated into the practice session.

In most instances of learning functional and skilled tasks, it has been shown that adults learn better from random practice situations. Adult learners' retention and transfer of motor skills is stronger following random practice (Figure 4-7).[53–57] Blocked practice may help someone improve form on a task in an isolated setting but does not seem to translate into performing that skill in a natural situation. For example, in learning to play tennis, it would be better to practice forehand and backhand strokes and volleying in a random order—similar to how they will really occur in a game—rather than practice forehand strokes for 50 trials, then backhand strokes for 50 trials. It has been suggested that in random practice, as the learner shifts from one task to

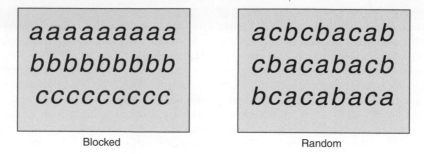

Blocked   Random

Figure 4-6 Sample practice schedules for reach to grasp activity illustrate blocked and random practice: a, reach and grasp for a paper cup; b, reach and grasp for a coffee mug; c, reach and grasp for a glass.

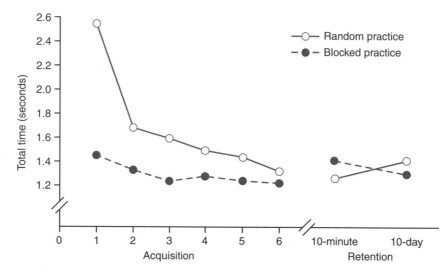

Figure 4-7 Effect of blocked versus random practice on acquisition and retention of a motor skill. Although blocked practice led to better performance during acquisition, random practice led to greater learning as measured by retention tests. (Adapted with permission from Shea JB, Morgan RL: Contextual interference effects on the acquisition, retention, and transfer of a motor skill, *J Exp Psychol* 5(2):179-187, 1979.)

another, she must think about the differences between tasks and focus on the different strategies that must be performed to complete each task.[58] Random practice seems to be best for skilled learners because it allows them to derive a range of solutions to the task that can be used at a later time.

Blocked practice does seem to have a place in the early stages of learning brand new skills that have never been done. Blocked practice may be most appropriate in the early cognitive stages of motor learning, for children, and for individuals with cognitive impairments.[59-61] Adolescents with Down syndrome appear to benefit more from blocked practice than random practice.[59] Impact of practice method on motor learning in children will be further discussed later in this chapter.

Constant Versus Variable Practice

Constant practice occurs when an individual practices one variation of a movement skill several times in a row. An example would be repeatedly practicing standing up from a wheelchair or throwing a basketball into a hoop. *Variable practice* occurs when the learner practices several variations of a motor skill during a practice session. For example, a rehabilitation patient may practice standing up from the wheelchair, standing up from the bed, standing up from the toilet, and standing up from the floor. A child might practice throwing a ball into a hoop, throwing a ball at a target on the wall, throwing a ball underhand, throwing a ball overhand, or throwing a ball to a partner all within the same session. Variable practice training is useful in helping the learner generalize a motor skill over a wide variety of environmental settings and conditions. Learning is felt to be enhanced by the variable practice because the strength of the general motor program rules, specific to the new task, would be increased. This mechanism is also considered one way that an individual can attempt a novel task because the person can incorporate rules developed for previous motor tasks to solve the novel task.

Whole Versus Part Task Training

A task can be practiced as a complete action (*whole task practice*) or broken up into its component parts (*part practice*). Continuous tasks such as walking, running, or stair climbing are more effectively learned with whole task practice. It has been demonstrated that if walking is broken down into part practice of a component, such as weight shifting forward over the foot, the learner demonstrates improvements in weight shifting behaviors but does not generalize this improvement into the walking sequence.[62]

Skills that can be broken down into discrete parts may be most effectively taught using part practice training. For example, a patient learning how to independently transfer out of a wheelchair might be first taught how to lock the brakes on the chair, then how to scoot forward in the chair. After these parts of the task are mastered, the patient might learn to properly place her feet, lean forward over the feet, and finally stand. Similarly, when learning a dressing task, a child might first be taught to pull a shirt over her head then push in each arm. Once these components are completed, the focus might be on learning how to fasten buttons or the zipper.

Feedback

Feedback is a critical component of motor learning. As discussed in the motor learning theory section, two types of feedback guide learning: intrinsic feedback and extrinsic feedback. When structuring the learning session, a therapist will want the learner to experience the type of intrinsic feedback that will best help the learner learn the task or general motor programs necessary for efficient performance of the skill. In structuring the motor learning session, the therapist must consider how to structure the extrinsic feedback provided to enhance learning.

Terminal Versus Concurrent Feedback

Information given during task performance is known as *concurrent feedback*. Coaches, therapists, and educators often use concurrent feedback by altering sensory input, providing manual cues, or giving verbal information to facilitate specific movements. Concurrent feedback has several purposes: to help guide the learner so she can feel the desired movement pattern, to enhance execution of a certain pattern of movement by encouraging activation of specific musculature, and to assist the individual in successfully accomplishing a goal. Similar to other types of extrinsic feedback, when concurrent feedback is used too frequently, it may actually impede learning because the learner may become dependent on it. Furthermore, the person providing the feedback becomes a part of the performer's environment. Thus the performer still needs to learn how to move effectively when the feedback is removed.

Feedback can also be provided less frequently. Feedback that is provided less than 100% of the time is called *intermittent feedback. Faded feedback* can also be given, in which the frequency of feedback is greater in the early stages of learning a task and then decreases as the learner progresses in learning the task. Another schedule of giving feedback is *summarized feedback*, in which feedback is given after several trials. These various feedback schedules decrease a performer's reliance on external feedback and may ultimately enhance learning of a motor skill.[63]

Feedback can also be given at the completion of a motor task and is called *terminal feedback*. Terminal feedback is usually categorized into two forms: knowledge of results and knowledge of performance (Table 4-2). *Knowledge of results* is information related to the outcome, whether successful or not. We know whether we have been successful in picking up a cup or walking across the room. Knowledge of results feedback appears to be most effective if provided in a faded or

---

Table 4-2

Examples of Feedback Given after Task Performance

Knowledge of Results	Knowledge of Performance
Outcome of Success or Failure	*Task Execution*
"You walked across the room!"	"You did not keep your elbow straight."
"That task took you 1 minute 30 seconds to complete."	"You are not bearing as much weight on your right side when you walk."
"You scored 5 points out of 8!"	"You were looking at your feet."

summary feedback schedule, with too much immediate feedback of performance outcome detrimental to learning.[49] *Knowledge of performance* pertains to information received regarding execution of the task and typically relates to the type or quality of the movement. Although knowledge of results is useful at any time during the learning process, knowledge of performance should be used selectively. Because a learner is thinking so hard about performing a task in the early stages of learning, providing detailed information can be confusing and may be detrimental to long-term learning.

Key concepts related to providing concurrent or terminal feedback for any population include (1) use of feedback that is specific to the task and the learner's needs; (2) minimizing use of excessive feedback; and (3) encouragement of active problem solving that allows time to self-assess, rather than rely on feedback.

DEVELOPMENTAL ASPECTS OF MOTOR LEARNING

Motor learning strategies, to most effectively meet the needs of the learner, vary based on learner characteristics. For example, children learn differently than adults. Nervous system development/maturation in children may influence a child's ability to learn and master some motor skills.[64] Cognitive development may influence how a child can receive and process information. When working with children, adults, and older adults, therapists need to consider the unique needs of each learner to design optimal motor learning sessions and provide the most useful extrinsic feedback. Both practice and feedback components of the motor learning tasks are important considerations in designing and implementing motor learning strategies for each individual patient.

Motor Learning and Children

Practice

When learning a brand new motor skill, children practice, practice, and practice. For example, when learning to walk, an infant covers a distance equal to 29 football fields daily.[65] A typical 14-month-old is reported to take more than 2000 steps per hour, which is equivalent to a distance of seven football fields.[66]

As young children are learning new gross motor tasks, blocked practice appears to lead to better transfer and performance of the skill. Del Rey and colleagues[61] had typically developing children (approximately 8 years old) practice an anticipation timing task at different speeds in either a blocked or random order and

then tested them on a transfer test with the new coordination pattern. The researchers found that blocked practice led to better performance on the transfer task than did random practice. In Frisbee throwing experiments, accuracy in throwing the Frisbee at a target was improved by blocked practice in children, although adults improved accuracy the most with random practice.[67,68] The contextual interference provided by random practice schedules does not appear to help children learn new motor skills.[69]

Although most of the literature on children supports a blocked or mixed schedule for learning whole body tasks, some researchers have found that typically developing children may learn skilled or sport-specific skills if a variable practice schedule is used.[70-72] This variable practice schedule combines blocked and random practice elements and allows the child to benefit from practicing the new skill with elements of contextual interference. Vera and associates[70] found that 9-year-old children performed the skill of kicking a soccer ball best following blocked or combined practice, but only children in a combined practice situation improved in dribbling the soccer ball. Similarly, Douvis[71] examined the impact of variable practice on learning the tennis forehand drive in children and adolescents. Adolescents did better than children on the task, reflecting the influence of age and development, but both age groups did the best with variable practice. The variable practice sessions allowed the tennis players to use the forehand drive in a manner that more resembled the actual game of tennis, where a player may use a forehand drive, then a backhand drive, etc.

Feedback

Feedback plays an important role in motor learning for infants and children. Infants in an imitation experiment demonstrated strongest responses when their mothers offered demonstration and verbal praise related to completion of play tasks. Infants as young as 10 months of age have demonstrated the use of intrinsic, proprioceptive input in learning new tasks.[73] In these experiments, infants were exposed to the task of using a cane to pull an out-of-reach toy closer. Infants who physically practiced the task appeared to perceive the cane could be used as a tool to reach a toy, but infants who only watched as someone else pulled the cane to obtain a toy did not seem to react to the cane as a tool that could be used to obtain a toy.

Children differ from adults in the type and frequency of feedback that best supports their motor learning. In children, if knowledge of results (KR) is too specific, it confuses the child and interferes with learning.[49,74] When learning a new motor task, it appears that children benefit more from more constant feedback than they do from reduced feedback. Ten-year-olds learning a new task in a 100% feedback group had better consistency in a retention test compared with 10-year-olds who received reduced (62% faded) feedback.[75] Because of developmental differences in information processing abilities and memory, children may require the increased level of feedback. In looking at the type of extrinsic feedback provided, children also appear to benefit from feedback addressing internal requirements of a task rather than external results. In a dart throwing learning situation, adults benefited more from feedback about the darts and target than about their form (e.g., hand position, elbow activity) during dart throwing. Children in this same experiment improved the most in dart throwing when they received feedback on specific hand, elbow, and arm activity to be used during dart throwing.[76] A child's ability to benefit from more internally focused, proprioceptive, or kinesthetic feedback than from information related to the task outcome may also reflect the child's developmental ability in processing sensory information and information processing.

Motor Learning and Older Adults

Very broadly speaking, aging affects motor learning. It is unclear exactly why this is the case. It is believed, however, to be at least partly related to age-related changes in the function of subsystems needed for motor task performance, such as force production and control, sensory capacity, and attentional demands.

Consensus information is lacking regarding the effect of age on motor learning. Results of studies must be evaluated carefully before making a global statement on motor learning in older adults. Studies often have small sample sizes of convenience, rarely examine motor learning in patient populations, and typically use a variety of motor tasks—some of which may not offer immediate clinical implications for learning or relearning functional activity within the clinical or home setting.

There are presently a handful of studies suggesting that older adults have:

- Deficits in sequence motor learning.
- Deficits in learning new technology but not in benefits of practice.
- Deficits in learning effortful bimanual coordination patterns with preserved or enhanced use of augmented feedback.

Sequential Learning

Performing learned or learning new motor sequences is important functionally. Clearly, linking motor acts such as rolling, sitting up, standing up, and walking play a major role in daily life. However, motor sequence learning is typically evaluated by the use of more rudimentary acts such as pointing to different targets on a computer screen or pressing different sets of buttons on a keypad. The relationship between the sensorimotor organization of sequences of actions like those performed during activities of daily living and those being tested in a motor learning experiment remains to be established. Irrespective of this issue, a recent well-designed laboratory-based study on sequential motor learning did find that older adults were slower to perform a novel sequential action and that it may have been due to how older persons organize subsequences of complex movements.[77]

At least one example of learning a functional sequence exists in the literature. Tunney and associates[78] provided healthy younger and older adults with a 10-step sequence for performing a car transfer using a standard walker. This sequence was practiced in (first) 4-step and (second) 6-step trials. Subjects were scored on a final trial and 48 hours later by a physical therapist based on the number of steps followed or completed. Older adults' scores were significantly lower immediately after practice and at 48 hours as compared with younger adults. The authors took this as evidence that older adults do not acquire and maintain a functional motor skill as accurately as younger adults. All subjects were healthy, did not need to use a walker to ambulate or transfer, and were equally successful in actually transferring into the car. It is unclear if the measure of learning matched the outcome of the to-be-learned task. Did the 10-step procedure map, in an ecologically valid way, onto the subjects' natural performance and, therefore, their learning? Was following the 10-step procedure actually necessary? In the section below, it will be shown that guided attention, such as attending to key aspects of a task, may be more useful for learning a complex motor sequence than using a guided action in which a person follows a specific step-by-step process.

Practice

It is clear that older adults are able to improve motor performance with practice.[79–81] For example, an early study suggested that benefits of blocked versus random practice were tied to a participant's general level of physical activity: those with higher levels of physical activity were able to benefit from random practice.[82] This suggests that individual differences may interact with practice schedules. Jamieson and Rogers[81] evaluated the effects of blocked and random practice on learning to use an ATM machine in younger and older adults. While older adults were slower and less accurate in menu selections and more likely to forget the receipt or cash, both younger and older adults benefitted from random practice. Random practice was also superior to blocked practice. Additionally, older adults were able to transfer learning to a novel ATM scenario.

More recently, Hickman and associates[83] studied guided action versus guided attention training in learning to use a new technology—a hydroponic garden control system. Both younger and older adults were able to follow the guided action information (step-by-step training materials), and this method offered benefits in performance. However, groups that originally received guided attention training, which assisted in remembering what to do more generally, benefited more when step-by-step training materials were not provided. This effect was found in both older and younger adults.

With respect to massed versus distributed practice, at least one study has demonstrated benefits of distributed over massed practice for older adults. Kausler and associates[84] had subjects perform a set of 16 motor tasks under distributed or massed practice conditions. Distributed practice resulted in better recall of these tasks. As with previously cited studies, older adults demonstrated performance decrements when compared with younger adults.

In summary, older adults tend to perform to-be-learned tasks with slower speeds and greater error, yet they seem to benefit equally, as compared with younger adults, from practice schedules conducive to motor learning.

Feedback

Knowledge of results (KR) has been shown to be equally effective in motor learning when younger and older adults are compared. For example, Swanson and Lee[85] had younger and older subjects learn a continuous movement comprising a three step spatial sequence with the upper extremity. While older adults exhibited decrements in movement accuracy and consistency during acquisition trials, both groups benefited from KR similarly. Wishart and Lee[86] expanded this result to include KR provided at 100% frequency of trials and in a fading fashion. They found that for this type of task, younger and older adults used KR in a similar way to learn. More recently, using an isometric force-production task, van Dijk and associates[87] found that KR or kinetic feedback was similarly beneficial to younger and older adults.

When tasks are complex and deviate from preferred patterns, there appears to be a difference with respect to how older adults use extrinsic information. In a series of studies,[88-90] an examination was undertaken to determine the role of feedback in assisting acquisition and maintenance of automatic versus effortful bimanual

coordination patterns with the upper extremities. First, so-called automatic (in-phase), bimanual coordination patterns are performed equally well by younger and older adults with only a small decrement in accuracy (error) and stability (standard deviation) with increasing pacing speeds.[89] On the other hand, effortful patterns (antiphase upper extremity movements) tended to show a greater decrement in accuracy and stability by older adults.

A 90-degree bimanual coordination pattern is considered complex and effortful because it is not purely in-phase (0-degrees difference between two limbs) and not purely antiphase (180 degrees "out-of-phase"). Swinnen and associates[88] examined the acquisition of this pattern in older and younger adults. During acquisition, both groups tended toward the less effortful patterns of in-phase and antiphase. However, older adults had more difficulty (greater absolute deviation from required phase) and exhibited greater variability in maintaining the 90-degree phase pattern by the end of the acquisition trials. Augmented visual feedback in real time benefitted both groups. These researchers also examined learning under blindfolded and normal vision (nonaugmented) conditions as a means to determine the extent to which subjects were dependent upon the augmented visual feedback. Older subjects exhibited more difficulties in these nonaugmented conditions, suggesting that they may have become more dependent on the augmented visual feedback. But this could also have been explained by the possible reduced quality of sensory information associated with aging.

A follow-up study by Wishart and associates[90] compared concurrent versus terminal feedback in this 90-degree phase bimanual coordination pattern. Older adults gained more from the concurrent feedback than younger adults relative to the terminal feedback condition. Taking this series of findings collectively, it appears older adults are able to use KR for learning new motor skills, but on the other hand, the utility of feedback in learning complex coordination patterns may lie in its nature and extent.

SUMMARY

Motor learning has occurred when a performance of a motor behavior has permanently changed as a result of practice. The process of motor learning occurs over time and individuals progress through stages of learning, from the stiff, awkward cognitive stage through the expert stage where fluid movement seems to occur automatically. Clinicians must make decisions as to how much practice is necessary, how practice sessions should be structured, and how to maximize the most effective forms of feedback. Motor learning of functional tasks is considered to be complete when an individual can easily perform the task in a variety of environments or situations (generalization) and can consistently perform the task over several sessions. The overall motor learning process is similar in individuals of all ages, but some differences exist in which forms of practice and feedback best enhance learning in children, adults, and older adults.

REFERENCES

1. James W: Habit. In Shoben EJ, Ruch F, editors: *Perspectives in psychology*, Fairlawn, NJ, 1963, Scott, Foresman & Co (Habit originally published in 1890).
2. Sherrington CS: *The integrative action of the nervous system*, New York, 1906, Cambridge University Press.
3. Denny-Brown D: Disintegration of motor function resulting from cerebral lesion, *J Nerv Ment Dis* 112:1–45, 1950.
4. Seyffarth H, Denny-Brown D: The grasp reflex and the instinctive grasp reaction, *Brain* 71:109–183, 1948.
5. Twitchell TE: The restoration of motor function following hemiplegia in man, *Brain* 74:443–480, 1951.
6. Schmidt RA, Wrisberg CA: *Motor learning and performance*, ed 3, Champaign, Ill, 2004, Human Kinetics.
7. Kandel ER, Schwartz JH, Jessell TM: *Principles of neural science*, ed 4, New York, 2000, McGraw-Hill.
8. Lashley KS: The problem of serial order in behavior. In Jeffress LA, editor: *Cerebral mechanisms in behavior*, New York, 1951, John Wiley & Sons, pp 112–136.
9. Gordon J: Assumptions underlying physical therapy intervention. In Carr JA, Shephard RB, editors: *Movement science: foundations for physical therapy in rehabilitation*, Rockville, Md, 1987, Aspen, pp 1–30.
10. Wing AM, Haggard P, Flanagan J: *Hand and brain: the neurophysiology and psychology of hand movements*, New York, 1996, Academic Press.
11. Schmidt R: *Motor control and learning*, Champaign, Ill, 1988, Human Kinetics.
12. Gabbard C: Studying action representation in children via motor imagery, *Brain Cogn* 234–239, 2009.
13. Shumway-Cook A, Woollacott M: *Motor control: translating research into clinical practice*, ed 3, Baltimore, 2007, Williams & Wilkins.
14. Horak B: Assumptions underlying motor control for neurologic rehabilitation. In Lister M, editor: *Contemporary management of motor control problems: proceedings of the II STEP conference*, Alexandria, Va, 1991, Foundation for Physical Therapy, pp 11–28.
15. Nowakowski RS: Basic concepts of CNS development. In Johnson MH, editor: *Brain development and cognition*, Cambridge, Mass, 1993, Blackwell, pp 54–92.
16. Carr J, Shepherd R: *Neurological rehabilitation: optimizing motor performance*, Oxford, UK, 1998, Butterworth Heinemann, pp 3–22.
17. Thelen E: Motor development: a new synthesis, *Am Psychol* 50:79–95, 1995.
18. Heriza C: Motor development: Traditional and contemporary theories. In Lister M, editor: *Contemporary Management of Motor Control Problems: Proceedings of the II STEP Conference*, Alexandria, Va, 1991, Foundation for Physical Therapy, pp 99–126.
19. Bernstein N: *The coordination and regulation of movements*, Oxford, UK, 1967, Pergamon.
20. Keele SW: Movement control in skilled motor performance, *Psychol Bull* 70:387–403, 1968.
21. Morris ME, Summers JJ, Matyas TA, et al: Current status of the motor program, *Phys Ther* 74:738–748, 1994.
22. Thelen E, Ulrich BD: Hidden skills: a dynamic systems analysis of treadmill stepping during the first year, *Monogr Soc Res Child Dev* 56(1, No. 223):1–104, 1991.
23. Gordon J: Current status of the motor program: invited commentary, *Phys Ther* 74:748–751, 1994.
24. Weiss PH, Jeannerod M, Paulignan Y, et al: Is the organization of goal-directed action modality specific? *Neuropsychologia* 38:1136–1147, 2000.
25. Kelso JAS: *Human motor behavior*, Hillsdale, NJ, 1982, Lawrence Erlbaum Associates.
26. Vereijken B, van Emmerik REA, Whiting HTA, et al: Freezing degrees of freedom in skill acquisition, *J Mot Behav* 24:133–142, 1992.
27. Spencer JP, Thelen E: A multimuscle state analysis of adult motor learning, *Exp Brain Res* 128:505–516, 1997.
28. Hay L, Redon C: The control of goal-directed movements in children: role of proprioceptive muscle afferents, *Hum Mov Sci* 16:433–451, 1997.
29. Goble DJ, Lewis CA, Hurvitz EA, et al: Development of upper limb proprioceptive accuracy in children and adolescents, *Hum Mov Sci* 24:155–170, 2005.
30. Goble DJ, Coxon JP, Wenderoth N, et al: Proprioceptive sensibility in the elderly: degeneration, functional consequences and plastic-adaptive processes, *Neurosci Biobehav Rev* 33:271–278, 2009.
31. Cruse H, Wischmeyer M, Bruwer P, et al: On the cost functions for the control of the human arm movement, *Biol Cybern* 62:519–528, 1990.
32. Nelson WL: Physical principles for economics of skilled movements, *Biol Cybern* 46:135–147, 1983.
33. Wolpert DM, Ghahramani Z, Jordan MI: Are arm trajectories planned in kinematic or dynamic coordinate? An adaptation study, *Exp Brain Res* 103:460–470, 1995.
34. Flash T, Hogan N: The coordination of arm movements: an experimentally confirmed mathematical model, *J Neurosci* 5:1688–1703, 1985.
35. Konczak J, Dichgans J: The development toward stereotypic arm kinematics during reaching in the first 3 years of life, *Exp Brain Res* 117:346–354, 1997.
36. Decety J, Grezes J: Neural mechanisms subserving the perception of human actions, *Trends Cogn Sci* 3:172–178, 1999.
37. Munzert J, Lorey B, Zentgraf K: Cognitive motor processes: the role of motor imagery in the study of motor representations, *Brain Res Rev* 60(2):306–326, 2009.
38. Frick A, Daum MM, Wilson M, et al: Effects of action on children's and adult's mental imagery, *J Exp Child Psychol* 194:34–51, 2009.

39. Funk M, Brugger P, Wilkening F: Motor processes in children's imagery: the case of mental rotation of hands, *Dev Sci* 8(5):402–408, 2005.

40. Caeyenberghs K, Tsoupas J, Wison PH, et al: Motor imagery development in children, *Dev Neuropsychol* 34(1):103–121, 2009.

41. Choudhury S, Charman T, Bird V, et al: Development of action representation during adolescence, *Neuropsychologia* 45:255–262, 2007.

42. Gerardin E, Sirigu A, Lehericy S, et al: Partially overlapping neural networks for real and imagined hand movements, *Cereb Cortex* 10:1093–1104, 2000.

43. Personnier P, Ballay Y, Papaxanthis C: Mentally represented motor actions in normal aging: III. Electromyographic features of imagined arm movements, *Behav Brain Res* 206(2):184–191, 2010.

44. Personnier P, Paizis C, Ballay Y, et al: Mentally represented motor action in normal aging: II. The influence of the gravito-inertial context on the duration of overt and covert arm movements, *Behav Brain Res* 186:273–283, 2008.

45. Skoura X, Personnier P, Vinter A, et al: Decline in motor prediction in elderly subjects: right versus left arm differences in mentally simulated motor actions, *Cortex* 44:1271–1278, 2008.

46. Skoura X, Papaxanthis C, Vinter A, et al: Mentally represented motor actions in normal aging: I. Age effects on the temporal features of overt and covert execution of actions, *Behav Brain Res* 165:229–239, 2005.

47. Adams JA: A closed-loop theory of motor learning, *J Mot Behav* 3:110–150, 1971.

48. Schmidt RA: A schema theory of discrete motor skill learning, *Psychol Rev* 82:225–260, 1975.

49. Schmidt RA, Lee TD: *Motor control and learning: a behavioral emphasis*, Champaign, Ill, 2005, Human Kinetics.

50. Fitts PM: Categories of human learning. In Melton AW, editor: *Perceptual-motor skills learning*, New York, 1964, Academic Press, pp 243–285.

51. Gentile AM: Skill acquisition: action, movement, and neuromotor processes. In Carr JA, Shepherd RB, Gordon J, et al: *Movement science: foundations for physical therapy in rehabilitation*, Rockville, Md, 1987, Aspen, pp 93–154.

52. Taub E, Miller NE, Novack TA, et al: Technique to improve chronic motor deficit after stroke, *Arch Phys Med Rehabil* 74:347–354, 1993.

53. Battig WF: Facilitation and interference. In Bilodeau ED, editor: *Acquisition of skill*, New York, 1966, Academic Press, pp 215–244.

54. Battig WF: The flexibility of human memory. In Cermak LS, Craik FIM, editors: *Levels of processing in human memory*, Hillsdale, NJ, 1979, Erlbaum, pp 23–44.

55. Magill RA, Hall KG: A review of the contextual interference effect in motor skill acquisition, *Hum Mov Sci* 9:241–289, 1990.

56. Shea JB, Morgan RL: Contextual interference effects on the acquisition, retention, and transfer of a motor skill, *J Exp Psychol* 5:179–187, 1979.

57. Hanlon RE: Motor learning following unilateral stroke, *Arch Phys Med Rehabil* 77:811–815, 1996.

58. Shea JB, Zimny ST: Context effects in memory and learning movement information. In Magill RA, editor: *Memory and control of action*, Amsterdam, 1983, Elsevier, pp 345–366.

59. Edwards IM, Elliot D, Lee TD: Contextual interference effects during skill acquisition and transfer in Down syndrome adolescents, *Adapt Phys Activ Q* 3:250–258, 1986.

60. Herbert EP, Landin D, Solmon MA: Practice schedule effects on the performance and learning of low- and high-skilled students: an applied study, *Res Q Exerc Sport* 67:52–58, 1996.

61. Del Rey P, Whitehurst M, Wughalter E, et al: Contextual interference and experience in acquisition and transfer, *Percept Mot Skills* 57:241–242, 1983.

62. Winstein CJ, Gardner ER, McNeal DR, et al: Standing balance training: effect on balance and locomotion in hemiparetic adults, *Arch Phys Med Rehabil* 70:755–762, 1989.

63. Winstein CJ, Pohl PS, Lewthwaite R: Effects of physical guidance and knowledge of results on motor learning: support for a guidance hypothesis, *Res Q Exerc Sport* 65(4):316–324, 1994.

64. Savion-Lemieux T, Bailey JA, Penhune VB: Developmental contributions to motor sequence learning, *Exp Brain Res* 195:293–306, 2009.

65. Adolph KE, Vereijken B, Shrout PE: What changes in infant walking and why, *Child Dev* 74:475–497, 2003.

66. Adolph KE: Learning to move, *Curr Dir Psychol Sci* 17(3):213–218, 2008.

67. Pinto-Zipp G, Gentile AM: Practice schedules in motor learning: children vs. adults, *Soc Neurosci Abstr* 21:1620, 1995.

68. Jarus T, Goverover Y: Effects of contextual interference and age on acquisition, retention and transfer of motor skill, *Percept Mot Skills* 88:437–447, 1999.

69. Perez CR, Meira CM, Tani G: Does the contextual interference effect last over extended transfer trials? *Percept Mot Skills* 10(1):58–60, 2005.

70. Vera JG, Alvarex JC, Medina MM: Effects of different practice conditions on acquisition, retention, and transfer of soccer skills by 9-year-old schoolchildren, *Percept Mot Skills* 106(2):447–460, 2008.

71. Douvis SJ: Variable practice in learning the forehand drive in tennis, *Percept Mot Skills* 101(2):531–545, 2005.

72. Granda VJ, Montilla MM: Practice schedule and acquisition, retention and transfer of a throwing task in 6-year-old children, *Percept Mot Skills* 96:1015–1024, 2003.

73. Sommerville JA, Hildebrand EA, Crane CC: Experience mattes: the impact of doing versus watching on infants' subsequent perception of tool use events, *Dev Psychol* 44(5):1249–1256, 2008.

74. Newell KM, Kennedy JA: Knowledge of results and children's motor learning, *Dev Psychol* 14:531–536, 1978.

75. Sullivan KJ, Kantak SS, Burtner PA: Motor learning in children: feedback effects on skill acquisition, *Phys Ther* 88:720–732, 2008.

76. Emanuel M, Jarus T, Bart O: Effect of focus of attention and age on motor acquisition, retention, and transfer: a randomized trial, *Phys Ther* 88(2):251–260, 2008.

77. Shea CH, Park JH, Braden HW: Age-related effects in sequential motor learning, *Phys Ther* 86(4):478–488, 2006.

78. Tunney N, et al: Aging and motor learning of a functional motor task, *Phys Occup Ther Geriatr* 21(3):1–16, 2003.

79. Salthouse TA, Somberg BL: Skill performance: effects of adult age and experience on elementary processes, *J Exp Psychol Gen* 111:176–207, 1982.

80. Hertzog CK, Williams MV, Walsh DA: The effect of practice on age differences in central perceptual processing, *J Gerontol* 31:428–433, 1976.

81. Jamieson BA, Rogers WA: Age-related effects of blocked and random practice schedules on learning a new technology, *J Gerontol B Psychol Sci Soc Sci* 55B(6):P343–P353, 2000.

82. Del Rey P: Effects of contextual interference on the memory of older females differing in levels of physical activity, *Percept Mot Skills* 55:171–180, 1982.

83. Hickman JM, Rogers WA, Fisk AD: Training older adults to use new technology, *J Gerontol B Psychol Sci Soc Sci* 62B(Special Issue I):77–84, 2007.

84. Kausler DH, Wiley JG, Phillips PL: Adult age differences in memory for massed and distributed repeated actions, *Psychol Aging* 5:530–534, 1990.

85. Swanson LR, Lee TD: Effects of aging and schedules of knowledge of results on motor learning, *J Gerontol* 47(6):P406–P411, 1992.

86. Wishart LR, Lee TD: Effects of aging and reducing relative frequency of knowledge of results on learning a motor skill, *Percept Mot Skills* 84:1107–1122, 1997.

87. van Dijk H, Mulder T, Hermens HJ: Effects of age and content of augmented feedback on learning an isometric force-production task, *Exp Aging Res* 33(3):341–353, 2007.

88. Swinnen SP, Verschueren SMP, Bogaerts H, et al: Age-related deficits in motor learning and differences in feedback processing during the production of a bimanual coordination pattern, *Cogn Neuropsychol* 15(5):439–466, 1998.

89. Wishart LR, Lee TD, Murdoch JE, et al: Effects of aging on automatic and effortful processes in bimanual coordination, *J Gerontol B Psychol Sci Soc Sci* 55B(2):P85–P94, 2000.

90. Wishart LR, Lee TD, Murdoch JE: Age-related differences and the role of augmented visual feedback in learning a bimanual coordination pattern, *Acta Psychol (Amst)* 110(2–3):247–263, 2002.

91. Wolf SL, Winstein CJ, Miller P, et al: Effect of constraint-induced movement therapy on upper extremity function 3 to 9 months after stroke: the EXCITE randomized clinical trial, *JAMA* 296:2095–2104, 2006.

92. Page S, Levine P, Peonard A: Modified constraint-induced therapy in acute stroke: a randomized controlled pilot study, *Neurorehabil Neural Repair* 9:27–32, 2005.

93. Lin KC: Effects of modified constraint-induced movement therapy on reach-to-grasp movements and functional performance after chronic stroke: a randomized controlled study, *Clin Rehabil* 21:1075–1086, 2007.

94. Gordon AM, Charles J, Wolf SL: Methods of constraint-induced movement therapy for children with hemiplegic cerebral palsy: development of a child-friendly intervention for improving upper-extremity function, *Arch Phys Med Rehabil* 86:837–844, 2005.

95. Naylor CE, Bower E: Modified constraint-induced movement therapy for young children with hemiplegic cerebral palsy: a pilot study, *Dev Med Child Neurol* 47:365–369, 2005.

96. Taub E, Ramey SL, DeLuca S, et al: Efficacy of constraint-induced movement therapy for children with cerebral palsy with asymmetric motor impairment, *Pediatrics* 113:305–312, 2004.

97. Liepert J, Bauder H, Wolfgant HR, et al: Treatment induced cortical reorganization after stroke in humans, *Stroke* 31:1210–1216, 2000.

98. Nudo RJ, Wise BM, SiFuentes F, et al: Neural substrates for the effects of rehabilitation training on motor recovery following ischemic infarct, *Science* 272:1791–1794, 1996.

Evaluation of Function, Activity, and Participation

OBJECTIVES

After reading this chapter, the reader will be able to:

1. Discuss the importance of evaluating a person's ability to participate in life roles.
2. Identify well-developed methods of evaluating function, activity, and participation.
3. Compare and contrast commonly used standardized assessment instruments of function, activity, and participation.

4. Discuss issues of reliability, validity, sensitivity, and responsiveness of standardized assessment instruments used to measure function, activity, and participation.
5. Explore the relationships between function, activity, participation in life roles, quality of life, and health status.

As discussed in Chapter 1, our success at meeting the challenges of everyday life reflects our functional independence and ability to participate in life roles. Is a small child capable of shopping for groceries, cooking, and managing finances? What about the older adult? Can an adult successfully balance the demands of work, home, family, and self? The answer to the first question is, of course, no. Within our society, we care for children until they are capable of these activities. Children do, however, develop skills in mobility, dressing, and hygiene that allow them some degree of functional independence. We hope that the answer to the latter two questions is yes. Adults and older adults want to live their lives as successfully and independently as possible. Occasionally, illness or injury may limit a person's ability to physically function as independently as she would wish, interfering with the ability to participate in important activities with family and friends. At this point, the individual may turn to the health care community for support and assistance in regaining a self-sufficient, satisfying lifestyle.

The primary task of health care professionals is to improve the health and functional independence of the client. As mentioned in Chapter 1, *health* is a state of complete physical, mental, and social well-being, not merely the absence of disease and infirmity.[1] In medical, surgical, psychosocial, and rehabilitation intervention, professionals strive to maintain or restore function. Health professionals in these areas of intervention hope

to improve a person's functional capacity.[2] As interventions improve a person's ability to function independently and participate in life roles, optimization of health and quality of life should also be supported.

For the physical or occupational therapist, the focus of intervention is on physical functioning. The area of physical function includes a person's ability to move through the environment, perform self-care activities, successfully complete job tasks, and enjoy recreational pursuits.[3] How well can the client move from place to place? Is she able to successfully perform the tasks related to a profession or job? Can she take care of basic daily tasks such as bathing, dressing, and eating? How about more difficult tasks, such as shopping, taking a bus, or cleaning the house? Can the client enjoy leisure and recreational activities? It is important for the young child to be able to play, not only for fun and leisure but also to learn more about the world. By focusing intervention in these areas, the physical and occupational therapist can improve a client's ability to live as independently as possible, participate in meaningful life activities, and improve her quality of life.

For health care professionals to best serve their clients, they must be able to clearly, efficiently, and reliably identify what activities are meaningful and necessary to each person. The therapist must determine at what level the client is able to perform these important everyday tasks. Functional evaluation has long been an effective method to identify a client's strengths and needs, develop appropriate treatment plans, and evaluate the effectiveness of that treatment over time. Functional evaluation consists of observing a client's ability to perform activities. When possible, these activities should be observed within the home and community setting. Function can be measured by noting the distance a person is able to walk or timing how long a person can balance in sitting. Standardized assessments are also available to measure the functional ability of children and adults. In addition to assessment of functional ability, a client's level of participation in home, work, and community activities should also be measured. Standardized instruments are also available that address participation and quality of life.

Comprehensive evaluation of function allows health care providers to develop meaningful treatment programs that will improve the quality of life for their clients.[4] When appropriate assessment instruments are used as a basis for intervention, therapists can measure success in achieving the primary goal of therapy—improvement of the functional independence and level of participation of their clients.

CHARACTERISTICS

An evaluation of functional performance can take many different forms and be implemented in many ways. Each individual incorporates a unique set of functional tasks into her day, based on self-care, work, and leisure activities. All of these activities relate to how well a person can complete the necessary tasks of everyday life and should be evaluated by the health care team. Self-care activities such as dressing, washing, eating, and ambulating are referred to as *basic activities of daily living* (BADL). More advanced activities that allow us to live independently in our communities, such as shopping, using transportation, cooking, and cleaning, are referred to as *instrumental activities of daily living* (IADL). Functional assessment needs to look at both of these categories of activities, as well as at abilities in job-related tasks and recreation. Assessment of IADL, work, and leisure activities in a person's natural environments, such as home, workplace, and community, provides a picture of the person's level of participation. By addressing all areas of a person's life, the evaluation reflects important aspects of how successfully the person can independently care for herself and enjoy life.

In evaluating function, the health care provider must be sure that the entire spectrum of activities performed during the client's day is represented. The evaluation must address issues related to emotional, social, and environmental issues, not just physical functioning. How does a person interact with the environment?

Can she easily commute to the workplace or get to the grocery store when necessary? Is it easy to move from place to place within the home regardless of whether the floor is carpeted or tiled? It must be clear that the goal of the functional assessment is to identify how the individual is able to perform everyday life activities, not to document the impairments specific to medical problems such as weakness, depression, or confusion. It is important to understand how the client reacts to her medical problems and how medical issues interfere with successfully meeting the demands of daily life. Identification of such barriers is helpful in modifying the task or the environment to enhance the client's level of participation. All in all, an assessment of function, activity, and participation must try to gauge an individual's maximal functional potential, encompassing all domains of function and health.

When assessing participation, self-report questionnaires are often used and can explore several dimensions of participation. These dimensions can include assessment of quality, quantity, and degree of satisfaction with one's own level of participation, as well as whether assistance is needed or an assistive device is used.[5] It is possible to evaluate not only if a person can participate in an event but also how often or with how much ease the person can participate. In addition, how satisfying was the level of participation. It is also important to consider an individual's level of satisfaction with an activity such as going to work, shopping at the mall, visiting relatives, cooking for the family, etc. When assessing participation, the dimension of participation that is important to the patient and relevant to the intervention being provided should be considered.[5] Especially with the dimension of satisfaction with participation, a relationship can be seen with the individual's perception of quality of life. It is sometimes difficult to differentiate between a measure of participation and quality of life.[6]

Examination Formats: Standardized Versus Nonstandardized

Both standardized and nonstandardized formats are important components of a comprehensive examination of functional activities and participation. *Standardized* assessment strategies use a formal functional assessment test/instrument, and the assessment is administered in the same way to everyone, every time it is used. The items included in a standardized assessment are carefully selected and very clearly defined so that the assessment instrument validly measures the construct that it purports to measure. Valid, reliable standardized assessment instruments undergo a rigorous developmental process to make the instrument useful within the clinical setting. *Nonstandardized* examination activities can be individualized to each client and include a review of activities that are important for the individual client. By identifying the activities necessary for a client to successfully participate in her daily home, work, and leisure activities, a therapist can most comprehensively examine the client's level of function and participation. This information is critical for development of effective, meaningful intervention plans. Nonstandardized examination strategies include observation of the client performing an activity. It is important to define these observations with objective measurements so that any changes in the client's ability to perform the activity can be clearly documented.

Several objective methods can be used to document performance of functional activities. A therapist can time how long it takes a person to walk from her bedroom to the bathroom. In watching a client walk in a home setting, with a variety of floor coverings, how many times does a patient lose her balance when transitioning from a tile floor to a carpeted surface? By using objective measures of observed behaviors, a therapist can easily measure how a client's performance has changed over time.

Whenever a therapist works with a client and evaluates how well that person can get out of bed, walk to the bathroom, or get dressed, the therapist is evaluating functional activities. When observing these tasks within the client's natural environment, a truer picture of participation is gained. When using this nonstandardized format, it is difficult to ensure that the evaluation is complete. Have all of the important aspects of the client's daily routine been included or just the activities important to the therapist? When it is time to reevaluate, the therapist can replicate the initial evaluation if objective, measurable descriptions of the task completion were used at initial examination. The use of objective descriptions allows the therapist to accurately note client progress and effectively communicate client status to the client, family, and health care team.

A comprehensive evaluation of functional ability, activity, and participation should contain both standardized and nonstandardized components. The use of a formal standardized assessment provides the therapist with a body of reliable, valid information for all clients. Alone, this assessment strategy may not represent all activities that the client feels are important and meaningful in her everyday life. By also including a more individualized, nonstandardized component within the functional evaluation, the therapist identifies important information unique to the client.[3]

Selection Considerations for Standardized Assessments of Function, Activity, and Participation

Several standardized assessment instruments are available today to measure function, participation, and quality of life. As clinicians, we must choose an instrument that best meets the needs of each individual client. For some clients, disease-specific factors may interfere with function, such as the pain of arthritis. Young children certainly participate in a different set of functional activities than do adults. Other individuals may perform functional tasks quite well only when using an assistive device or may require the assistance of a caregiver. We need to consider all of these issues when selecting the best assessment instrument to assist in design and implementation of effective intervention plans. Factors that contribute to the selection of the most appropriate standardized measures for evaluation of a specific client include the focus/purpose of the assessment, the age range or patient population for whom the tool was developed, the psychometric properties of the assessment (i.e., reliability, validity, responsiveness), and the design of the assessment (i.e., survey, observational). The therapist must also keep in mind whether the instrument measures activity, participation, or quality of life.

Measurement Issues

Several characteristics of assessment instruments affect their ability to accurately measure functional skills. Well-developed assessment strategies incorporate the principles of measurement science into their format. Measurement science involves the use of specific rules to evaluate a situation. By adhering to rules in the evaluation process, several important properties of measurement science are supported, including (1) reliability, (2) validity, (3) responsiveness, and (4) precision. Information regarding the reliability and validity of published standardized assessments should be reported in assessment manuals or research reports. The health care professional should use the reported information to determine whether the tool has been proved to be reliable and valid.

Reliability refers to the ability of the test instrument to report findings in a consistent and repeatable fashion. The assessment should yield very similar results when administered to the same client by two different therapists (*interrater reliability*) or when administered by the same therapist on two separate occasions within a short time frame (*intrarater reliability*). Consistency between two administrations of the same test within a short period is also called *test-retest reliability*.

Validity implies that the assessment is achieving its intended function and truly measuring what it is supposed to measure. *Construct validity* reflects the extent to which the test measures the construct or trait it is meant to measure. For example, does the measure validly measure activity, participation, or function? *Content validity* reflects if the test content fully measures the behaviors that should be included. In this case, does a functional test include items that reflect all the important functional activities for a child, an adult, or an older adult? *Concurrent validity* reflects how closely a standardized assessment scores compare with the scores on a well-established assessment measuring the same construct. For example, does a new functional assessment measure function in a similar manner to a well-established functional assessment.

Precision and responsiveness of an instrument are also considerations if therapists anticipate that the use of a standardized functional assessment will allow them to document changes in a client's status over time, as a result of either therapy or progression of disease or secondary to development. *Precision* refers to the ability to detect appropriate levels of change.[2] For example, consider the client with poor endurance who has a spinal cord injury and must learn to walk with bilateral lower extremity orthoses and crutches. If an assessment tool contains only one item to assess walking that requires the client to walk 50 yards independently, this client will not be able to pass the item for a very long time. A more precise test for this client may have several items related to the ability to walk (i.e., for 10 feet, 10 yards, 25 yards, and so on). *Responsiveness* to change refers to a test's ability to measure an aspect of performance that is anticipated to change as a result of therapy. For example, consider a client who has had an injury that makes it impossible to use the right hand in functional activities. In therapy, you are working with the client to help her learn to use the left hand to feed herself and to write. A responsive assessment tool will measure her ability to perform these activities with her left hand. An unresponsive tool will measure the return of function of the right hand.

It is also important to consider if an assessment evaluates performance discreetly enough to document changes that may occur as a result of therapy. How many points must a score improve until there is minimally significant change? Several different terms are used to address different aspects of this issue. *Minimal detectable change* in assessment scores reflects a change that is greater than that which could be due to measurement error.[7] A *minimally clinically important difference* is the smallest difference that a patient finds to be beneficial.[8]

Rating Performance

Standardized assessments vary in how they rate an individual's performance. In the simplest rating format, a skill is noted as being present or absent, thereby documenting whether something can be done. Checklist-type assessments favor this type of rating format but do not address the quality of that performance. It cannot be determined whether the skill is accomplished efficiently, consistently, or to the degree necessary for functional independence within a wide variety of environments. For example, if the client can walk 20 to 30 feet with a cane and ascend the stairs in the therapy department, she would certainly pass a checklist assessment that includes these tasks. What happens if the individual then goes home and encounters thick, plush carpeting or a steeper flight of stairs than those in the therapy department? Her ability to get into her apartment and walk from room to room may be very different from the performance seen in the therapy department. From another perspective, if while an individual walks with a cane the other arm becomes stiff and the hand clenches, the quality of ambulation may not be sufficient for her to perform daily tasks such as carrying a plate to the table or bringing in the newspaper. By checking off how many items a person can complete on a functional task checklist, ordinal data is obtained. If on initial assessment a person completes 10 items on a checklist and on discharge the person can complete 20 items on the checklist, it is clear that the person can do more activities, but it is not implied that the patient is twice as accomplished on discharge as she was on the initial exam.

Another type of rating system uses a visual analog scale. A client is asked to rate her performance on a linear scale, on which one end of the line reflects one extreme and the other end the other extreme of performance. She responds by placing a mark on the line at the point she feels best represents her performance. This system allows her to express a level of skill in a functional task at some point between being fully dependent and fully independent. An example of this type of scale is given in Figure 5-1. Again, this type of rating system yields ordinal data, with a higher score reflecting better performance than a lower score.

Other scales use a summative rating system, in which different items are weighted so that independent completion of all tasks represented in the assessment results in a total score of 100. In the development of this type of scale, weighting of items is generally based on professional judgment. Therefore, this scale reflects the developer's values about the importance of different functional skills, not necessarily how important certain skills are to a client's life. The performance of each task is evaluated and scored to reflect total or partial

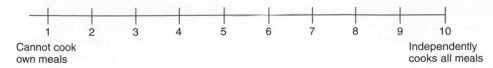

Figure 5-1 Linear rating scale for ability to prepare meals.

completion of the task independently. Scores for all tasks are added and compared with a perfect total score of 100. A score of 100 does not necessarily reflect normal performance, just as a score of 85 does not mean that someone is functioning within 15% of typical performance. Another confusing aspect of summative scale formats is how the scores can be compared mathematically. When an individual achieves a score of 10 on the initial assessment and a score of 50 on a subsequent assessment, it is not necessarily true that she is performing five times better than initially. It is only known that 50 reflects more points than 10. We must remember that the score can be compared only within the context of the assessment instrument. This type of rating scale is good for measuring whether change has occurred over time or with intervention.

As standardized assessments have been revised or developed over the past 20 years, the fit of items within the construct of the assessment and level of difficulty of items has been appraised. By using the item response theory, assessment instruments have been developed that yield interval-level data. With interval-level data, data points are equidistant from one another. For example, a score of 10 really does reflect performance that is twice as good as a score of 5. By developing instruments that measure functional performance and participation with interval-level data, improved outcome data can be obtained and provide more effective interpretation of outcomes.

Focus

An initial consideration when selecting an assessment instrument is to consider what needs to be measured. Measurement of a patient's ability to perform a functional task reflects the patient's *capacity* to complete the task, while measurement of the patient's actual use of the task within daily activity gives a measure of *performance* of the skill. Capacity is considered to reflect the activity level of the International Classification of Functioning, Disability and Health (ICF),[9] and performance reflects the participation level.

The type of setting in which the assessment is taking place and the client status are taken into consideration when considering the focus of the assessment strategy that is necessary. For example, in an inpatient setting it may be important to examine how independently a patient can perform BADL such as bed mobility, eating, dressing, and hygiene. Level of independence in these skills will assist the team in determining how much assistance for self-care a patient needs, which is important when considering possible discharge options. As a patient is completing rehabilitation or living at home with a chronic condition, it may be most appropriate to examine a patient's ability to function within her home and community. Can she shop, cook, clean, or commute to work? An assessment focusing on participation level activities would be most appropriate for these individuals. Through the rehabilitation or habilitation course, it is important to examine how the level of independence in functional activities and the level of participation contribute to a patient's quality of life. Depending on patient status and setting, assessment instruments addressing functional status or participation might be most appropriate, but assessments of the quality of life provide valuable information at any time within the health care course.

Many of the formal functional assessment instruments in use were developed to meet the needs of specific client populations and focus on factors influencing activity and participation of that group. For example, the Arthritis Impact Measurement Scale, 2nd edition (AIMS-2), is a questionnaire addressing health status of adults with rheumatoid arthritis. It examines physical, psychological, and social function, as well as pain.[10] As originally developed, it was not optimal for use with children, older adults, or individuals with other medical problems. A functional assessment tool for children with juvenile rheumatoid arthritis, the Juvenile Arthritis Functional Assessment Scale,[11] was developed. The GERI-AIMS (an adaptation of the AIMS) was designed for use with older individuals with osteoarthritis or rheumatoid arthritis. It also assesses functional impairments related to other common medical problems of older adults, independent of the arthritis-specific functional impairment.[12]

Other types of instruments are available for individuals who demonstrate neurological involvement. Several functional assessment instruments have been developed for use with adults who have had a cerebral vascular accident (CVA). Examples include the Stroke Impact Scale (SIS),[13] Stroke Rehabilitation Assessment of Movement (STREAM),[14] and the Rivermead Motor

Assessment.[15] The Gross Motor Function Measure (GMFM) was developed specifically for use with children with cerebral palsy.[16] This instrument has also been shown to be valid for individuals with Down syndrome,[17] traumatic brain injury,[18] and spinal muscular atrophy.[19]

Care must be taken to choose the appropriate assessment instrument. Instruments that are developed for specific client populations can focus on issues particular to a disease process that limits function, such as the pain of the arthritic client. These instruments, however, are not necessarily appropriate for use with other client populations because they may not be sensitive enough to other problem areas affecting performance. Also, instruments developed for use with a specific age group may not address issues important for older or younger individuals. In general, functional assessment instruments may not be valid for use in client populations other than those for which they were developed.

Design

Once clinicians decide which assessment instrument best assesses a specific client's functional skills and limitations, they must also decide which type of assessment can best be used with the client. The two basic types of functional assessment designs are assessments in which information is self-reported by the client and performance-based assessments in which the examiner observes the performance of the activity.

Self-report types of assessments can be completed by either interview or by self-administered, client completion of a questionnaire or survey. The *interview assessment* is completed by a trained interviewer who asks the client a set of standard questions and records the answers in a standardized format. The information gleaned from this type of assessment is most useful when the interviewer has had training in how to administer and score the assessment. It is important that the interviewer not expand on questions or prompt answers to avoid influencing the client. *Self-administered assessments* are generally presented as questionnaires. The directions for completion of the questionnaire and questions themselves must be clearly written, so the client can understand what is being asked. It is also important to ensure that the way questions are asked or focused does not bias the answers. The accuracy of these types of assessments depends on the quality of the instrument itself and the person's ability to complete the questionnaire. In some instances, a caregiver or family member may complete the questionnaire for the client. When working with children, a parent will fill out the information for a young child. As the child becomes old enough to independently answer the questions, information

may be collected from both the child and the parents/caregivers.

Both interview and self-administered assessments are based on a client's self-report of her functional status or level of participation. Studies that compare the validity of the self-report with direct observation assessments have shown that agreement between the client's report and the direct observation is good to excellent in BADL. Research has shown that skill in IADL was slightly underreported in client self-reports.[20] The validity of self-report measures makes them attractive for use in health care settings, especially because they are easy and relatively inexpensive to administer.

Performance-based assessments are those in which an evaluator observes the client's performance in functional tasks. This type of assessment does report someone's ability to complete BADL but is not as easily applied to the evaluation of IADL. Because the assessment is completed in a structured test environment, performance in the home environment may not be reflected. Direct observation assessment is also time-consuming and therefore an expensive process.

Summary

When choosing an assessment instrument, a therapist must consider all of the factors that have been discussed. Does an instrument measure the capacity to complete an activity or performance of the activity during participation in daily routines? For what client population is the assessment appropriate? What type of assessment best and most accurately measures a person's functional skills? How does the assessment rate the performance? Is an instrument measuring whether a skill can be performed, how often a skill is performed, or how satisfied the client is with the performance? What type of assessment and rating system provides the best information to identify clients who require services, to develop treatment plans, or to assess the effectiveness of intervention? Even after answering all of these questions, the therapist must consider additional aspects of assessment instruments that contribute to their effectiveness as measurement tools and affect the interpretation of the data they provide. These aspects include the reliability, validity, and responsiveness of the instrument.

SURVEY OF MEASUREMENT INSTRUMENTS

In this section, we review a sample of standardized functional assessment instruments; only a small number of the assessment tools available to clinicians are discussed. These specific instruments were chosen because they are assessment instruments appropriate for individuals of different ages or because they are commonly used in clinical practice.

Pediatric Assessment Tools of Function, Activity, and Participation

Functional Independence Measure for Children

The WeeFIM™ instrument is an adaptation of the Functional Independence Measure (FIM™ [1] instrument) designed to measure the acquisition of functional skills in children with disability from 6 months through 7 years of age (Figure 5-2). The WeeFIM™ instrument measures the severity of the child's disability and evaluates outcomes of pediatric rehabilitation. It can be used in both inpatient and outpatient settings, and it can be administered by a variety of health and education professionals to measure the child's actual performance of functional tasks. Like the FIM™ instrument, the WeeFIM™ instrument focuses on BADL with three domains: self-care, mobility, and cognition. A seven-point ordinal scale is used to reflect the level of independence in these tasks. A score of 7 indicates the ability to perform a task independently, and a score of 1 indicates a need for total assistance. Scores of 1 to 5 are used when caregiver assistance is necessary, and a score of 6 indicates modified independence (e.g., need for assistive device).[21]

The skills included in the WeeFIM™ are typical of children at 6 years of age who do not have disabilities. For this reason, the tool has demonstrated a ceiling effect when used with a child with a disability living in the community with higher levels of function.[22,23]

The Wee-FIM™ measures function at the activity level of the ICF. It has been recommended that multiple instruments should be used to comprehensively measure outcomes for children with physical disabilities. Measures of health status or health-related quality of life, such as the PedsQL or Child Health Questionnaire, complement the WeeFIM™ in measurement of the child's health and outcomes.[22,24]

The WeeFIM™ instrument has demonstrated good reliability whether administered via direct observation or structured interview.[25,26] Instrument validity was originally determined for children in the United States but has also been accepted for Japanese children.[27] The WeeFIM™ has been found to be reliable and valid for children with cerebral palsy in Turkey, although under 4 years of age, some floor effect was found.[28] Reported limitations for

---

[1]FIM™ is a trademark of the Uniform Data System for Medical Rehabilitation, a division of U B Foundation Activities, Inc.

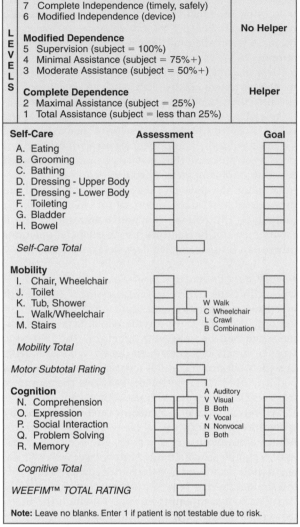

Figure 5-2 WeeFIM™ instrument. (From *WeeFIM Systems clinical guide: version 5.01*, Buffalo, NY, 2002, Center for Functional Assessment Research and UDSMR, State University of New York at Buffalo.)

the WeeFIM™ instrument concern its use of an ordinal scoring scale and the sensitivity of the scale.[29]

To address concerns about the ability of the WeeFIM™ to measure function in children under the age of 3 years, a new scale, the WeeFIM™ 0-3 module, has been developed. This family-centered questionnaire looks at precursor skills needed for functional tasks such as self-feeding. The WeeFIM™ 0-3 includes 35 items, divided into 3 domains (motor, cognitive, and behavioral perceptions). The behavioral perceptions section is meant to identify areas where the caregiver may be having difficulty with interaction or care of the infant (e.g., cuddling, bathing, dressing). Infant behaviors are scored on a three-point ordinal scale indicating if an action rarely/never (1), sometimes (2), or usually (3) occurs. Initial studies of psychometric properties indicate that the WeeFIM™ 0-3 can differentiate between children with and without a disability. A child's functional skill development can be tracked longitudinally using the WeeFIM™ 0-3 module followed by the WeeFIM™ and FIM™.[30]

Gross Motor Function Measure

The Gross Motor Function Measure[31] is a criterion-referenced assessment designed to be used with children with cerebral palsy. It evaluates the child's ability to complete motor functions, such as rolling, crawling, sitting, standing, walking, running, stair use, and jumping. A four-point ordinal scale of measurement is used to assess each item. A score of 0 indicates the task cannot be done, 1 indicates the task can be initiated (<10% completion), 2 indicates partial completion of the task (10% to <100% completion), and 3 indicates the task can be completed. Two forms of the GMFM are available: the GMFM-88 and GMFM-66. The GMFM-66 provides a version of the instrument yielding interval-level data and expands upon the scoring options and uses of the instrument.[32] The GMFM measures function at the activity level of the ICF.

Test-retest reliability, interrater, intrarater, and internal reliability have all been found to be excellent (>0.99) for both GMFM-88 and GMFM-66.[31,33,34] Content and construct validity are also reported to be good. Longitudinal construct validity has been demonstrated for both the GMFM-88 and GMFM-66 scoring formats.[35] Concurrent validity with the PEDI has been found.[36] GMFM construct validity for children with diplegic cerebral palsy during a 12- to 24-month period also has been demonstrated.[37] The measure is considered to be sensitive to changes in performance in functional tasks, making it an effective tool for documenting change in the motor performance of children with cerebral palsy.[16,31]

Pediatric Evaluation of Disability Index

The Pediatric Evaluation of Disability Index (PEDI) assesses the capability and performance of functional skills by children between the ages of 6 months and 7.5 years in the areas of self-care, mobility, social function, and household chores (per Box 5-1). Aspects of the PEDI measure function at the activity level and other components measure function at the participation level of the ICF. The index is meant to be used to detect

---

Box 5-1

Types of Activities Assessed in Pediatric Evaluation of Disability Index

Self-care
- Eating—types of food, use of utensils, use of drinking containers
- Hygiene—toothbrushing, hair brushing, nose care, hand washing
- Dressing—pullovers, fasteners, pants, shoes/socks
- Toileting tasks

Mobility
- Transfers—toilet, tub, chair, car, bed
- Indoor locomotion
- Outdoor locomotion
- Stairs

Social Function
- Comprehension of language
- Functional use of communication
- Problem resolution
- Peer interaction
- Play
- Orientation to self, time

Household Chores
- Function in community

---

functional deficits of individual children with disabilities, to monitor the child's progress in rehabilitation, and to assist in program evaluation. The PEDI can be administered in a structured interview format with the child's parents (which is reported to take 45 to 60 minutes) or by recording the judgment of therapists and teachers about the child's abilities (which is reported to take 20 to 30 minutes). Three different aspects of the child's functional performance are assessed: (1) the child's functional skill level, (2) the need for modification or adaptive equipment to achieve the task, and (3) the amount of physical assistance the child requires.[38]

The PEDI was used to assess 412 nondisabled children from New England. This normative sample represented all age groups for whom the test is appropriate and attempted to reflect demographics of the U.S. census in 1980.[39] Results from this study have provided some information on the development of functional skills in children and permit comparisons between children with and without disabilities. The normative scores also allow the nominal data recorded in the PEDI to be converted to ratio scales that reflect item difficulty.

Good reliability and validity of the PEDI have been demonstrated. High internal consistency has been reported.[39,40] Using a structured interview administration format, researchers have documented good inter-rater reliability. Nichols and Case-Smith[41] suggested that reliability is increased when both the parents and primary therapist complete the PEDI. The PEDI demonstrated the ability to correctly discriminate between disabled and normal populations and to detect change over time with intervention. Minimally clinically important difference (MCID) has been explored for children in rehabilitation settings.[42] Concurrent validity of 0.70 to 0.73 between the PEDI and Battelle Developmental Inventory Screening Test (BDIST) has been demonstrated, implying that the two tests address similar but not identical issues. Good concurrent validity between the PEDI, BDIST, and Functional Independence Measure for Children (WeeFIM™) instrument has also been demonstrated with a population of children with severe disabilities. Concurrent validity with the WeeFIM™ has also been reported in children with traumatic brain injury.[43] Construct validity is achieved because the PEDI supports the assumptions that functional behaviors change with age and that attainment of a functional skill precedes independence in that skill. The latter assumption implies that the degree of caregiver assistance is an important changeable dimension to monitor in a functional assessment framework.[38,39]

In 2011 a new edition of the PEDI, the PEDI-CAT, is expected to be available and will use a computer adaptive testing format to more efficiently assess function in children up to 15 years of age. A 4-point scoring system will be used to rate performance in self-care, mobility and social function. The original caregiver assistance scale will be replaced by a scale entitled "responsibilities," which will be scored on a 5-point scale. The new responsibilities section will more broadly address skills needed to live independently, with new content focusing on citizenship, safety, and community mobility.[44]

School Function Assessment

The School Function Assessment (SFA) is intended to assess how well an elementary school student with disabilities who attends kindergarten through sixth grade can meet the functional demands of the school setting. The SFA is administered as a judgment-based questionnaire, documenting a student's typical behavior compared with same-age or same-class peers. Criterion-referenced scoring represents the student's interaction within the school context, and criterion-referenced cutoff scores compare the

Table 5-1

Types of Activities Assessed in the School Function Assessment

Category	Activities Assessed
Social participation in school activities	Classroom
	Recess or playground
	Transportation
	Bathroom or toileting
	Transition to or from class
	Mealtime or snack time
Activity performance in school-related function: physical	Travel
	Maintain or change position
	Set up or clean up
	Hygiene
	Clothing management
	Stairs
Activity performance in school-related function: cognitive or behavioral	Communication
	Computer or equipment use
	Behavior regulation
	Memory or understanding

student's performance with grade-level expectations.[45] The SFA measures function both at the activity and participation level of the ICF.

The SFA consists of three separately scored sections: (1) social participation in school activities, (2) task supports necessary to participate in activities, and (3) activity performance in school-related functional activities (Table 5-1). Raw scores from each of the three sections are converted into criterion scores using a Rasch analysis statistical model. Tables of criterion scores and standard error of measurement are provided in the test manual. The participation and task support scales can be used as a screening device to identify students who demonstrate functional limitations in the school setting.[45] Selective scales can also be assessed individually to address specific areas of concern for intervention. In addition, the SFA can be used to support the individualized education plan development and document progress or effects of intervention.

In development of the SFA, a standardization sample of 363 students with disabilities was used. The criterion cutoff scores reflect the performance of 318 nondisabled peers. The test manual reports good internal reliability of each item (0.92 to 0.98) and test reliability (0.82 to 0.98 in a study with 23 participants; 0.80 to 0.99 in a study with 29 participants). Content validity is supported by expert review during the development and piloting of the SFA.

Concurrent validity has been demonstrated with the Vineland Adaptive Behavior Scales–classroom edition (VABS-C).[46] Construct validity is supported with the SFA successfully differentiating between children in regular education and elementary school students with disabilities.[46,47] Internal construct validity was further confirmed with Rasch analysis.[48]

Assessment of Life Habits (LIFE-H)

The LIFE-H[49] was originally designed for both children and adults with neurological dysfunction, such as stroke, spinal cord injury (myelomeningocele), traumatic brain injury, and cerebral palsy. Life habits are defined as the regular activities and social roles or values of a person in her life. The LIFE-H measures the degree of difficulty someone has with a task, their satisfaction with the task, and type of assistance needed. Among the domains included in the LIFE-H are activities in fitness, personal care, communication, housing, and mobility. Social roles are also included. such as education, employment, recreation, interpersonal relations, and responsibilities. The LIFE-H measures function at the participation level of the ICF. Upon review of participation measures for children, the LIFE-H addresses all domains of the ICF for children. Acceptable levels of test-retest reliability and internal consistency have been demonstrated for respondent interview, but no data is available for self-assessment.[50,51] Content validity was established by panels of parents, therapists, and researchers, while concurrent validity is reported between domains of the PEDI, WeeFIM™, and LIFE-H.[52]

Pediatric Quality of Life Inventory (Peds QL™)

The Peds QL™ examines the health and roles of children between 2 and 18 years old, measuring both health status and participation.[53] Physical, emotional, social, and school function are included. Different forms of the assessment are available for children of different ages and in most age categories both a parent form and child form are available. The Peds QL™ has been shown to have good reliability.[54-57] The assessment has also been shown to discriminate between children with a variety of health conditions and children without the health condition (e.g., cerebral palsy, asthma, cancer, arthritis).[54-56,58]

Children's Assessment of Participation and Enjoyment (CAPE) and Preference for Activity of Children (PAC)

The CAPE/PAC[59] was developed to measure participation in leisure activities by looking at recreational, physical, social, skill-based, and self-improvement activities. Multiple dimensions of participation are measured, such as the diversity of activities in which a child participates, with whom the child participates, where the child participates, and how much the child enjoys the participation. The CAPE/PAC is designed for children between the ages of 6 and 21 years. Limited reliability and validity information is available for the published version of the CAPE/PAC. Original reliability and validity studies were done on an earlier version of the tool, which had fewer items than the current published tool.

Adult Assessment Tools of Function Activity and Participation

Barthel Index

The Barthel Index was developed to measure improvement in clients with chronic disability who were participating in rehabilitation (Table 5-2). BADL are assessed, including toileting, bathing, eating, dressing, continence, transfers, and ambulation. Clients receive numerical scores based on whether they require physical assistance to perform the task or can complete it independently. Items are weighted according to the professional judgment of the developers. A client scoring 0 points would be dependent in all assessed activities of daily living, whereas a score of 100 would reflect independence in these activities.[60] The Barthel Index measures function at the activity level of the ICF.

Specific reliability and validity studies have not been reported, but Barthel Index scores of adult clients who have had a stroke or have severe disabilities correlate with clinical outcomes and functional status.[61,62] Specific, detailed instructions are provided, supporting standardized use of the measure.[63]

The Barthel index was one of the earliest standardized functional assessments. The FIM™ instrument was developed to be a more comprehensive tool. Research shows a relationship between the two instruments because a Barthel Index score can be derived from FIM™ instrument motor item scores.[64] The Barthel Index, total FIM™ instrument score, and motor FIM™ instrument score all demonstrate similar responsiveness in the evaluation of inpatient rehabilitation clients with multiple sclerosis and stroke.[65]

Functional Independence Measure

The FIM™ instrument was developed as part of the Uniform Data System for Medical Rehabilitation at the State University of New York at Buffalo,[66] and Version 5.1 of the FIM System™ was published in 1997.[67] The FIM™ instrument assesses the functional

Table 5-2

Barthel Index: A Functional Evaluation Tool to Assess a Client's Level of Independent Activity

Activity	Independent Function	Dependent Function
Feeding	Independent = 10. The client can feed herself a meal from a tray or table when someone puts the food within her reach. She must put on an assistive device if this is needed, cut up the food, use salt and pepper, spread butter, etc. She must accomplish this in a reasonable time.	Some help is necessary (with cutting up food, etc.) = 5.
Moving from wheelchair to bed and return	Independent in all phases of this activity = 15. Client can safely approach the bed in her wheelchair, lock brakes, lift footrests, move safely to bed, lie down, come to a sitting position on the side of the bed, change the position of the wheelchair (if necessary) to transfer back into it safely, and return to the wheelchair.	Either some minimal help is needed in some step of this activity or the client needs to be reminded or supervised for safety of one or more parts of this activity = 10. Client can come to a sitting position without the help of a second person but needs to be lifted out of bed, or she transfers with a great deal of help = 5.
Doing personal toilet	Client can wash hands and face, comb hair, clean teeth, and shave = 5. The client may use any kind of razor but must put in blade or plug in razor without help as well as get it from drawer or cabinet. Female clients must put on own makeup, if used, but need not braid or style hair.	With help = 0.
Getting on and off toilet	Client is able to get on and off toilet, fasten and unfasten clothes, prevent soiling of clothes, and use toilet paper without help = 10. She may use a wall bar or other stable object for support if needed. If it is necessary to use a bed pan instead of a toilet, she must be able to place it on a chair, empty it, and clean it.	Client needs help because of imbalance or in handling clothes or in using toilet paper = 5.
Bathing	Client may use a bathtub or a shower or take a complete sponge bath = 5. She must be able to do all the steps involved in whichever method is used without another person being present.	With help = 0.
Walking on a level surface	Client can walk at least 50 yards without help or supervision = 15. She may wear braces or prosthesis and use crutches, canes, or a walkerette, but not a rolling walker. She must be able to lock and unlock braces if used, assume the standing position and sit down, get the necessary mechanical aids into position for use, and dispose of them when she sits.	Client needs help or supervision in any of the above but can walk at least 50 yards with a little help = 10.

Table 5-2—cont'd

Barthel Index: A Functional Evaluation Tool to Assess a Client's Level of Independent Activity

Activity	Independent Function	Dependent Function
Propelling a wheelchair	If a client cannot ambulate but can propel a wheelchair independently = 5*. She must be able to go around corners, turn around, maneuver the chair to a table, bed, toilet, etc. She must be able to push a chair at least 50 yards. *Do not score this item if the client gets score for walking.	With help = 0*.
Ascending and descending	Client is able to go up and down a flight of stairs safely without help or supervision = 10. She may and should use handrails, canes, or crutches when needed. She must be able to carry canes or crutches as she ascends or descends stairs.	Client needs help with or supervision of either ascending or descending stairs = 5.
Dressing and undressing	Client is able to put on and remove and fasten all clothing, and tie shoelaces (unless it is necessary to use adaptations for this) = 10. The activity includes putting on and removing and fastening corset or braces when these are prescribed. Such special clothing as suspenders, loafer shoes, or dresses that open down the front may be used when necessary.	Client needs help in putting on and removing or fastening any clothing = 5. She must do at least half the work herself. She must accomplish this in a reasonable time.
Continence of bowels	Client is able to control her bowels and have no accidents = 10.	Client needs help in using a suppository or taking an enema or has occasional accidents = 5.
Controlling bladder	Client is able to control her bladder day and night = 10. Clients who wear an external device must be able to care for it independently.	Client has occasional accidents or cannot wait for the bed pan or get to the toilet in time or needs help with an external device = 5.

The best possible score is 100. A score of 0 indicates that the client cannot meet the criteria as defined for each function.
Adapted from Mahoney FI, Barthel DQ: Functional evaluation: the Barthel Index, *Md State Med J* 14:61-65, 1965.

skills of individuals over 7 years old (Figure 5-3). This data set has been used widely in the United States and internationally; it consists of more than 1 million records.[29] It is used in inpatient rehabilitation settings, as well as in long-term care, subacute rehabilitation, and home care environments to measure the activity level of function.

The FIM™ instrument is meant to reflect an individual's usual performance rather than her best performance. The assessment can be completed by direct client observation or interview. Six domains of function are evaluated: self-care, sphincter control, transfers, locomotion, communication, and social cognition. Self-care activities include dressing, eating, grooming, and bathing. Transfers from the bed to chair, to the toilet, and to the tub or shower are included in the mobility section. Locomotion includes walking, managing stairs, and propelling a wheelchair. Items are scored on a 7-point ordinal scale, with 7 reflecting complete independence and 1 reflecting total dependence. Scores of 1 to 5 indicate a need for caregiver assistance. Scores in all domains are added to obtain a total FIM™ instrument score; motor and cognitive scores can be calculated separately.

Reliability and validity of the FIM™ instrument are generally reported to be good, with very good interrater

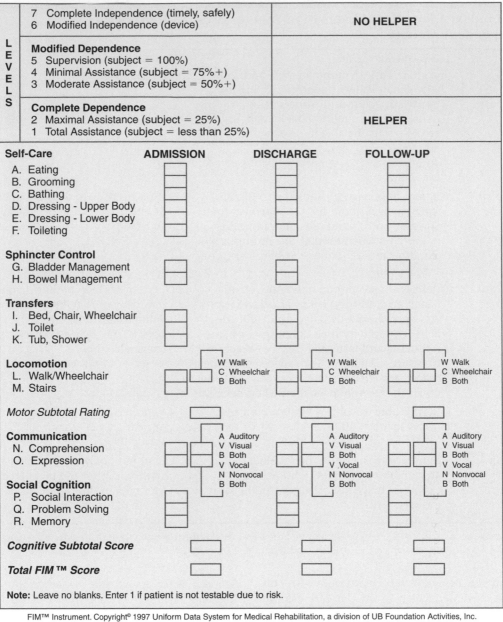

FIM™ Instrument

LEVELS		NO HELPER
	7 Complete Independence (timely, safely) 6 Modified Independence (device)	NO HELPER
	Modified Dependence 5 Supervision (subject = 100%) 4 Minimal Assistance (subject = 75%+) 3 Moderate Assistance (subject = 50%+)	
	Complete Dependence 2 Maximal Assistance (subject = 25%) 1 Total Assistance (subject = less than 25%)	HELPER

	ADMISSION	DISCHARGE	FOLLOW-UP
Self-Care			
A. Eating			
B. Grooming			
C. Bathing			
D. Dressing - Upper Body			
E. Dressing - Lower Body			
F. Toileting			
Sphincter Control			
G. Bladder Management			
H. Bowel Management			
Transfers			
I. Bed, Chair, Wheelchair			
J. Toilet			
K. Tub, Shower			
Locomotion	W Walk / C Wheelchair / B Both	W Walk / C Wheelchair / B Both	W Walk / C Wheelchair / B Both
L. Walk/Wheelchair			
M. Stairs			
Motor Subtotal Rating			
Communication	A Auditory / V Visual / B Both	A Auditory / V Visual / B Both	A Auditory / V Visual / B Both
N. Comprehension	V Vocal / N Nonvocal / B Both	V Vocal / N Nonvocal / B Both	V Vocal / N Nonvocal / B Both
O. Expression			
Social Cognition			
P. Social Interaction			
Q. Problem Solving			
R. Memory			
Cognitive Subtotal Score			
Total FIM™ Score			

Note: Leave no blanks. Enter 1 if patient is not testable due to risk.

Figure 5-3 FIM instrument. (From *Guide for the uniform data set for medical rehabilitation [including the FIM instrument], version 5.1*, Buffalo, NY, 1997, Center for Functional Assessment Research and UDSMR, State University of New York at Buffalo.)

reliability to the total score (0.96), motor score (0.96), and cognitive score (0.91). Some individual subtest inter-rater reliability scores are weaker, such as the memory subtest, which depends on the training of the examiner (0.53, untrained; 0.69, trained).[67] Kohler and colleagues[68]

reflect that most reliability studies have been conducted with individuals who have been trained in use of the FIM™ and in controlled settings. In a study looking at agreement between FIM™ scores when a patient is transferred from one setting to a different rehabilitation setting, only low agreement between the paired FIM™ scores was found.[68] These findings suggest that in general clinical settings where therapists may not have gone through specific FIM™ training that the reliability of the FIM™ scores cannot be assumed.

Concurrent validity has been reported with the Barthel Index.[69] Construct validity research summarized by Deutsch and colleagues[29] and a study with clients with multiple sclerosis[70] indicate good FIM™ instrument construct validity. Functional independence is a multidimensional entity and may be better reflected by the subscores.[71] The responsiveness of the FIM™ instrument also has been reported to be good; scores can differentiate client populations and improve over the course of rehabilitation.[29] The FIM™ was found to be more responsive to change than the Barthel Index in a group of patients with stroke.[72]

The Assessment of Life Habits (LIFE-H)

The LIFE-H assessment is described in the section on pediatric assessment tools. The instrument was originally developed for children and adults, with the only difference being simplified language for children. Test-retest reliability of the LIFE-H satisfactions scale is high in older adults with functional disabilities.[73] For individuals with stroke, similar levels of participation were documented by both patients and their proxies, reflecting that proxy respondents can be used when patients are unable to respond.[74] The LIFE-H has been found to be a measure of social participation in individuals who have had a stroke that is responsive to change.[75]

Short Form-36 (SF-36)

The SF-36[76] is a health status profile originally designed to measure health status of patients and outcomes of patients. Health status could be compared between groups of patients by type of intervention, disease, or type of health insurance. The original target population was individuals living in the community. The SF-36 is used today in outpatient settings and with community-dwelling older adults.

The 36 questions on the SF-36 are meant to reflect 8 domains of health, including physical functioning, physical role, pain, general health, vitality, social function, emotional role, and mental health. The categories of physical role and emotional role reflect performance at the activity and participation levels.[77]

The SF-36 has been found to be reliable and valid for measuring health-related quality of life of individuals with several chronic health conditions and in several countries.[78-81] Especially the physical functioning domain of the SF-36 measures mobility disability in several patient populations.[78,82,83]

SUMMARY

The desire to identify positive outcomes is directly related to the importance of evaluating a client's ability to perform functional tasks and participate in meaningful activities. The primary goal of physical and occupational therapy intervention is to improve the client's functional abilities and participation. Functional outcome measures can guide the therapist in the development of meaningful, functional goals for the client. By emphasizing functional outcomes, intervention focuses on the client's independence rather than on attainment of normality.[4] A client with a spinal cord injury may not be able to walk in the community but with a wheelchair may have independent community mobility. This client may also be able to participate in work- and leisure-related activities when using the wheelchair. Focus on functional outcomes contributes to improved quality of life and overall health.

Evaluation of a client's functional abilities can include both standardized and nonstandardized components. A functional assessment should encompass activities that are important throughout a client's day and should consider social, emotional, environmental, and cognitive issues relevant to that client. The spectrum of tasks assessed must reflect those necessary for the client to function in her environment. For example, the School Function Assessment will better assess how a first-grader is functioning in school than the Pediatric Evaluation of Disability Index. Likewise, the Barthel Index may adequately reflect the functional ability of a client in a long-term care facility but will not address the IADL necessary for that client's discharge to a home setting.

Use of standardized assessment instruments increases the reliability and validity of the evaluation, assists in objectively documenting outcomes, and improves communication between professional caregivers. The mode of administration, scoring format, and measurement characteristics of a standardized assessment are important to consider, as noted in the descriptions of the instruments reviewed in this chapter.

Establishing a client's level of function and participation is the first step to designing interventions that address that person's individual needs. The clinician must work with the client to identify the activities that define the client's participation in family, work, and leisure activities throughout the day. Once important activities are identified, the therapist can further explore which components of function are limiting performance based on an evaluation of functional skills. Strength, endurance, balance, mobility, or coordination may be the factors that limit physical performance. Specific therapeutic programs can be designed to address any of those components of the functional task. The client should then be encouraged to practice the important functional activities, using any necessary assistive devices or environmental modifications. As functional activities are mastered, the client is progressing on the path to improved participation in meaningful activities, health, and quality of life.

REFERENCES

1. World Health Organization: *The first ten years of the World Health Organization*, Geneva, 1958, World Health Organization.
2. Liang MH, Jette AM: Measuring functional ability in chronic arthritis: a critical review, *Arthritis Rheum* 24:80–86, 1981.
3. Guccione AA: *Geriatric physical therapy*, ed 2, St Louis, 2000, Mosby.
4. Haley SM, Coster WJ, Ludlow LH: Pediatric functional outcome measures, *Phys Med Rehabil Clin N Am* 2:689–723, 1991.
5. Resnik L, Plow MA: Measuring participation as defined by the international classification of functioning, disability and health: an evaluation of existing measures, *Arch Phys Med Rehabil* 90:856–966, 2009.
6. Noonan VK, Kopec JA, Noreau L, et al: A review of participation instruments based on the international classification of functioning, disability and health, *Disabil Rehabil* 31(23):1–19, 2009.
7. Haley SM, Fragala-Pinkham MA: Interpreting change scores of tests and measures used in physical therapy, *Phys Ther* 86:735–743, 2006.
8. Copay AG, Subach BR, Glassman SD, et al: Understanding the minimum clinically important difference: a review of concepts and methods, *Spine* 7(5):541–546, 2007.
9. World Health Organization: *International classification of functioning, disability, and health*, Geneva, 2001, World Health Organization.
10. Meenen RF, Mason JH, Anderson JJ, et al: AIMS2. The content and properties of a revised and expanded Arthritis Impact measurement Scales Health Status Questionnaire, *Arthritis Rheum* 35(1):1–10, 1992.
11. Lovell DJ, Howe S, Shear E, et al: Development of a disability measurement tool for juvenile rheumatoid arthritis: the Juvenile Arthritis Functional Assessment Scale, *Arthritis Rheum* 32:1390–1395, 1989.
12. Hughes SL, Edelman P, Chang RW, et al: The GERI-AIMS: reliability and validity of the Arthritis Impact Measurement Scales adapted for elderly respondents, *Arthritis Rheum* 34:856–865, 1991.
13. Duncan PW, Wallace D, MinLai S, et al: The Stroke Impact Scale version 2.0: evaluation of reliability, validity, and sensitivity to change, *Stroke* 30:2131–2140, 1999.
14. Daley K, Mayo NE, Wood-Dauphinee SL, et al: Verification of the Stroke Rehabilitation Assessment of Movement (STREAM), *Physiother Can* 49:269–278, 1997.
15. Lincoln NB, Leadbitter D: Assessment of motor function in stroke patients, *Physiotherapy* 65:48–51, 1979.
16. Russell DJ, Rosenbaum PL, Cadman DT, et al: The Gross Motor Function Measure: a means to evaluate the effects of physical therapy, *Dev Med Child Neurol* 31:341–352, 1989.
17. Gemus M, Palisano R, Russell D, et al: Using the Gross Motor Function Measure to evaluate motor development in children with Down syndrome, *Phys Occup Ther Pediatr* 21(2/3):69–79, 2001.
18. Linder-Lucht M, Othmer V, Walther M, et al: Validation of the Gross Motor Function Measure for use in children and adolescents with traumatic brain injuries, *Pediatrics* 120(4):880–886, 2007.
19. Nelson L, Owens H, Hynan LS, et al: The Gross Motor Function Measure is a valid and sensitive outcome measure for spinal muscular atrophy, *Neuromuscul Disord* 16:374–380, 2006.
20. Harris BA, Jette AM, Campion EW, et al: Validity of self-report measures of functional disability, *Top Geriatr Rehabil* 1:31–41, 1986.
21. Msall ME, DiGaudio KM, Duffy LC: Use of functional assessment in children with developmental disabilities, *Phys Med Rehabil Clin N Am* 4:517–527, 1993.
22. Thomas-Stonell N, Johnson P, Rumney P, et al: An evaluation of the responsiveness of a comprehensive set of outcome measures for children and adolescents with traumatic brain injuries, *Pediatr Rehabil* 9(1):14–23, 2006.
23. Serghiou MH, Rose MW, Pidcock FS, et al: The WeeFIM [R] instrument—a paediatric measure of functional independence to predict longitudinal recovery of paediatric burn patients, *Dev Neurorehabil* 11(1):39–50, 2008.
24. Grilli L, Feldman DE, Majnemer A, et al: Associations between a Functional Independence Measure (WeeFIM) and pediatric quality of life inventory (PedsQL4.0), *Qual Life Res* 15:1023–1031, 2006.
25. Ottenbacher KJ, Taylor ET, Msall ME, et al: The stability and equivalence reliability of the Functional Independence Measure for children (WeeFIM), *Dev Med Child Neurol* 38:907–916, 1996.
26. Sperle FA, Ottenbacher KJ, Braun SL, et al: Equivalence reliability of the Functional Independence Measure for Children (WeeFIM) administration methods, *Am J Occup Ther* 51:35–41, 1997.
27. Liu M, Toikawa H, Seki M, et al: Functional Independence Measure for Children (WeeFIM): a preliminary study in nondisabled Japanese children, *Am J Phys Med Rehabil* 77:36–44, 1998.
28. Tur BS, Kucukdeveci AA, Kutlay S, et al: Psychometric properties of the WeeFIM in children with cerebral palsy in Turkey, *Dev Med Child Neurol* 51:732–738, 2009.
29. Deutsch A, Braun S, Granger C: The Functional Independence Measure (FIM Instrument) and the Functional Independence Measure for Children (WeeFIM Instrument): ten years of development, *Crit Rev Phys Rehabil Med* 8:267–281, 1996.
30. Niewczyk PM, Granger CV: Measuring function in young children with impairments, *Pediatr Phys Ther* 22:42–51, 2010.
31. Russell DJ, Rosenbaum PL, Avery LM, et al: *Gross Motor Function Measure (GMFM-66 & GMFM-88) user's manual*, Hamilton, Ontario, Canada, 2002, MacKeith Press.

32. Avery L, Russell D, Raina P, et al: Rasch analysis of the Gross Motor Function Measure: validating the assumptions of the Rasch model to create an interval-level measure, *Arch Phys Med Rehabil* 84:697–705, 2003.

33. Russell DJ, Avery LM, Rosenbaum PL, et al: Improved scaling of the Gross Motor Function Measure for Children with cerebral palsy: evidence of reliability and validity, *Phys Ther* 80(9):873–885, 2000.

34. McCarthy M, Silberstein CE, Atkins EA, et al: Comparing reliability and validity of pediatric instruments for measuring health and well-being of children with spastic cerebral palsy, *Dev Med Child Neurol* 44:468–476, 2002.

35. Josenby AL, Jarnlo GB, Gummesson C, et al: Longitudinal construct validity of the GMFM-88 total score and goal total score and the GMFM-66 score in a 5-year follow-up study, *Phys Ther* 89(4):342–350, 2009.

36. Vos-Vormans DC, Ketelaar M, Gorter JW: Responsiveness of evaluative measures for children with cerebral palsy: the Gross Motor Function Measure and the Pediatric Evaluation of Disability Inventory, *Disabil Rehabil* 27(20):1245–1252, 2005.

37. Bjornson KF, Graubert CS, Buford VL, et al: Validity of the Gross Motor Function Measure, *Pediatr Phys Ther* 10:43–47, 1998.

38. Feldman AB, Haley SM, Coryell J: Concurrent and construct validity of the Pediatric Evaluation of Disability Inventory, *Phys Ther* 70:602–610, 1990.

39. Haley SM, Coster WJ, Ludlow LH, et al: *Pediatric Evaluation of Disability Inventory (PEDI)*, Boston, 1992, New England Medical Center Hospital and PEDI Research Group.

40. Berg M, Jahnsen R, Froslie KF, et al: Reliability of the Pediatric Evaluation Disability Inventory (PEDI), *Phys Occup Ther Pediatr* 24(3):51–77, 2004.

41. Nichols DS, Case-Smith J: Reliability and validity of the Pediatric Evaluation of Disability Inventory, *Pediatr Phys Ther* 8:15–24, 1996.

42. Iyer LV, Haley SM, Watkins MP, et al: Establishing minimal clinically important differences for scores on the Pediatric Evaluation of Disability Inventory for inpatient rehabilitation, *Phys Ther* 83(10):888–898, 2003.

43. Ziviani J, Ottenbacher KJ, Shephard K, et al: Concurrent validity of the Functional Independence Measure for Children (WeeFIM) and the Pediatric Evaluation of Disabilities Inventory in children with developmental disabilities and acquired brain injuries, *Phys Occup Ther Pediatr* 21(2/3):91–101, 2001.

44. Haley SM, Coster WI, Kao YC, et al: Lessons from use of the Pediatric Evaluation of Disability Inventory: Where do we go from here? *Pediatr Phys Ther* 22:69–75, 2010.

45. Coster W, Deeney T, Haltiwanger J, et al: *The School Function Assessment*, San Antonio, Tex, 1998, Therapy Skill Builders.

46. Hwang JL, Davies PL, Taylor MP, et al: Validation of School Function Assessment with elementary school children, *OTJR: Occupation, Participation and Health* 22(2):48–58, 2002.

47. Davies PL, Soon PL, Young M, et al: Validity and Reliability of the School Function Assessment in elementary school students with disabilities, *Phys Occup Ther Pediatr* 24(3):23–43, 2004.

48. Hwang JL, Davis PL: Rasch analysis of the School Function Assessment provides additional evidence for internal validity of the activity performance scales, *Am J Occup Ther* 63:369–373, 2009.

49. Noreau L, Fougeyrollas P, Vincent C: The LIFE-H: assessment of the quality of social participation, *Technol Disabil* 14(3):113–118, 2002.

50. Morris C, Kurinczuk JJ, Fitzpatrick F: Child or family assessed measures of activity performance and participation for children with cerebral palsy: a structured review, *Child Care Health Dev* 31(4):397–407, 2005.

51. Noreau L, Lepage C, Boissiere L, et al: Measuring participation in children with disabilities using the Assessment of Life Habits, *Dev Med Child Neurol* 49:666–671, 2007.

52. Sakzewski L, Boyd R, Ziviani J: Clinimetric properties of participation measures for 5- to 13-year-old children with cerebral palsy: a systematic review, *Dev Med Child Neurol* 49:232–240, 2007.

53. Varni JW: *The PedsQL™ Measurement Model for Pediatric Quality of Life Inventory™*, 1998 (website) http://www.pedsql.org/.

54. Varni JW, Limbers CA, Burwinkle TM: How young can children reliably and validly self-report their health-related quality of life? An analysis of 8,591 children across age subgroups with the Peds QL 4.0 Generic Core Scales, *Health Qual Life Outcomes* 5:1, 2007.

55. Varni JW, Burwinkle TM, Seid M: The Peds QL 4.0 as a school population health measure: feasibility, reliability and validity, *Qual Life Res* 15(2):203–215, 2006.

56. Varni JW, Limbers CA, Burwinkle TM: Parent proxy-report of their children's health-related quality of life: an analysis of 13,878 parents' reliability and validity across age subgroups using the Peds QL 4.0 Generic Core Scales, *Health Qual Life Outcomes* 5:2, 2007.

57. Cremens J, Eiser C, Blades M: Factors influencing agreement between child self-report and parent proxy-reports on the Pediatric Quality of Life Inventory 4.0 (Peds QL) Generic Core Scales, *Health Qual Life Outcomes* 4(5):1–8, 2006.

58. Varni J, Burwinkle T, Rapoff M, et al: The Peds QL in pediatric asthma: reliability and validity of the Pediatric Quality of Life Inventory Generic Core Scales and asthma module, *J Behav Med* 27(3):297–318, 2004.

59. King GA, Law M, King S, et al: *Children's Assessment of Participation and Enjoyment and Preferences for Activities of Kids*, San Antonio, TX, 2004, PsychCorp.

60. Mahoney FI, Barthel DW: Functional evaluation: Barthel Index, *Md State Med J* 14:61–65, 1965.

61. Granger CV, Albrecht GL, Hamilton BB: Outcome of comprehensive medical rehabilitation: measurement by PULSES Profile and Barthel Index, *Arch Phys Med Rehabil* 60:145–154, 1979.

62. Granger CV, Dewis LS, Peters NC, et al: Stroke rehabilitation: analyses of repeated Barthel Index measures, *Arch Phys Med Rehabil* 60:14–17, 1979.

63. Jette AM: State of the art in functional status assessment. In Rothestein J, editor: *Measurement in physical therapy*, New York, 1985, Churchill Livingstone, pp 137–168.

64. Nyein K, McMichael L, Turner-Stokes L: Can a Barthel score be derived from the FIM? *Clin Rehabil* 13:56–63, 1999.

65. van der Putten JJ, Hobart JC, Freeman JA, et al: Measuring change in disability after inpatient rehabilitation: comparison of the responsiveness of the Barthel Index and the Functional Independence Measure, *J Neurol Neurosurg Psychiatry* 66:480–484, 1999.

66. Uniform Data System for Medical Rehabilitation at the State University of New York at Buffalo, 1990. *Guide for Uniform Data Set for Medical Rehabilitation*, 1997.

67. Hamilton BB, Laughlin JA, Fiedler RC, et al: Interrater reliability of the 7-level Functional Independence Measure (FIM), *Scand J Rehabil Med* 26(3):115–119, 1994.

68. Kohler F, Dickson H, Redmond H, et al: Agreement of Functional Independence Measure item scores in patients transferred from one rehabilitation setting to another, *Eur J Phys Rehabil Med* 45(4):479–485, 2009.

69. Kidd D, Stewart G, Baldry J, et al: The Functional Independence Measure: a comparative validity and reliability study, *Disabil Rehabil* 17:10–14, 1995.

70. Brosseau L: The inter-rater reliability and construct validity of the Functional Independence Measure for multiple sclerosis subjects, *Clin Rehabil* 8:107–115, 1994.

71. Ravaud JF, Delcey M, Yelnik A: Construct validity of the Functional Independence Measure (FIM): questioning the unidimensionality of the scale and the "value" of FIM scores, *Scand J Rehabil Med* 31:31–41, 1999.

72. Dromerick AW, Edwards DF, Direnger MN: Sensitivity to changes in disability after stroke: a comparison of four scales useful in clinical trials, *J Rehabil Res Dev* 40:1–8, 2003.

73. Poulin V, Desrosiers J: Reliability of the LIFE-H satisfaction scale and relationship between participation and satisfaction of older adults with disabilities, *Disabil Rehabil* 31(16):1311–1317, 2009.

74. Poulin V, Desrosiers J: Participation after stroke: comparing proxies' and patients' perceptions, *J Rehabil Med* 40:28–35, 2008.

75. Figueiredo S, Komer-Bitensky N, Rochette A, et al: Use of the LIFE-H in stroke rehabilitation: a structured review of its psychometric properties, *Disabil Rehabil* 32(9):705–712, 2010.

76. Ware JE, Kosinski M, Gandek B: *SF-36 Health survey: manual and interpretation guide*, Lincoln, RI, 2000, Quality Metric.

77. Perenboom RJM, Chorus AMJ: Measuring participation according to the International Classification of Functioning, Disability and Health (ICF), *Disabil Rehabil* 25(11/12): 577–587, 2003.

78. Brown CA, Cheng EM, Hays RD, et al: SF-36 includes less Parkinson disease (PD)-targeted content but is more responsive to change than two PD-targeted health-related quality of life measures, *Qual Life Res* 18:1219–1237, 2009.

79. Guilfoyle MR, Seeley H, Laing RJ: The short form 35 health survey in spine disease–validation against condition-specific measures, *Br J Neurosurg* 23(4):401–405, 2009.

80. Wang R, Wu C, Zhao Y, et al: Health related quality of life measured by SF-36: a population based study in Shanghai, China, *BMC Public Health* 8:292, 2008.

81. Lim LL, Seubsman SA, Sleigh A: Thai SF-36 health survey: tests of data quality, scaling assumptions, reliability and validity in healthy men and women, *Health Qual Life Outcomes* 6:52, 2008.

82. Syddall HE, Martin HJ, Harwood RH, et al: The SF-36: a simple, effective measure of mobility-disability for epidemiological studies, *J Nutr Health Aging* 13(1):57–62, 2009.

83. Bohannon RW, DePasquale L: Physical Functioning Scale of the Short-Form (SF) 36: internal consistency and validity with older adults, *J Geriatr Phys Ther* 33:16–18, 2010.

BODY SYSTEMS CONTRIBUTING TO FUNCTIONAL MOVEMENT

CHAPTER 6

Skeletal System Changes

OBJECTIVES

After studying this chapter, the reader will be able to:

1. Describe the structures and components of the skeletal system.
2. Identify the function of bone and cartilage in supporting posture and movement.
3. Discuss unique structural and functional characteristics of the skeletal system in the developing fetus, infant, child, adolescent, adult, and older adult.
4. Relate the age-related characteristics of the skeletal system to functional movement abilities and risk factors.
5. Incorporate consideration of life span development of the skeletal system into patient assessment and treatment planning.

The ability to walk, run, lift, and manipulate objects is influenced by the strength and resilience of the skeletal system. A young infant cannot walk, climb stairs, push a stroller, or tie shoes. Not only do infants lack the experience and practice necessary for these tasks, their immature skeleton does not provide a structural framework on which these movements can take place. Older adults may not have the spring in their step, power in their tennis serve, or manual dexterity they enjoyed when they were younger. The changes in the skeletal system that occur with aging may contribute to decreased efficiency of movement. Across the life span, the skeletal system evolves and influences our ability for unrestricted movement.

The skeletal system, as discussed in this chapter, consists of the bony skeleton and cartilage. The skeleton provides a structure on which muscles can work. The size and shape of the bones, mechanics of joint articulations, and location of muscular attachments form an efficient system of levers and struts. Joints allow bones to articulate with each other, and the shape of the joint contributes to efficiency of movement. Cartilage acts as a shock absorber and protects joint surfaces from wear and tear. We better appreciate the contribution of the skeletal system to functional movement when we understand the role of its components and their changing properties throughout development.

COMPONENTS OF THE SKELETAL SYSTEM

Cartilage

Cartilage, a type of connective tissue, can tolerate mechanical stress and acts as a supporting structure in the body. It provides a mechanism for shock absorption, acts as a sliding surface for the joints, and plays a role in the development and growth of bone. During fetal development, a cartilage model is laid down from which the long bones of the body will develop. The ends of immature long bones and some sites of muscular attachment also contain cartilage plates, which are sites of bone growth.

Three types of cartilage exist, each meeting different functional needs (Figure 6-1). *Hyaline cartilage* is the most abundant and rigid. It is found at the articular

HYALINE CARTILAGE

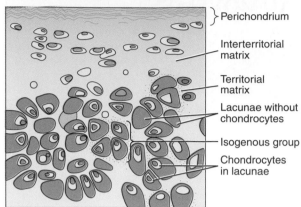

- Perichondrium
- Interterritorial matrix
- Territorial matrix
- Lacunae without chondrocytes
- Isogenous group
- Chondrocytes in lacunae

FIBROCARTILAGE

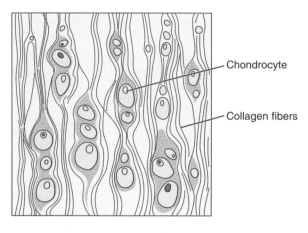

- Chondrocyte
- Collagen fibers

ELASTIC CARTILAGE

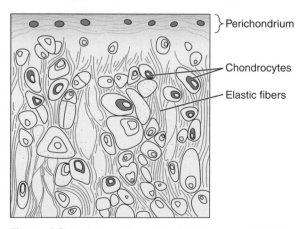

- Perichondrium
- Chondrocytes
- Elastic fibers

Figure 6-1 Diagram of the types of cartilage. (From Gartner LP, Hiatt JL: *Color textbook of histology*, ed 2, Philadelphia, 2001, WB Saunders, p 130.)

surfaces of joints and the walls of respiratory passages, such as the trachea and bronchi. Hyaline cartilage also makes up the fetal model of the future long bones and can be found at the epiphyseal growth plates of immature bone. *Fibrocartilage* is found at the acetabulum, intervertebral disks, menisci, and tendinous insertions. It is more pliable than hyaline cartilage but still provides strength and support to the skeletal system. Fibrocartilage fibers are arranged parallel to the stress forces that the tissue experiences. *Elastic cartilage* is the most pliable cartilage and can be found at the larynx, ear, and epiglottis, where it provides support with flexibility.

Hyaline cartilage covers the ends of the bones that make up synovial joints, and in this capacity, it is called *articular cartilage*. It is responsible for facilitating motion at the joints and can tolerate a variety of loading forces. Synovial fluid and the compression of fluids from within the surface of the articular cartilage contribute to lubrication of the joint. Articular cartilage provides a low friction surface and allows joints to move freely through older adulthood.[1,2] Years of microtrauma, isolated instances of more severe joint trauma, and aging of the cartilaginous tissue eventually result in a breakdown of articular cartilage, which contributes to the development of *osteoarthritis* for many older adults.

Properties

Cartilage consists of water, proteoglycans, collagen fibers, and cartilage cells (*chondrocytes*). The proteoglycans and collagen fibers make up the extracellular collagen matrix surrounding the chondrocytes. Differences in the extracellular matrix and amount of water in the tissue help to differentiate the three types of cartilage. For example, the water content of articular cartilage is 60% to 80%[2] but that of fibrocartilage is only 50%.[1] The collagen matrix contributes to the stiffness and resilience of the collagen and helps to bind water within the cartilage.[3]

Cartilage has no nerve supply and no vascular supply of its own. Oxygen and nutrients must be obtained from surrounding tissues. Most cartilage is covered by a layer of dense connective tissue called the *perichondrium*. The perichondrium is vascularized and supplies nutrients to the cartilage via diffusion. Articular cartilage is not covered with perichondrium and depends on diffusion of nutrients from synovial fluid and subchondral bone. In articular cartilage, periods of compression and decompression facilitate the exchange of fluids: during decompression, osmotic forces allow nutrients to diffuse into the cartilage, and during compression, fluids and waste products can be squeezed out.[1,4] Both processes are necessary to maintain adequate nutrition of the cartilage. Health of the articular cartilage is promoted through use, or the loading of the cartilage.[5]

In the absence of mechanical loading, atrophy of the articular tissue may be seen. The atrophied articular cartilage may be less able to withstand weight-bearing and movement forces, leading to further degeneration of the cartilage.[3,5]

Formation

Cartilage is derived from embryonic mesoderm, as is other connective tissue. Cartilage growth occurs through two different processes: interstitial growth and appositional growth. Interstitial growth occurs within the cartilage through mitotic division of the existing chondrocytes. It occurs in the early phases of cartilage development to increase tissue mass, at the epiphyseal plates of long bones, and at articular surfaces. In appositional growth, new cartilage is laid down at the surface of the perichondrium. In this process, chondroblasts of the perichondrium, which are precursors to chondrocytes, form an extracellular matrix and develop into mature chondrocytes. Nonarticular cartilage loses the capacity for interstitial growth early and then undergoes only appositional growth.

In the formation of articular cartilage, collagen fibers of the extracellular matrix weave together and form a loop parallel to the joint surface. These collagen fibers are embedded in the subchondral bone or deep cartilage tissue. This structural arrangement helps the cartilage to retain water and to maintain its shape.[1,4]

With use and age, cells of the articular surface are worn away, the cartilage thins, and eventually the surface changes. Cartilage repair depends on interstitial growth and the ability of chondrocytes to synthesize and maintain the extracellular matrix. Articular cartilage has the ability to repair itself, undergo limited mitosis, metabolize nutrients, and maintain its matrix even during aging. Aging cartilage is more limited than younger cartilage in its ability to repair because of a decrease in the number of cartilage cells with aging[6] and possibly because of a decreased ability to synthesize a new extracellular matrix.[3,5,6] For example, with rest, a young individual with chondromalacia is able to recover from articular cartilage damage. In the older individual, similar cartilage degeneration cannot be repaired, and osteoarthritis results.

The factors that limit healing in cartilage are the limited ability of mature chondrocytes to divide and the avascularity of cartilage. Some repair can occur only in cartilage with perichondrium where limited new cartilage cells are produced.[2] Damaged articular cartilage is replaced by dense connective tissue or fibrocartilage, whose mechanical properties are not optimal for providing low friction joint motion under high mechanical loads. The effects of aging and wear and tear over time result in a worn, less efficient articular surface.

Aging

The composition of articular cartilage changes with age. The primary changes seen in cartilage with aging are changes in the composition of the cellular matrix of the chondrocyte, less effective chondrocyte repair ability, cross-linkage of protein and collagen, increased calcification of cartilage, loss of water concentration, and increased fibrillation.[3] The cellular matrix changes include changes in water concentration and loss of some of the protein molecules that contribute to the stiffness and resilience of articular cartilage. As cartilage loses its stiffness and tensile strength, it is more susceptible to injury.[7]

Increased cross-linkage of collagen fibers, elastin fibers, and protein causes the extracellular matrix to become more rigid and eventually calcify, making diffusion of nutrients more difficult. If cartilage nutrition cannot be maintained, chondrocytes die. Calcification is seen when calcium phosphate crystals enter the cartilage matrix.[2,3] When cartilage is damaged in the adult, blood vessels also develop at the site of injury to assist in healing, but this blood supply leads to calcification rather than repaired cartilage.[2] Decreased numbers of cells are seen throughout the cartilage, especially at weight-bearing surfaces. Repeated exposure to mechanical loading wears away the cartilage and compromises its ability to protect the articulating bony surfaces. The extracellular matrix of the articular cartilage becomes hard and brittle, resulting in decreased resiliency, strength, and efficiency. Friction increases during joint movement with the thinning, fraying, and cracking of articular cartilage.

With age, cartilage becomes dehydrated, poorly nourished, and thinner. It is less able to withstand stresses placed upon it, and when damage occurs, the cartilage cannot repair itself effectively. Over time this is one mechanism that is thought to lead to osteoarthritis.[5] Another theory relates the cause of osteoarthritis to wear and tear on the articular cartilage from lifelong stresses.[7]

Bone

The bony skeleton accounts for 14% of older adult weight, 15% of the weight of the newborn, and 17% of young adult weight. It also accounts for 97% to 98% of total height. Intervertebral disks contribute to the remaining height. In humans, bone has several functions, including (1) protection of vital organs, (2) support of body weight, (3) storage for minerals, (4) structural leverage for movement, and (5) bone marrow storage.[8]

Bony protection of the central nervous system is provided by the skull, which forms a vault around the brain, and by the vertebral column, which encases the spinal cord. The rib cage protects the lungs and heart. The bones of the vertebral column, shoulder girdle, pelvic girdle, upper extremities, and lower extremities are arranged to effectively support the body weight in upright postures. Joints functionally connect the bones, enhancing their support functions or fostering efficient articulations. Muscles are strategically attached to this bony framework, allowing efficient movement to occur with muscular contraction.

In addition to providing protection and support, bone is a storage site for materials used by the body. Bone marrow, which is important in the formation of blood cells, is stored in bone. Calcium, phosphate, and other ions are stored in bone as crystalline salts. These salts contribute to the strength of the bone and its ability to withstand the compressive forces of weight bearing. The stored minerals are also used to maintain blood mineral levels when changes in diet or metabolic demand occur. If the blood levels of calcium and phosphate drop, these minerals are accessed from the bone. Likewise, after a meal, calcium is deposited in bone or excreted rather than increased in blood levels.

The structure of bone, as well as its stiffness and strength, allows it to meet the functional demands of everyday activities. Throughout development, bone must be produced and maintained in sufficient quantity to withstand a lifetime of weight bearing, movement, and functional activity.

General Structure and Form

Bone is a connective tissue composed of bone cells and bone matrix. These elements are held together by a ground substance. The bone matrix is a hard, calcified substance made up of collagen fibers and mineral salts. It surrounds the primary bone cell, the *osteocyte,* which functions to maintain the nutrition and mineral content of the bone matrix. Two other types of bone cells are the *osteoblast,* which is active in the formation of new bone, and the *osteoclast,* which is associated with resorption of bone. Osteoblasts are found on the surface of bone and synthesize new bone matrix. As they are encased in sufficient bone matrix, they become osteocytes. Osteoclasts are found in areas of bone resorption, where they break down the bone matrix and release minerals into the circulation.[8]

The external surface of bone, except at articular surfaces, is covered with periosteum. The periosteum is made up of collagen fibers and bone-forming cells, which provide a source of osteoblasts. The internal surface of bone, the *endosteum,* is thinner than the periosteum but also supplies osteoblasts for bone growth and repair. Both surfaces are vascularized and play a role in nutrition of bone.

All bones are made up of two types of bone tissue: *compact bone* (also called *cortical bone* or *lamellar bone*) and *cancellous bone* (also called *trabecular or spongy bone*) (Figure 6-2). Compact bone, which is hard and dense, represents the majority of bone in the human skeleton. It makes up the shaft of long bones and provides a thin outer covering for areas of cancellous bone. Compact bone is dense and stiff, which allows it to resist bending and torsional forces. Cancellous bone, made up of loosely woven strands of bone tissue (*trabeculae*), represents only about 20% of bone in the human skeleton. It is found at the ends of the long bones and surrounds the inner bone marrow cavity of the shaft. The open spaces of the cancellous bone house the bone marrow, minerals, and vessels that nourish the bone. The structure of the trabeculae of the cancellous bone provides more flexibility than compact bone, making the cancellous (trabecular) bone more responsive to compressive forces.[9]

Compact bone is formed when thin plates of bone (*lamellae*) are arranged concentrically around a channel containing blood vessels and nerves (*haversian canals*). This vascular channel is formed when new bone matrix surrounds existing blood vessels. Four to twenty lamellae surround a haversian canal, making up an osteon (*haversian system*). Osteons provide a mechanism to maintain nutrition of the bone. They are continuously being destroyed and rebuilt throughout the life span.

Figure 6-2 shows compact bone surrounding a portion of cancellous bone within one of the long bones of the human skeleton. The shaft of the long bones contains a marrow cavity. This structure allows the load-bearing compact bone to form the outer ring of the shaft of the bone and moves the load-bearing function away from the center of the bone. Because of this structure, the long bones provide a light weight structure that can effectively resist bending, torsional, and compressive forces. In adulthood, through the activity of osteoclasts and osteoblasts, the size of this central canal increases (see Figure 6-7), which mechanically increases the ability of bones to resist forces placed on it.[9]

Bones of the spine, wrist, and hip are made up of a high proportion of cancellous bone. As we age, loss of cancellous bone occurs earlier than that of cortical bone. It is not surprising then that the wrist, spine, and hip are frequent sites of fracture in older adults with osteoporosis.

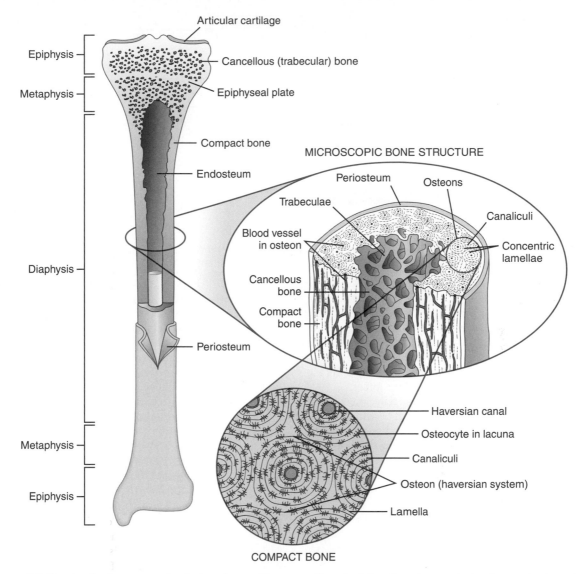

Figure 6-2 The structural components of a long bone with cross sections depicting the microscopic structure and enlarged view of compact bone with haversian system.

The general form of each bone, its muscular attachments, and its anatomic relationships are all genetically determined. Heredity and the mechanical stresses placed on developing bone dictate the shape, size, and structure of the mature bone. Bone mass, girth, cortical thickness, curvature, density, and arrangement of trabeculae are influenced by the mechanical stresses produced during functional activities. Heredity also appears to influence bone mass as evidenced by the racial differences in skeletal weight, bone size, and bone mineral content of adults of different races. Bone size, bone mineral density, and bone strength of black children, adolescents, and adults are greater than in white individuals.[10-13] Racial and ethnic differences in bone size and density become apparent in childhood in non-Hispanic white, non-Hispanic black, and Hispanic populations in the United States.[13,14]

The development and maintenance of bone shape, thickness, and size appear to be related to the forces placed upon the bone and influenced further by hormonal and nutritional factors. In considering the influences of mechanical loads upon bone tissue development, two theoretical models should be considered: Wolff's law and the mechanostat theory.[15] The relationship between bone structure and the mechanical loads it experiences was

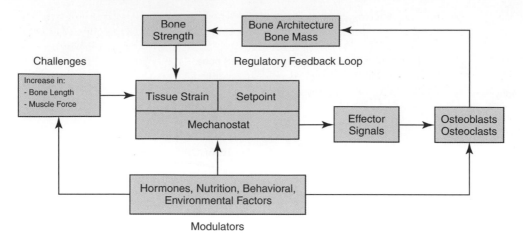

Figure 6-3 A functional model of bone development based on the mechanostat theory. (From Rauch F and Schoenau E: The developing bone: slave or master of its cells and molecules? *Pediatr Res* 50[3]:309-314, 2001.)

identified by J. Wolff in 1892. According to *Wolff's law* of bone transformation, the structure of bone will change in response to the mechanical loads placed on it, according to certain mathematical laws. Weight bearing and the pull of muscular attachments on bone during activities direct the arrangement of collagen fibers within bone trabeculae in the same direction as the stress forces.

The *mechanostat theory* explains how mechanical input is used to develop effective load-bearing bones.[16] As mechanical strain is placed upon the bone by muscle pull or the pull of gravity in weight-bearing positions, the bone adapts to effectively support the body. As mechanical forces are placed on the bone, osteoblast function is stimulated, and new bone is laid down on the periosteal surface and in the trabeculae. Likewise, when bone is not exposed to mechanical strain, because of bed rest, space flight, or immobility, osteoclast activity is favored, and bone is resorbed from the endosteal surface and the trabeculae. It is thought that the osteoclast is the cell that detects the mechanical forces placed on the bone because the osteoclast is surrounded by fluid and displaced by compression. The osteoclast and its dendrites then trigger the response by the osteoblasts. If insufficient compression is placed upon the osteoclast, it is thought that nutrition to the osteocyte is compromised and the cell dies, triggering the osteoclast function.[17] In addition to the mechanical forces on the bone, the mechanostat theory also considers the hormonal and nutritional influences on bone growth (Figure 6-3).[16-18] Based on the mechanostat theory, mechanical strain, and hormonal and nutritional factors all influence the shape, size, and density of bone. These theories support the importance of physical activity, especially in weight bearing, on optimizing bone development, bone density, and bone strength.

As discussed before, nutrition and hormones are important factors in the growth and development process of bone. During childhood, nutritional deficiencies contribute to conditions such as scurvy and rickets. Throughout life, nutrition also influences the effectiveness with which bone can be formed and maintained. People who do not have sufficient protein, calcium, vitamin D, and vitamin C in their diet experience abnormal bone growth. In vitamin C deficiency, the cartilage formed for bone growth lacks collagen. In severe vitamin C deficiency (scurvy), decreased rate of growth at the cartilage growth plates of the long bones results in deficient bone formation. Vitamin D deficiency in children causes rickets. In this disorder, growth in the region of the cartilage growth plate is distorted because calcification of the cartilage is deficient.[19] Vitamin D is also important in the absorption of calcium in the gastrointestinal tract. Across the life span, inadequate dietary protein interferes with collagen production by the osteoblasts, leading to poor calcification of the bone matrix. Protein deficiency can result in bone absorption from the endosteal surface and thinning of trabecular bone.[18]

The role of hormones, such as growth hormone (GH), insulin-like growth factor-1 (IGF-1), thyroid hormones, and sex hormones in bone development, is evident both before and after puberty. Before puberty, thyroid function, GH, and IGF-1 hormonal activity regulate bone growth.[20] During and after puberty, the sex steroid hormones begin playing a major role.[16,20] A rapid growth period accompanies the hormonal changes of adolescence. Low levels of estrogen are needed for the pubertal growth spurt of bone in both boys and girls.[21] During puberty, girls also demonstrate greater growth in cortical bone than boys, which may be related to increased sensitivity to estrogen, providing girls with increased bone storage to support gestational and lactation roles.[9,16] In contrast, accelerated loss of bone mineral content occurs immediately after menopause, again related to hormonal changes in the body. Estrogen loss plays a major role in the accelerated rate of bone loss for women in the 4 to 8 years after menopause.[20,22] Decreases in both circulated estrogen and testosterone play a role in bone loss for men.[20,22] Parathyroid hormone and calcitonin also influence bone resorption because they respond to serum calcium levels. Because bone serves as the storage site for calcium, as the concentration of calcium in the blood changes, calcium in the bone is accessed through stimulation of calcium-regulating hormones. The parathyroid hormone is sensitive to serum calcium levels. If the serum calcium level gets low, then the parathyroid hormone signals for bone resorption, which will increase the amount of circulating calcium. If serum calcium levels get too high, calcitonin will signal that no further calcium needs to be resorbed from the bone, and osteoblast activity will decrease.

Development

In embryological development, bone forms from the mesoderm. Fetal bone is made of *primary* or *woven bone tissue*. Woven bone consists of an irregular array of collagen fibers and is less mineralized than mature bone. As osteons form, mineralization of the bony matrix increases, and mature bone tissue replaces woven bone. A similar process can be seen throughout development as new, woven bone is laid down and other bone tissue is resorbed. Therefore, woven bone, mature bone, and areas of bone resorption are all found in adult bone tissue.

Bone develops through one of two different processes: intramembranous ossification or endochondral ossification. *Intramembranous ossification* takes place directly within mesenchyme tissue, beginning near the end of the embryonic period and proceeding rapidly. Mesenchymal cells produce an organic matrix called *osteoid,* which is composed of collagen fibers. Calcium phosphate crystals accumulate on the collagen fibers, resulting in ossification. In this process, numerous ossification centers are formed, which fuse into cancellous bone tissue. With time, some of this cancellous bone will become compact bone. The skull, carpals, tarsals, and part of the clavicle are formed by intramembranous ossification.

In *endochondral ossification,* a hyaline cartilage model of the bone is laid down first and then replaced by bone in an orderly fashion. Endochondral bone growth is seen in the long bones of the body and is the method by which bones increase in length (see Figure 6-2). The parts of the long bone are defined as the following:

- Diaphysis: the shaft of the long bone; the portion of bone formed by the primary center of ossification
- Epiphysis: the ends of the long bone; the portions formed by secondary centers of ossification
- Epiphyseal plate: the bone's growth zone, which is composed of hyaline cartilage
- Metaphysis: the wider part of the shaft of the long bone, adjacent to the epiphyseal plate, that consists of cancellous bone during development; in adulthood, it is continuous with the epiphysis

Endochondral bone development is illustrated in Figure 6-4. Primary centers of ossification form at the center of the diaphysis. First, a bony collar is laid down around the center of the diaphysis via intramembranous ossification of the perichondrium. Cartilage cells in the central diaphysis then become hypertrophied and are destroyed. As the remaining cartilage matrix becomes calcified, the area is infiltrated by osteoblasts and capillaries. The osteoblasts lay down ossified bone matrix. Ossification proceeds toward the ends of the diaphysis. Secondary ossification centers form in the epiphysis. Ossification radiates in all directions from the secondary ossification center. Endochondral ossification is also seen in the vertebrae, as depicted in Figure 6-5.

A growth (epiphyseal) plate, composed of hyaline cartilage, is formed between the diaphyses and epiphyses. This is the site of longitudinal bone growth. Interstitial growth of the hyaline cartilage continues at the surface of the epiphysis. The new cartilage undergoes endochondral ossification in the metaphysis. As the bone approaches its adult length, chondrocyte formation slows while endochondral ossification at the metaphysis continues. The epiphyseal plate narrows and eventually closes.

Mechanical loading of the epiphyseal plate affects longitudinal bone growth. The growth plate is usually aligned perpendicular to the load that crosses it, and formation of new bone is stimulated as tension or compression forces are applied.[8] Unequal forces along the epiphyseal plate may stimulate a change of direction of bone growth, whereas torsional forces at the growth plate may result in rotational changes. The changes in angle of inclination between the femoral neck and shaft—from approximately 135 to 145 degrees in infancy to 125 degrees in the adult and 120 degrees in the older adult—provide an example of directional change in normal bone development (Figure 6-6).[23] The torsional changes in the femur, from retroversion prenatally to 25 to 30 degrees of anteversion at birth and 10 to 15 degrees of anteversion in the adult,[23] are also illustrated in Figure 6-6. Table 6-1 summarizes some of these changes in lower extremity structure. It should

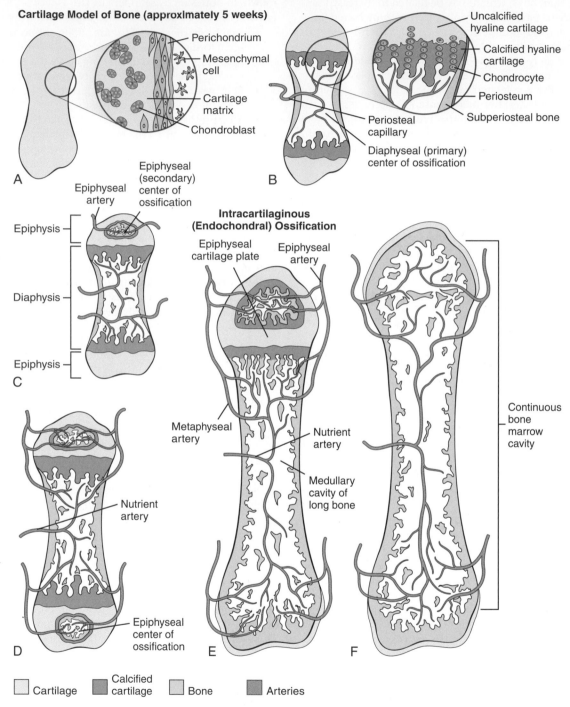

Figure 6-4 Stages in endochondral ossification of a long bone. **A,** Cartilage model. **B,** Periosteal stage; cartilage begins to calcify. **C,** Vascular mesenchyme enters the calcified cartilage matrix and divides the cartilage matrix into two zones of ossification; blood vessels and mesenchyme enter the upper epiphyseal cartilage. **D,** The epiphyseal center of ossification develops in the cartilage. A similar center of ossification develops in the lower epiphyseal cartilage. **E,** Intracartilaginous ossification; the lower epiphyseal plate disappears. **F,** Next, the upper epiphyseal plate disappears, forming a continuous bone marrow cavity.

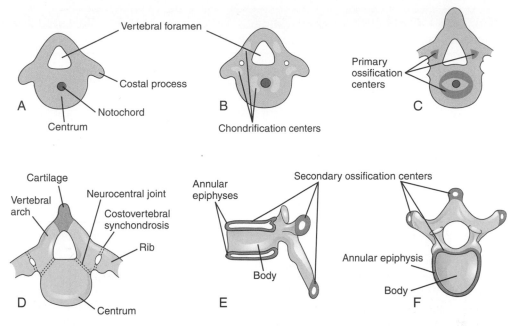

Figure 6-5 Stages of vertebral development. **A,** Precartilaginous vertebra at 5 weeks. **B,** Chondrification centers in a mesenchymal vertebra at 6 weeks. **C,** Primary centers of ossification in a cartilaginous vertebra at 7 weeks. **D,** A thoracic vertebra at birth, consisting of three bony parts. Note the cartilage between the halves of the vertebral neural arch and between the arch and the centrum. **E and F,** Two views of a typical thoracic vertebra at puberty showing the location of the secondary centers of ossification. (From Moore KL, Persaud TVN: *The developing human*, ed 6, Philadelphia, 1998, WB Saunders, p 413.)

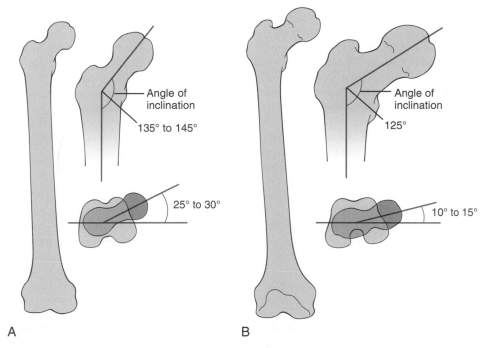

Figure 6-6 Comparison of the newborn (**A**) and adult (**B**) femoral angle of inclination (top) and femoral angle of torsion (bottom). The enlarged views of the femoral angle of torsion show a superior perspective, looking down from the head/neck of femur to the femoral condyles.

Table 6–1

Developmental Changes in Lower Extremity Alignment

	Birth	3 Yr	Adult
Acetabular roof	7 degrees from vertical	17 degrees from vertical	
Femur			
Angle of inclination	135-145 degrees		125 degrees
Angle of torsion	25- to 30-degree anteversion		10- to 15-degree anteversion
Tibial torsion	5- to 10-degree internal tibial torsion		20- to 25-degree external tibial torsion
Calcaneus	22-degree varus		0- to 3-degree varus

Data from Bernhardt DB: Prenatal and postnatal growth and development of the foot and ankle, *Phys Ther* 68:1831-1839, 1988.

also be noted that shearing forces applied across the epiphyseal plate may contribute to displacement of the growth plate. Therapeutically, this is an important consideration when working with individuals whose skeleton has not reached maturity because displacement of the epiphyseal plate interferes with normal growth.

Cartilaginous growth plates are found not only at the ends of long bones but also at points of muscular attachment, where they are called traction *epiphyses,* or *apophyses.* Muscle contraction places a traction force on the bone and stimulates bone growth. This is demonstrated at the proximal femur. Figure 6-7 reflects the effects of muscle pull on the greater trochanter and lesser trochanter of the femur. The greater trochanter has broad muscular attachments, whereas the lesser trochanter has only one muscular attachment. The traction force exerted by the muscular activity stimulates varying degrees of bone growth at these locations, helping shape the developing bone into its mature form. Muscle weakness can affect bone growth, as demonstrated in Figure 6-7, as well as bone length. Children with brachial plexus injuries at birth and with childhood onset hemiplegia demonstrate less bone growth of the involved upper extremity as compared with the upper extremity without neurological impairment, resulting in limb length inequality.[24-26]

Bones grow not only in length but also in diameter. New bone is laid down on the outer surface of the bone and is absorbed from the inner surface, determining the thickness of bone and size of the marrow cavity within the bone. This process is called *appositional growth* and continues throughout life, but the proportion of bone formation to resorption varies. In childhood and adolescence, formation is greater than resorption, increasing bone diameter and thickness. Throughout early and middle adulthood, equilibrium between the two

processes maintains bone size. In later adult life, resorption exceeds formation, resulting in loss of bone mass. Because resorption occurs at the inner surface of the bone, the marrow cavity becomes larger, and the bony shell surrounding it becomes thinner (Figure 6-8). Muscle weakness can also affect appositional bone growth.

Bone is an adaptable tissue, responding to hormonal demands and the mechanical stresses placed on it. To maintain bone mass and architecture, a balance must be achieved between these two processes. Good nutrition and exercise are important throughout the life span to build and maintain maximal bone mass and structural competence of the skeleton. Many studies of the effect of exercise on bone mass suggest that increased functional loading results in increased bone mass, whereas decreased functional loading results in bone loss.[27-32] The role of exercise on bone development at various stages of the life span will be discussed later in this chapter.

Aging

As discussed, adaptation of bone through remodeling continues throughout life. Skeletal maturity, however, as measured by closure of the epiphyseal plate, occurs within the first 2 decades of life. Maximal bone mass, which is the total bone growth in length and thickness, is thought to be obtained during the late 20s or early 30s.[30-33] Time of peak bone mass is difficult to specify because factors such as sex and race influence when peak bone mass is reached[10,31] and peak bone mass is attained at different sites at different times.[34] The age at which bone resorption begins to exceed bone formation is also not consistently reported in the literature. Some authors state that bone mass begins to decrease in the third to fourth decade,[35] but others feel bone mineral density does not decrease until the fifth

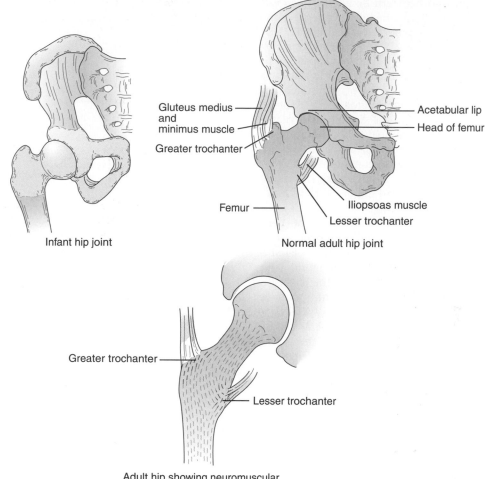

Infant hip joint

Gluteus medius
and
minimus muscle

Greater trochanter

Femur

Acetabular lip

Head of femur

Iliopsoas muscle

Lesser trochanter

Normal adult hip joint

Greater trochanter

Lesser trochanter

Adult hip showing neuromuscular
weakness and underdeveloped trochanters

Figure 6-7 The muscular attachments to an immature bone help to shape bone growth. Compared with the hip joint of a normal adult, a hip joint of an adult with neuromuscular weakness shows an underdeveloped trochanter.

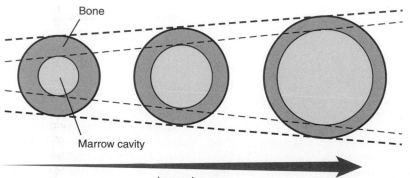

Bone

Marrow cavity

Increasing age

Figure 6-8 Schematic approximates the effect of appositional bone growth over time, which leads to an increase in the diameter of bone. Bone thickness decreases, and the width of the marrow cavity increases because resorption is greater than production.

decade for women and the sixth decade for men.[31] It also appears that cancellous bone loss may begin in the fourth decade, while cortical bone loss begins later.[20,22,36] Bone loss also appears to vary between racial groups[10,11] and with gender.[20,22,36] Although such loss appears to be less severe in black adults than it is in white adults, this may be reflective of the greater bone mass attained during the bone growth in this racial group.[10–13,37] Women also appear to lose more bone mass than men, related to accelerated loss during menopause, loss of estrogen's impact on slowing bone resorption, and the testosterone level of men enhancing calcium absorption.[20,22,36] A decrease in mass eventually results in a more fragile bone, which is less able to withstand mechanical forces such as compression and bending.

Other changes involved in the aging of bone include cross-linkage, architectural rearrangement of collagen fibers, and excessive mineralization of trabecular bone. Fibrils are arranged more longitudinally. Osteons become shorter and narrower as the haversian canals become wider. Excessive mineralization of bone occurs as bone matrix deteriorates, because as the bone becomes more porous, more sites for mineral deposition are provided. These changes increase the brittleness of bone and compromise its ability to withstand mechanical loads.

Throughout life, the body must maintain the necessary serum calcium level. Intestinal absorption of calcium declines with age, increasing the amount of calcium that must be retrieved from bone to meet the needs of the body. As a result, bone mass is gradually lost because bone resorption frequently occurs faster than new bone can be formed. The loss of bone tissue during remodeling leaves the bone thinner and more susceptible to injury. The increased brittleness due to internal changes in bone structure also increases the risk of fracture.

Joints

The joints provide the functional connection between bones. The primary purpose of most joints is to enable a wide range of movement. Within the joint, bones can be connected by ligaments, tendons, muscles, other connective tissue structures, and the joint capsule. Two types of joints are found in the mature skeletal system: synarthroses and diarthroses.

Synarthrosis joints allow minimal to no movement and provide areas of stability to the skeleton. The sutures of the skull and tibiofibular joint are examples of this type of joint. The articulation between the bones consists of connective tissue, which may be replaced by bone during aging.

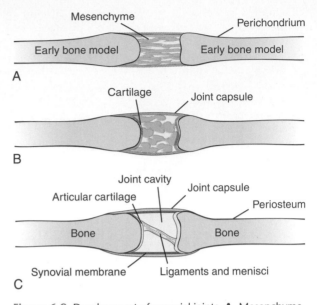

Figure 6-9 Development of synovial joints. **A,** Mesenchyme collects in the space between early bone models. **B,** Differentiation of mesenchyme into cartilage and joint capsule; beginning of cavitation. **C,** Formation of joint cavity and structure.

Diarthrosis joints allow movement. The joint capsule functionally connects two adjoining bones to form a cavity that is filled with synovial fluid, which bathes the joint surfaces with nutrition and provides a cushion between the bones (Figure 6-9). Diarthrodial joints are found in several shapes and sizes; their shape and form help define the type of movement that can be produced at the joint. For example, hinge joints, such as the elbow, allow movement in one axis only, whereas a ball-and-socket type of joint, such as the hip, allows a wide range of motion in multiple axes.

SKELETAL SYSTEM DEVELOPMENT

Skeletal system development follows a pattern of maturation that begins before birth and continues through the last decades of life.

Prenatal Period

As discussed earlier, bone and cartilage are differentiated from the mesoderm layer early in the gestational period. Development of bone, via either intramembranous or endochondral ossification, begins in the embryonic period (third to eighth gestational weeks). By the fifth week of gestation, mesenchymal models of bones appear in the extremities, with upper extremity development preceding lower extremity development. In the sixth week, mesenchymal cells have differentiated into chondroblasts, which form the cartilage model of the long bones. Primary centers of ossification appear as early as the seventh to eighth week (Figure 6-10); by the twelfth week of gestation, they have appeared in almost all bones of the extremities.[38] The diaphyses are fairly well ossified by birth, but the epiphyses remain cartilaginous. A few secondary ossification centers begin to appear late in fetal development (Figures 6-10 and 6-11).

Vertebral development also begins in the embryonic period. Cartilage models of the vertebrae are formed from mesenchymal cells located around the notochord. By the seventh to eighth gestational week, three ossification centers have formed in the vertebrae model. These bony parts remain connected by cartilage at birth (see Figure 6-5).[38]

After the early models of bone are present, joint formation occurs, and by the early fetal period, most joints have been formed. In articular joints, mesenchyme differentiates into the joint capsule, ligaments, tendons,

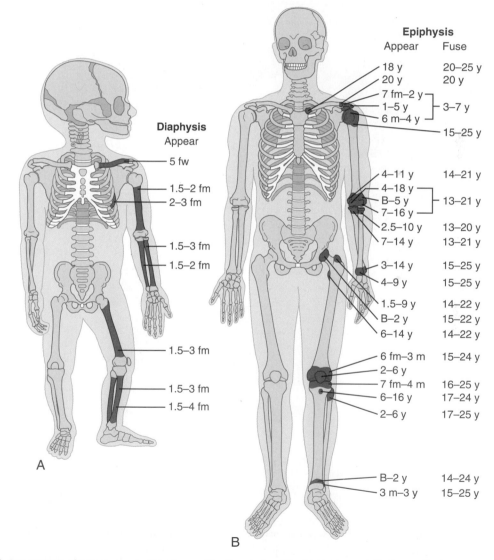

Figure 6-10 Appearance of primary and secondary ossification centers. **A,** Appearance of diaphyses. **B,** Appearance and fusion of epiphyses (*fw*, fetal weeks; *fm*, fetal months; *m*, postnatal months; *y*, years; *B*, birth). (Graca JC, Noback CR: Revised on the basis of Augier, 1931.)

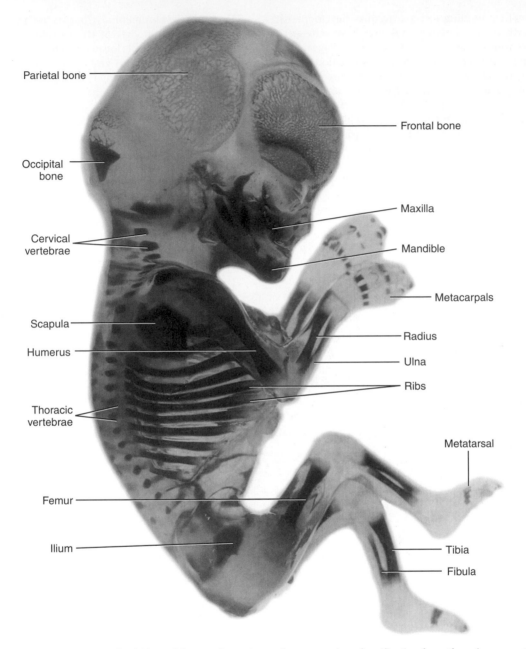

Parietal bone

Frontal bone

Occipital bone

Maxilla

Mandible

Cervical vertebrae

Metacarpals

Scapula

Radius

Humerus

Ulna

Ribs

Thoracic vertebrae

Metatarsal

Femur

Ilium

Tibia

Fibula

Figure 6-11 Electron micrograph of 12-week human fetus shows the progression of ossification from the primary centers that are endochondral in the appendicular and axial parts of the skeleton except for most of the cranial bones. (From Moore KL, Persaud TVN: *Before we are born: essentials of embryology and birth defects*, ed 5, Philadelphia, 1998, WB Saunders, p 395.) Courtesy of Dr. Gary Geddes, Lake Oswego, Ore.

and menisci. Depressions then begin to form in the mesenchyme, resulting in formation of the joint cavity and bursae (see Figure 6-9). Once the joint is formed, intrauterine movement is important for ongoing joint development.

The confined intrauterine environment in the later weeks of gestation limits the positioning options of the fetus and applies forces to the fetal skeletal system. Intrauterine molding of the developing skeletal system can occur and results in deformities such as congenital hip dislocation, tibial bowing, metatarsus adductus, calcaneus varus, and extreme ankle dorsiflexion. Some of these deformities will spontaneously improve in the first few years of life. Others, such as congenital hip dislocation, require early orthopedic management, applying corrective mechanical forces to the skeleton during infancy.[39]

Functionally, early intramembranous ossification of the skull serves to protect the developing brain. The bones of the skull are not fused, as evidenced by the "soft spots," called *fontanelles*. Expansion and molding of the cranium accommodate brain growth. The lack of fusion of the bones of the skull also allows adaptation of the cranium to the intrauterine environment and passage through the birth canal.

Infancy and Childhood

Infancy and childhood are times of bone growth, modeling, and remodeling. Two periods of rapid growth in bone mineral density are seen in childhood, first from 1 to 4 years of age and again at puberty, preceded by similar growth spurts in body mass.[31] Bone mineral content increases more in the 2 to 3 years surrounding peak height velocity than at any other time in life, with 20% to 30% of peak bone density and bone mineral content reported in this time frame.[9,30,31,36,40] Children attain 50% to 60% of their peak bone mass by puberty and up to 90% (in boys) and 95% (in girls) before age 20.[31,33] Before puberty, both boys and girls demonstrate similar, linear increases in peak bone mineral density and bone mineral content,[16] but after peak height velocity is reached, increases are greater for boys than girls (Figure 6-12).[9,31,40,41] The increased testosterone levels in boys contributes to the increased level of bone formation.[36] Both bone mineral density and bone mineral content are influenced by height and weight in childhood, with bone mineral content most influenced by these factors.[31,41] Factors that may contribute to the sex differences in bone mineral content and density are related to differences in bone shape and geometry, calcium intake and absorption, hormone production, and physical activity levels.

Dynamic Bone Growth

Through childhood, both endochondral and appositional bone growth are dynamic processes. As mentioned, the diaphyses of the long bones are fairly well ossified at birth. Secondary ossification centers in the epiphyses continue to appear through adolescence (see

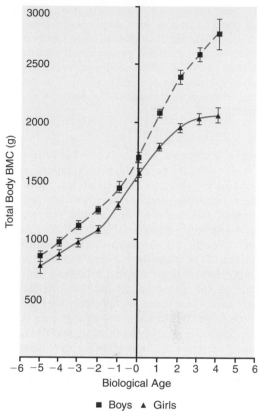

Figure 6-12 Total bone mineral content (g) of subjects in yearly age increments; younger than (negative) and older than (positive) age of peak bone velocity. (From Whiting SJ, et al: Factors that affect bone mineral accrual in the adolescent growth spurt, *J Nutr* 134[3]:696S–700S, 2004.)

Figure 6-10). Throughout infancy and early childhood, bone growth occurs rapidly. Factors such as genetic makeup, nutrition, general health, and hormonal levels affect the rate of bone growth and time of appearance of the secondary ossification centers.[39] Physical activity has also been demonstrated to increase bone mineral content and bone mineral density in prepubertal children.[30,31,34,40,42-44] Participation in physical activity, especially high-impact activities, is most beneficial in children in the years immediately preceding peak height velocity.[30,34,40] Participation in physical activity before puberty fosters growth in both muscle and bone mass. As children then continue to be active, especially in high-impact activities such as jumping, bone growth is stimulated both by weight-bearing forces and the mechanical pull of the muscles. Physical activity and sports place forces on the growing bone that impact length, size, curvature, and shape of the bone, all of which are important for optimal bone function across the life span.[34,40] Exercise programs, including high-impact activities such as jumping and soccer, have been shown to increase site-specific bone mineral density in children through early stages of puberty,[45,46] regardless of ethnicity.[47]

Areas of Bone Growth

During infancy and childhood, many changes are seen in the size, shape, angulation, rotation, and proportions of the skeleton. The head and trunk of the newborn infant make up a proportionally larger part of the total skeleton than in the adult. During childhood, the growth of the axial skeleton does not contribute as much to a child's increasing height as does the growth of the lower extremities. The lower extremities and pelvis undergo angular, rotational, and length changes as the infant learns to move. At birth, the ilia and sacrum are more upright than they are in the adult. Once the infant starts walking, the curvature of the sacrum increases, the ilia thicken, and the acetabular depth increases.[48] The acetabular roof rotates from a relatively vertical position to one of more forward inclination (Bernhardt, 1988). Bernhardt describes changes throughout the developing lower extremity (see Table 6-1). The femoral angle of inclination decreases (see Figure 6-6), creating a better lever arm for force production of the hip abductors. The femoral angle of torsion also changes (see Figure 6-6), decreasing the amount of anteversion from birth to adulthood. Different rates of growth in the three epiphyseal zones of the proximal femur contribute to the angular and rotational changes of the bone.[49] By 8 years of age, the proximal femur has attained its adult form.[50]

Angular and torsional changes also take place in the tibia and ankle/foot complex. External tibial torsion increases from the newborn period to adulthood. The relationship between the femur and tibia changes from a position of genu varum (bow-legged) in infancy to one of genu valgus (knock-knee) by 3 years of age. The degree of valgus then decreases to 5 to 6 degrees.[51] In adolescence, girls have demonstrated a stable valgus angle of approximately 5.5 degrees, while in boys the valgus angle decreases slightly to approximately 4.5 degrees.[52] The newborn's foot also is in a position of varus at the calcaneous and forefoot, which slowly decreases until adult values are reached. Slight forefoot varus may persist until 2 years of age. Weight bearing and the torsional forces of muscles actively contracting during creeping (four-point), standing, and walking contribute to these changes.

Not only does the lower extremity skeleton undergo transformation as the infant develops functional movement skills, but changes are also seen in the spine. In the newborn, the anteroposterior spinal curve is relatively concave. The cervical lordosis is present at birth, possibly because of early ossification of the occipital bone, but it becomes more evident by 3 months of age, when the infant has developed head control. The lumbar lordosis develops as the infant learns to sit. Iliopsoas muscle tightness from fetal positioning combined with antigravity work in prone, four-point, and kneeling positions may contribute to development of the lumbar lordosis.[13,53] When spinal deformities occur, such as scoliosis and kyphosis, bracing the immature skeleton places mechanical forces upon the growing spine to assist in correcting or minimizing the problem.

Adolescence

During adolescence, bone continues to grow and remodel in response to mechanical-loading stresses. Physical activity, body weight, and caloric and calcium intake contributes to the growth of bone, formation of bone matrix, and bone mineralization.[31,32,40,41,54] Calcium absorption is also more efficient during puberty, especially in black teens.[30] The adolescent experiences sudden increases in height and weight, with growth of the trunk exceeding the lower extremities. The adolescent growth spurt of girls begins at an average of 12 years of age, preceding that of boys by approximately 2 years. A growth spurt in bone width is seen through adolescence in boys and up to age 14 in girls.[8] In general, boys enter puberty later than girls, and their pubertal growth spurt lasts longer than girls, contributing to greater height, bone mass and bone size in boys as compared with girls.[36] Lean body mass is related to increases in cortical bone mass in both boys and girls, while fat mass is only related to increased cortical bone mass in girls.[55] Rapid bone growth frequently outpaces increases in muscle length, resulting in decreased flexibility. Injuries can result if adolescents do not modify their activities to accommodate these changes in flexibility.

Hormonal influences on growing bone change with puberty as the sex hormones, androgens and estrogen influence bone growth and bone mineral acquisition.[30] Hormones, nutrition, and physical activity all affect the mechanostat and therefore influence bone growth during adolescence.[9] Androgens increase bone size by stimulating appositional growth in boys, while estrogen may contribute to increased cortical bone density in girls.[9,16] Estrogen appears to reduce bone resorption at the endosteal surface, while allowing bone to be laid down at the periosteal surface.[55] Hormonal influences also appear to impact growth of cancellous (trabecular) bone. As mentioned earlier, cortical bone growth is seen through childhood and adolescence and is related to height, weight, weight bearing, and mechanical forces. Cortical bone growth is more sensitive to body height than weight, whereas cancellous bone growth is more sensitive to weight.[31] Cancellous bone growth also becomes more apparent in later puberty, suggesting that hormonal influences are also key to growth.[9,31] High-impact physical activity such as jumping has also been found to increase site-specific bone mineral density in early puberty[56] and adolescence.[57]

Attainment of Skeletal Maturity

Skeletal maturity is attained when the epiphyseal plates close. Epiphyseal closure begins in childhood and is usually complete by 25 years of age (see Figure 6-10). Fusion of the vertebral arches is seen in the cervical spine in the first year of life and in the lumbar spine by 6 years of life. Fusion of the vertebral arch and centrum occurs between 5 and 8 years of age. Secondary centers of ossification in the vertebrae do not unite until the twenty-fifth year.[38] Fusion of the epiphyses occurs earlier in girls than in boys and has been linked to the fact that estrogen levels are higher in girls than in boys.[21] When skeletal maturity is reached, 95% of peak bone mass is present. The remaining 5% of peak bone mass is attained through appositional bone growth and continued thickening of the trabeculae.[36]

Adulthood

After the epiphyses have closed, the bones no longer lengthen. Throughout adulthood, only bone remodeling occurs. Weight bearing and muscle contraction continue to stimulate bone remodeling and to increase bone density.[58] Adequate nutritional and calcium intake also supports appropriate mineralization of the remodeled bone. Both men and women attain their maximal bone mass by their late 20s or early 30s.[33,59] Bone formation and resorption remain balanced until 30 to 50 years of age in men and 38 to 48 years of age in women, with the variation reported based on ethnicity.[60] After that time, bone loss is greater than bone replacement. In the adult skeleton, cortical bone loss has been reported to begin in the fourth decade and cancellous bone loss to begin in the third decade of life.[20,36]

Several different estimates of the amount of bone loss with aging are reported in the literature. Women lose 1% of bone mass per year before menopause.[59,61] For the 4 to 8 years after menopause, bone loss is accelerated in women, but after this time, the rate of loss returns to 0.5% to 1% per year.[59] Men are reported to lose 0.5% of bone mass per year. This loss translates into

a decline in bone strength, which increases the risk for spontaneous fractures and functional motor deficits.

Physical activity also plays a role in bone mass during adulthood. Individuals who have been physically active through childhood and adolescence have a greater peak bone mass as they enter adulthood and these individuals also show greater bone mass through adulthood than their peers who were not as active in childhood and adolescence. Participation in exercise programs does increase muscle mass in adulthood and therefore muscles can generate greater force on bone. Appositional bone growth is stimulated by weight-bearing and strength-training exercise programs, especially those that include high impact activities.[62-65]

Fibrous cartilage changes also become apparent in adulthood. The intervertebral disk begins to undergo changes at approximately 30 years. The nucleus pulposus loses ability to absorb water and becomes dehydrated, impacting on ability to function effectively in shock absorption. Structurally, small tears also appear around the annulus fibrosis, and the structural integrity of the intervertebral disc is compromised. Water loss continues slowly in older adulthood, during which the annulus fibrosus also undergoes further fibrotic changes. The intervertebral disc becomes flattened and less resilient. Considering the early changes in the disc, it is not surprising that a high incidence of back pain is reported between the ages of 30 and 50 years.[59,66]

Older Adulthood

With aging, the skeletal system becomes progressively more compromised. Loss of bone mass continues in older adulthood and can be related to osteopenia, osteomalacia, or osteoporosis. *Osteopenia* occurs when either organic or inorganic components of bone fail to develop. *Osteomalacia* refers to abnormal mineralization of the bone matrix because of calcium and phosphate deficiencies. It affects both recently formed and well-established bone, decreasing the amount of mineral per unit of bone matrix. *Osteoporosis* refers to a reduction in bone mass because of decreased formation of new bone or increased resorption while bone chemistry is normal. Age-related bone, which limits both the mechanical loading of bone and circulation, loss may be related to hormonal changes, dietary changes, and the decreased activity level of older adults. Decreased estrogen levels in both women and men are primarily responsible for loss of bone mineral density in older adults.[20] Estrogen and testosterone also appear to enhance calcium absorption from the intestine, minimizing the signaling of bone resorption in response to serum calcium levels. In women, the ability of estrogen to decrease bone resorption at the endosteal surface is also lost. Deficiencies in vitamin D also contribute to bone loss in older adults, possibly related to development of hyperparathyroid levels.[20] Vitamin D metabolism is also affected by decreased levels of calcitonin. In addition, the diet may contain lower amounts of calcium, vitamins, and minerals.[67]

Maintaining physical activity levels and participation in weight-bearing and strength-training exercise programs can help maintain levels of bone mineral density for older adults.[27,63,64,68–71] Continued functional loading of the skeletal system appears to help balance bone formation and resorption. Site-specific increases in bone mineral density have been demonstrated in older adults participating in exercise programs.[62,63,72,73] As with other age groups, weight-bearing activities were more effective than non-weight-bearing activities in bone growth. Strength training was also effective, but power training, which included both a speed and resistance component was the most effective at improving bone density.[74]

FUNCTIONAL IMPLICATIONS OF SKELETAL SYSTEM ISSUES

Changes in the skeletal system affect its effectiveness at all age levels, requiring special concern with relation to functional activities (Table 6-2). In infants,

Table 6–2

Age-Related Skeletal System Concerns Related to Physical Activity

Age Period	Skeletal System Concern
Prenatal	Intrauterine molding late in gestation Congenital hip dysplasia Congenital limb deficiency
Newborn	Epiphyseal infection
Childhood	Epiphyseal injury; growth plate fracture Apophyseal avulsion Greenstick fracture
Adolescence	Scoliosis Epiphyseal injury Apophyseal avulsion Stress fracture
Adulthood	Back pain secondary to disc changes
Older adulthood	Osteoporosis Osteoarthritis

congenital bone malformations or positional deformities may occur and impact development of an efficient, effective skeleton. In adolescence, not only do conditions such as idiopathic scoliosis impact on posture and functional ability, but rapid growth of the skeleton may also leave the teen vulnerable to avulsion fractures or injury to the cartilage growth plates in the bone. Osteoporosis and osteoarthritis are common problems for older adults. When therapists understand the processes underlying these two disorders, they can develop individualized prevention programs that will help limit the functional losses experienced by older adults (see Clinical Implications Box 6-1: Osteoporosis Prevention: a Lifelong Process).

Childhood and Adolescence

The dynamic quality of bone growth in childhood is also very useful in the management of skeletal abnormalities. Mechanical forces can contribute to the spontaneous correction of some skeletal abnormalities and the responsiveness of others to orthopedic treatment in children. The infant born with congenital bony deformities, such as congenital hip dysplasia, metatarsus adductus, or club foot, may benefit greatly from early orthopedic intervention. Corrective forces can be applied with casting or taping procedures, which when combined with muscle activity will correct bony alignment. Congenital plagiocephaly, which may occur secondary to positioning or torticollis (where the head is turned persistently to the side), may also self-correct as the infant develops head control and spends quality play time in a prone position. New parents are often given information on the importance of "tummy time" to enhance muscular control of the head and neck and development of symmetrical skull shape. If plagiocephaly is more severe, infants often wear orthotic helmets to help mold the skull into a more symmetrical shape.

Abnormal skeletal development also occurs if unbalanced muscle action around a joint is present, as in cerebral palsy or spina bifida. For example, bone growth will proceed in response to the strong adduction and internal rotation forces exerted by muscles at the hip of the child with cerebral palsy. This abnormal force interferes with normal development of the acetabulum, femoral torsion, and the femoral neck/shaft angle. The hip can become unstable, and the risk for dislocation is increased.

The epiphysis is an active site for new bone formation and plays an important role in early skeletal development. During periods of rapid growth, forces acting on the epiphysis can have dramatic effects. Injury or infection to the epiphysis can result in abnormal bone growth and limb length deficiencies.[39] The newborn

CLINICAL IMPLICATIONS Box 6-1

Osteoporosis Prevention: A Lifelong Process

Osteoporosis is a common, costly condition of older adults that results in bone fracture, pain, and disability. The best way to prevent or minimize risk for osteoporosis is to maximize the amount of bone tissue present in adulthood. Peak bone mass is attained in young adulthood and can be enhanced by several factors throughout childhood. These factors include dietary intake of adequate amounts of calories, calcium, and vitamin D; physical activities that provide weight-bearing and mechanical strain stimuli to the bone and muscle; and maintenance of appropriate body weight. Research has shown that the effects of increased physical activity in increasing bone mineral concentration and bone mineral density are greatest in prepubertal children.* For this reason, it is important to begin preventive measures for osteoporosis early. Such programs should continue across the life span. Health care providers can guide their patients of all ages to the most effective methods that will optimize bone growth and minimize the risk of osteoporosis.

Osteoporosis prevention strategies for individuals of all ages include the following:
- Regular, ongoing physical activity that begins in childhood and continues throughout adulthood
- Participation in a variety of diverse movement activities that provide different patterns of mechanical strain. Moderate- to high-impact activities are recommended for children and adolescents. Low to moderate-impact activities are recommended for middle aged and older adults.
- Participation in weight-bearing exercise at least 3 to 5 times per week, for 10 to 45 minutes per session
- Exercise that increases strength, flexibility, and coordination. Muscle strength gains positively influence bone density, and improved flexibility and coordination also decrease the likelihood of falls in older adults.
- Eating a well-balanced diet to support the energy demands of the growing body and to provide appropriate vitamins and minerals for bone growth and maintenance
- Intake of appropriate levels of calcium from the diet to enhance mineralization of the developing bone and to maintain appropriate levels of blood calcium
- Maintaining optimal body weight. Increased body weight, especially of lean muscle mass, has been associated with increased bone mass.
- Ensuring optimal hormonal function, periods of amenorrhea should be avoided and delayed puberty should be managed medically. Appropriate levels of estrogen are necessary to trigger the adolescent growth spurt and to optimize bone growth.
- Avoiding periods of immobilization when bone density is rapidly lost.

*References 9,31,34,40,63,80–83.

---

infant is especially susceptible to infection of the epiphysis because the epiphyseal plate is very thin at this age and does not provide a significant barrier between the metaphysis and the epiphysis. Blood vessels easily cross the growth plate, allowing infection to be spread from the metaphysis to the epiphysis. As the epiphyseal plate becomes thicker, the blood vessels can no longer cross it, eliminating the possibility for transmission of infection. Fractures of the epiphyseal plate are also seen in children because the cartilaginous growth plates within the bone are not as resistant to stress as adult bone. The growth plate is also weaker than the surrounding tissue. Even though many of these fractures heal well with rest and medical management, those injuries where the growth plate alignment is altered leave the child at risk for growth abnormalities and development of bone deformities. Children are most susceptible to growth plate fractures as they enter the period of peak height velocity growth.[75] During this rapid growth spurt, the epiphysis is less stable than the

joints, making epiphyseal injury likely when the joint area is involved. Apparent joint sprains in this age group should be critically evaluated to rule out involvement of the epiphysis.

Structural differences between growing and adult bone also make children more susceptible to injuries such as plastic deformation of the bone, greenstick fractures, and apophyseal avulsion (avulsion of muscle tendon from its insertion). In general, growing bone is less dense and more porous than adult bone. As a result, it is more sensitive to both compressive and tensile stress. The cortex of the metaphysis is also thinner than that of the diaphysis, making it less resistant to compressive forces. The periosteum, however, is thicker than in adult bone and less readily torn, resulting in fewer displaced fractures.

Skeletal system problems such as scoliosis often become obvious and may progress rapidly during adolescence. Idiopathic scoliosis, which is a lateral curvature of the spine of unknown origin, can occur through childhood but is most common in adolescence. Mild scoliosis of 5 degrees or less is seen in 10% of children during puberty; boys and girls are equally represented. Only a small percentage of scoliotic curves progress to greater than 15 degrees.[76]

Stress fractures and apophyseal avulsion fractures are also seen, especially in the adolescent athlete when activity or training level changes. These injuries are related to overuse and stress on the system beyond the ability for self-repair. Common sites for growth plate injury and stress fracture in the adolescent are the proximal humerus, distal radius, lumbar spine, tibia, and fibula. Young baseball players or those children who play overhead sports are at risk for humerus or shoulder injuries.[75] Gymnasts or individuals performing repetitive activities that place an axial load on an extended spine are at risk for lumbar spondylolysis, a stress fracture of the pars interarticularis.[77] Gymnasts also frequently report distal radius fractures.[75] Long-distance runners frequently have fractures at the tibia or fibula.[78]

Apophyseal avulsion fractures occur when traction forces are applied at the apophysis and it is pulled away from the bone. Common sites for avulsion fractures are the anterior superior iliac spine, anterior inferior iliac spine, lesser trochanter, and ischium.[77] Osgood-Schlatter disease may also be associated with avulsion of the apophysis at the tibial tuberosity after a traction injury. The definite cause of this disease is unknown, but it affects adolescent boys (10 to 15 years of age) and girls (8 to 13 years of age).[78] Physical conditioning programs, thorough preseason screening examinations, and appropriate supervision during athletic activities are important to prevent these stress-related injuries.

Cartilage injury can also be seen in adolescence. Chondromalacia of the patella, with softening and fibrillation of the cartilage, results from stress on the kneecap. Rotational or angular malalignment of the patella is usually seen. Restriction of overactivity allows the cartilage to repair itself.

Osteoporosis

Osteoporosis is defined as having bone density more than 2.5 standard deviations below that of a reference range for young women and leaves the older adult at risk for bone fracture. Both older men and older women can develop osteoporosis, but it is more common in women. As previously discussed, primary prevention against development of osteoporosis and fractures in older adulthood is thought to be development of the maximum possible peak bone mass through childhood and young adulthood. Participation in load-bearing physical activity and good nutrition contribute to maximizing peak bone mass and maintaining bone health across the life span. Physical inactivity related to aging, long periods of bed rest, and exposure to weight-less environments have been identified as factors that contribute to osteoporosis. The individual most at risk for the development of osteoporosis is a white woman who has gone through menopause.

The clinical features of osteoporosis are pain, loss of height, kyphosis, and decreased function, because bone is unable to withstand the compression forces of weight bearing. MacKinnon[79] reports that 40% of normal bone strength should be adequate to withstand normal mechanical loading. When the amount of bone mass is no longer sufficient to support the body during activity, spontaneous fracture may result (Figure 6-13). The most frequent sites for spontaneous fracture secondary to osteoporosis are the spine, proximal femur, and wrist. These sites are also made up of primarily

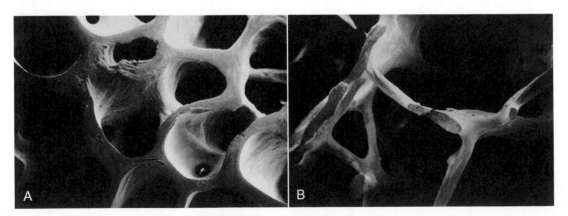

Figure 6-13 Electron micrograph of normal (**A**) and osteoporotic (**B**) bone. (From Dempster DW, Shane E, Horbert W et al: A simple method for corrective light and scanning electron microscopy of human iliac crest bone biopsies, *J Bone Miner Res* 1:16-21, 1986, with permission of the American Society of Bone and Mineral Research.)

cancellous (trabecular) bone, which loses bone mineral density, especially immediately after menopause.[36] Anterior compression fractures of the vertebrae result in wedge-shaped vertebrae and lead to kyphotic posturing. Central collapse of adjacent vertebra lead to fish-shaped vertebrae, decreasing the disk space and skeletal height. In general, the microfractures related to osteoporosis cause pain and lead to a flexed posture.

Osteoporosis caused by the progressive loss of bone mass with aging is referred to as *senile*, or *involutional*, *osteoporosis*. Two categories of involutional osteoporosis exist. One category, related to decreased intestinal absorption of calcium, occurs in both men and women and affects both cortical and cancellous bone. The second category of involutional osteoporosis occurs in the 4 to 8 years after menopause[22] and affects primarily cancellous bone.[36] When estrogen secretion decreases with menopause, the bone is thought to become more sensitive to the parathyroid hormone, increasing the rate of bone resorption.

Good nutrition and a lifelong commitment to exercise may influence the maximum bone mass attained in early adulthood and maintenance of that bone mass. Participation in moderate- to high-impact physical activities (jumping, skipping, dancing) appears to have the greatest impact on bone growth in the prepubertal years.* Exercise programs may effectively slow or prevent the bone loss associated with aging or even slightly increase the bone mass at sites of bone loading (such as the lumbar spine or femoral neck).† In the planning of exercise programs, weight-bearing and strengthening activities should be included.[68] The most effective type of exercise program for maintaining bone health in adults and older adults includes low- to moderate-impact weight-bearing activities, such as walking, jogging, and stair climbing.[80,82] A program that includes this variety of weight-bearing activity places a variety of stresses on the bone and is more effective than just walking. Resistance training, a form of strengthening exercise, has also been found to be effective in maintaining bone health in adults.[64,80,82] Power training, in which resistance training is performed with fast movements rather than slow movements, appears to be most effective in maintaining bone mineral density.[74] Spinal extension exercises should be emphasized because flexion exercises may be problematic, contributing to anterior wedging and compression fractures of the vertebrae.[79] For older adults, the exercise program should also focus on balance and flexibility to help decrease risk for falls.

---

*References 9,31,34,40,63,80–83.
†References 27,63,72,73,79,80,82,84.

Osteoarthritis

Osteoarthritis is an age-related condition characterized by joint pain during movement and weight bearing, limited joint range of motion, and loss of physical function, which ultimately limits participation in important life activities. Development of osteoarthritis is related to the degeneration of articular cartilage, which occurs with age. It affects 70% of people at some point in their life and most adults older than 70 years.[1] The cartilage thins, and clefts and cracks form, leaving the surface uneven and unable to efficiently provide frictionless joint motion. Calcification of the cartilage is also seen with age and in response to injury.[2] Underlying bone, which is innervated, becomes exposed to mechanical stress, resulting in pain. Bony spurs or outgrowths covered with hyaline cartilage may also develop in the joint. The individual with osteoarthritis experiences pain with movement and limited range of motion.

Treatment for osteoarthritis is limited to the protection of affected joints from undue stress, minimization of joint range-of-motion limitations, and relief of pain. Antiinflammatory medications offer some relief. Weight loss in overweight individuals will also help decrease pain by lessening the loading of the joint. Individuals with osteoarthritis benefit from participation in exercise programs that emphasize balanced loading of the joint surface. The exercises should address improvement in muscle strength, preservation of joint range of motion, and improved efficiency when performing everyday tasks so that loading forces on the cartilage are equalized. Prolonged jogging or impact exercises should be avoided because they put high loads on the cartilage and may increase tissue destruction. When conservative treatment approaches do not relieve symptoms, surgical debridement of the joint surface or joint replacement is considered.

SUMMARY

Cartilage, bones, and joints are the essential components of the skeletal system that develop over a lifetime and have the capacity to increase or limit physical ability to function. Together, these elements provide a structural base on which movement can take place. Optimal, healthy development of the skeletal system depends not only on genetics and nutrition but also on an active lifestyle. The mechanical stresses of everyday functional activities and exercise help the system achieve its most efficient form and maintain its stability. The time period in which physical activity and exercise can make the most impact upon peak bone mass development is in the 2 to 3 years before peak height velocity. Lifelong commitment to good nutrition and exercise helps the attainment of maximal bone mass and maintenance of a strong skeletal system well into older adulthood.

REFERENCES

1. Gradisar IA, Porterfield JA: Articular cartilage: structure and function, *Top Geriatr Rehabil* 4:1–9, 1989.

2. Ross MH, Kaye GI, Pawlina W: *Histology: a text and atlas*, ed 4, Baltimore, 2003, Lippincott Williams & Wilkins.

3. Ahmed MS, Matsumura B, Cristian A: Age-related changes in muscles and joints, *Phys Med Rehabil Clin N Am* 16:19–39, 2005.

4. Pickles B: Biological aspects of aging. In Jackson O, editor: *Physical therapy of the geriatric patient*, ed 2, New York, 1989, Churchill Livingston, pp 27–76.

5. Bullough PG: The role of joint architecture in the etiology of arthritis, *Osteoarthritis Cartilage* 12:S2–S9, 2004.

6. Bobacz K, Erlacher L, Smolen J, et al: Chondrocyte number and proteoglycan synthesis in the aging and osteoarthritic human articular cartilage, *Ann Rheum Dis* 63:1618–1622, 2004.

7. Martin JA, Buckwalter JA: Aging, articular cartilage chondrocyte senescence and osteoarthritis, *Biogerontology* 3:257–264, 2002.

8. Malina RM, Bouchard C, Bar-Or O: *Growth, maturation and physical activity*, ed 2, Champaign, Ill, 2004, Human Kinetics.

9. Kontulainen SA, Hughes JM, Macdonald HM, et al: The biomechanical basis of bone strength development during growth, *Med Sport Sci* 51:13–32, 2007.

10. Berenson AB, Rahman M, Wilkinson G: Racial difference in the correlates of bone mineral contensity/density and age at peak among reproductive-aged women, *Osteoporos Int* 20:1439–1449, 2009.

11. Melton LJ III, Marquez MA, Achenbach SJ, et al: Variations in bond density among persons of African heritage, *Osteoporos Int* 13:551–559, 2002.

12. Pollock NK, Laing EM, Taylor RG, et al: Comparisons of trabecular and cortical bone in late adolescent black and white females, *J Bone Miner Metab* 22(2):655–665, 2011.

13. Walker J: Musculoskeletal development: a review, *Phys Ther* 71:878–889, 1991.

14. Wetzsteon RJ, Hughes JM, Kaufman BC, et al: Ethnic differences in bone geometry and strength are apparent in childhood, *Bone* 44:970–975, 2009.

15. Frost HM: Bone "mass" and the "mechanostat": a proposal, *Anat Rec* 219:1–9, 1987.

16. Schoenau E: From mechanostat theory to development of the "Functional Muscle-Bone-Unit", *J Musculoskelet Neuronal Interact* 5(3):232–238, 2005.

17. Hughes JM, Petit MA: Biological underpinnings of Frost's mechanostat thresholds: the important role of osteocytes, *J Musculoskelet Neuronal Interact* 10(3):128–135, 2010.

18. Bass SL, Eser P, Daly R: The effect of exercise and nutrition on the mechanostat, *J Musculoskelet Neuronal Interact* 5(3):239–254, 2005.

19. Smith DW: Recognizable patterns of human deformation: identification and management of mechanical effects on morphogenesis, *Major Probl Clin Pediatr* 21:1–151, 1981.

20. Riggs BL, Khosla S, Melton LJ III: Sex steroids and the construction and conservation of the adult skeleton, *Endocr Rev* 23(3):279–302, 2002.

21. Cutler GB: The role of estrogen in bone growth and maturation during childhood and adolescence, *J Steroid Biochem Mol Biol* 61(3–6):141–147, 1997.

22. Khosla S, Riggs L: Pathophysiology of age-related bone loss and osteoporosis, *Endocrinol Metab Clin North Am* 34:1015–1030, 2005.

23. Bernhardt DB: Prenatal and postnatal growth and development of the foot and ankle, *Phys Ther* 68:1831–1839, 1988.

24. Bae DS, Ferretti M, Waters PM: Upper extremity size differences in brachial plexus birth palsy, *Hand* 3:297–303, 2008.

25. Demir SO, Oktay F, Uysal H, et al: Upper extremity shortness in children with hemiplegic cerebral palsy, *J Pediatr Orthop* 26(6):764–768, 2006.

26. Uysal H, Demir SO, Oktay F, et al: Extremity shortness in obstetric brachial plexus lesion and its relationship to root avulsion, *J Child Neurol* 22(12):1377–1383, 2007.

27. Bouxsein MS, Marcus R: Overview of exercise and bone mass, *Rheum Dis Clin North Am* 20:787–802, 1994.

28. Lanyon LE: Strain-related bone modeling and remodeling, *Top Geriatr Rehabil* 4(2):13–24, 1989.

29. Lanyon LE: Using functional loading to influence bone mass and architecture objectives, mechanisms, and relationship with estrogen of the mechanically adaptive process in bone, *Bone* 18(Suppl 1):37S–43S, 1996.

30. Loud KJ, Gordon CM: Adolescent bone health, *Arch Pediatr Adolesc Med* 160:1026–1032, 2006.

31. Ondrak KS, Morgan DW: Physical activity, calcium intake and bone health in children and adolescents, *Sports Med* 37(7):587–600, 2007.

32. Welten DC, Kemper HC, Post GB, et al: Weight-bearing activity during youth is a more important factor for peak bone mass than calcium intake, *J Bone Miner Res* 9:1089–1096, 1994.

33. Anderson J: Calcium, phosphorus, and human bone development, *J Nutr* 126:1153S–1158S, 1996.

34. Greene DA, Naughton GA: Adaptive skeletal responses to mechanical loading during adolescence, *Sports Med* 35(9):723–732, 2006.

35. Thibodeau GA, Patton KT: *Anatomy and physiology*, ed 4, St Louis, 1999, Mosby.

36. Riggs BL, Melton LJ III, Robb RA, et al: Population-based study of age and sex differences in bone volumetric density, size, geometry, and structure at different skeletal sites, *J Bone Miner Res* 19:1945–1954, 2004.

37. Parfitt AM: Genetic effects on bone mass and turnover: relevance to black/white differences, *J Am Coll Nutr* 16:325–333, 1997.

38. Moore KL, Persaud TVN: *Before we are born: essentials of embryology and birth defects*, ed 7, Philadelphia, 2008, WB Saunders.

39. Hensinger RN, Jones ET: Developmental orthopedics, I: the lower limb, *Dev Med Child Neurol* 24:95–116, 1982.

40. Vincente-Rodriguez G: How does exercise affect bone development during growth? *Sports Med* 36(7):561–569, 2006.

41. Whiting SJ, Vatanparast H, Baxter-Jones A, et al: Factors that affect bone mineral accrual in the adolescent growth spurt, *J Nutr* 134:696S–700S, 2004.

42. Bradney M, Pearce G, Naughton G, et al: Moderate exercise during growth in prepubertal boys: changes in bone mass, size, volumetric density and bone strength–a controlled prospective study, *J Bone Miner Res* 13:1814–1821, 1998.

43. Cooper C, Cawley M, Bhalla A, et al: Childhood growth, physical activity and peak bone mass in women, *J Bone Miner Res* 10:940–947, 1995.

44. Courteix D, Lespessailles E, Peres SL, et al: Effect of physical training on bone mineral density in prepubertal girls: a comparative study between impact-loading and non-impact-loading sports, *Osteoporos Int* 8:152–158, 1998.

45. Hind K, Burrows M: Weight-bearing exercise and bone mineral accrual in children and adolescents: a review of controlled trials, *Bone* 40:14–27, 2007.

46. MacKelvie KJ, Petit MA, Khan KM, et al: Bone mass and structure are enhanced following a 20-year randomized controlled trial of exercise in prepubertal boys, *Bone* 34:755–764, 2004.

47. MacKelvie KJ, McKay HA, Petit MA, et al: Bone mineral response to a 7-month randomized controlled, school-based jumping intervention in 121 prepubertal boys: associations with ethnicity and body mass index, *J Bone Miner Res* 17:834–844, 2002.

48. Sinclair D, Dangerfield P: *Human growth after birth*, ed 6, New York, 1998, Oxford University Press.

49. Bernhardt DB: Prenatal and postnatal growth and development of the foot and ankle, *Phys Ther* 68:1831–1839, 1988.

50. Ogden JA: Development and growth of the hip. In Katz JF, Siffert RS, editors: *Management of hip disorders in children*, Philadelphia, 1983, JB Lippincott.

51. Salenius P, Vankka E: The development of the tibiofemoral angle in children, *J Bone Joint Surg Am* 57(2):259–61, 1975.

52. Cahuzac JP, Vardon D, Sales de Gauzy J: Development of the clinical tibiofemoral angle in normal adolescents. A study of 427 normal subjects from 10 to 16 years of age, *J Bone Joint Surg Br* 77(5):729–732, 1995.

53. LeVeau BF, Bernhardt DB: Developmental biomechanics, *Phys Ther* 64:1874–1882, 1984.

54. Barr SI, McKay HA: Nutrition, exercise and bone status in youth, *Int J Sport Nutr* 8:124–142, 1998.

55. Sayers A, Tobias JH: Fat mass exerts a greater effect on cortical bone mass in girls than boys, *J Clin Endocrinol Metab* 95(2):699–706, 2010.

56. Petit MA, McKay HA, MacKelvie KJ, et al: A randomized school-based jumping intervention confers site- and maturity-specific benefits on bone structural properties in girls: a hip structural analysis study, *J Bone Miner Res* 17(3):363–372, 2002.

57. DeBar LL, Ritenbaugh C, Ickin M, et al: A health plan-based lifestyle intervention increases bone mineral density in adolescent girls, *Arch Pediatr Adolesc Med* 160:1269–1276, 2006.

58. Whitbourne SK: *The aging body–physiological changes and psychological consequences*, New York, 1985, Springer-Verlag.

59. Goodman CC, Fuller KS: *Pathology: implications for the physical therapist*, ed 3, Philadelphia, 2009, WB Saunders.

60. Malkin I, Karasik D, Lifshits G, et al: Modelling of age-related bone loss using cross-sectional data, *Ann Hum Biol* 29(3):256–270, 2002.

61. Raab DM, Smith EL: Exercise and aging: effects on bone, *Top Geriatr Rehabil* 1:31–39, 1985.

62. Bailey CA, Kukuljan S, Daly RM: Effects of lifetime loading history on cortical bone density and its distribution in middle aged and older men, *Bone* 47:673–680, 2010.

63. Guadalupe-Grau A, Fuentes T, Guerra B, et al: Exercise and bone mass in adults, *Sports Med* 39(6):439–468, 2009.

64. Kelley GA, Kelley KS, Tran ZV: Resistance training and bone mineral density in women: a meta-analysis of control trials, *Am J Phys Med Rehabil* 80:65–77, 2001.

65. Nikander R, Kannus P, Rantalainen T, et al: Cross-sectional geometry of weight-bearing tibia in female athletes subjected to different exercise loadings, *Osteoporos Int* 21(10):1687–1694, 2010.

66. Koeller W, Muehlhaus S, Meier W, et al: Biomechanical properties of human intervertebral discs subjected to axial dynamic compression: influence of age and degeneration, *J Biomech* 19:807–816, 1986.

67. Spirduso WW: *Physical dimensions of aging*, Champaign, Ill, 1995, Human Kinetics.

68. Cousins JM, Peti MA, Paudel ML, et al: Muscle power and physical activity are associated with bone strength in older men: the osteoporotic fractures in men study, *Bone* 47:205–211, 2010.

69. Hamilton CJ, Swan VJD, Jamal SA: The effects of exercise and physical activity participation on bone mass and geometry in postmenopausal women: a systematic review of pQCT studies, *Osteoporos Int* 21:11–23, 2010.

70. Hamilton CJ, Thomas SG, Jamal SA: Associations between leisure physical activity participation and cortical bone mass and geometry at the radius and tibia in a Canadian cohort of postmenopausal women, *Bone* 46:774–779, 2010.

71. Souminen H: Physical activity and health: musculoskeletal issues, *Adv Physiother* 9:65–75, 2007.

72. Bravo G, Gauthier P, Roy PM, et al: Impact of a 12-month exercise program on the physical and psychological health of osteopenic women, *J Am Geriatr Soc* 44:756–762, 1996.

73. Prior JC, Barr SI, Chow R, et al: Physical activity as therapy for osteoporosis, *Can Med Assoc J* 155:940–944, 1996.

74. Stengel SV, Kemmler W, Pintag R, et al: Power training is more effective than strength training for maintaining bone mineral density in postmenopausal women, *J Appl Physiol* 99:181–188, 2005.

75. Caine D, DiFiori J, Maffulli N: Physeal injuries in children's and youth sports: reasons for concern? *Br J Sports Med* 40:749–760, 2006.

76. Staheli LT: Orthopedics in adolescence, *Dev Med Child Neurol* 25:806–818, 1983.

77. Smith AD: Children and sports. In Scoles P, editor: *Pediatric orthopedics in clinical practice*, ed 2, Chicago, 1988, Year Book.

78. Wojtys EM: Sports injuries in the immature athlete, *Orthop Clin North Am* 18:689–708, 1987.

79. MacKinnon JL: Osteoporosis: a review, *Phys Ther* 68: 1533–1540, 1988.

80. Beck BR, Snow CM: Bone health across the lifespan – exercising our options, *Exerc Sport Sci Rev* 31(3):117–122, 2003.

81. Corteix D, Lespessailles E, Peres SL, et al: Effect of physical training on bone mineral density in prepubertal girls: a comparative study between impact loading and non-impact loading sports, *Osteoporosis Int* 8:152–158, 1998.

82. Nikander R, Sievanen H, Heinonen A, et al: Targeted exercise against osteoporosis: a systematic review and meta-analysis for optimising bone strength throughout life, *BMC Med* (serial online): www.biomedcentral.com/1741-7015/8/47.

83. Snow CM: Exercise and bone mass in young and premenopausal women, *Bone* 18(Suppl 1):51S–55S, 1996.

84. Martin AD, Brown E: The effects of physical activity on the human skeleton, *Topics Geriatr Rehabil* 4:25–35, 1989.

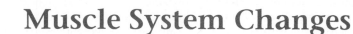

7

Muscle System Changes

After studying this chapter, the reader will be able to:

1. Define the basic characteristics of skeletal muscle morphology and organization.
2. Describe the basic physiology of skeletal muscle contraction.

3. Discuss the development changes in skeletal muscle across the life span.
4. Identify the functional implications of age-related changes in skeletal muscles.

Muscle is the largest tissue mass in the body. There are three types of muscles: voluntary (skeletal), involuntary (smooth), and cardiac. These three types of muscle are further divided into two subtypes of muscle: striated and nonstriated. Smooth muscle is the single example of the nonstriated type and is found in the walls of the digestive system, urinary bladder, and blood vessels. Smooth muscle contraction in these structures decreases their diameter. The cells are 10 to 600 μm in length and 2 to 12 μm in diameter. They are spindle shaped and have a single, centrally placed nucleus.

Cardiac and skeletal muscles are composed of striated muscle. Cardiac muscle is a special form of striated muscle found only in the heart. Its arrangement of contractile proteins is identical to that of skeletal muscle, but the arrangement of fibers is different. Cardiac cells are joined together by specialized intercellular junctions that are visible in the light microscope as dark heavy lines between the cells. The cells are irregularly shaped and usually contain a single, centrally placed nucleus.

Skeletal muscle, the focus of this chapter, is generally considered the main energy-consuming tissue of the body and provides the propulsive force to move about and to perform physical activities. Skeletal muscle is also known as voluntary, striated, striped, or segmental muscle. Approximately 20% of the energy produced during muscle contraction is used to produce movement; the remainder is lost as heat.

There are more than 500 skeletal muscles in the body. On a microscopic level, muscle cells are considered to be cylindrical. They range from 1 to 40 μm in length and from 10 to 100 μm in diameter. The cells are multinucleated, with the nuclei located at the periphery of the cell or just beneath the *sarcolemma*,

or plasma membrane. External to the sarcolemma is a highly glycosylated layer of collagen fibers called the *external lamina;* it is the external lamina that completely ensheathes each cell. This layer also contains proteins that function as enzymes.

ORGANIZATION OF MATURE SKELETAL MUSCLE

Skeletal muscle is organized from macroscopic to microscopic levels. A muscle's architecture is the "arrangement of muscle fibers within a muscle relative to the axis of force generation.[1]" Muscle function is determined in large part by the muscle architecture. "Architectural differences between muscles are the best predictors of force production.[2]" There are many different muscle designs.[3] Muscles are usually categorized into one of three types: longitudinal, pennate, and multipennate. In one type, called the parallel or longitudinal architecture, muscle fibers are arranged parallel to the force generating axis such as seen in the biceps. In a second type called the pennate architecture, the fibers are arranged at a single angle relative to the force generating axis, such as is present in the vastus lateralis. In the third type, the multipennate, fibers are arranged at varying angles relative to the force generating axis, such as seen in the gluteus medius. Muscle architecture also includes the length of the fibers within the muscle and the cross-sectional area of the muscle.[2] Muscle design reflects the functional use pattern of that muscle.

The entire muscle is encased in a thick connective sheath of collagen fibers called the *epimysium.* Extensions of this sheath extend into the interior of the muscle, subdividing it into small bundles or groups of myofibers called fascicles. Each bundle or fascicle is surrounded by a layer of connective tissue called the *perimysium*. Within the fascicle, each individual muscle myofiber is surrounded by a layer of connective tissue called the *endomysium*. The endomysium is rich in capillaries and, to a lesser extent, nerve fibers. All connective tissue coverings ultimately come together at the tendinous junction; the tendon transmits all contractile forces generated by the muscle fibers to the bone.

Each individual myofiber is filled with cylindric bundles of myofibrils that are made up of myofilaments. Myofibrils are the contractile structures of muscle. Filaments of actin and myosin are arranged in parallel groupings. Actin and myosin are contractile proteins. Actin, the thinner filament, originates at the Z disk; myosin is the thicker filament. During muscle contraction, as two Z disks move closer together, the actin and myosin filaments slide over each other. The area from one Z disk to the next Z disk constitutes a sarcomere, which is the basic contractile unit of the muscle fiber (Figure 7-1). Striations, the alternating light and dark pattern in the sarcomere seen under a light microscope, reflect the amount of overlap of the actin and myosin filaments. Myofibrils also contain the regulatory proteins tropomyosin and troponin and accessory proteins, titin and nebulin. Titin and nebulin maintain the alignment of the actin and myosin filaments within the sarcomere. Tropomyosin and troponin are both involved in muscle contraction. Troponin is a Ca^{2+} binding protein complex attached to tropomyosin.

A sagittal section of a muscle bundle depicted in Figure 7-2 shows the arrangement of the *sarcoplasmic reticulum* (SR), a system of membranous anastomosing channels intimately associated with the surface of each myofibril. At the feet of the SR are voltage sensitive receptor proteins: the ryanodine receptor (RyR) and calcium-ATPase (Ca-ATPase). Calcium (Ca^{2+}) stored in the SR is necessary for muscle contraction. RyR senses an action potential and opens the calcium channels to allow calcium to be released into the region of the myofilament. The *transverse tubular system* (T tubules) contains tubules that are extensions of the sarcolemma going deep into the interior of the muscle fiber. The function of the T tubules is to extend the wave of depolarization that initiates muscle contraction throughout all the myofibrils of the muscle. The Ca-ATPase pumps calcium back into the SR, allowing the muscle to relax. RyR and Ca-ATPase are two key calcium regulatory proteins involved in the excitation-contraction coupling process.

Excitation-Contraction Coupling

Excitation-contraction coupling is the mechanism that links plasma membrane stimulation with cross-bridge force production. The muscle receives a neural signal and converts that signal into mechanical force after synapsing at the *neuromuscular junction*. Figure 7-3 illustrates the expansion of an axon into a motor end plate that comes to rest in a depression of the surface of the myofiber. The chemical signal comes from the release of acetylcholine (ACh).

Muscle action potentials produced by the excitation-contraction coupling initiate calcium signals. The calcium signals activate a contraction-relaxation cycle. *Contraction* refers to activation of the cross-bridge cycle. Ca^{2+} activates the attractive forces between the filaments of actin and myosin by binding to troponin (Figure 7-4). However, the process of contraction will only continue if there is energy; this energy is derived from the high-energy bonds of adenosine triphosphate (ATP), which are degraded to adenosine diphosphate (ADP). In the presence of Ca^{2+} and ATP, the heads of the myosin molecules form cross-bridges with active sites on the thin filaments of actin (see Figure 7-4). The resulting energy produces a conformational change in the myosin head region that exerts a directional force on the actin filament. As a result, the actin filaments are drawn toward the center of the sarcomere, overlapping the myosin filament. The net result is shortening of the sarcomere, or contraction of the muscle. One ATP is needed for each cross-bridge cycle. After cross-bridge formation during the contraction phase of excitation-contraction coupling, relaxation occurs. Ca-ATPase pumps the calcium back into the SR, lowering the calcium levels and producing muscle relaxation. The concentration of calcium must drop to allow the unbinding of Ca^{2+} from troponin. The filaments slide back to their initial position assisted by elastic connective tissues within the muscle and titin. In summary, acetylcholine initiates the excitation-contraction coupling, and calcium binding to troponin initiates muscle contraction. A muscle twitch is synonymous to a single contraction-relaxation cycle in a skeletal muscle fiber.

Muscle Fiber Types

Muscle fibers can be described based on speed as type I or type II. Muscle fibers can also be classified according to their metabolic abilities. All human muscles are a mixture of three fiber types: I, IIa, IIx.[4] *Type I muscle fibers* are classified as slow oxidative because they use slow glycolysis and oxidative phosphorylation to produce ATP. Slow-twitch, type I fibers have a small diameter, with large amounts of oxidative enzymes and an extensive capillary density. Type I fibers are best suited for activities required in repetitive, lower-force contractions and are considered fatigue resistant. Only slow fibers are found in extraocular and middle ear muscles. Most "postural" muscles, such as those associated with the spinal column or the lower extremities,

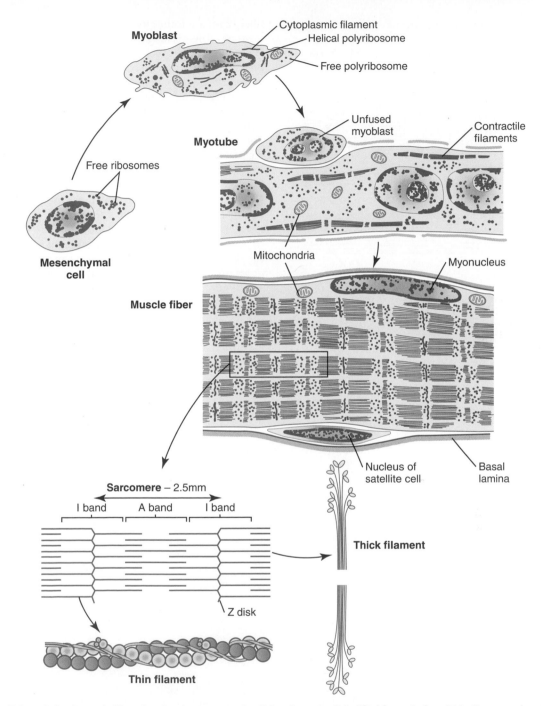

Figure 7-1 A skeletal muscle fiber showing important subcellular elements. (Modified from Carlson BM: *Human embryology and developmental biology*, ed 4, St Louis, 2009, Mosby.)

are composed predominantly of slow-twitch, or type I, fibers. Force is maintained economically by having lower myosin CA-ATPase activity than the fast-twitch fibers. The soleus muscle has a preponderance of slow-twitch muscle fibers and therefore is considered a postural muscle used for prolonged lower extremity activity to support the body against gravity.

Type II muscle fibers are classified as fast oxidative-glycolytic fibers. Type IIa fibers use both oxidative (aerobic) and glycolytic (anaerobic) metabolism. These

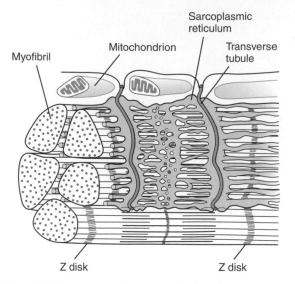

Figure 7-2 Transverse tubule sarcoplasmic reticulum system. (From Porterfield JA, DeRosa C: *Mechanical low back pain: perspectives in functional anatomy,* ed 2, Philadelphia, 1998, WB Saunders, p 57.)

fiber types are found in some ocular muscles and demonstrate fine, fast movements almost continuously. When glucose is quickly broken down without oxygen present, large amounts of lactate are produced along with ATP. Type IIx fibers[1] have a high capacity for glycolytic metabolism and can rapidly shorten. Fast-twitch fibers are suited for short bursts of powerful activity, although the type IIa fibers are more fatigue resistant. The contractile speed and twitch duration of type IIa are between those of type I and type IIx fibers. The gastrocnemius muscle has a preponderance of fast-twitch fibers. This gives the muscle its capacity for very forceful and rapid contractions, which are used for jumping. The reader is advised that because much of the muscle research related to aging was done before the change in nomenclature of the subcategories of type II fibers, therefore references continue to be made to type IIb fibers instead of type IIx in some of the cited studies.

Motor Unit

The functional unit of a muscle is the *motor unit,* which is defined as a single nerve cell body and its axon plus all muscle fibers innervated by the axon's branches.

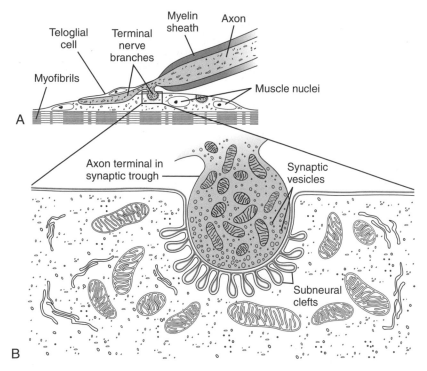

Figure 7-3 Neuromuscular junction: different views of the motor endplate. **A,** Longitudinal section through the endplate. **B,** Electron micrographic appearance of the contact point between one of the axon terminals and the muscle fiber membrane, representing the rectangular area shown in **A.** (Modified from Fawcett DW: *Bloom and Fawcett: textbook of histology,* ed 11, Philadelphia, 1986, WB Saunders, p 290.)

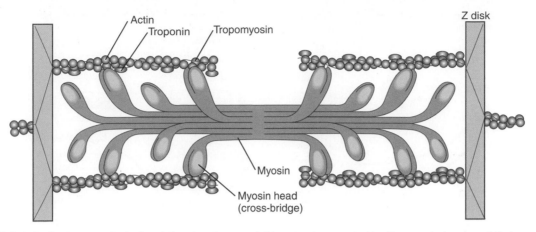

Figure 7-4 A single sarcomere is depicted showing the cross-bridge structure created by the myosin heads and their attachment to the actin filaments. The proteins troponin and tropomyosin are also shown. Troponin is responsible for exposing the actin filament to the myosin head, thereby allowing cross-bridge formation, that is, a contraction. (Modified from Berne RM, Levy MN: *Principles of physiology*, ed 2, 1996, Mosby.)

All the muscle fibers of a motor unit are of the same fiber type. Each muscle fiber receives innervation from one neuron. The intensity of a muscle contraction is graded by the number of motor units recruited and the rate of firing. The number of muscle fibers in a motor unit varies according to the muscle. For example, in the large muscles of the lower limb, motor units range in size from approximately 500 to 1000 fibers. In contrast, the small muscles in the hand or the extraocular muscles have motor units that range in size from approximately 10 to 100 fibers. These muscles are capable of producing very fine movements, such as typing, tying a bow, or making small adjustments of the eye.

Recruitment is the process of increasing the number of motor units contracting within a muscle at a given time.[4] The process of recruitment follows the size principle, with the small motor units being recruited before the larger motor units. The small motor neurons innervated by slow oxidative type I fibers are fired first, followed by fast oxidative-glycolytic, type IIa, and, finally, the fast glycolytic type IIx fibers.

SKELETAL MUSCLE DEVELOPMENT

Prenatal

To understand some of the age-related changes in skeletal muscle, it is important to study the events of skeletal muscle development. The muscular system develops from mesoderm, except for the muscles of the iris, which develop from neuroectoderm.[5]

The events of mesenchymal tissue differentiation into muscle fiber are depicted in Figure 7-5. The important cell types to be considered are myogenic precursor cells, myoblasts, myotubes, myofibers, fibroblasts, and satellite cells.[6,7]

Myogenic precursor cells are derived from the myotome of the somite. Muscle specific genes in these premuscle mesenchymal cells are turned on by regulatory factors. Exposure to growth factors produce *myoblasts*, which are spindle-shaped cells with centrally placed elongated nuclei. While these cells do begin to produce actin and myosin, their biggest role developmentally is to fuse together to form large, multinucleated cylinders called myotubes. They align into chainlike configurations parallel to the long axis of the limb. Each syncytium (the multinucleate mass of protoplasm produced by cell merging) contains a varying number of nuclei ranging up to several hundred. Cellular fusion via disintegration of the plasma membranes of adjacent myoblasts and myotubes is at present the explanation for how striated muscle cells become multinucleated.[8]

Myotubes are immature multinucleated muscle cells. Nuclei are centrally located in these elongated cylindrical cells. Contractile proteins actin and myosin are rapidly synthesized and become evident as striated fibrils in the peripheral cytoplasm. Other regulatory proteins, such as troponin and tropomyosin, are also synthesized. There are two types of myotubes: primary and secondary. Primary myotubes are the first to develop prenatally at 5 weeks of gestation. A few weeks later, the secondary myotubes develop. By 20 weeks of gestation,

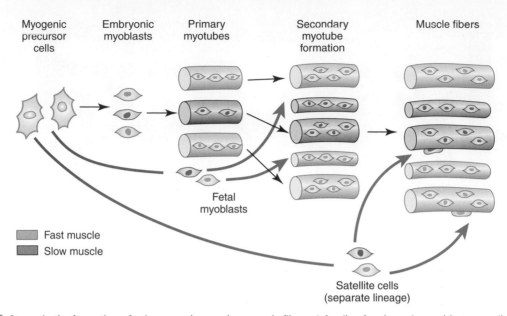

Myogenic precursor cells — Embryonic myoblasts — Primary myotubes — Secondary myotube formation — Muscle fibers

Fetal myoblasts

Fast muscle
Slow muscle

Satellite cells
(separate lineage)

Figure 7-5 Stages in the formation of primary and secondary muscle fibers. A family of embryonic myoblasts contributes to the formation of the primary myotubes, and fetal myoblasts contribute to secondary myotubes. The origin of satellite cells is still unresolved. (From Carlson BM: *Human embryology and developmental biology*, ed 4, St Louis, 2009, Mosby, p 250.)

the majority of myotubes have fused to form *myofibers*.[9] *Myofibers* are mature multinucleated muscle cells more commonly called muscle fibers. Myofibers contain the characteristic striations, or sarcomeres, of skeletal muscle. The peripheral migration of the nuclei marks the differentiation of the myotube into a muscle fiber.

Fibroblasts are the flattened, irregularly shaped cells found in association with the developing myofibers. During the early stages of development, these cells provide an extracellular matrix on which the connective tissue framework of a muscle is developed. Fibroblasts form the perimysium and epimysium.

The last cell type to be discussed is the *satellite cell*. These mononucleated, spindle-shaped cells are closely associated with the surface of the myofibers. They are found between the basal lamina and the muscle fiber and can be positively identified only with the electron microscope (see Figures 7-1 and 7-5). Satellite cells play an integral role in normal muscle growth during the postnatal period and in the repair of muscle following injury. At birth, satellite cell nuclei account for more than 30% of the total myofiber nuclei.[10]

The role of the satellite cells during normal postnatal growth is to supply nuclei to the enlarging fibers. Although myoblasts constitute a rapidly proliferating cell population during embryonic development, once incorporated into the syncytium of a myofiber, they no longer replicate DNA or divide. The nuclei are permanently postmitotic once they become part of the syncytium. Nevertheless, when myofibers increase in size

during growth, the number of nuclei increases, in some cases more than 100 times. This increase in myonuclei depends on the satellite cells associated with the fiber. These cells are continually dividing. After a mitotic division, one or both of the daughter cells fuse with the fiber, thereby injecting an additional nucleus into the syncytium. Likewise, in the event of massive injury to the muscle, myofibers usually die. New muscle fibers can be formed by surviving satellite cells. Activated by stress, the satellite cells repeat the embryonic events leading to muscle formation.[11] The damaged muscle is repaired or replaced. Although the ability of the satellite cells is significant, the damaged muscle may not fully regain its strength. The muscle compensates for residual loss of tissue by increasing the size of the remaining fibers.

As stated previously, muscle tissue develops from primitive cells called myoblasts, which are derived from mesenchymal cells. The muscles (myotomes) and bony segments (sclerotomes) of the vertebral column and overlying skin (dermatomes) are derived from somites, paired masses of mesoderm that lie on either side of the neural tube. Each segmental myotome separates into an epaxial and a hypaxial division. Myoblasts from the epaxial division become the extensor muscles of the neck and vertebral column (Figure 7-6). Myoblasts from the hypaxial division become the accessory muscles of the neck and the lateral and ventral trunk muscles. The muscles of the extremities develop from myoblasts located within the limb region that surrounds the developing bones

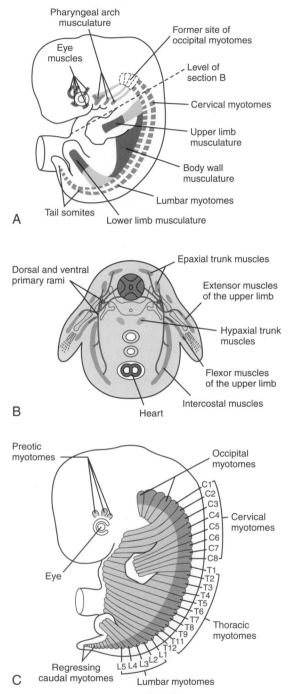

A

B

C

Figure 7-6 **A,** Sketch of an embryo (about 41 days), showing the myotomes and developing muscular system. **B,** Transverse section of the embryo, illustrating the epaxial and hypaxial derivatives of a myotome. **C,** Six-week embryo showing the myotome regions of the somites that give rise to most skeletal muscles. (From Moore KL, Persaud TVN: *Before we are born: essentials of embryology and birth defects*, ed 5, Philadelphia, 1998, WB Saunders, pp 401-402.)

(in situ). Some of the precursor myogenic cells in the limb buds come from somites.[12]

Control of Muscle Development and Differentiation

Primary myotubes are developed from embryonic myoblasts and can differentiate into both slow (type I) and fast fiber types (type II). This differentiation occurs before the motor nerve axons have contacted the newly formed muscle. Early motor neurons are present by the time the secondary myotubes are formed because they are derived from fetal myoblasts. Therefore, it is thought that the secondary myotubes require nervous input for their formation and differentiation.[7] The composition of contractile proteins determines the phenotype of muscle fibers. There are qualitative differences in contractile proteins between slow and fast muscle fibers, with different forms (isoforms) of those proteins being present from the fetal to neonatal periods and on to maturity.[7]

Differentiation into fiber types occurs about the same time as fibers are being innervated. The primary myotubes are innervated first. The formation of the myoneural junction is initiated with the development of ACh receptors in the periphery of the myotubes at approximately 8 weeks of gestation. This coincides with the earliest fetal movement observed in the intercostal muscles.[13] Prenatally, each motor end plate receives multiple axons. This polyneuronal innervation ensures that there will be at least one axon for every muscle fiber. Between 16 and 25 weeks of gestation, there is a dying back of extra connections and thus a transition to mononeuronal innervation indicative of the classic motor unit.[13] During the last half of gestation, there is also a tremendous increase in the number and size of muscle fibers. The increase in number is primarily from secondary myotubes. Fifteen percent of the body mass in the fetus midway through pregnancy is attributable to muscle. Muscle mass accounts for 25% of a person's body weight at birth.

Changes in Fiber Types

Muscle is developed from two distinct lineages: the primary and secondary myotubes. Primary myotubes develop and differentiate into muscle fibers without neural input; however, secondary myotubes require neural input for development. Generally, primary myotubes become type I fibers, and secondary myotubes become type II fibers. Because type I fibers are innervated before type II fibers, they are the first ones to be seen in the fetus. Type II fibers are generally not identified until 30 or 31 weeks of gestation.[14] Studies have concluded that between 31 and 37 weeks of gestation, type II fibers constitute about 25% of the muscle fibers present in the fetus.[15] Innervation by motor nerve fibers is necessary for the full differentiation of muscle fibers.[7]

Development and Migration of Fibers

Nearly all skeletal muscles are present and in essence exhibit a mature form at the end of the embryonic period (8 weeks of gestation). Approximately six fundamental processes occur during the first 8 weeks of development. The formation of a muscle is the result of one or more of these processes. The six fundamental processes as described by Crelin[16] are as follows:

1. The direction of the muscle fibers may change from the original cephalocaudal orientation in the myotome. Only a few muscles retain their initial fiber orientation (parallel to the long axis of the body); examples of these are the rectus abdominis and the erector spinae.
2. Portions of successive myotomes commonly fuse to form a single composite muscle. An example of this process is the rectus abdominis. This muscle is formed by the fusion of the ventral portions of the last six or seven thoracic myotomes.
3. A myotome may split longitudinally into two or more parts that become separate muscles; examples of this process are the trapezius and the sternocleidomastoid muscles.
4. The original myotome masses may split into two or more layers. The intercostal muscles are the derivatives of single myotomes, which split into two layers: the external and the internal intercostal muscles.
5. A portion of the muscle or all of the muscle may degenerate. The degenerated muscle leaves a sheet of connective tissue known as an *aponeurosis*. The epicranial aponeurosis connecting the frontal and occipital portions of the occipitofrontalis muscle is an example of this particular process.
6. The last process involves muscle migration of a myotome from its site of formation to a more remote region. The formation of the muscles of the upper chest is an example of this process. The serratus anterior muscle migrates to the thoracic region and attaches ultimately to the scapula and the upper eight or nine ribs. This muscle migration takes with it the fifth, sixth, and seventh cervical spinal nerves for innervation. The migration of the latissimus dorsi muscle is even more extensive. This migration carries with it its seventh and eighth cervical spinal nerve innervations to attach ultimately to the humerus, the lower thoracic and lumbar vertebrae, the last three or four ribs, and the crest of the ilium of the pelvis. In

muscle development, a wide range of variation of these six processes can occur without interfering with an individual's normal functional ability.

Infancy to Adolescence

The growth of skeletal muscles in the first year of life is the result of an increase in the size of the individual fibers and possibly the number of muscle fibers. Although the greatest increase in the number of muscle fibers occurs before birth, an increase in muscle fiber number does occur during the first year of postnatal development. The increase in fiber number is achieved by the differentiation of myoblasts into secondary myotubes or by division of already existing cells.[9] After birth, the growth of the muscle comes mainly from an increase in size of the individual fibers. The average muscle fiber size at birth is around 12 μm.

Differentiation of muscle fibers continues into postnatal life. At birth, the distribution of type I fibers ranges from 28% to 41% in various skeletal muscles. Intercostal and diaphragm muscles demonstrate adultlike distribution of type I fibers by 2 and 7 months, respectively.[17] The soleus achieves its type I predominance by 8 to 10 months of age.[18] Proportions of different types of fibers also vary considerably among individuals for a given skeletal muscle. For example, a standard deviation of about 15% is observed in the percentage of type I fibers in the vastus lateralis muscle of young men (the mean is about 50%) according to Malina, Bouchard, and Bar-Or.[15] Lexell and colleagues[19] did not find adult distribution of type I fibers in the vastus lateralis muscle of children from 5 to 15 years of age. However, a later study observed the adult distribution in 16 year olds, which might suggest a change occurs relative to puberty.[18] Changes in fiber type differentiation continue postnatally, even into the period preceding young adulthood.

The changes in contractile properties of skeletal muscle follow the differentiation of fiber types. The contractile properties of certain muscles slow postnatally, somewhere between 6 weeks and 3 years of age.[20] Whether the slowing of the contractile properties is caused by this differentiation is not certain.[18] The muscles that become postural muscles develop adult slow-twitch characteristics as motor development proceeds. Some characteristics of slow-twitch fibers are their slow speed of contraction and longer relaxation times.

Muscle maturation occurs in childhood. Contractile properties of muscle are measured by maximal twitch tension, time to peak tension, and half-relaxation times. Soleus muscle relaxation time was studied as a measure of muscle dynamics in children 3 to 10 years of age.[21] Researchers found that a child's muscles are initially slow to relax after contraction but that relaxation speed doubles between 3 and 10 years of age. These values reach adult rates at age 10. In further examination of this phenomenon, the investigators found that the speed of contraction improved because of the ability of the muscle to relax more quickly.[22] A possible mechanism for the change in muscle dynamics with age may be a change in the calcium reuptake mechanism of the SR. Furthermore, the change to an adult muscle phenotype of relaxation appears complete at age 10, the same time at which fiber diameter differences are apparent in males and females.[23]

Strength gains in children follow a typical growth curve for height and weight. Changes in strength are associated with increases in muscle size and muscle maturation. There are several characteristics of strength that may determine how strong someone will be at a given age, including the cross-sectional area of the muscle, the age of the individual, the gender of the individual, the body size or type, and the fiber type and size of the muscle being assessed. Muscle mass is gained before strength.[24] Muscle makes up only 25% of the total body mass at birth. However, between 5 and 17 years of age, muscle as a proportion of total body mass increases from 41% to 53% in males. During the same time period the values for females, 41% and 42%, do not change significantly.[15] Children are stronger than infants, and adolescents are stronger than children. In absolute terms, whether assessed cross-sectionally or longitudinally, muscle strength increases linearly with chronological age from childhood to age 12 or 13[25] and is mainly determined by the muscle's cross-sectional area. Tonson and associates[26] demonstrated that maximal isometric strength of the forearm flexors of three age groups—children, adolescents, and adults—was found to be proportional to the size of the muscle regardless the age of the subject.

Mean levels of isometric strength increase gradually between 3 and 6 years of age. Small gender differences are present.[25] Static strength in boys continues to increase linearly from 6 to 13 years, followed by a spurt that continues through the late teens. Wiggin and associates[27] recently reported normative data of quadriceps and hamstring strength as measured by isokinetic dynamometry in children 6 to 13 years old. Height was considered the best predictor of strength. Isokinetic dynamometry is being shown to be the most valid clinical means of measuring strength in children.[27]

Adolescence and Adulthood

Puberty marks an increase in growth of the musculoskeletal systems. As the skeleton grows, the muscles have to lengthen to reestablish the appropriate length-tension relationship. The resting length of a muscle affects the amount of tension that can be generated. At rest, the majority of skeletal muscles are near the optimal length for force production. Separation of the attachments of the muscles as the skeleton grows appears to be a strong stimulus for muscle growth.[28] Muscles add sarcomeres and fibrils to achieve a new length.[24] Greater muscle growth is seen in males than females because of the effects of steadily rising levels of testosterone.

Strength in Relation to Age and Muscle Mass

Strength is seen to increase linearly between the ages of 6 and 18 years (Figure 7-7). Boys have a strength spurt during the adolescent years, which is due to a rise in hormone production. The rise in testosterone begins 1 year before peak height velocity (PHV). This spike occurs at the same time as the divergence of strength between boys and girls.[29] Although testosterone is the most likely reason why males increase muscle mass and strength more than do females, other hormones play a role. Growth hormone, insulin, and thyroid hormones are important for somatic and muscle growth. With increasing age, the percentage of girls whose performance on strength tests equals or exceeds that of boys declines considerably. After age 16, the strength of an average boy is greater than that of a very strong girl. Peak strength velocity occurs about a year after PHV.[29] Although growth studies generally stop at age 18, strength continues to increase into the 20s, especially for men.

Strength appears to peak during young adulthood (in the 20s and early 30s).[30] Beginning at age 30, an estimated 5% of muscle mass is lost per decade.[31,32] While there is some slowing of contraction during middle adulthood (the 40s and 50s), it is not until the sixth decade (the 50s) that muscle strength begins a more steady decline and begins to effect function.[33,34] There is a 30% decline in muscle strength from age 50 to 70 years and a more rapid decline after 70 years of age.[35] The decrease is evident in both isometric and dynamic strength, but relatively speaking, eccentric strength is better maintained in older adults than is concentric strength.[36] Loss of strength in older men and women is greater than can be explained by loss of muscle mass alone.[37]

Firing Rate and Contractile Properties

The maximum force a muscle can produce is determined by the size of the muscle and the ability of the nervous system to generate a contraction. Muscles develop the ability to generate faster contractions, that is speed up, during the first 20 years of life with a documented decline seen in the proportion of type I muscle fibers

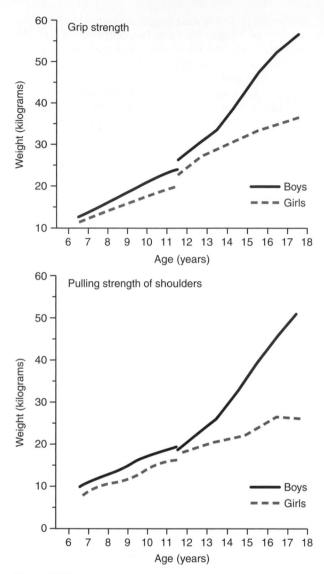

Figure 7-7 Mean grip strength and pulling strength between 6 and 18 years of age. (From Malina RM, Bouchard C, Bar-Or O: *Growth, maturation and physical activity*, ed 2, Champaign, Ill, 2004, Human Kinetics, p 219.)

(fast-twitch) fibers in the vastus lateralis increases from approximately 35% at age 5 to 50% at age 20.[19] The muscles of the body that are predominantly fast-twitch muscles do not exhibit adult proportions of type II fibers until young adulthood.

Motor neurons control the biochemical and physiological properties of the skeletal muscle they innervate. Once muscle fiber differentiation has occurred, neural input makes a tremendous difference in the way the muscle functions (muscle phenotype). Studies conducted on adults reveal that by switching a nerve (cross-innervation) from a fast-twitch (type II) glycolytic muscle to a slow-twitch (type I) oxidative muscle, the oxidative muscle becomes glycolytic. The reverse is also true. The expression of muscle fiber type in adults is dependent on innervation regardless of whether that muscle fiber was originally derived from a primary or a secondary myotube.

Older Adulthood

Sarcopenia

Loss of muscle mass begins in early adulthood with more loss occurring in older adulthood. The age-related loss of muscle called *sarcopenia* literally means "loss of flesh." While there is no one accepted definition of sarcopenia, individuals are considered sarcopenic if their lean body mass is less than 2 SD below the mean compared with a sample of healthy young adults. Using this definition, Baumgartner and associates[38] found that 19% of men and 34% of the women over 70 were sarcopenic. In individuals over 80, the percentages of men and women with sarcopenia were found to be even higher, 55% and 52%, respectively. Iannuzzi-Sucich, Prestwood, and Kenny[39] found similar rates in a population of older, community-dwelling adults. They concluded that sarcopenia is common in adults over 65, with BMI being a strong indicator of muscle mass. A larger BMI was associated with less lean muscle mass. Sarcopenia is a commonly recognized cause of loss of strength and functional abilities in older adults.

Janssen and associates[40] reported that more muscle mass is lost in the lower body in men and women with sarcopenia. While the age-related decline in muscle mass begins in the 30s, the loss does not reach functional significance until the sixth decade. Higher rates of physical disability have been demonstrated in those individuals with sarcopenia. Baumgartner and associates[38] found a fourfold higher rate of disability in men and a 3.6 higher rate of disability in women in their study compared to those with more muscle mass. Janssen, Heymsfield, and Ross[41] found a higher

in the vastus lateralis.[19] The increase of muscle cross-sectional area is associated with the relative proportion of fast type II fibers and with an increase in mean fiber size.[34] Elder and Kakulas[18] postulated that over the course of development from infancy to childhood and into adulthood, muscles undergo a fast-slow-fast phenotype change to meet the demands of motor development. The phenotype of a muscle reflects its functional use, not necessarily its developmental characteristics or genotype. For example, the proportion of type II

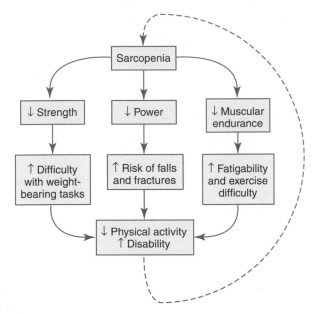

Figure 7-8 A model of the functional consequences of age-related sarcopenia and positive feedback loop by which the end result of reduced physical activity further exacerbates progression of the disorder. ↓ indicates decrease; ↑ indicates increase. (From Hunter GR, McCarthy FP, Bamman MM: Effects of resistance training on older adults, *Sports Med* 34(5):329-348, 2004.)

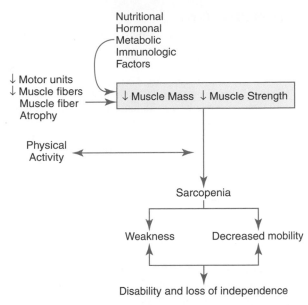

Figure 7-9 Factors contributing to sarcopenia. This figure summarizes the influences of multiple factors that lead to age-associated declines in muscle mass and strength and the subsequent impact on disability and loss of independence. (From Doherty TJ: Invited review: aging and sarcopenia, *J Appl Physiol* 95:1717-1727, 2003.)

prevalence of severe sarcopenia in women than men over 60 years of age, which was then associated with a greater amount of impairment and disability. The degree of muscle loss associated with aging may be partially related to the activity level of the individual. A model of the potential functional consequences of age-related sarcopenia is seen in Figure 7-8.

Mechanism of Muscle Loss

The etiology of sarcopenia is multifactorial[42–45] as seen in Figure 7-9. Loss of muscle mass has been associated with muscle disuse, changes in the nervous system (especially the motor unit), hormonal changes, inflammatory effects, diminished caloric intake, and changes in muscle structure and function. Functional decline in older adults has a strong inverse relationship with physical activity.[46] Starting around the age of 30, strength declines 10% to 15% per decade in the absence of physical training.[47] In those older adults who are lifelong trained, muscle mass and strength may be relatively preserved but not to the extent that loss of muscle mass and strength can be prevented with aging.[48]

The ability of muscle to rapidly produce force and therefore exhibit maximum strength declines with age

due to a loss of both muscular and neural function. A motor unit is composed of an alpha motor neuron and all the muscle fibers it innervates. The number of motor units remains constant from 10 to 60 years of age.[49] However, after age 60 there is an increase in rate of loss with a 70% reduction seen by the age of 90.[50] Loss of motor neurons orphans muscle fibers. Abandoned muscle fibers are partially reinnervated by surviving motor neurons. As a result, there is a decline in functional motor units and an increase in the innervation ratio. The process of denervation and reinnervation is called *motor unit remodeling.* For example, if the motor unit originally consisted of 1 motor nerve and 50 muscle fibers, after motor unit remodeling, the ratio would be 1 motor nerve to 75 or 100 fibers. As a result of motor unit remodeling, the number of fibers innervated by a motor neuron increases so that the remaining motor units exert, on average, greater amounts of force. With aging, a selective denervation of type II fibers occurs with reinnervation by slow motor neurons.[51] Physiologically, they become slow motor units. The functional significance of the reorganization is that the nervous system may have to alter its strategies for controlling muscle force.

Inflammatory Effects

Loss of muscle mass and strength may result from the inflammatory effect of exercise. Physical exercise can result in free radical-mediated damage to muscle tissue. While low levels of reactive oxygen species (ROS) are needed for normal force production, higher levels are detrimental and can result in weakness and fatigue.[52] Exercise is thought to be protective. The increase in inflammatory mediators that normally occurs with exercise is transient. Chronically elevated levels of these inflammatory mediators because of age and disease are not beneficial. The mechanism whereby inflammation contributes to the overall loss of muscle mass and strength with aging continues to be investigated. Higher levels of inflammatory markers (interleukin 6 and C-reactive protein) have been found to be associated with a greater risk of losing muscle strength in older women and men.[53] The risk is 2 to 3 times greater for more than a 40% loss over a 3-year period of time. Inflammatory factors may play a role in the onset and progression of sarcopenia.[54]

Diminished Caloric Intake

Changes in the quality and quantity of dietary protein could contribute to a loss of muscle with advanced aging. Many older adults do not ingest the recommended daily allowance (RDA) for protein, which is 0.8 g/kg/day. Evans[55] suggests that this minimum RDA may not be sufficient to maintain muscle mass with exercise. Boirie[56] suggested that dietary supplementation with certain amino acids, institution of changes in patterns of protein ingestion, as well as increases in the amount of dietary protein could counteract some of the age-related loss of muscle in older adults.

Structural Changes

Structural changes also occur in the muscle itself. There are changes in the mitochondria, T tubules, and the SR.[57] Connective tissue increases in the area of the endomysium, the location of the capillary bed. In addition, the basement membrane increases in thickness around both the capillary and the myofiber. The net result of these changes (all mainly at the level of the endomysium) is an increase in diffusion distances, possibly producing an age-related hypoxia. It is unknown whether chemical changes in the basement membrane, for example, may produce a selective barrier to certain essential molecules required by the muscle fibers.

Changes in Muscle Protein Synthesis

Muscle protein synthesis rates decline in muscle with old age. This decline affects three processes involved in muscle contraction: ATP production, excitation-contraction coupling, and cross-bridge cycling.[42] A decline in mitochondrial protein production and activity results in decreased oxidative capacity by limiting the amount of ATP available for muscle contraction. The decline in muscle proteins has been associated with age-related loss in muscle strength and aerobic exercise tolerance.[32] The decline in protein synthesis in muscle has been related to declines in insulin-like growth factor, testosterone, and dehydroepiandrosterone (DHEA) sulfate.[42] The degradation of excitation-contraction coupling that occurs with age also contributes to the loss of strength seen in sarcopenia. Uncoupling occurs because two key proteins are altered, resulting in a slower release of calcium through the ryanodine receptor. The functional result is that it takes longer to produce a contraction and longer to relax after a contraction in older adults. The cross-bridging cycle is unable to produce as much strength with age due to structural and chemical changes in myosin, the muscle protein that contributes most to muscle mass.[42]

Changes in Contractile Properties

The ability of muscle to generate force is reduced with age. Older adults do not develop force as rapidly as young adults because of a loss of type II muscle fibers. Type II muscles can intrinsically develop more force because they have a larger cross-sectional area and a fast cross-bridge cycling rate compared with type I muscles.[58] Older adults have less difficulty with eccentric contractions than with concentric contractions. A selective loss of type II fibers could explain why muscles generate force more slowly but also relax more slowly. Also if the loss of type I motor units is compensated for by hypertrophy of smaller, slower motor units, the resultant change in fiber type could also explain why slower muscle is preserved with aging. Motor unit firing rates appear to generally be reduced with aging, but the changes seem to be task and muscle specific. Not all muscles are equally affected by age.

Rate of Force Development

Force control is lessened in the older adult because of the greater number of low threshold (type I) motor units compared with the number found in younger adults. The force-velocity curve is shifted secondary to aging (Figure 7-10). This occurs because the older muscle is less able to generate force at all contraction speeds. Concentric actions decline the greatest with eccentric contractions and eccentric strength being relatively preserved. Loss of eccentric strength is 10% to 30% less than concentric strength.[59] Healthy older adults were found to be significantly less steady when performing dynamic contraction than young adults.[60] When comparing fallers and nonfallers, the same researchers

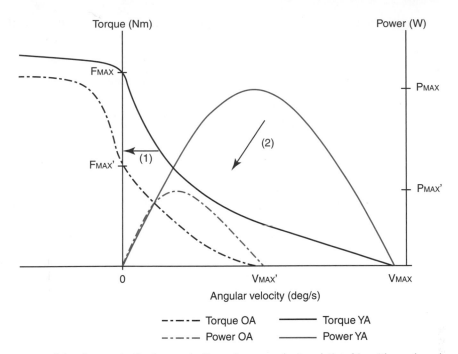

Figure 7-10 A summary of the changes to the force-velocity and power-velocity relationship with age based on data from the studies referenced in this review. *OA,* older adults; *YA,* young adults; P$_{max'}$, older adults maximal power; $V_{max'}$, older adults' maximum contraction velocity; F_{max}, young adults' peak isometric torque; $F_{max'}$, older adults' peak isometric torque. With increased age, the force-velocity and power-velocity curves shift downward and to the left. (From Raz IS, Bird SR, Shield AJ: Aging and the force-velocity relationship of muscles, *Exp Gerontol* 45:81-90, 2010.)

found that the fallers were less steady during eccentric contractions than nonfallers. Functional capacity can be impacted by the age-related decline in force production and speed of force production (power).

The effect of age on strength is seen in Figure 7-11. For an excellent review of aging and force-velocity relationship of muscles, the reader is referred to Raz, Bird, and Shield.[59]

Other Changes Associated with Age

Collagen As we age, the amount of connective tissue increases, mostly at the level of the endomysium. Collagen obtained from old muscle is less soluble and exhibits increased resistance to degradative enzymes such as collagenase. Changes in the collagen are consistent with increased cross-linking or additional bonds between the collagen molecules and would explain the increase in stiffness of old muscle. This stiffness and altered connective tissue content may contribute to the preservation of eccentric strength in older adults by providing increased passive resistance during muscle lengthening.[44,61] As muscle fibers are lost and replaced by fat and collagen, the volume or girth of the muscle as measured anthropometrically may not demonstrate an actual reduction in muscle mass.

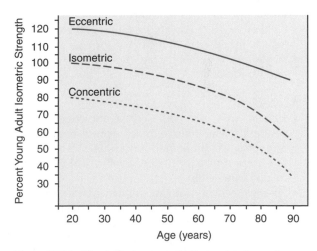

Figure 7-11 Effect of age on maximal strength throughout the human life span. The shape and height of the schematic curves are based on Vandervoort's gerontology research and depend on the type of strength being measured: isometric, concentric (muscle allowed to shorten while contracting), or eccentric (active muscle being lengthened by external load). (From Vandervoort AA: Aging of the human neuromuscular system, *Muscle Nerve* 25:17-25, 2002.)

Motor End Plate   Changes in one part of the motor unit affect other parts of the motor unit. Motor end plates remodel continuously during normal aging, with changes seen in presynaptic and postsynaptic components.[62] The number of synaptic vesicles is increased with age, but they are found in tight clusters, suggesting that they have undergone agglutination. The synaptic cleft becomes enlarged, and the enlarged area is filled with thickened basal lamina. In addition, the functional folds appear unfolded, and the plasma membrane of the muscle fiber appears thickened.

FUNCTIONAL IMPLICATIONS

Changes occurring in the development of skeletal muscle tissue across the life span have functional and clinical implications for muscle strength, endurance, power, and function. Clinical Implications Box 7-1: Muscle

CLINICAL IMPLICATIONS Box 7-1

Muscle Strength Acquisition Across the Life Span

Strength acquisition follows a general growth curve as seen in other anthropometric measures, such as height and weight. Children at or after puberty demonstrate changes in muscle mass and muscle strength.

Children
- Static strength and power in children may be determined more by genetic factors than is muscle endurance.
- Children can increase strength and endurance as a result of regular participation in a program of progressive resistance training.
- A properly designed resistive exercise program does not negatively impact the growth and development of youth.[74]
- Recommendations regarding resistance training in children and adolescents are found in the Canadian Society for Exercise Physiology's position paper.[77]
- A position statement from the National Strength and Conditioning Association is also available.[99]

Adolescents
- Muscle mass in adolescence increases before strength. Peak muscle mass occurs during and after peak weight gain, but maximal strength does not occur until after the peak velocity of growth in height and weight.
- Preadolescent and adolescents can increase strength and power after participating in a well-designed and properly supervised resistance training program.[99]
- Adolescents have an increased risk for musculoskeletal injury such as apophyseal avulsion during periods of rapid growth. This risk can be countered with a good stretching program.
- Physiological mismatching is possible between 13 and 17 years of age and may increase the risk of injury resulting from differences in body size, age, and maturity status.

- The health benefits from participation in a well-designed and appropriately supervised resistance training program far outweigh the potential risks.

Adults
- Maximal strength is achieved in the 30s and maintained until the 50s.[30]
- Strength training results in improved performance in trained and untrained individuals.
- Strength training needs to be specific to the task, such as speed, power, and endurance.
- If strengthening is performed throughout middle and older adulthood, age-related strength loss is mitigated but *not* eliminated.[48,100]

Older Adults
- Progressive resistance training is an effective and safe way to increase strength in older adults.[94,101,102]
- Women may respond differently to strength training.[103,104]
- Frailty and advanced age are not a contraindication to exercise.[102,105] A sedentary lifestyle is far more dangerous than activity in the older adult.
- Participation in a regular progressive resistive exercise can combat the functional declines associated with aging.[87,90,94,106]
- Training for power may be more important than training for strength because of the carryover to functional activities, such as rising from a chair or climbing stairs.[97,106]
- Gait speed is positively affected by progressive resistance strength training.[96,107] Gait speed is a powerful predictor of health.[108]
- Recommendations for strength training in older adults can be found in the position stand of the American College of Sports Medicine[81] and the Canadian Journal of Public Health.[109]

Strength Acquisition Across the Life Span outlines markers for promoting strength and related training and exercise programs along the developmental continuum.

Muscle strength is an expression of muscular force, or the individual's capacity to develop tension against an external resistance. The literature defines several types of strength: static, power, and dynamic.[25] *Static, or isometric, strength* is the maximal voluntary force produced against an external resistance without any change in muscle length. It is generally measured in specific muscle groups, such as those in the hand, by grip strength or isokinetically in the quadriceps or hamstrings. *Power* is explosive strength or the ability of muscles to produce a certain amount of force in the shortest amount of time. It is measured as a function of strength. *Dynamic strength* is the force generated by repetitive contractions of a muscle. Therefore, it is closely linked to muscular endurance. Dynamic strength is also known as functional strength in the physical fitness literature.

Muscle endurance is the ability to repeat or maintain muscular contractions over time. It is believed that the capacity of a muscle to increase in muscular endurance is related to the ability of the muscle to use oxygen, or the *oxidative metabolism* of the muscle. This ability is related to the individual's maximal oxygen uptake, or VO_{2max}, levels. This is defined as the transport of oxygen from the atmosphere for use by the mitochondria of the muscle and is related to individual cardiovascular efficiency (see Chapter 15).[63] Muscle fatigue is the reduced ability to achieve the same amount of force output. Fatigue is related to endurance but is not the same thing. Although endurance is related to the aerobic capacity of the muscle, fatigue may be the result of a failure of motor unit recruitment or altered excitation-contraction coupling. There are many central and peripheral factors that can be responsible for muscle fatigue.

Muscle fatigue is the loss of force and power, which leads to reduced task performance.[64] It is task specific and manifests differently in men and women.[65,66] Furthermore the response to exercise and production of fatigue may change over the life span. The origin of fatigue is multifactorial as are the different domains of fatigue.[67] Some of the same factors implicated in the causation and progression of sarcopenia have been identified as contributing to fatigue, such as the decline in mitochondrial function, oxidative stress, and inflammation. The time to task failure, or the inability to continue a task because of fatigue, is different between young and old and women and men as seen in Figure 7-12. Factors affecting fatigue include the muscle groups involved, the type and intensity of the contraction, whether the limb is supported, and the environment in which the task is performed.[65]

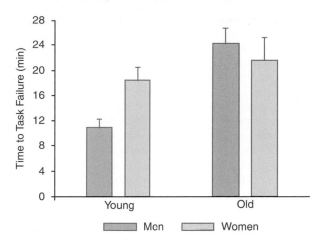

Figure 7-12 Time to task failure for a sustained isometric fatiguing contraction performed with elbow flexor muscles with young and old men and women. The time to failure was longer for the young women compared with the young men but similar for older men and women. (From Hunter SK, Critchlow A, Enoka RM: Influence of aging on sex differences in muscle fatigability, *J Appl Physiol* 97:1723-1732, 2004.)

Childhood and Adolescence

Information on normative strength values is not very extensive for early childhood; more information is available for the middle childhood and adolescent years. It is clear that muscular strength increases gradually during early infancy and early childhood. Longitudinal studies show that the adolescent growth spurt in isometric strength occurs within a year before the age at peak height velocity and may coincide with peak weight velocity.[29] In girls, there is improvement in strength through about 15 years of age.[15] Boys experience a longer growing period of almost 2 years, which along with a sharper acceleration of growth accounts for the gender difference in growth during puberty. Strength and body size and muscle mass are related. Because boys are usually bigger than girls and have more muscle mass, boys are stronger. When strength is measured per unit body size, boys are stronger in the upper body and trunk than girls. Power as measured by the ability to perform a vertical jump or a standing long jump shows increases in boys and girls from 6 to 12 or 13 years old. After 13, boys continue to improve while girls' scores level off. This age-related trend is seen in the development of strength, aerobic power, and motor performance.[15]

Children typically participate in short bursts of highly intense activity. During short intense bouts of exercise, children have a lesser ability to generate mechanical energy from chemical energy sources.[68] These exercise needs can more easily be met by anaerobic energy production. Anaerobic function in children improves faster than can be accounted for by growth alone.[69] Genetics, fiber type differentiation, hormonal influences, and improved coordination all contribute to the development of anaerobic muscle function.[68,70]

"Energy for skeletal muscle contraction in activities lasting more than several minutes is derived from aerobic metabolism.[71]" Muscular endurance improves linearly with age from 5 to 13 or 14 years in boys, followed by a spurt similar to that for static muscular strength. Muscular endurance also increases with age in girls, but there is no clear evidence of a spurt like that seen in boys.[72] Faigenbaum and associates[73] compared the effect of two exercise prescriptions on a small group of children ranging in age from 5.2 to 11.8 years. The children exercised in a community youth center twice a week for 8 weeks. One group performed low repetitions against a heavy load, and the other performed high repetitions against a moderate load. The control group did no resistance training. Strength and endurance of leg extension increased in both exercise groups. Endurance increased to a significantly greater degree in the group performing high repetitions against a moderate load.

Genetic factors contribute to muscle strength development and performance. Static strength and power in children may be determined more by genetic factors than muscle endurance. During growth, the genetic influence on strength development is strong. Body mass and height are most directly related to strength. Genes seem to play a greater role in strength development in males than in females.[25] At puberty, the interaction between height, body mass, and biological maturity explains the majority of strength differences seen with age.

Strength can be increased in children before puberty through the use of resistance training. However, the increase in muscle strength occurs without much increase in muscle size.[69] Strength gains are related to quality changes in the way that the nervous system functions. Malina[74] summarized that twice-a-week resistance training was able to produce significant strength gains during childhood and adolescence with minimal injuries reported. Benson and colleagues[75] demonstrated strength and endurance gains beyond typical maturation using a high-intensity training program. There is consensus that resistance training is beneficial to children and adolescents[76,77] because it can lead to improved muscular function and health benefits.

Adulthood and Aging

Strength in men is greatest between the ages of 30 and 35 years. Larsson and co-workers[30] reported an increase in quadriceps strength up to 30 years of age

and a decline after age 50. Generally, strength declines between 30% to 50% from the ages of 30 to 80.[46] Physiologically, a loss of 30% of a body system's (such as the muscular system) reserve capacity limits function and a decrease of 70% results in system failure.[78] The loss of muscle mass and strength with age significantly affects function. Beginning at age 30, an estimated 5% of muscle mass is lost, which is paralleled by a loss of strength.[31,32] A person 80 years of age may have lost so much strength that she may have barely enough strength to get out of a chair.

Adults have the ability to improve strength by resistance training.[79] Training needs to be specific to how the muscle is expected to function, statically for holding, for power or for endurance, in order to see improvements. Training also needs to be specific to the type of task being performed. Once a strength base is established, specific power or endurance training can be followed. The variability of motor performance between young and old adults appears to be the result of muscle force production fluctuations.[80] Fluctuations in muscle force production during a voluntary contraction are influenced by the architecture or shape of the muscle, the type of contraction the muscle is undergoing, the intensity of the contraction, and the properties of the motor units involved. The rate at which a muscle develops force (acceleration) during a slow concentric or eccentric contraction can fluctuate around a mean. Healthy older adults were found to demonstrate greater force fluctuations during submaximal contractions than younger adults. Depending on the muscle group involved, these fluctuations could be decreased by either increased physical activity or strengthening.[80] The researchers determined that the motor unit discharge rate to both the agonist and antagonist muscles was most likely responsible for the difference seen between young and older adults.

Researchers agree that the rate of decline in muscular strength with age appears greater in the lower body than the upper body.[81] Larsson and colleagues[30] evaluated 114 males, ages 11 to 70 years, for both static and dynamic lower extremity strength. Both strength and speed of contraction were found to decline with age. Studies of women indicate similar findings that muscle strength, both static and dynamic, decreases with age.[36] Women are weaker than men in muscular strength.[36] Women also demonstrate the decrement in strength earlier than do men.[82] There is a curvilinear relationship between maximum voluntary isometric strength and age in healthy adults (Figure 7-13).[83] Some of the strength loss in individuals may be related to activity or fitness level of the individual. If an individual remains active, the amount of muscle strength lost may be less (Table 7-1).

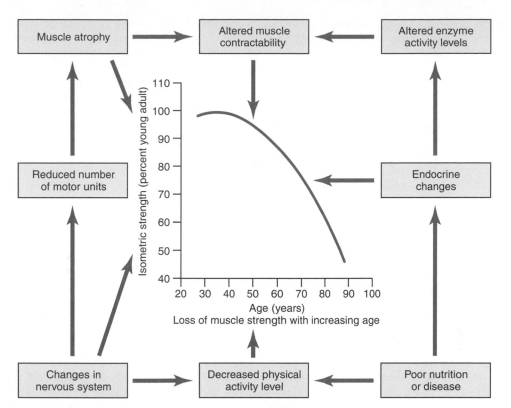

Figure 7-13 Relationship between age and maximal isometric muscle strength in healthy adults. The decline with age does not become apparent until the sixth decade. Note the curvilinear pattern, which is steeper for concentric strength (muscle shortening during contraction) but less affected by age for eccentric strength (active muscle is lengthened by external resistance). Many mechanisms contribute to the loss of muscle strength with aging, including muscle atrophy that is likely genetically controlled and muscle loss due to inactivity in sedentary individuals. (Modified from Vandervoort AA: Biological and physiological changes. In Pickles B, Compton A, Cott CA, contractability et al, editors: *Physiotherapy with older people,* Philadelphia, 1995, WB Saunders, p 73.)

Table **7-1**
Strength Changes In Older Adulthood

Better Relative Maintenance	Greater Relative Decline
Muscles used in activities of daily living	Muscles used infrequently in specialized activities
Isometric strength	Dynamic strength
Eccentric contractions	Concentric contractions
Slow-velocity contractions	Rapid-velocity contractions
Repeated low-level contractions	Power production
Strength using small joint angles	Strength using large joint angles
Strength in males	Strength in females

From Spirduso WW: *Physical dimensions of aging,* Champaign, Ill, 1995, Human Kinetics.

Loss of muscle strength is associated with a loss of function in older adults. The strength-function relationship is also curvilinear. As noted by Buchner and de Lateur,[84] there appears to be a minimum amount of strength required for a given task; this threshold may vary from task to task. Strong correlations between strength and function may exist only in individuals who have less than the "threshold" amount of strength. The amount of strength and the mode of muscle contraction—isometric, concentric, or eccentric—are specific to the task to be performed. For example, isometric hip abductor strength may be more representative of the force that needs to be generated during single limb stance than a concentric contraction of the same muscle group. By using the best measure of strength for a particular task, Chandler and co-workers[85] were able to predict the relative strength of the correlations between muscle strength and certain functional activities.

Strength of the quadriceps has been studied as it relates to falls and steadiness in standing. Sarcopenia can result in force generation fluctuations that might hinder the prevention of falling. After 16 weeks of resistance training, older adults improved in their use of tripping reactions.[86] Maximum push-off force improved in the trained group. Faller and nonfallers were distinguished by increased unsteadiness during eccentric quadriceps contractions.[60] Symons and associates[87] found that after a 12-week strength training program, older adults improved their performance of stair ascent and descent.

Muscle power also relates to the ability to perform functional skills. As stated earlier, power diminishes with age; in fact, power declines faster than strength.[59] The decline in power is related to the loss of the fast-twitch, type II muscle fibers that occurs with age. Men appear to be affected more by the loss of power with age than do women. The loss of power can be as much as 10% greater than the loss of strength.[88]

Declines in strength and power are the result of a decline in the amount of muscle, sarcopenia, and altered muscle quality. Muscle quality is the relationship between muscle mass, strength, and speed. It encompasses all the factors governing rapid force development (RFD), such as motor unit firing rate, amount of type II fibers, and pennation angle of the muscle fibers. Decline in RFD in older adults occurs because of the preferential decline in cross-sectional area of type II muscle fibers.[33] Additionally, there is a slowing of motor unit firing rates, a decrease in the pennation angle of the muscle fibers and reduced tendon stiffness.[48]

Lifelong trained older adults have been found to be stronger than age-matched untrained older adults.[48] The greater decline in strength relative to decline in muscle mass seems to be accounted for by the significant decline in the quality of muscle.[37]

In 2000, Kraemer and Newton[89] recommended velocity-specific resistance training for improvement in power. Puthoff and Nielsen[90] studied the relationships between impairments in strength and power of the lower extremities and function in older adults. Their regression analysis showed that power had a stronger indirect effect on function than strength. Peak power measurements explained more of the variance in functional activities than strength measurements. The researchers concluded that older adults would benefit from velocity-specific resistance training, that is, work at both low and high velocities in addition to strength training.

Endurance is related to the "use it or lose it" concept and can be assessed by looking at muscle fatigue. As previously defined, muscle fatigue "develops gradually soon after the onset of sustained physical activity.[65]" Baudry and associates[91] demonstrated more fatigability in older adults than younger adults with maximal

concentric and eccentric contractions of the dorsiflexor muscles. They attributed the fatigue in the older adults to impaired neuromuscular propagation and to changes in control of excitation-contraction coupling by Ca^{2+}. The latter change in excitation-contraction coupling was given as a reason for the fatigue in the young adults.

Endurance exercises may help normalize mitochondrial function in older individuals.[92] In a cross-sectional study, researchers measured insulin sensitivity and mitochondrial function in two groups of endurance-trained and sedentary young and older adults. Endurance training ameliorated the age-related decline in mitochondrial oxidative capacity in the older adults. Both the older and younger adults who underwent endurance training had higher levels of insulin sensitivity than the sedentary adults, but the amount of difference did not reach statistical significance.

Strength Training in Older Adults

Older adults can improve muscular strength and endurance and substantially increase their functional capacity. Strength training helps offset the loss of muscle and the decline in strength seen with normal aging, according to the American College of Sports Medicine's position stand.[81] Older adults should participate in aerobic activities, strength training, and exercises for postural stability and flexibility. Vandervoort[93] states that the benefits and guidelines for strength training in older individuals can be summed up by, again, the old adage "use it or lose it."

Exercise is efficacious even in the oldest old. Physical frailty can be delayed by increasing the activity level of the older adult. Resistance exercise training and aerobic exercise training has been found to increase muscle strength and aerobic capacity by at least 20% to 30% in older adults.[81] In a recent Cochrane review,[94] progressive resistive training was shown to produce functional improvements in mobility and performance. Older adults were able to improve in activities such as getting up from a chair and stair climbing. These improvements were generally greater than improvements in walking speed, a very powerful predictor of health. Interestingly, the older adults were also able to improve their performance of more complex activities, such as preparing a meal and taking a bath, with progressive strength training.

Eccentric loading of muscles is recommended for older adults so that they take advantage of their relatively higher eccentric strength.[83] The eccentric part of the training program, as they describe, is implemented after a strength base has been established. Eventually, the eccentric training involves using weights that are greater than what the person can lift and lengthening the time it takes to eccentrically "let go" of the muscle. Although eccentric exercise has been found to improve strength,[95] concentric training demonstrated the greatest gains when compared with isometric or eccentric training.[87] Eighteen men and twelve women with mean ages of 73 participated in a 12-week training program using a Biodex. They were divided into three groups: isometric, concentric, and eccentric. All three exhibited increases in strength: peak isometric, isokinetic concentric, and eccentric of the knee extensors. The strength improvement manifested as functional improvement in stair climbing.

Progressive resistive exercise is the most common type of exercise used with older adults and has been shown to be very effective for increasing their strength.[96] In a meta-analysis, Steib, Schoene, and Pfeifer[97] concluded that there was strong evidence for training at high intensities for maximizing strength adaptations compared with moderate to lower intensities. However, the ability to maximize strength does not necessarily carry over to functional improvement. In fact, low to moderate exercise intensity was shown to have considerable effects on function and strength measures of older adults. Specific exercises related to activities of daily living are seen as a promising strategy for enhancing function in older adults. Interestingly, studies using power training showed improved chair rising and stair climbing but did not provide an advantage to performing a timed up and go test or positively impact walking speed. More research is recommended to establish appropriate recommendations for resistive training in older adults.

Aerobic exercise and endurance training can increase VO_{2max}, which typically declines with age. Aerobic exercise improves the ability of the muscle to use oxygen. Endurance training increases VO_{2max} by increasing cardiac output or by widening the arterial-to-venous oxygen difference.[98] For example, the maximum amount of oxygen available to a 75-year-old master athlete may be 85 mL/min/kg compared with 15 mL/min/kg for a debilitated 75-year-old person. If 12 mL/min/kg is required to walk at 3 miles per hour, walking would "cost" the athlete 14% of VO_{2max} compared with 80% for the debilitated older adult. However, Aagaard and colleagues[48] recommended long-term strength training over aerobic training to counter the age-related loss of muscle mass and subsequent strength with increasing age, reinforcing the ACSM guidelines, which include multiple forms of exercise for older adults to maximize function. Ideally, muscles need to produce force at all contraction velocities (eccentric and concentric). The optimal contraction velocity needs to be correlated with the functional demands of the task. If loads are varied, it may improve

functional performance. Traditional resistance training does not improve eccentric force production, which is important for fall prevention and for many ADL activities.[60,80] (For additional discussion on cardiovascular changes with aging and fitness issues, see Chapters 8 and 15.)

SUMMARY

Many factors can influence muscle development both before and after birth, including genetics, nutrition, and activity levels. Muscle maturation occurs in childhood, and the rate of that maturation may limit the speed and dexterity with which a child can perform motor tasks. Strength development in childhood and adolescence increases with age.[26,29] Anaerobic function also improves during the same time period.[68] Physiological mismatching can occur in adolescence, when skeletal growth temporarily outstrips the ability of limb muscles to lengthen. Strength gains increase with age to maturity and then decline in middle adulthood.

After the age of 50, the loss of muscle mass, known as sarcopenia, can affect strength and functional abilities. As we age, maintaining functional independence has a great deal to do with remaining physically active. During the last decade, key research has been published on the effects of strength training in older adults. Knowledge of how and why weakness occurs is far more abundant than in previous decades. Age-related changes in muscle cannot be stopped, but they can be slowed. The only known way to slow them is to maintain a healthy nutritional status and to exercise on a regular basis. Exercise needs to be resistive in nature and include power training, eccentric loading, and functional activities. Human muscle remains responsive to these factors throughout the life span. Even aged muscle is trainable with the appropriate endurance and resistance goals. As part of our role as advocates for healthy aging, we refer you to the National Institutes of Health website http://nihseniorhealth.gov/exerciseforolderadults/toc.html, which is designed to motivate older adults to exercise.

REFERENCES

1. Lieber RL: *Skeletal muscle structure and function: implications for rehabilitation and sports medicine*, Baltimore, 1992, Williams & Wilkins.
2. Lieber RL, Friden J: Functional and clinical significance of skeletal muscle architecture, *Muscle Nerve* 23:1647–1666, 2000.
3. Lieber RL: *Skeletal muscle structure, function, and plasticity*, Philadelphia, 2010, Wolters Kluwer/Lippincott Williams & Wilkins.

4. McArdle WD, Katch FI, Katch VL: *Exercise physiology: energy, nutrition and human performance*, ed 7, Philadelphia, 2010, Wolter Kluwer/Lippincott Williams & Wilkins.

5. Uusitalo M, Kivela T: Development of cytoskeleton in neuroectodermally derived epithelial and muscle cells of human eye, *Invest Ophthalmol Vis Sci* 36:2584–2591, 1995.

6. Colling-Saltin AS: Skeletal muscle development in the human fetus and during childhood. In Berg K, Eriksson BO, editors: *Children and exercise IX*, Baltimore, 1980, University Park Press, pp 193–207.

7. Carlson BM: *Human embryology and developmental biology*, ed 4, St Louis, 2009, Mosby.

8. Minguetti G, Mair WG: Ultrastructure of developing human muscle: The problem of multinucleation of striated muscle cells, *Arq Neuropsiquiatr* 44:1–14, 1986.

9. Mastaglia FL: The growth and development of the skeletal muscles. In Davis JA, Dobbing J, editors: *Scientific foundations of paediatrics*, Philadelphia, 1974, WB Saunders, pp 348–375.

10. Schultz E, Lipton BH: Skeletal muscle satellite cells: changes in proliferation potential as a function of age, *Mech Ageing Dev* 20:377–383, 1982.

11. Le Grand F, Rudnicki M: Satellite and stem cells in muscle growth and repair, *Development* 134:3953–3957, 2007.

12. Moore KL, Persaud TVN: *The developing human: clinically oriented embryology*, ed 7, Philadelphia, 2003, WB Saunders.

13. Hesselmans LF, Jennekens FG, Van Den Oord CJ, et al: Development of innervation of skeletal muscle fibers in man: relation to acetylcholine receptors, *Anat Rec* 236:553–562, 1993.

14. Grinnell AD: Dynamics of nerve-muscle interaction in developing and mature neuromuscular junctions, *Physiol Rev* 75:789–834, 1995.

15. Malina RM, Bouchard C, Bar-Or O: *Growth, maturation and physical activity*, ed 2, Champaign, Ill, 2004, Human Kinetics.

16. Crelin ES: Development of the musculoskeletal system, *Clin Symp* 33:2–36, 1981.

17. Keens TG, Bryan AC, Levison H, et al: Developmental pattern of muscle fiber types in human ventilatory muscles, *J Appl Physiol* 44:909–913, 1978.

18. Elder GC, Kakulas BA: Histochemical and contractile property changes during human muscle development, *Muscle Nerve* 16:1246–1253, 1993.

19. Lexell J, Sjostrom M, Nordlund A, et al: Growth and development of human muscle: a quantitative morphological study of whole vastus lateralis from childhood to adult age, *Muscle Nerve* 15:4040–4049, 1992.

20. Gatev V, Stamatova L, Angelova B: Contraction time in skeletal muscles of normal children, *Electromyogr Clin Neurophysiol* 17:441–452, 1977.

21. Lin JP, Brown JK, Walsh EG: Physiological maturation of muscles in childhood, *Lancet* 343:1386–1389, 1994.

22. Lin JP, Brown JK, Walsh EG: The maturation of motor dexterity, or why Johnny can't go any faster, *Dev Med Child Neurol* 38:244–254, 1996.

23. Brooke MH, Engel WK: Histographic analyses of human muscle biopsies with regard to fiber types: 4. Children's biopsies, *Neurology* 19:591–605, 1969.

24. Malina RM: Growth of muscle and muscle mass. In Faulkner R, Tanner JM, editor: *Human growth: a comprehensive treatise, vol. 2: postnatal growth*, New York, 1986, Plenum Press, pp 77–99.

25. Beunen G, Thomis M: Muscular strength development in children and adolescents, *Pediatr Exerc Sci* 12:174–197, 2000.

26. Tonson A, Ratel S, Le Fur Y, et al: Effect of maturation on the relationship between muscle size and force production, *Med Sci Sports Exerc* 40(5):918–925, 2008.

27. Wiggin M, Wilkinson K, Habetz S, et al: Percentile values of isokinetic peak torque in children six through thirteen years old, *Pediatr Phys Ther* 18:3–18, 2006.

28. Sinclair D, Dangerfield P: *Human growth after birth*, ed 6, Oxford, UK, 1998, Oxford University Press.

29. De Ste Croix M: Advances in paediatric strength assessment: changing our perspective on strength development, *J Sport Sci Med* 6:292–304, 2007.

30. Larsson L, Grimby G, Karlsson J: Muscle strength and speed of movement in relation to age and muscle morphology, *J Appl Physiol* 46:451–456, 1979.

31. Greenlund LJS, Nair KS: Sarcopenia - consequences, mechanisms, and potential therapies, *Mech Age Dev* 124:287–299, 2003.

32. Nair KS: Aging muscle, *Am J Clin Nutr* 81:953–963, 2005.

33. Vandervoort AA: Aging of the human neuromuscular system, *Muscle Nerve* 25:17–25, 2002.

34. Suominen H: Physical activity and health: musculoskeletal issues, *Adv Physiother* 9:65–75, 2007.

35. Connelly DM: Resisted exercise training of institutionalized older adults for improved strength and functional mobility: a review, *Top Geriatr Rehabil* 15:6–28, 2000.

36. Lexell J: Human aging, muscle mass, and fiber type composition, *J Gerontol* 50A(special issue):11–16, 1995.

37. Goodpaster BH, Park SW, Harris TB, et al: The loss of skeletal muscle strength, mass, and quality in older adults: the health, aging and body composition study, *J Gerontol A Biol Sci Med Sci* 61A:1059–1064, 2006.

38. Baumgartner RN, Koehler KM, Gallagher D, et al: Epidemiology of sarcopenia among the elderly in New Mexico, *Am J Epidemiol* 147:755–763, 1998.

39. Iannuzzi-Sucich M, Prestwood KM, Kenny AM: Prevalence of sarcopenia and predictors of skeletal muscle mass in healthy, older men and women, *J Gerontol A Biol Sci Med Sci* 57A:M772–M777, 2002.

40. Janssen I, Heymsfield SB, Wang AM, et al: Skeletal muscle mass and distribution in 468 men and women ages 18–88 yr, *J Appl Physiol* 89:81–88, 2000.

41. Janssen I, Heymsfield SB, Ross R: Low relative skeletal muscle mass (sarcopenia) in older persons is associated with functional impairment and physical disability, *J Am Geriatr Soc* 50:889–896, 2002.

42. Jones TE, Stephenson KW, King JG, et al: Sarcopenia - mechanisms and treatments, *J Geriatr Phys Ther* 32:39–45, 2009.

43. Di Orio A, Abate M, Di Renzo D, et al: Sarcopenia: age-related skeletal muscle changes form determinants to physical disability, *Int J Immunopathol Pharmacol* 19(4):703–719, 2006.

44. Doherty TJ: Invited review: aging and sarcopenia, *J Appl Physiol* 95:1717–1727, 2003.

45. Marcel TJ: Sarcopenia: causes, consequences, and prevention, *J Gerontol A Biol Sci Med Sci* 58A(10):911–916, 2003.

46. Eynon N, Yamin C, Ben-Sira D: Optimal health and function among the elderly: lessening severity of ADL disability, *Eur Rev Aging Phys Act* 6:55–61, 2009.

47. Doherty TJ: The influence of aging and sex on skeletal muscle mass and strength, *Curr Opin Clin Nutr Metab Care* 4:503–508, 2001.

48. Aagaard P, Magnusson PS, Larsson B, et al: Mechanical muscle function, morphology, and fiber type in lifelong trained elderly, *Med Sci Sports Exerc* 39(11):1989–1996, 2007.

49. McComas AJ: Invited review: motor unit estimation: methods, results, and present studies, *Muscle Nerve* 14:585–597, 1991.

50. Thomlinson BE, Irving D: The numbers of limb motor neurons in the human lumbosacral cord throughout life, *J Neurol Sci* 34:213–260, 1977.

51. Roos MR, Rice CL, Vandervoort AA: Age-related change in motor unit function, *Muscle Nerve* 20:679–690, 1997.

52. Powers SK, Jackson MJ: Exercise-induced oxidative stress: cellular mechanisms and impact on muscle force production, *Physiol Rev* 88:1243–1276, 2008.

53. Schaap LA, Saskia MF, Deeg DJH, et al: Inflammatory markers and loss of muscle mass (sarcopenia) and strength, *Am J Med* 119:526.e9–526.e17, 2009.

54. Roth SM, Metter EJ, Ling S, et al: Inflammatory factors in age-related muscle wasting, *Curr Opin Rheumatol* 18(6):625–630, 2006.

55. Evans WJ: Protein nutrition, exercise and aging, *J Am Coll Nutr* 23(6):601S–609S, 2004.

56. Boire Y: Physiopathological mechanism of sarcopenia, *J Nutr Health Aging* 13(8):717–723, 2009.

57. Guttman E, Hazlikova V: Fast and slow motor units and aging, *J Gerontol* 22:280–300, 1976.

58. Metzger JM, Moss RL: Calcium-sensitive cross-bridge transitions in mammalian fast and slow skeletal muscle fibres, *Science* 247:1088–1090, 1990.

59. Raz IS, Bird SR, Shield AJ: Aging and the force-velocity relationship of muscles, *Exp Gerontol* 45:81–90, 2010.

60. Carville SF, Perry MC, Rutherford OM, et al: Steadiness of quadriceps contractions in young and older adults with and without a history of falling, *Eur J Appl Physiol* 100:527–533, 2007.

61. Hortobagyi T, Zheng DH, Weidner M, et al: The influence of aging on muscle strength and muscle fiber characteristics with special reference to eccentric strength, *J Gerontol A Biol Sci Med Sci* 50:B399–B406, 1995.

62. Lexell J: Evidence for nervous system degeneration with advancing age, *J Nutr* 127:1011S–1013S, 1997.

63. Frontera WR, Evans WJ: Exercise performance and endurance training in the elderly, *Top Geriatr Rehabil* 2:17–32, 1986.

64. Fitts RH: Mechanisms of muscular fatigue. In Poortmans JR, editor: *Principles of exercise biochemistry*, ed 3, New York, 2004, Karger, pp 279–300.

65. Enoka RM, Duchateau J: Muscle fatigue: what, why and how it influences muscle function, *J Physiol* 586:11–23, 2008.

66. Hunter SK: Sex differences and mechanisms of task-specific muscle fatigue, *Exerc Sport Sci Rev* 37(3):113–122, 2009.

67. Alexander NB, Taffet GE, Horne FM, et al: Bedside-to-Bench conference: research agenda for idiopathic fatigue and aging, *J Am Geriatr Soc* 58:967–975, 2010.

68. Van Praagh E: Anaerobic fitness tests: what are we measuring? *Med Sport Sci* 50:26–45, 2007.

69. Rowland TW: *Children's exercise physiology*, ed 2, Champaign, Ill, 2005, Human Kinetics.

70. Van Praagh E: Development of anaerobic function during childhood and adolescence, *Pediatr Exerc Sci* 12:150–173, 2000.

71. Rowland TW: *Developmental exercise physiology*, Champaign, Ill, 1996, Human Kinetics.

72. Malina RM, Bouchard C: *Growth, maturation and physical activity*, Champaign, Ill, 1991, Human Kinetics.

73. Faigenbaum AD, Westcott WL, Loud RL, et al: The effects of different resistance training protocols on muscular strength and endurance development in children, *Pediatrics* 104:e5, 1999, (website) http://www.pediatrics.org/cgi/content/full/104/1/e5.

74. Malina RM: Weight training in youth - growth, maturation, and safety: an evidence-based review, *Clin J Sport Med* 16:478–487, 2006.

75. Benson AC, Torode ME, Fiatrarone Singh MA: A rationale and method for high-intensity progressive resistance training with children and adolescents, *Contemp Clin Trials* 28:442–450, 2007.

76. Faigenbaum AD: Resistance training for children and adolescents: are there health outcomes? *Am J Lifestyle Med* 1:190–200, 2007.

77. Behm DF, Faigenbaum AD, Falk B, et al: Canadian society for exercise physiology position paper: resistance training in children and adolescents, *Appl Physiol Nutr Metab* 33:547–561, 2008.

78. Bortz WM II: A conceptual framework of frailty: a review, *J Gerontol A Biol Sci Med Sci* 50:897–904, 2002.

79. Lowndes J, Carpenter RL, Zoeller RF, et al: Association of age with muscle size and strength before and after short-term resistance training in young adults, *J Strength Cond Res* 234(7):1915–1920, 2009.

80. Enoka RM, Christou EA, Hunter SK, et al: Mechanisms that contribute to differences in motor performance between young and old adults, *J Electromyogr Kinesiol* 13:1–12, 2003.

81. American College of Sports Medicine: Position stand: exercise and physical activity for older adults, *Med Sci Sports Exerc* 41(7):1510–1530, 2009.

82. Phillips BA, Lo SK, Mastaglia FL: Muscle force measured using "break" testing with a hand-held myometer in normal subjects aged 20–69 years, *Arch Phys Med Rehabil* 81:653–661, 2000.

83. Krishnathasan D, Vandervoort AA: Eccentric strength training prescription for older adults, *Top Geriatr Rehabil* 15:29–40, 2000.

84. Buchner DM, de Lateaur BJ: The importance of skeletal muscle strength to physical function in older adults, *Ann Behav Med* 13:91–98, 1991.

85. Chandler JM, Duncan PW, Kochersberger G, et al: Is lower extremity strength gain associated with improvement in physical performance and disability in frail, community-dwelling elders? *Arch Phys Med Rehabil* 79:24–30, 1998.

86. Pijnappels M, Reeves ND, Maganaris CN, et al: Tripping without falling: lower limb strength, a limitation for balance recovery and a target for training in the elderly, *J Electromyogr Kinesiol* 18:188–196, 2008.

87. Symons TB, Vandervoort AA, Rice CL, et al: Effects of maximal isometric and isokinetic resistance training on strength and functional mobility in older adults, *J Gerontol A Biol Sci Med Sci* 60A(6):777–781, 2005.

88. Metter EF, Conwit R, Tobin J, et al: Age-associated loss of power and strength in the upper extremities in women and men, *J Gerontol A Biol Sci Med Sci* 52:B267–B276, 1997.

89. Kraemer WJ, Newton RU: Training for muscular power, *Phys Med Rehabil Clin N Am* 11:341–368, 2000.

90. Puthoff ML, Nielsen DH: Relationships among impairments in lower-extremity strength and poser, functional limitations, and disability in older adults, *Phys Ther* 87:1334–1347, 2007.

91. Baudry S, Klass M, Pasquet B, et al: Age-related fatigability of the ankle dorsiflexor muscles during concentric and eccentric contractions, *Eur J Appl Physiol* 100:515–526, 2007.

92. Lanza IR, Short DK, Raghavakaimal S, et al: Endurance exercise as a countermeasure for aging, *Diabetes* 57(11):2933–2943, 2008.

93. Vandervoort AA: Introduction, *Top Geriatr Rehabil* 15:vi–viii, 2000.

94. Lui CJ, Latham NK: Progressive resistance strength training for improving physical function in older adults, *Cochrane Database Syst Rev* 3:CD002759, 2009.

95. Hortobagyi T, DeVita P: Favorable neuromuscular and cardiovascular responses to 7 days of exercise with an eccentric overload in elderly women, *J Gerontol A Biol Sci Med Sci* 55(8):B401–B410, 2000.

96. Latham NK, Anderson C, Bennett D, et al: Progressive resistance strength training for physical disability in older people, *Cochrane Database Syst Rev* 2:CD002759, 2003.

97. Steib S, Schoene D, Pfeifer K: Dose-response relationship of resistance training in older adults: a meta-analysis, *Med Sci Sports Exerc* 42(5):902–914, 2010.

98. Thompson LV: Physiological changes associated with aging. In Guccione AA, editor: *Geriatr Phys Ther*, ed 2, St Louis, 2000, Mosby, pp 28–55.

99. Faigenbaum AD, Kraemer WJ, Blimkie CJR, et al: Youth resistance training: updated position statement paper from the National Strength and Conditioning Association, *J Strength Cond Res* 23(Suppl 5):S60–S80, 2009.

100. Deschenes MR: Effects of aging on muscle fibre type and size, *Sports Med* 34(12):809–824, 2004.

101. Hunter GR, McCarthy FP, Bamman MM: Effects of resistance training on older adults, *Sports Med* 34(5):329–348, 2004.

102. Seynnes O, Fiatarone Singh MA, Hue O, et al: Physiological and functional responses to low-moderate versus high-intensity progressive resistance training in frail elders, *J Gerontol A Biol Sci Med Sci* 59(5):503–509, 2004.

103. Hakkinen K, Pakarinen A, Kraemer WJ, et al: Selective muscle hypertrophy, changes in EMG and force, and serum hormones during strength training in older women, *J Appl Physiol* 91:569–580, 2001.

104. Mueller M, Breil FA, Vogt M, et al: Different response to eccentric and concentric training in older men and women, *Eur J Appl Physiol* 107:145–153, 2009.

105. Fiatarone MA, O'Neill EF, Ryan ND, et al: Exercise training and nutritional supplementation for physical frailty in very elderly people, *N Engl J Med* 330:1769–1775, 1994.

106. Henwood TR, Riek S, Taaffe DR: Strength versus muscle power-specific resistance training in community-dwelling older adults, *J Gerontol A Biol Sci Med Sci* 63A(1):83–91, 2008.

107. Barry BK, Carson RG: Transfer of resistance training to enhance rapid coordinated force production by older adults, *Exp Brain Res* 159(2):225–238, 2004.

108. Cesari M, Pahor M, Lauretani F, et al: Skeletal muscle and mortality results from the InCHIANTI study, *J Gerontol A Biol Sci Med Sci* 64A(3):377–384, 2009.

109. Paterson DH, Jones GR, Rice CL: Ageing and physical activity: evidence to develop exercise recommendations for older adults, *Can J Public Health* 98(Suppl 2):S69–S108, 2007.

CHAPTER 8

Cardiovascular and Pulmonary Systems Changes

OBJECTIVES

After studying this chapter, the reader will be able to:

1. Describe structural and functional characteristics of the cardiovascular and pulmonary systems as they relate to physical functioning.
2. Discuss age-related structural and functional characteristics of the cardiovascular and pulmonary systems.

3. Relate age-related changes in the cardiovascular and pulmonary systems to physical functioning, activity, and participation.

Together, the cardiovascular and pulmonary systems deliver necessary nutrients and oxygen to body tissues, as well as remove waste products. Blood circulating through the vascular system provides the transport system for these substances. Oxygen is delivered to the blood via the pulmonary system. An understanding of the structure, function, and development of these two systems as they relate to how well a person can participate in daily activities is important to assess and promote functional movement and wellness across the life span.

COMPONENTS OF THE CARDIOVASCULAR AND PULMONARY SYSTEMS

Cardiovascular System

Components

The cardiovascular system is made up of the heart and the vascular network. Its purpose is to pump blood and to deliver it throughout the body. The blood is pumped from the heart through a high-pressure arterial system to the target organs. There, nutrients and waste products are exchanged between capillaries and tissues. The low-pressure venous system then returns blood to the heart. *Heart rate* refers to the number of times the heart beats per minute; *stroke volume* refers to the amount of blood that is pumped from the ventricle with each

heartbeat. By multiplying heart rate by stroke volume, one can determine the amount of blood pumped from the ventricles in 1 minute, which is referred to as *cardiac output.*

The Heart The heart is made up of four chambers and acts as the pump of the cardiovascular system. The cardiovascular pump works very differently before and after birth. Figure 8-1 depicts the prenatal circulation that permits most of the oxygenated blood to bypass the liver and lungs via 3 shunts: (1) ductus venosus, (2) foramen ovale, and (3) ductus arteriosus. Poorly oxygenated blood returns to the placenta for oxygen and nutrients from the umbilical arteries.[1] Dramatic changes occur in the cardiovascular and pulmonary systems at birth when the infant's lungs fill with air. The shunts are no longer needed and immediately start to close. Figure 8-2 illustrates postnatal circulation of blood through the heart, lungs, and periphery. After birth, the atria move blood into the ventricles, which then pump with sufficient force to deliver blood to the lungs and the periphery. The chambers of the right side of the heart receive blood from the periphery and pump it to the lungs to be oxygenated. The chambers on the left side of the heart then receive the oxygenated blood and pump it through the aorta to the systemic circulation. Valves in the heart ensure unidirectional blood flow. The tricuspid and mitral valves, found between the atria and ventricles, prevent blood from flowing back into the atria during ventricular contraction. The aortic and pulmonary valves,

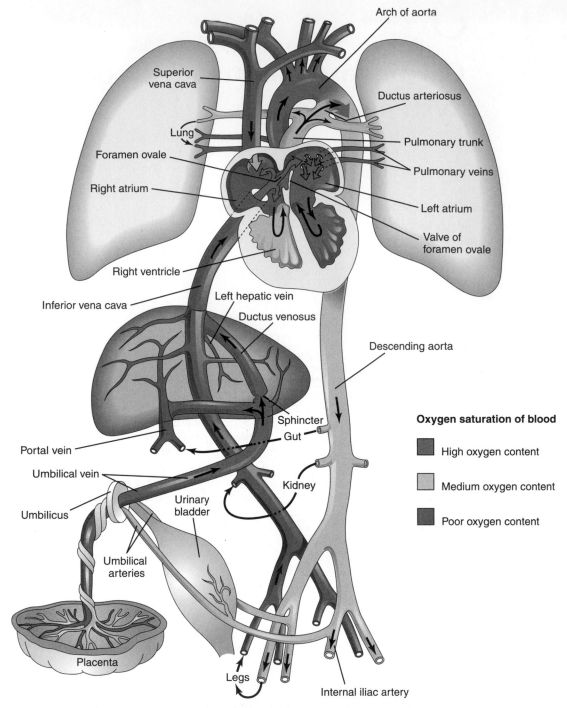

Figure 8-1 Schematic of the fetal circulation. The shades of blue (dark to light) indicate the oxygen saturation of the blood, and the arrows show the course of the blood from the placenta to the heart. The organs are not drawn to scale. Three shunts: (1) ductus venosus, (2) foramen ovale, and (3) ductus arteriosus permit most of the blood to bypass the liver and lungs. The poorly oxygenated blood returns to the placenta for oxygen and nutrients through the umbilical arteries. (From Moore KL, Persaud TVN: *Before we are born: essentials of embryology and birth defects,* ed 5, Philadelphia, 1998, WB Saunders, p 370.)

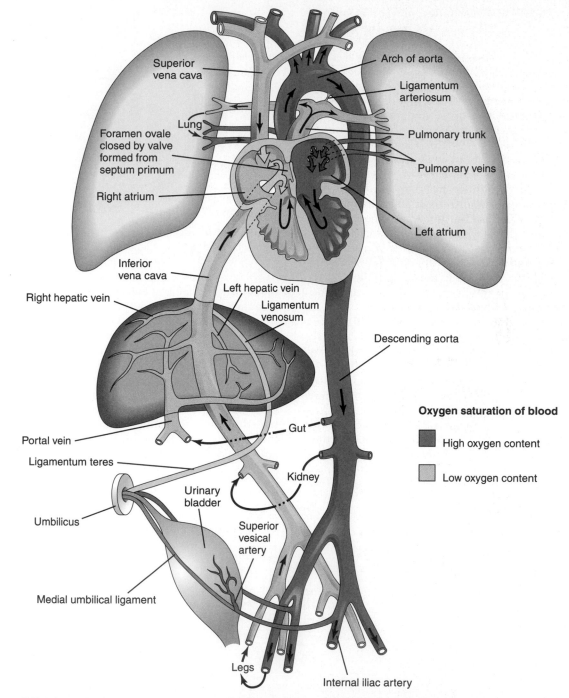

Figure 8-2 Schematic of the neonatal circulation. The adult *derivatives* of the fetal vessels and structures that become nonfunctional at birth are also shown. The arrows indicate the course of the blood in the infant. The organs are not drawn to scale. After birth, the *three shunts* that short-circuited the blood during fetal life cease to function, and the pulmonary and systemic circulations *separate*. (From Moore KL, Persaud TVN: *Before we are born: essentials of embryology and birth defects*, ed 5, Philadelphia, 1998, WB Saunders, p 371.)

also called the *semilunar valves,* prevent blood from flowing back into the ventricles from the aorta and pulmonary artery.

Structurally, the heart is made up of three layers, which are also called *tunics* (Figure 8-3). The inner layer, the *endocardium,* is made up of a single layer of squamous endothelial cells and a layer of connective tissue. The connective tissue contains blood vessels, nerves, and branches of the conducting system of the heart. The middle layer, the *myocardium,* is the thick muscular layer of the heart and is richly supplied with capillaries. Cardiac muscle cells in the myocardium are able to conduct electricity, but they also have a long refractory period, allowing them to maintain rhythmic heart contraction. The outer layer, the *epicardium,* is made up of loose connective tissue and fat that is covered by simple squamous epithelium. Large blood vessels, such as the coronary arteries, and nerves that supply the heart are found in the epicardium.

Contraction of the heart muscle is controlled by the cardiac conducting system, which consists of the sinoatrial node, atrioventricular node, and atrioventricular bundle of His (Figure 8-4). The conduction system contains specialized cardiac muscle cells that carry impulses faster than other myocardial cells. The stimulus for cardiac contraction originates in the sinoatrial node, the pacemaker of the heart. Autonomic nerve and ganglion cells are also found near and in the node. These cells influence the circulatory and nervous system and help regulate heart rate and contractility. The atrioventricular node receives the impulse from

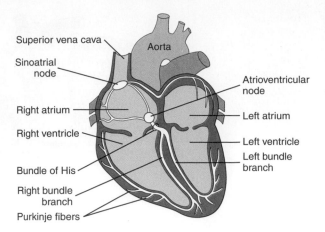

Figure 8-4 The conducting system of the heart. (From Gartner LP, Hiatt JL: *Color textbook of histology,* ed 2, Philadelphia, 2001, WB Saunders, p 267.)

the sinoatrial node and delays it slightly, allowing the atria time to empty before the ventricles contract. The atrioventricular bundle of His and its branches then carry the stimulus to the ventricles. From there, the contractile stimulus is transmitted from one cardiac muscle fiber to another, resulting in a wave of cardiac contractions. The conduction system of the heart is a coordinating system. Each part of it can conduct or initiate an impulse on its own, but the rhythm is controlled because the sinoatrial node fires first. When the sinoatrial node is not functioning properly, cardiac arrhythmias occur.

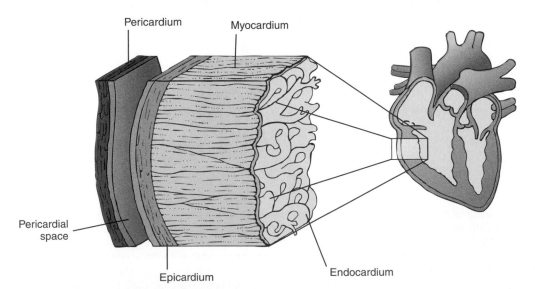

Figure 8-3 Layers of the heart. (From Black JM, Matassarin-Jacobs E: *Medical-surgical nursing: clinical management for continuity of care,* ed 5, Philadelphia, 1997, WB Saunders, p 1192.)

The Vascular System Three main types of vessels make up the vascular system: *arteries, capillaries,* and *veins.* Arteries and veins are structurally similar to the heart in that they are made up of three concentric layers (Figure 8-5). The inner layer, *tunica intima,* is made up

of a layer of endothelial cells and a subendothelial layer of elastic connective tissue. Some smooth muscle cells are also found in the subendothelial layer. The middle layer, *tunica media,* consists of concentric layers of smooth muscle cells, elastic fibers, collagen fibers, and

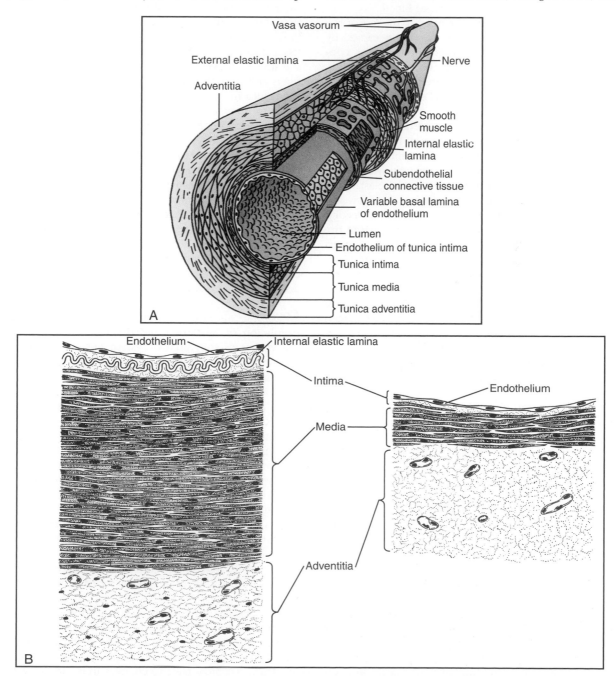

Figure 8-5 A, Diagram of a typical artery showing the three layers: tunica intima, tunica media, and tunica adventitia. **B,** Comparison of muscular artery (*left*) and accompanying vein (*right*). (**A** From Gartner LP, Hiatt JL: *Color textbook of histology,* Philadelphia, 1997, WB Saunders, p 213; **B** from Junqueira LC, Carneiro J, Kelley RO: *Basic histology,* ed 10, Large Medical Books McGraw-Hill. Medical Pub Division, 2003.)

proteoglycans. The outer layer, *tunica adventitia,* is made up of fibroelastic connective tissue. Small blood vessels, *vasa vasorum,* are found in the media and adventitia layers of large vessels. They nourish the thicker layers of the vessel, where sufficient nutrition cannot be supplied by diffusion from the circulating blood.

Arteries carry blood from the heart to the rest of the body and minimize fluctuations in pressure caused by the heartbeat. For instance, when the ventricles contract, the arteries are stretched, decreasing pressure. When the ventricles relax, the arteries return to their original size and maintain the level of pressure.

Arteries can be divided into three groups. The large elastic arteries, called *conducting arteries,* include the aorta and its main branches. The tunica media of these vessels is made up of layers of elastic membrane, which makes them efficient at absorbing the pressure changes that accompany each heartbeat. Almost no elastin layers are present in the aorta at birth, but this increases to 40 to 70 layers in the adult.[2] The second category, the *muscular,* or *distributing arteries,* are branches of the large elastic arteries that supply blood to the organs and extremities. The tunica media of the distributing arteries is made of up to 40 layers of smooth muscle cells that regulate blood flow in response to nervous system or hormonal input. Connective tissue, including elastic and collagen fibers, can be found between the muscular layers. The third category of arteries, the *arterioles,* are small vessels that deliver blood to the capillaries. The tunica intima of the arteriole consists of a layer of endothelium and an internal elastic membrane. The tunica media is made of one to five layers of smooth muscle cells and a few elastic fibers. Vasoconstriction and vasodilation of the arterioles control the systemic blood pressure so that only a slow steady stream of blood enters the capillaries. The arterioles are innervated by the autonomic nervous system and can quickly react to functional needs of the tissue.

Capillaries provide a site for the exchange of nutrients and waste products between the blood and the tissue, connect the arterial and venous systems, and contain a large volume of the blood in the body. The capillary itself is a small vessel, made up of a single layer of endothelial cells surrounded by a thin layer of collagen fibers. Areas of the body with high metabolic needs, such as the lungs, liver, kidneys, cardiac muscle, and skeletal muscle, have large capillary networks.

Veins are responsible for carrying blood back to the heart and for the transport of waste products from the tissue. Veins have larger diameters and thinner walls than do arteries. Because of their size and the large number of veins that make up the venous system, blood flows back to the heart slowly and at low pressure.

Veins can be divided into three major categories by size. *Venules,* the smallest veins, receive blood from the capillaries. The diameter of the venule is greater than that of the capillary and serves to slow the rate of blood flow. As the venule size increases, layers of connective tissue and then smooth muscle cells are added. When the size of the venule is approximately 50 μm, elastic fibers and smooth muscle fibers can be found between the tunica intima and the tunica adventitia. The next category of *small to medium-sized* veins includes most named veins in the body and their branches. These veins contain valves that maintain unidirectional flow of blood. The tunica intima and tunica media are thin, whereas the tunica adventitia is thick. The *large veins* make up the third category of veins and include the superior vena cava, inferior vena cava, portal vein, pulmonary veins, abdominal veins, and main tributaries. The tunica adventitia is the thickest and most developed component of these veins, containing longitudinal bundles of smooth muscle fibers. These muscle cells strengthen the venous wall and help to prevent distention.

Control

Regulation of heart rate and dilation/constriction of the vessels of the vascular system are influenced by the autonomic nervous system and by the presence of chemicals in the circulation. Nervous system control originates in the medulla and is carried via the sympathetic and parasympathetic branches of the autonomic nervous system.

Autonomic fibers are found within the cardiac conducting system. Sympathetic input to the heart increases the rate and strength of cardiac contraction via the release of catecholamines (epinephrine and norepinephrine). Sympathetic innervation of smooth muscle cells in the tunica media of the arteries and the tunica media and tunica adventitia of the veins stimulates vasoconstriction. Parasympathetic input to the heart is received via the vagus nerve and slows the heart rate by releasing acetylcholine. Skeletal muscle arteries also dilate in response to parasympathetic input.

The vascular system relates sensory information to the nervous system through the stretch-sensitive *baroreceptors,* found in the aorta and carotid sinus, and the *chemoreceptors,* found in the carotid and aortic bodies. These receptors react to changes in blood pressure, levels of oxygen and carbon dioxide in the circulating blood, and acidity (pH) of the blood.

Mechanics of Circulation

Blood flow is regulated by pressures exerted by the various structures in the system. Within the heart, *preload* is the amount of pressure necessary to stretch the ventricles during cardiac filling. *Afterload* is the amount of pressure that must be exerted by the ventricles to overcome aortic pressure, open the aortic valve, and push the blood out toward the periphery. The vessels then continue to control blood flow, not only because of the neural and chemical influences described here but also because of their physical properties. Length and diameter of the vessels help to determine peripheral vascular resistance and to influence the speed of blood flow. Blood pressure is actually the pressure exerted by the blood on the vessels as it flows through them.

For efficient mechanical control of blood flow, the blood pressure must be sufficient for blood to flow through the system and must stretch the ventricles during preload. It must likewise not be so high that afterload is increased, making the ventricles work harder to overcome aortic pressure and to empty. In individuals with *hypertension* (high blood pressure), the chronic increased aortic pressure eventually leads to left ventricular hypertrophy because the ventricle has been working so hard to maintain adequate stroke volume. This can eventually contribute to congestive heart failure.

Pulmonary System

Components

The pulmonary system consists of the lungs and the structures that connect the lungs to the external environment. It is a closed system, open to the external environment only at the nose and mouth.

The system can be divided into two major structural parts: the conducting portion and the respiratory portion (Figure 8-6). Functionally, the pulmonary system can be divided into the ventilatory pump and the respiratory component.

Conducting Portion　When considering the structural components of the pulmonary system, the conducting portion of the pulmonary system provides a pathway for air to travel between the environment and the lungs. In this portion, no gas exchange takes

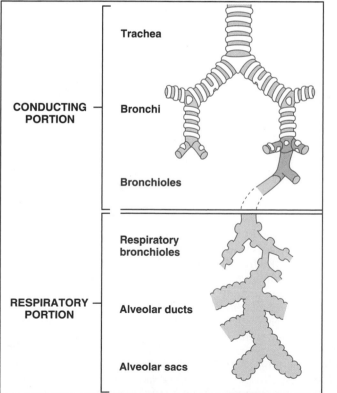

Figure 8-6 The main divisions of the pulmonary system: the conducting portion and the respiratory portion. (From Costanzo LS: *Physiology*. Philadelphia, 1998, WB Saunders, 164.)

place, but the air is cleaned, moistened, and warmed. The conducting portion of the pulmonary system includes the nose, pharynx, larynx, and trachea and portions of the bronchial tree in the lungs. The conducting portion of the bronchial tree includes the two main bronchi, bronchi to the main lobes and to the segments of the lungs, and bronchioles. The diameter of these conducting tubes decreases with each successive branching, helping to regulate the flow of air during inspiration and expiration. The *bronchi* are made up of hyaline cartilage and smooth muscle cells. The muscle cells are arranged in spirals and increase in number closer to the respiratory portion of the pulmonary system. The *bronchioles* are made up of smooth muscle cells and elastic fibers. Sympathetic nervous system input via the vagus nerve influences contraction of the smooth muscle cells and changes in length and diameter of the conducting vessels in the bronchial tree.

Respiratory Portion   The respiratory portion of the pulmonary system includes the remaining branches of the bronchial tree, alveolar ducts, alveolar sacs, and alveoli. As air is moved through these structures, gas exchange takes place. Respiratory bronchioles differ from conducting bronchioles because they have alveoli along their walls. At the alveolar level, only a very thin barrier is found between the air and the circulating blood. Alveoli are not only found in the respiratory bronchioles; large numbers of alveoli branch off of the alveolar ducts and alveolar sacs. *Alveolar sacs* (clusters of alveoli) and alveoli branch off of alveolar ducts, which contain smooth muscle cells, elastic fibers, and collagen fibers. Elastic and reticular fibers are found where the alveoli arise from the respiratory bronchioles, alveolar ducts, or alveolar sacs. The elastic fibers help to open the alveoli during inspiration and allow recoil during exhalation. Reticular fibers help maintain the shape of the alveoli.

Alveolar epithelium is made up of two types of cells. *Type I* alveolar cells are flat and thin respiratory epithelial cells, providing a large surface area for gas exchange. *Type II* cells are responsible for the production of surfactant, the detergent-like substance that mixes with water to decrease the alveolar surface tension. The decreased surface tension allows the alveoli to open more easily during respiration. Without surfactant, alveolar collapse can occur. This is especially important for the newborn. Lack of surfactant in the premature infant results in respiratory distress. Surfactant is constantly produced and turned over throughout life.

Air can also move from one part of the respiratory system to another via collateral ventilation mechanisms. Two mechanisms of collateral ventilation are pores of Kohn and Lambert canals. *Pores of Kohn* are gaps in the alveolar walls that provide an opening from one alveolus and its neighbor. *Lambert canals,* or *channels,* are small pathways from the respiratory bronchi to nearby alveoli. The pores of Kohn also help with distribution of surfactant over the alveolar surface, which helps maintain the surface tension and prevent atelectasis.[3]

Functional Components of the Pulmonary System
The pulmonary system can also be divided into 2 functional components: the ventilator pump and the respiratory component. The ventilatory pump component controls the flow of gases. It is made up of the respiratory muscles, thorax, diaphragm, and abdominal compartments.

The respiratory component is the site of gas exchange and consists of the lungs, intrapulmonary airways, and intrapulmonary vessels.

Control and Regulation

Ventilation is controlled by input from the respiratory center of the central nervous system, located in the brain stem. Chemoreceptors detect changes in blood levels of oxygen and carbon dioxide, as well as the pH of the blood, stimulating appropriate respiratory changes. Proprioceptive input from stretch receptors in the lungs also stimulates respiration.

The pulmonary system is innervated by the parasympathetic and sympathetic branches of the autonomic nervous system. Parasympathetic input results in bronchial constriction, whereas sympathetic input results in bronchodilation. Sensory and motor nerve fibers are found in the lung to the level of the terminal bronchioles.

Mechanics of Ventilation

The lungs, thorax, intercostal muscles, and diaphragm provide a pumping action that transports gas between the environment and the alveoli. During inspiration, the intercostal muscles contract to elevate the rib cage. The diaphragm also contracts, increasing the diameter of the thoracic cavity. This muscle activity expands the pleural cavity and results in increased negative pressure in the thoracic cavity. Atmospheric air rushes in, and the lungs expand. Bronchi and bronchioles increase in diameter. The expansion of the lungs activates stretch receptors, inhibiting inspiration. Exhalation occurs passively, with muscle relaxation and elastic recoil of the chest wall. Inhibitory input to inspiration is decreased, once again activating inspiration.

The ability of the musculoskeletal pump to transport inspiratory and expiratory gases is influenced by the compliance and resistance of the chest wall and lungs. Flexibility of the joints of the thoracic cavity contributes to achieving optimal expansion of the space. Resistance and elasticity of the pulmonary tissues must be overcome by contraction of the respiratory muscles, diaphragm, intercostal muscles, and accessory muscles of respiration. Resistance of the conducting airways also affects the amount of work necessary to deliver air to the respiratory system.

The amount of air contained in the lungs is defined by various functional volumes (Figure 8-7). The maximal amount of air that can be contained in the lungs is referred to as the total lung capacity. The amount of air moved during resting inspiration and exhalation is referred to as the tidal volume (TV). The additional inspired air that can be taken into the lungs with a deep breath is called the inspiratory reserve volume (IRV); the additional air that can be pushed out of the lungs with forced exhalation is called the expiratory reserve volume (ERV). The sum of these three volumes is called the vital capacity (VC). The residual volume (RV) is the amount of air that is left in the lungs after exhalation. Minute ventilation (MV) is the total amount of air exchanged by the pulmonary system in 1 minute. Forced expiratory volume (FEV) can also be measured, and the amount of gas expired in the first second of a forced vital capacity test is referred to as FEV1. The FEV1 is used to measure airway resistance.

Resistance and compliance factors, the breathing rate, and the amount of air being moved with each breath determine the energy cost of breathing. The pulmonary system itself requires oxygen to fuel the work of breathing. The source of that oxygen is the bronchial arteries, which deliver blood from the aorta to the lung tissue. Blood is then returned to the heart via the pulmonary and bronchial veins.

DEVELOPMENT OF THE CARDIOVASCULAR AND PULMONARY SYSTEMS ACROSS THE LIFE SPAN

Prenatal Period

Cardiovascular System

The cardiovascular system is the earliest system of the body to function in the developing embryo, with blood circulation starting in the third week of gestation. Functionally, this circulation is necessary because the embryo has grown, and simple diffusion of nutrients and waste products across cell membranes can no longer meet nutritional demands.

By the end of the third week of gestation, a primitive heart tube has been formed from clusters of mesoderm cells. As this tube elongates, a series of dilations and constrictions differentiate the vessel into an atrium, a ventricle, the truncus arteriosus, and the sinus venosus. The sinus venosus functions early as the pacemaker of the conducting system of the heart and is the precursor to the sinoatrial node, atrioventricular node, and bundle of His. At approximately 4 weeks of gestation, areas of swelling form on the walls of the atrioventricular canal. These swellings, called *endocardial cushions,* grow together during the fifth week of gestation and begin to divide the heart into left and right chambers.

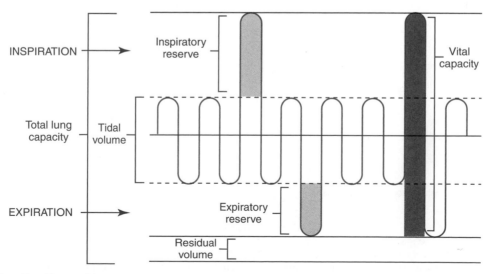

Figure 8-7 Functional lung volumes.

The primitive atrium is also divided into two chambers by the formation of the septum primum and the septum secundum. An oval opening left between the interatrial septae, called the *foramen ovale,* is important for fetal circulation. Near the end of the fourth week of gestation, contractions of the heart coordinate unidirectional flow of blood. By the seventh week, the heart tube has become a four-chambered vessel.

The embryo's primitive heart tube establishes links with its blood vessels and with the placenta as early as 13 to 15 days of gestation. Circulation is then established between the mother and the embryo, ensuring the exchange of nutrients and waste products. Maternal nutrients and oxygen are transported to the fetus via the umbilical vein; waste products and carbon dioxide are removed via the umbilical artery. By the fifth week of development, embryonic vessel formation is underway.

Vascular development begins with the differentiation of mesodermal cells into vessels, which then form larger vascular networks in organs such as the liver and endocardium of the heart. Further development of the vessels occurs as branches are formed from existing vessels. This process is called *angiogenesis* and can occur in embryonic development, as well as throughout the life span.

The fetus receives all necessary oxygen from the mother; little blood flow is necessary through the lungs. Fetal hemoglobin levels are higher than postnatal hemoglobin levels. This is necessary because the oxygen saturation of blood coming to the fetus from the umbilical vein is only 70% compared with an arterial blood oxygen saturation of 97% after birth. By having an increased hemoglobin level, the fetus has a greater capacity to carry oxygen to the tissues.

Pulmonary System

The pulmonary system of the embryo arises from both endodermal and mesodermal germ cells and first appears in the fourth week of gestation. Endodermal cells from the primitive pharynx form the epithelial lining of trachea, larynx, bronchi, and lungs. Mesoderm surrounding the developing lung buds contributes to the development of smooth muscle, connective tissue, and cartilage within these structures.

Early development of the fetal pulmonary system is shown in Figure 8-8. At 28 days of gestation, *bronchial buds* have developed at the end of the laryngotracheal tube and have divided into the right and left lung buds. At 35 days, secondary bronchi have appeared. By 42 days, all of the branches of the conducting airways have been formed. Between 42 and 56 days of

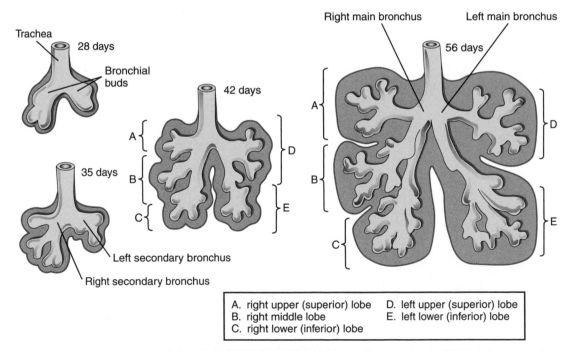

A. right upper (superior) lobe   D. left upper (superior) lobe
B. right middle lobe   E. left lower (inferior) lobe
C. right lower (inferior) lobe

Figure 8-8 Successive stages in the development of bronchi and lungs. (From Moore KL, Persaud TVN: *Before we are born: essentials of embryology and birth defects,* ed 5, Philadelphia, 1998, WB Saunders, p 247.)

gestation, branching has continued to the level of at least two respiratory bronchioles. Formation of the pulmonary arterial tree accompanies the branching of the respiratory tree.

The bronchial epithelium thins and flattens, increasing the diameter of the bronchi and terminal bronchioles. Capillaries also appear in the epithelium. From 24 weeks of gestation until birth, development of the *terminal respiratory units* continues. These may also be referred to as *terminal sacs* or *primitive alveoli*. Type II epithelial cells appear in the lining of the primitive alveoli. Primitive alveoli continue to multiply in the last few weeks of the normal gestational period. The structure of the primitive alveoli becomes more complex, and the number of alveoli continues to increase after birth until approximately 8 years of age.[1]

Type II epithelial cells begin producing surfactant at approximately 24 weeks of gestation.[1,4] Surfactant is necessary for maximum lung expansion after birth. Once surfactant is produced, the amniotic fluid begins to contain lecithin, a phospholipid. The ratio of two types of phospholipids, lecithin and sphingomyelin (L/S ratio), is used as an index of lung maturity. A ratio of 2:1 or greater indicates that the lungs are mature and that the risk of development of respiratory distress syndrome in the fetus is minimal.[5,6] By 26 to 28 weeks of gestation, the fetus has sufficient vascularized terminal sacs and surfactant to survive if born prematurely.

The intrauterine lung is not responsible for gas exchange. Weak attempts at fetal breathing appear to be in preparation for respiration after birth. Instead, the lung tissue secretes liquid that is swallowed or added to amniotic fluid. This fluid production slows shortly before birth so that the lungs are only 50% filled with fluid at birth.[1] This fluid has to be removed as the lungs inflate after birth. Like the cardiovascular system, the pulmonary system undergoes dramatic change in the moments after birth.

Infancy and Young Childhood

Cardiovascular and Pulmonary Adjustments at Birth

Immediately after birth, blood must be circulated to the lung tissue, and the lungs must inflate. Much of the fluid that fills the lungs is pushed out through the nose and mouth as a result of pressure on the thorax during the birth process; remaining fluid can be drained by the pulmonary vasculature and lymphatic system.[1] With each of the first breaths, more and more air is retained in the lungs, building up the newborn's functional residual capacity (residual volume plus expiratory reserve volume). With inspiration, alveolar expansion occurs, delivering oxygenated air to the alveoli.

After birth, blood must be shunted into the pulmonary circulation to receive oxygen from the alveoli. As the lungs expand, pulmonary vascular resistance decreases, and blood flow to the lungs increases. With the occlusion of the umbilical cord, the ductus venosus, which had delivered blood from the umbilical vein to the inferior vena cava, closes. This results in decreased pressure in the inferior vena cava and right atrium. As left atrial pressure becomes greater than right atrial pressure, the foramen ovale closes. Another circulatory change occurs as increased systemic and aortic pressures pump the blood toward the pulmonary artery, reversing the direction of blood flow through the ductus arteriosus. The ductus arteriosus constricts and eventually closes (see Figures 8-1 and 8-2).

Cardiovascular System

The newborn heart lies horizontally in the chest cavity, but a more vertical position is assumed as the lungs expand and the chest cavity grows. Irregularity in the electrocardiogram of the newborn is not unusual because stabilization of the autonomic nervous system, conductivity of cardiac muscle fibers, heart position, and hemodynamics are not yet completed.[7]

Through infancy and childhood, heart size increases at a rate similar to that of the increase in fat-free body weight. Heart volumes are approximately 40 mL at birth, 80 mL at 6 months, and 160 mL by 2 years of age. The ratio of heart volume to body weight remains constant at approximately 10 mL/kg of body weight.[7] Although there is no increase in the number of cardiac muscle fibers (myocytes) as the heart grows, the cross-sectional area of the fibers increases.

Several changes in the myocyte are noted during development, allowing the mature myocyte to contract with more force than the immature myocyte. Immature myocytes are spherical, whereas mature myocytes are more rectangular. As myocytes mature, the number of myofibrils per cross-sectional area increases, and with increased myofibrils, the contractile properties of the myocyte increase. Myofibrils in immature myocytes are also randomly arranged, but as myocytes mature, the myofibrils assume a parallel orientation and increase their force-generating potential.[8]

The vascularization of the heart muscle increases from one vessel for six muscle fibers in the newborn to one vessel for each muscle fiber, as seen in the adult. At birth, the thicknesses of the right and left ventricle walls are equal, but as the left ventricle starts pumping against increased pressure, the left ventricular wall increases in size and becomes approximately twice as thick as the right ventricular wall by adulthood.[9]

Arteries and veins also increase in size as body weight and height increase. The thickness of the vessel wall increases as increased functional demands are placed on the vessels. Development of smooth muscle within the walls of the vessels occurs more slowly. No muscle cells are present at birth in the alveolar blood vessels. Muscle cells can be seen in pulmonary vasculature at the level of the respiratory bronchiole by 4 months of age and at the alveolar ducts by 3 years of age. Some alveolar arteries have muscle cells in their walls at 10 years, but others do not complete this process until 19 years of age.[10]

The heart rate and stroke volume of infants and young children are very different from those of adults. Because stroke volume is related to heart size, the smaller the heart, the less blood that can be pumped with each heart beat. At birth, stroke volume is only 3 to 4 mL, whereas it may be 40 mL in the preadolescent and 60 mL in the young adult. To compensate for smaller stroke volumes, children demonstrate higher heart rates than adults. Table 8-1 provides both mean resting heart rates and normal ranges of heart rate. Boys and girls younger than 10 years have similar heart rates, but after puberty, girls' heart rates are 3 to 5 beats per minute (bpm) higher than those of boys.[7]

Blood pressure also changes from infancy through childhood. These changes are related to ongoing development of (1) the autonomic nervous system, (2) peripheral vascular resistance, and (3) body mass. Blood pressure increases in children are strongly related to increases in height and weight. Over the past decade, population-based increases have been seen in both population norms of blood pressure in children and in incidence of hypertension.[11-13] Pediatric hypertension is discussed in more detail in Clinical Implications Box 8-1.

Table 8-1

Measures of Cardiovascular and Pulmonary Function Across the Life Span

Age	Resting Heart Rate (mean beats/min)	Resting Heart Rate (range, beats/min)	Systolic Blood Pressure (mean mm Hg)	Systolic Blood Pressure (range, mm Hg)	Diastolic Blood Pressure (mean mm Hg)	Diastolic Blood Pressure (range, mm Hg)	Respiratory Rate (range, breaths/min)
Newborn	120–125	70–190	73	54–92	55	38–72	30–40
1 yr	120	80–160	90	71–109	56	39–73	20–40
2 yr	110	80–130	91	72–110	56	39–72	25–32
6 yr	100	75–115	96	77–115	57	41–74	21–26
10 yr	90	70–110	102	84–121	62	45–79	20–26
16 yr	80 (girls) 75 (boys)	60–100 (girls) 55–95 (boys)	117	98–136	67	49–85	16–20
Adult	74–76	60–100	120–125 (20–45 yr) 135–140 (45–65 yr)	*	80 (20–45 yr) 85 (45–65 yr)	*	10–20
Older adults (>65 yr)	74–76	60–100	150	*	85	*	*

*Data unavailable.

Data from Jarvis C: *Physical examination and health assessment*, ed 3, Philadelphia, 1996, WB Saunders, pp 186–187; Paz JC, Panik M: *Acute care handbook for physical therapists*, Woburn, Mass, 1997, Butterworth–Heinemann, p 370 (source: Bullock B: *Pathophysiology: adaptations and alterations in function*, ed 4, Philadelphia, 1996, Lippincott) Wong DL, Perry SE: *Maternal child nursing care*, St Louis, 1998, Mosby, pp 1790–1791 (sources: Gillette PC: Dysrhythmias. In Adams FH et al, editors: *Moss' heart disease in infants, children, and adolescents*, ed 4, Baltimore, 1989, Williams & Wilkins; Rosner B: *Data from second task force on blood pressure control in children*, Bethesda, Md, 1987, National Heart, Lung and Blood Institute).

CLINICAL IMPLICATIONS Box 8-1

Hypertension: An Issue for Children and Adults

Hypertension (HTN) has long been identified as a serious health problem for adults, increasing the risk for development of heart disease, stroke, renal disease, etc. In the past decade, increased attention has been paid to the prevalence of hypertension in children and its related outcomes. It is projected that the global prevalence of hypertension will increase by at least 25% by 2025, but some population-based studies indicate that the increase may be even greater.[47]

Hypertension in Adults

Blood pressure does appear to increase with age and has also been linked to obesity, reduced levels of physical activity, elevated sodium intake, and other dietary choices.[48] Other medical conditions, such as renal disease, diabetes mellitus, sleep apnea, and thyroid disease, can also contribute to development of hypertension. In older adults, vascular stiffness, age-related changes in sympathetic nervous system control of the vasculature,[35] and increased salt sensitivity (especially in women) contribute to prevalence of HTN in 60% of individuals between 60 and 69 years of age and greater than 75% of individuals over 80 years of age.[38,48]

Diagnosis is based on values of systolic and diastolic blood pressure as normal, prehypertensive, hypertension stage 1, or hypertension stage 2. If blood pressure values are above 140/90 mm Hg on two separate clinic visits, a diagnosis of hypertension is made.

Table 8-1A Diagnostic Table

	Systolic Blood Pressure	Diastolic Blood Pressure
Normal	<120 mm Hg	<80 mm Hg
Pre-HTN	120-135 mm Hg	80-89 mm Hg
HTN 1	140-159 mm Hg	90-99 mm Hg
HTN 2	>160 mm Hg	>100 mm Hg

From National Institutes of Health (NIH): *The 7th report of the Joint National Committee on Prevention, Detection, Evaluation and Treatment of High Blood Pressure*, NIH Publication No. 04-5230, August, 2004, US Department of Health and Human Services.

Risks/outcomes of HTN in adults:
• Stroke
• Cardiovascular disease/mortality
• Kidney damage
• Cognitive changes

Intervention for HTN in Adults

Intervention to control hypertension in adulthood focuses on lifestyle modifications that will support weight loss, increase level of physical activity, and dietary changes. A diet that includes fresh fruits and vegetables, low-fat foods, and low salt is recommended (see Table 8-1B). Medications are also used to control factors contributing to HTN. Several categories of medications have been demonstrated to effectively control hypertension. Pharmaceutical management of hypertension is beyond the scope of this text. A useful reference is *the 7th Report of the Joint National Committee on Prevention, Detection, Evaluation and Treatment of High Blood Pressure*.[48]

Hypertension in Children

Prevalence of hypertension in children has increased over the past decade in several countries. Estimates of HTN in children range from 2% to 5%.[11–13,49–52]

Both primary and secondary hypertension is seen in children. Prevalence of hypertension is strongly associated with prevalence of obesity in children. Secondary hypertension, resulting from other conditions such as renal, heart, and endocrine disease or use of medications or nutritional supplements, is more common in children than adults.

Diagnosis

It is recommended that children over the age of 3 years have routine screening of blood pressure, using a blood pressure cuff appropriate for child size. Normal, prehypertensive, hypertension stage 1, or hypertension stage 2 are identified based on comparing systolic and diastolic blood pressure with pediatric blood pressure tables. These tables identify the 50th, 90th, 95th, and 99th percentiles of blood pressure for children, referenced to age in years and percentile of height. If blood pressure is above the 90th percentile or 95th percentile on three separate clinic visits, a diagnosis of prehypertension or hypertension is made. Guidelines are also provided for when to consult the pediatric blood pressure tables (see Table 8-1C).

(Continued)

CLINICAL IMPLICATIONS Box 8-1—Cont'd

Hypertension: an Issue for Children and Adults—Cont'd

Table 8-1B Lifestyle Modifications to Prevent and Manage Hypertension in Adults*

Modification	Recommendation	Approximate SBP Reduction (Range)†
Weight reduction	Maintain normal body weight (body mass index 18.5-24.9 kg/m²)	5-20 mm Hg/10 kg
Adopt DASH eating plan	Consume a diet rich in fruits, vegetables, and low-fat dairy products with a reduced content of saturated and total fat	8-14 mm Hg
Dietary sodium reduction	Reduce dietary sodium intake to no more than 100 mmol per day (2.4 g sodium or 6 g sodium chloride)	2-8 mm Hg
Physical activity	Engage in regular aerobic physical activity such as brisk walking (at least 30 minutes per day, most days of the week)	4-9 mm Hg
Moderation of alcohol consumption	Limit consumption to no more than two drinks (e.g., 24 oz beer, 10 oz wine, or 3 oz 80-proof whiskey) per day in most men and to no more than one drink per day in women and lighter-weight persons	2-4 mm Hg

DASH, Dietary Approaches to Stop Hypertension; *SBP,* systolic blood pressure.
*For overall cardiovascular risk reduction, stop smoking.
†The effects of implementing these modifications are dose and time dependent and could be greater for some individuals.
From National Institutes of Health (NIH): *The 7th report of the Joint National Committee on Prevention, Detection, Evaluation and Treatment of High Blood Pressure,* NIH Publication No. 04-5230, August, 2004, US Department of Health and Human Services.

Table 8-1C Simplified Blood Pressure (BP) Table that Indicates when Provider Should Consult Reference Standards for Identifying Pediatric Hypertension

Look up blood pressure if...

Age in Yr	Systolic BP (mm Hg)	Diastolic BP (mm Hg)
3 to <6	≥100	>60
6 to <9	≥105	>70
9 to <12	≥110	>75
12 to <15	≥115	>75
≥15	≥120	≥80

From Mitchell CK, Theroit JA, Sayat JG, et al: A simplified table improves the recognition of paediatric hypertension, *J Paediatr Child Health* 47(1-2):22-26, 2010.

Risks/outcomes of HTN in children and adolescents:
Studies have shown that children and adolescents with HTN have an increased prevalence of:
• Left ventricular hypertrophy
• Thickening of the carotid artery intima
• Arterial stiffness
• Cognitive changes

Intervention
Intervention to control hypertension in children focuses on lifestyle modifications that support weight loss, increase level of physical activity, and dietary changes. A diet that includes fresh fruits and vegetables, low-fat foods, and low salt is recommended. Diagnostic and intervention information related to children and adolescence is summarized in Table 8-1D.

CLINICAL IMPLICATIONS Box 8-1—Cont'd

Hypertension: An Issue for Children and Adults—Cont'd

Table 8-1D Diagnostic Table and Intervention Table for Hypertension in Children

	SBP or DBP Percentile	Frequency of BP Measurement	Therapeutic Lifestyle Changes	Pharmacological Therapy
Normal	<90th	Recheck at next scheduled physical examination	Encourage healthy diet, sleep, and physical activity	—
Pre-hypertension	90th to <95th or if BP exceeds 120/80 mm Hg even if below 90th percentile up to <95th percentile*	Recheck in 6 mo	Weight-management counseling if overweight, introduce physical activity, and diet management†	None unless compelling indications such as CKD, diabetes mellitus, heart failure, or LVH exist
Stage 1 hypertension	95th percentile to 99th percentile plus 5 mm Hg	Recheck in 1-2 wk or sooner if the patient is symptomatic; if persistently elevated on two additional occasions, evaluate or refer to source of care within 1 month	Weight-management counseling if overweight, introduce physical activity, and diet management†	Initiate therapy based on indications or if compelling indications as above
Stage 2 hypertension	>99th percentile plus 5 mm Hg	Evaluate or refer to source of care within 1 wk or immediately if patient is symptomatic	Weight-management counseling if overweight, introduce physical activity, and diet management†	Initiate therapy‡

BP, blood pressure; *CKD*, chronic kidney disease; *DBP*, diastolic blood pressure; *LVH*, left ventricular hypertrophy; *SBP*, systolic blood pressure.
*This occurs typically at 12 years old for SBP and 16 years old for DBP.
†Parents and children trying to modify the eating plan to the Dietary Approaches to Stop Hypertension (DASH) eating plan could benefit from consultation with a registered or licensed nutritionist to get them started.
‡More than one drug may be required.
From National Institutes of Health (NIH): *The 4th report on the diagnosis, evaluation and treatment of high blood pressure in children and adolescents*, NIH Publication No. 05-5267, revised May 2005, US Department of Health and Human Services.

Blood volume also increases with body size; the total blood volume of the newborn is 300 to 400 mL, whereas the adolescent or young adult has approximately 5 L of blood. Hemoglobin levels in the blood vary with age, affecting the oxygen-carrying capacity of the blood. In the newborn, hemoglobin levels are high (20 g/100 mL), but they fall to 10 g/100 mL by 3 to 6 months of age. Hemoglobin values then slowly increase with age to adult levels of 16 g/100 mL for men and 14 g/100 mL for women.[7] As discussed, the newborn's hemoglobin level is high due to the lower oxygen saturation of the blood in the umbilical vein.

Pulmonary System

Ventilatory Pump Development From a mechanical point of view, the shape of the chest wall and limitations in posture and movement affect the infant's breathing efficiency. At birth, the infant maintains a posture of shoulder elevation, limiting the cervical dimensions of the thorax. The ribs are made up primarily of cartilage

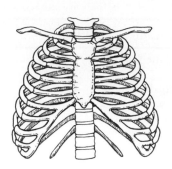
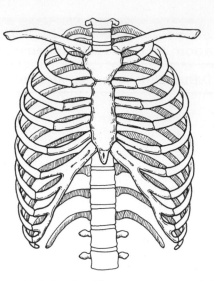

Figure 8-9 Comparison of the infant thorax (*left*) with the mature thorax (*right*). A major difference between the infant and mature adult thorax, other than the size, is the orientation of the ribs. The ribs are oriented horizontally in the infant thorax but are angled downward in the adult.

and are in a horizontal position, giving the lower thorax a circular dimension (Figure 8-9). This results in a relatively flexible thorax and affects the alignment of the diaphragm. The diaphragm and other ventilatory muscles of the newborn are made up of more type IIa muscle fibers than type I muscle fibers, affecting muscle strength and endurance.[14] The structural immaturity of the thorax, combined with a lack of development and control of the ventilatory muscles, prevents the infant from stabilizing the rib cage and effectively using the diaphragm to breathe. The pliancy of the infant's thorax both minimizes inspiratory forces of the rib cage and makes the infant susceptible to paradoxical movement during inspiration.[15]

As the infant learns to move the head and upper body against gravity and to reach in the first 3 to 6 months, muscular development allows increased expansion and use of the upper chest in breathing. In the second half of the first year, the infant learns to sit, stand, and walk, systematically overcoming the force of gravity. As the upright sitting position is assumed, the force of gravity and forces from developing abdominal musculature will pull the ribs downward into a more angular position. This not only expands the thoracic cavity but also increases spacing between the ribs, allowing the intercostal muscles to work more efficiently. Throughout childhood, the rib cage becomes more rigid as osteophytes are laid down to replace cartilage. With growth, the diaphragm is pulled into a dome shape that improves the length-tension relationship of the muscle and improves function. Active use of the

abdominal muscles stabilizes the rib cage within the more rigid thorax, providing a stable base for diaphragmatic action.[15,16]

Respiratory System Development   Only a small percentage of the total number of alveoli to be developed are present at birth. From birth to 3 years of age, some of the nonrespiratory bronchioles in the conducting airway system that were formed prenatally are converted to respiratory bronchioles. This increases the gas exchange capacity of the lungs. New alveoli continue to develop until approximately 8 years of age, when the adult number of 300 million alveoli is attained.[1,7] The size and complexity of the alveoli increase throughout infancy and childhood, increasing the available surface area for air exchange. The growth of the alveolar surface appears to be related to the increased oxygen demand of working tissue. The pulmonary arterial and venous vasculature develops concurrently with the development of alveoli.

The conducting and respiratory airways increase in length and diameter until growth of the thoracic cavity is complete. Children under 5 years of age have a larger number of small airways that are less than 2 mm in diameter. For example, 50% of airways in the neonate and 20% of airways in the adult have diameters of less than 2 mm.[17] Small airways can be problematic in two ways. First, they offer increased resistance to airflow, thereby increasing the work of breathing. Second, they are very easily obstructed by foreign objects.

The bronchioles and alveoli of infants and young children are weaker and less efficient than those of adults. Smooth muscle in the walls of the bronchioles does not develop until the child is 3 to 4 years old. As a result, the airway is more susceptible to collapse, thus trapping air. The development of elastic tissue in the alveoli may be incomplete until after adolescence; this means decreased lung compliance and distensibility for infants and young children. This makes it harder for the infant and small child to fully inflate their lungs and maintain lung volume. In children younger than 7 years, decreased elastic recoil causes the airways to close at a greater lung volume than in older children and adults. When combined with small airway size, this relative lack of recoil places young children more at risk for complications from small airway diseases such as bronchiolitis.[17]

One other structural difference between the pulmonary systems of children and adults is the absence of collateral ventilation mechanisms in children. This decreased collateral circulation may increase the risk of respiratory infection and atelectasis in children. Pores of Kohn have not been seen in children younger than 6 years. Lambert canals are not thought to develop until at least 6 to 8 years of age.[18,19]

In summary, the development of the lungs into their adult form continues well into childhood. Lung volume increases proportionally with increases in body size and increases as the number of alveoli increases.[7] Vital capacity values are related to height. Size of the conducting airways is related to stature, and the total number of alveoli an individual develops is proportional to height, which reinforces the relationship between lung volume and body size.[10] In the first year of life, the infant has little pulmonary reserve and must increase breathing frequency to meet demands for increased oxygen. Inspiratory and expiratory reserve volumes sufficient to meet increased needs are evident at about 1 year of age.

Differences between the child's and the adult's pulmonary function are seen in breathing pattern and in breathing frequency. The newborn infant undergoes dramatic changes in intrathoracic pressure, lung inflation, and pulmonary circulation. It is not unusual to observe irregular breathing patterns, including periods of apnea, during this time. Small airway size, together with the limited number of developed alveoli, leave the young infant with a small lung volume. As a result, the newborn's respiratory rate is higher than at any other time in the life span (Table 8-1).

Adolescence

Growth and functional changes of the cardiovascular and pulmonary systems continue through childhood and into adolescence. During the adolescent growth spurt, gender differences in cardiovascular and pulmonary function become apparent. Left ventricular mass increases in parallel with body mass equally for boys and girls until 9 to 12 years of age. In adolescence, the left ventricular mass of boys is greater than that of girls. Adolescents who participate in endurance-type sports also have a greater left ventricular mass than their peers who do not participate in this type of activity.[7] By adolescence, blood volume of boys is also greater than that of girls.

The amount of muscle in the heart increases, resulting in increased blood pressure and decreased heart rate.[9] Increased blood pressure is primarily related to increased body weight. In girls, blood pressure increases during their prepubertal growth spurt and then levels off. In boys, blood pressure gradually increases with lean body mass through 18 years of age. By the end of adolescence, systolic blood pressures of boys become slightly greater than those of girls, while no gender difference is seen for diastolic blood pressure.[7] It should be noted that more recently, increases in blood pressure for both boys and girls have been linked to body weight and increasing levels of obesity (see Clinical Implications Box 8-1). Gender differences in heart rate are also reported: the basal heart rate of girls is 3 to 5 beats per minute faster than that of boys. Stroke volume also increases but does not appear to be related only to heart size.

In the year preceding the peak height velocity, stroke volume changes appear to be related to an increased arterial-venous oxygen difference. This implies that more oxygen is being extracted by the tissues, which may be due to age-related changes in muscle mass, muscle enzyme profusion, and the ratio of capillaries to muscle fiber. In the year after peak height velocity, increased stroke volume may be related to an increased cardiac preload condition with increased venous return.[20]

The adolescent growth spurt is also reflected in lung size and lung volume. Proximal airways and vasculature increase in size. Alveoli become larger, and greater amounts of elastic fiber can be found in the alveolar wall. The capillaries in the alveolar region also become larger, supporting increased gas exchange. By age 19, muscle is developed in the walls of the arteries found at the alveoli, increasing the efficient control of blood flow by vasodilation and vasoconstriction.[21]

Adulthood and Aging

Normal function of the cardiovascular and pulmonary systems in early and middle adulthood is described in the beginning of this chapter. Heart size and weight may continue to increase in adulthood, primarily because of fat deposition.[9] Some gender differences in function of the cardiovascular and pulmonary systems do exist. During submaximal exercise, the cardiac output of women is 5% to 10% greater than that of men. This may be related to stroke volume differences and the fact that women have slightly less hemoglobin (14 g/100 mL blood) than men (15 to 16 g/100 mL blood).[3] Age-related changes in mean heart weight are not demonstrated in men, but in women, the mean heart weight increases between the fourth and seventh decades of life.[22] Women may also experience greater aortic stiffening after menopause.[23]

With increasing age, anatomical and physiological changes are seen in the cardiovascular and pulmonary systems. At least initially, these age-related changes do not seem to significantly interfere with function. Functional losses are more evident beginning in the seventh decade of life.[24] It is also difficult to differentiate cardiovascular and pulmonary changes related purely to aging from those caused by asymptomatic disease or deconditioning. As discussed in Chapter 15, it is thought that physically active adults can minimize the impact of aging on cardiovascular and pulmonary function.

Cardiovascular System

The Heart Structural changes are seen in the heart and cardiac cells with aging. In general, the number of myocytes decreases, whereas their size increases. In the myocardium, increasing amounts of elastic tissue, fat, and collagen contribute to increased stiffness and decreased compliance of the ventricles. Cross-linkage of collagen in the myocardium also contributes to increased stiffness. Accumulation of lipofuscin, a waste product associated with oxidative damage, is also seen in the cardiac muscle cells, resulting in a darkening of the myocardium. Lipofuscin deposits interfere with mitochondrial turnover in the cardiac myocyte and contribute to cellular aging and cell death.[25,26]

Thickening of the left ventricular wall is seen in both men and women and seems to be related to age, body mass index (BMI), smoking history, diabetes, and blood pressure. Increases are greater in women than men, especially when estrogen levels decrease. Over a 10-year period, men demonstrated a 15% increased risk for left ventricular hypertrophy, whereas women demonstrated a 67% increase in risk.[27] Some of this thickening may be related to hypertrophy of the myocytes secondary to the increased demand on the heart necessary to pump blood through a less compliant vascular system. The decreased compliance in the vasculature contributes to systolic hypertension, which predominates in older adulthood, raising the pulse pressure and therefore the work of the left ventricle.[23,28] The volume of the left ventricle is slightly decreased, and the left atrium is slightly dilated. In the endocardium, thickened areas of elastic and collagen fibers can be noted, especially in the atria. Fragmentation and disorganization of elastic, collagen, and muscle fibers also occur.[25,29] Increased fat is found within the epicardium, especially over the right ventricle and in the atrioventricular groove.[22]

With aging, changes are also seen in the heart valves and in the conduction system. The valves become thickened and calcified. Collagen and lipid accumulation, as well as calcification, within the aortic and mitral valves impairs the ability of the valves to completely close. Valvular changes contribute to the increased incidence of heart murmur in the older adult population. Collagen and fat are also laid down in the left bundle branches of the conduction system. By age 60, the number of pacemaker cells in the sinoatrial node begins to decrease; by age 75, less than 10% of the number of sinoatrial node cells found in the adult heart are seen.[29,30] Cellular loss is also noted in the atrioventricular node and bundle of His. These changes in the conduction system may contribute to the increased incidence of premature ventricular complexes and differences seen on the older adult's electrocardiogram. The QRS wave shifts to the left, and ST segment depression is seen.

The Vasculature The vasculature undergoes change throughout life, with vessels becoming thicker, more rigid, and more dilated. In general, the vascular course becomes more tortuous. Changes attributed to aging are initially seen in the coronary arteries at approximately 20 years of age and in the remainder of the arterial system after 40 years of age. Dilation occurs in proximal arteries such as the aorta, whereas thickening of the arterial wall predominates in the peripheral arteries. Elastic arteries change more than muscular arteries, with irregular thickening of elastic tissue, fragmenting of elastic fibers, lipid infiltration, and calcification. These changes are seen earliest in the proximal portions of the large arteries.[29] The older vessel is thickened and less elastic, which results in less compliance. Arteriosclerosis refers to decreased compliance of the arteries, which is a normal consequence of age-related changes in the arterial walls.[31] This is contrasted to atherosclerosis, a pathological deposition of fatty plaques on the inner layer of the vessel, which also results in increased resistance to blood flow through the vessel. Research has shown that regular aerobic, endurance exercise can minimize the age-related changes in central arterial compliance. This possibly reflects the mechanism by which exercise decreases the risk of cardiovascular disease in older adults.[28,32]

Functional Changes The changes in the cardiovascular system associated with aging functionally affect the heart rate, blood pressure, stroke volume, and adaptability of the system to stress. The structural changes of the left ventricular wall reduce the ability of the ventricle to fill and contract. These changes do not have much effect on an individual at rest or during light exercise, but maximal exercise capacity decreases.

The sensitivity of regulatory mechanisms, such as the baroreceptors, is diminished in the older individual, affecting adaptability of the cardiovascular system to stressful situations such as cough, the Valsalva maneuver, and orthostasis. In older adults, the effectiveness of the sympathetic nervous system response to drops in blood pressure appears to be reduced due to stiffening of the vascular system.[33] This may help explain why older adults more often experience orthostatic hypotension than younger adults.[34,35] Increased plasma catecholamine levels and decreased end-organ responsiveness to adrenergic stimulation also affect the ability of the system to increase heart rate, contractility of the heart, and vasodilation of the vessels in response to stress. Because of decreased adaptability, the heart takes longer to reach a steady state or to recover from exercise. Older adults who are physically active appear to have improvements of the baroreflex control of heart rate than their sedentary peers, reflecting the role of exercise in improving vagal control of the heart.[34]

The resting heart rate changes minimally with aging, but maximum heart rate decreases. Because heart rate varies with several factors, including level of fitness, a wide range of resting heart rates is within normal limits for the older adult (see Table 8-1). The decrease in the maximum heart rate may be related to (1) decreased activity of the cardiac pacemaker, (2) decreased sensitivity to catecholamines, and (3) increased ventricular filling time. Increased ventricular filling time results from decreased ventricular compliance. Contraction time and diastole may also be increased because of slowed calcium uptake in the sarcoplasmic reticulum of the cardiac cells. Because of poor calcium transport and storage, the heart muscle will take longer to reach peak tension and to relax. Decreased venous tone, slowed relaxation of the ventricles, thickening of the mitral valve, and left ventricular stiffness may result in a decreased preload condition. The filling rate of the 65- to 80-year-old heart has been shown to be 50% of that of 25- to 40-year-old subjects.[36] Stiffening of the aorta and major arteries, increased systemic blood pressure, and poor perfusion of the skeletal muscle contribute to an increase in afterload.[28,37,38]

At rest and during exercise, blood pressure increases through adulthood and older adulthood. Blood pressure remains significantly related to adiposity through adulthood.[39] Systolic blood pressure rises in older adults, while diastolic blood pressure may decrease after the sixth decade (see Table 8-1).[38] The widening difference between systolic and diastolic blood pressure results in an increased pulse pressure, which can stress the heart and vasculature. The increase in systolic blood pressure is related to reduced loss of smooth muscle cells in the arterial wall, increased collagen content and cross-linkage within the vessels, thinning of the arterial wall, and calcium deposition in the vessel. These changes lead to increased stiffness in the vessels.[38] Moderate-intensity aerobic exercise appears to lower resting systolic blood pressure.[28] Low-intensity aerobic training in older adult hypertensive patients has also been shown to lower blood pressure, with these patients returning to a pre-training level of blood pressure when exercise was discontinued.[40] This finding seems to reflect that lifestyle factors also play a role in determining the blood pressure of the older adult. Even with attention to lifestyle choices that maintain appropriate body weight and regular physical activity, it appears that aging of the cardiovascular system leaves the older adult susceptible to development of hypertension (see Clinical Implications Box 8-1).

Delivery of oxygen to the peripheral tissues is altered with aging. The efficiency of oxygen extraction from the blood at the tissue level decreases with age, narrowing the arterial-venous oxygen difference. Loss of muscle strength, decreased muscle enzyme levels, and diminished size of the capillary network that perfuse muscle limit oxygen extraction from the circulating blood. Other vascular changes with aging, obstruction of major vessels, and decreased levels of hemoglobin are also factors. With increasing age, increased obesity, and decreased efficiency of sweating, blood is shunted away from the muscles and to the skin, assisting in body cooling. This also reduces blood flow to the tissues and contributes to the decreased efficiency of oxygen extraction.

Pulmonary System

Both the ventilatory pump and respiratory system are affected by aging. Because of this, older adults are at increased risk for respiratory failure because of changes in the lungs. Risk of ventilatory failure also increases because of changes in the ventilatory pump.[41]

Ventilatory Pump Changes Structural changes occur with aging and create a stiffer, bony thorax, which increases the work of breathing. The thorax becomes shortened vertically and larger in the anterior-posterior dimension. Thoracic kyphosis and decreased mobility of the joints allow rib rotation. Rib decalcification, increased calcification of the rib cartilage, and changes in the articulation between the ribs and vertebrae may also contribute to increased stiffness. Elasticity of cartilage and collagen in the annulus fibrosus decreases, and loss of fluid from the nucleus pulposus results in a flattened, less resilient disk. Because of the resting position of the thorax, the intrathoracic pressure at end-expiration is higher, again increasing airway resistance and effort during breathing. Functionally, these changes result in decreased chest wall expansion during breathing. In a young adult, a 40% change in lung volume is noted with thoracic expansion, but only a 30% change is seen in older adults.[41]

Elasticity and compliance are also decreased within the lung because of changes in collagen and elastin. Cross-linkage of collagen is seen, and there is a loss of elastin in the airways and blood vessels. This results in decreased recoil of the lung, especially at higher lung volumes.[41] In the conducting airways, elasticity of bronchial cartilage is diminished. This results in a slightly increased diameter of the large airways. Hyaline cartilage structures in the trachea may become ossified. Bronchial mucous glands increase in number, thickening the mucus layer in the airway and offering more resistance to airflow. The number and thickness of elastic fibers in the walls of smaller airways decrease, again increasing the resistance to airflow and diminishing elastic recoil of the lungs. As elastic recoil of the lungs is diminished, residual volume increases and vital capacity is reduced. Lungs, alveoli, and alveolar ducts enlarge with age. As a result, more time is needed for inspired air to reach the alveolar area. Decreased elasticity of the alveoli makes them susceptible to collapse on expiration.

Respiratory muscles become less efficient with age. Inspiratory muscle strength and endurance appear to decrease.[41] Structural changes in the thoracic cavity alter the length-tension relationship of the respiratory muscles, increasing the work of breathing. For example, the resting position of the diaphragm changes as the thoracic height decreases and diameter increases. Increased residual volume of the aging lung will also affect the resting position of the diaphragm. The abdominal muscles become less effective at stabilizing the diaphragm. Because of these changes, the older adult has to increase breathing rate rather than tidal volume to increase minute ventilation. This also increases the work of breathing.[42]

Respiratory System Changes   Many changes are noted in the aging lung. The loss of elastic recoil of the lung, as mentioned earlier, decreases effectiveness of the ventilatory pump. The alveolar surface area also changes. A loss of surface area results from a decrease in the actual number of alveoli per unit of lung volume; loss of alveolar wall tissue; and increased size of the respiratory bronchioles, alveolar sacs, and alveolar ducts.

The pulmonary vasculature undergoes the same changes within its vascular wall that were discussed earlier. The capillary bed at the alveolar interface becomes smaller, which, when combined with increased alveolar size, limits the diffusing capacity of the system. Pulmonary blood flow and blood volume within the capillary bed decrease. As a result, pulmonary gas exchange is affected. The alveolar-to-arteriole oxygen gradient increases as the arterial Po_2 decreases. The decrease in Po_2 with age has been well documented,[10] but recent references note a decrease in Po_2 until the age of 70 to 75 years, after which Po_2 plateaus.[41] Arterial Pco_2 remains constant throughout adulthood.

Functionally, the impact of these changes is reflected in lung volumes and arterial blood gas values at rest and during exercise. Although total lung capacity does not change, vital capacity decreases while functional residual capacity and residual volume increase. By 70 years of age, vital capacity is reported to decrease to 75% of earlier values, and residual volume increases by 50%.[10] Inspiratory and expiratory reserve volumes also decrease because of the decreased elasticity of the lung. The loss of elasticity causes the airways to close at a higher volume during expiration, which affects the amount of oxygenated air that is distributed to the tissue. The pulmonary system works harder to deliver less oxygen to the tissues in older adults.

FUNCTIONAL IMPLICATIONS OF CHANGES IN THE CARDIOVASCULAR AND PULMONARY SYSTEMS

Because of anatomical and physiological differences in the cardiovascular and pulmonary systems of the infant, child, adolescent, and adult, function and efficiency differ in each age group. Through childhood, most changes are related to changes in body size. Gender differences become apparent in adolescence. In adulthood and older adulthood, effects of environment and normal aging alter the efficiency and capacity of the cardiovascular and pulmonary systems. Lifestyle habits that affect respiratory system function in older adults include nutrition, smoking habits, and exercise. In the presence of protein malnutrition, muscle atrophy may be seen in the respiratory muscles. Smoking has a negative effect on both the cardiovascular and pulmonary systems.

Efficiency of the cardiovascular and pulmonary system is reflected in measures such as cardiac output, minute ventilation, and maximal aerobic capacity. *Cardiac output* is a measure of the efficiency of the cardiovascular system. *Minute ventilation,* the volume of air moved into the lungs in 1 minute, is a measure of the efficiency of the pulmonary system. These two measures, when considered with the ability of working tissue to use oxygen for energy production, indicate an individual's *maximal aerobic capacity,* or level of cardiovascular and pulmonary fitness.

Cardiac output varies with an individual's age. The cardiac output of children is less than that of adults both at rest and during exercise. Small heart size limits stroke volume to such a degree that even the increased heart rate of children cannot compensate. Functionally, the lower cardiac output does not affect a child's level of activity because even with less hemoglobin than an adult, the child efficiently extracts oxygen from the blood. In addition, the small body size of children and their ability to easily dissipate heat over their relatively large body surface area enables them to function with a smaller cardiac output. Cardiac output increases as the body grows. In older adults, cardiac output declines because the heart must pump harder to overcome increased stiffness of the vessels, stiffness of the ventricular wall increases, and diastolic filling becomes more difficult.[28] With aging, both maximal heart rate and maximal stroke volume are decreased. Because cardiac output during maximal exercise is the product of these two values, it also decreases with age.[3]

Oxygen transportation to working tissues is another important factor in determining an individual's maximal aerobic capacity. Efficient ventilation carries inspired air to a well-developed and expanded alveolar network. Efficient circulation provides sufficient oxygenated blood to the pulmonary capillary network and to the capillaries of working tissues. Factors such as airway resistance, compliance of the thorax, functioning of the respiratory muscles, and compliance/elasticity of the lung and airways affect efficiency. The functional volumes of air in the lungs, such as the tidal volume, vary with the demands placed on the pulmonary system. As more oxygen is required during light to moderate exercise, tidal volume increases.[10]

Cardiorespiratory fitness in older adults is impacted by changes in cardiac factors and diminished ability of the peripheral tissues to extract oxygen. Beginning at age 30 to 40, declines in peak VO_2 begin to be seen. The decline is 3% to 6% per decade initially. Although the rate of decline increases after age 45, the decline accelerates even more after the age of 70 years when a decline of 20% per decade.[43,44] Cardiorespiratory fitness of both men and women decrease to approximately 65% of peak aerobic capacity.[44] Both the decrease in cardiac output and the diminished ability of the peripheral tissues (muscle) to extract oxygen contribute to the decrease

in maximal oxygen uptake.[45,46] It appears that the rate of decline in cardiorespiratory fitness is greater in older men than women, but when adjusted for fat-free body mass, the changes in aerobic capacity are similar in men and women.[43] Individuals who have maintained high levels of physical activity through their lifetime and have higher levels of peak oxygen uptake as they enter older adulthood maintain higher cardiorespiratory fitness than their more sedentary peers but still have accelerated decreases in cardiorespiratory fitness with increasing age.[43,44]

Changes in the functional lung volumes and decreased efficiency of the respiratory muscles reduce an older individual's ability to increase tidal volume and minute ventilation in response to exercise. The pulmonary system is less able to adapt to stress because of (1) the loss of elastic recoil and chest wall compliance, (2) changes in central nervous system control, (3) innervation of respiratory muscles, and (4) impaired perception of carbon dioxide levels. Breathing frequency is increased in an attempt to provide necessary oxygen transport. The inability of the pulmonary system to meet needs is also thought to limit exercise in the older individual.[30,37] These changes are minimized in the healthy, active, nonsmoking older adult, and endurance training is thought to improve inspiratory muscle strength and lung function.[3]

SUMMARY

The cardiovascular and pulmonary systems work closely together to provide the food and fuel necessary for physical function. Changes in these systems over the life span can alter the functional ability of the systems and those of the individual. Some of these changes appear to be the result of normal development, whereas others may be determined by lifestyle choices. Research shows that regular physical activity can have a positive impact on function and health and that exercise at any age is important to maintain these two important systems at maximal efficiency.

Cardiovascular and pulmonary efficiency contributes to an individual's level of physical fitness. Fitness is a measure of a person's functional ability and health. Clinically, cardiovascular disease is a significant problem for adults. Risk factors for cardiovascular disease can sometimes be identified in young children. It is important to consider cardiovascular and pulmonary development and function across the life span as clinicians work with their clients to prevent cardiovascular disease and to minimize the effects of aging on these systems. A more extensive discussion of fitness issues across the life span, including the effects of exercise and training on the body systems, can be found in Chapter 15.

REFERENCES

1. Moore KL, Persaud TVN: *Before we are born: essentials of embryology and birth defects*, ed 7, Philadelphia, 2008, WB Saunders.
2. Ross MH, Kaye GL, Pawlina W: *Histology: a text and atlas*, ed 4, Baltimore, 2003, Lippincott, Williams & Wilkins.
3. McArdle WD, Katch FL, Katch VL: *Exercise physiology: energy, nutrition and human performance*, ed 7, Philadelphia, 2010, Lippincott, Williams & Wilkins.
4. Carlson BM: *Human embryology and developmental biology*, ed 4, Philadelphia, 2009, Mosby Elsevier.
5. Luo G, Norwitz ER: Revisiting amniocenteses for fetal lung maturity after 36 weeks' gestation, *Rev Obstet Gynecol* 1(2):61–68, 2008.
6. Burgess WE, Chernick V: *Respiratory therapy in newborn infants and children*, ed 2, New York, 1986, Thieme.
7. Malina RM, Bouchard C, Bar-Or O: *Growth, maturation and physical activity*, ed 2, Champaign, Ill, 2004, Human Kinetics.
8. Anderson PAW: The heart and development, *Semin Perinatol* 20:482–509, 1996.
9. Sinclair D, Dangerfield P: *Human growth after birth*, ed 6, New York, 1998, Oxford University Press.
10. Murray JF: *The normal lung*, ed 2, Philadelphia, 1986, WB Saunders.
11. Flynn JT: Pediatric hypertension update, *Curr Opin Nephrol Hypertens* 19:292–297, 2010.
12. Feber J, Ahmed M: Hypertension in children: new trends and challenges, *Clin Sci* 119:151–161, 2010.
13. Liang YJ, Xi B, Hu YH, et al: Trends in blood pressure and hypertension among Chinese children and adolescents: China Health and Nutrition Surveys 1991–2004, *Blood Press* 20(1):45–53, 2010.
14. Bourgeois MS, Zadai CC: Impaired ventilation and respiration in the older adult. In Guccione AA, editor: *Geriatric physical therapy*, ed 2, St Louis, 2000, Mosby, pp 226–244.
15. Reilly KJ, Moore CA: Respiratory movement patterns during vocalizations at 7 and 11 months of age, *J Speech Lang Hear Res* 52:223–239, 2009.
16. Massery M: Chest development as a component of normal motor development: implications for pediatric physical therapists, *Pediatr Phys Ther* 3:3–8, 1991.
17. DeCesare JA, Graybill CA: Physical therapy for the child with respiratory dysfunction. In Irwin S, Tecklin JS, editors: *Cardiopulmonary physical therapy*, ed 2, St Louis, 1990, Mosby, pp 417–460.
18. Boyden EA: Development and growth of the airways. In Hodson WA, editor: *Development of the lung*, New York, 1977, Marcel Dekker, pp 3–35.
19. Meyrick B, Reid LM: Ultrastructure of alveolar lining and its development. In Hodson WA, editor: *Development of the lung*, New York, 1977, Marcel Dekker, pp 135–214.
20. Cunningham DA, Paterson DH, Blimke CJR: The development of the cardiorespiratory system with growth and physical activity. In Boileau RA, editor: *Advances in pediatric sport science, vol 1: biological issues*, Champaign, Ill, 1984, Human Kinetics, pp 85–116.
21. Davis JA, Dobbings J: *Scientific foundations of pediatrics*, Baltimore, 1981, University Park Press.
22. Kitzman DW, Edwards WD: Minireview: age-related changes in the anatomy of the normal human heart, *J Geriatr Med Sci* 45:33–39, 1990.
23. Lee HY, Oh BH: Aging and arterial stiffness, *Circ J* 71:2257–2262, 2010.
24. Cunningham DA, Paterson DH: Discussion: exercise, fitness and aging. In Bouchard C, Shephard RJ, Stephens T, et al, editors: *Exercise, fitness and health: a consensus of current knowledge*, Champaign, Ill, 1990, Human Kinetics, pp 699–704.
25. Terman A, Gustafsson B, Brunk UT: Autophage, organelles and ageing, *J Pathol* 211(2):124–143, 2007.
26. Terman A, Kurz T, Gustafsson B, et al: The involvement of lysosomes in myocardial aging and disease, *Curr Cardiol Rev* 4(2):107–115, 2008.
27. Lieb W, Xanthakis V, Sullivan LM, et al: Longitudinal tracking of left ventricular mass over the adult life course: clinical correlates of short- and long-term change in the Framingham offspring study, *Circulation* 119(240):3085–3092, 2009.
28. Sattelmair JR, Pertman JH, Forman DE: Effects of physical activity on cardiovascular and noncardiovascular outcomes in older adults, *Clin Geriatr Med* 25:677–702, 2009.
29. Wei JY: Cardiovascular anatomic and physiologic changes with age, *Top Geriatr Rehabil* 2:10–16, 1986.
30. Tecklin JS: Cardiopulmonary changes with aging. In Irwin S, Tecklin JS, editors: *Cardiopulmonary physical therapy: a guide to practice*, ed 4, St Louis, 2004, Mosby, pp 102–120.
31. Zadai CC: Cardiopulmonary issues in the geriatric population: implications for rehabilitation, *Top Geriatr Rehabil* 2:1–9, 1986.
32. Tanaka H, Dinenno FA, Monahan KD, et al: Aging, habitual exercise and dynamic arterial compliance, *Circulation* 102:1270–1275, 2000.
33. Hart EC, Joyner MJ, Wallin BG, et al: Age-related differences in the sympathetic-hemodynamic balance in men, *Hypertension* 54(1):127–133, 2009.
34. Shi X, Schaller FA, Tierney N, et al: Physically active lifestyle enhances vagal-cardiac function but not central autonomic neural interaction in elderly humans, *Exp Biol Med* 233:209–218, 2008.
35. Studinger P, Goldstein R, Taylor JA: Age- and fitness-related alterations in vascular sympathetic control, *J Physiol* 587:2049–2057, 2009.
36. Gerstenblith G, Frederiksen J, Yin FCP, et al: Echo-cardiographic assessment of a normal adult aging population, *Circulation* 56:273–278, 1977.
37. Shephard RJ: The cardiovascular benefits of exercise in the elderly, *Top Geriatr Rehabil* 1:1–10, 1985.
38. Acelajado MC, Oparil S: Hypertension in the elderly, *Clin Geriatr Med* 25:391–412, 2009.
39. Gerber LM, Stern PM: Relationship of body size to blood pressure: sex-specific and developmental influences, *Hum Biol* 71(4):505–528, 1999.
40. Motoyama M, Sunami Y, Kinoshita F, et al: Blood pressure lowering effect of low-intensity aerobic training in elderly hypertensive patients, *Med Sci Sports Exerc* 30:818–823, 1998.

41. Rossi A, Ganassini A, Tantacci C, et al: Aging and the respiratory system, *Aging Clin Exp Res* 8:143–161, 1996.

42. Frontera WR, Evans WJ: Exercise performance and endurance training in the elderly, *Top Geriatr Rehabil* 2:17–32, 1986.

43. Fleg JL, Morrell CH, Bos AG, et al: Accelerated longitudinal decline of aerobic capacity in healthy older adults, *Circulation* 112:674–682, 2005.

44. Jackson AS, Sui X, Hebert JR, et al: Role of lifestyle and aging on longitudinal change in cardiorespiratory fitness, *Arch Intern Med* 169(19):1781–1787, 2009.

45. McGuire DK, Levine BD, Williamson JW, et al: A 30-year follow-up of the Dallas bed rest and training study: I. Effect of age on the cardiovascular response to exercise, *Circulation* 104:1350–1357, 2001.

46. McGavock JM, Hastings JL, Snell PG, et al: A forty-year follow-up of the Dallas bed rest and training study: the effect of age on the cardiovascular response to exercise in men, *J Gerontol A Biol Sci Med Sci* 64A(2):293–299, 2009.

47. Tu K, Chen Z, Lipscombe LL: Prevalence and incidence of hypertension from 1995 to 2005: a population-based study, *CMAJ* 178(11):1429–1435, 2008.

48. National Institutes of Health (NIH): *The 7th report of the Joint National Committee on Prevention, Detection, Evaluation and Treatment of High Blood Pressure*, NIH Publication No. 04-5230, August, 2004, US Department of Health and Human Services.

49. National Institutes of Health (NIH): *The 4th report on the diagnosis, evaluation and treatment of high blood pressure in children and adolescents*, NIH Publication No. 05-5267, revised May 2005, US Department of Health and Human Services.

50. Andrade H, Antonio N, Rodrigues D, et al: High blood pressure in the pediatric age group, *Rev Port Cardiol* 29(3):413–432, 2010.

51. Falkner B: Hypertension in children and adolescents: epidemiology and natural history, *Pediatr Nephrol* 25:1219–1224, 2010.

52. Mitchell CK, Theroit JA, Sayat JG, et al: A simplified table improves the recognition of paediatric hypertension, *J Paediatr Child Health* 47(1–2):22–26, 2010.

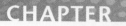

Nervous System Changes

OBJECTIVES

After studying this chapter, the reader will be able to:

1. Describe the role and functions of the nervous system.
2. Discuss unique structural and functional changes of the nervous system in the developing fetus, infant, child, adolescent, adult, and older adult.
3. Relate nervous system changes over time to functional differences in movement, cognition, and motivation.
4. Incorporate issues of life-span development of the nervous system into patient examination and intervention.

The nervous system is frequently referred to as the *command center for human function.* It not only receives information but also integrates all incoming messages to orchestrate fluid, appropriate responses. The nervous system truly oversees other body systems as they cooperate to perform day-to-day activities and controls the major functions of moving, thinking, and feeling.

Movement is controlled when the nervous system functions as an initiator, a modulator, and a comparator, activating the muscular and skeletal systems. Movement is not the product of any one system, nor does one system act in isolation from the others to produce movement. Attention is necessary for motor function. Abnormal movement might result from a problem in the skeletal, muscular, cardiopulmonary, or nervous system. For example, in either muscle disease (e.g., muscular dystrophy) or peripheral nerve injury, the end result is movement dysfunction.

A unique role of the nervous system is thought processing, that is, cognition and intelligence. Psychological theorists such as Erikson[1] have little to say about how the brain "thinks." Physiologists believe that the ability of the brain to form memories is a mechanism for intelligence. Memory formation is contingent on an individual's level of alertness and ability to focus attention. Memory formation occurs in an area of the brain called the *hippocampus.*[2] The frontal area of the brain has been linked to abstract thought and personality. Its protracted development in adolescence is what finally allows a teenager to become a thinking adult. After head trauma, a patient's sensory, motor, and cognitive deficits can be attributed to damage to a specific area of the brain. In other areas of the brain, called *association*

areas, sensory input is connected to meaning. For example, in the visual association areas, visual input is connected with the memory and names of shapes.

Another important aspect of nervous system control is its role in motivation and emotions. One of the oldest parts of the brain, called the *limbic system,* is responsible for attending to sensory and motor cues; monitoring basic drives for food, water, and sexual gratification; and attaching emotional meaning to actions. The ability of the nervous system to react to these cues is not well understood. Emotions can provide powerful motivation for movement. The affective component of movement dysfunction is often the most difficult to deal with, as when trying to motivate a person to perform better physically.

COMPONENTS OF THE NERVOUS SYSTEM

At the cellular level, the nervous system is made up of two different types of cells: neurons and glial cells. Both cell types are derived from embryonic ectoderm. *Neurons* and their processes allow the nervous system to communicate and to direct movement activities. *Glia* provide guidance, support, and protection for neurons. On a larger scale, structures such as the brain, spinal cord, and cranial and peripheral nerves make up the functional infrastructure of the nervous system.

Neurons

Neurons are complex structures that form the major communication system of the body. A typical neuron is composed of a cell body, an axon which carries impulses to other neurons, and multiple dendrites that receive incoming stimuli from other neurons. Neurons communicate via electrical impulse conduction down axons and across synapses to other neurons, muscles, or glands. Neurons vary in size and shape according to their function. For example, pyramidal neurons found in the cerebral cortex and Purkinje cells in the cerebellum (Figure 9-1) are the major output cells for their respective areas. Pyramidal cell axons make up projection, association, and commissural fibers. They travel to the spinal cord, to other areas of the brain, and from one hemisphere to the other. Purkinje cells send information from the cerebellum to the cerebellar nuclei and vestibular nuclei. The structure often reflects the role the neuron plays in the communications network of the nervous system.

Dendrites are branched to receive multiple inputs from other neurons. The pattern of branching indicates the purpose of the neuron. The neuron communicates by initiating a signal, called an *action potential.* The axon or nerve fiber terminates in an end bulb that synapses with a target cell. Many axons can converge on a single target. Axons can also branch to transmit signals to more than one target cell or more than one location on a target cell. Information from one source, such as the visual system can be conveyed to many different sites through divergence. These convergent or divergent impulses can be summated in time or space

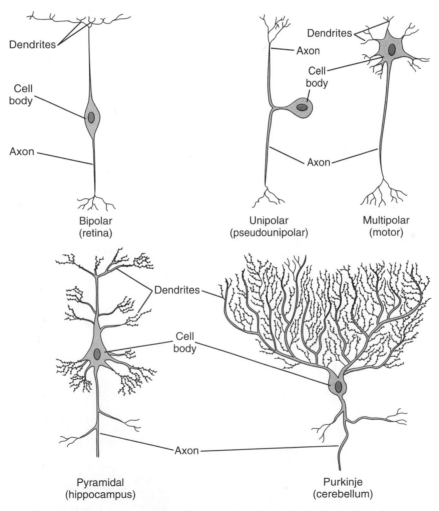

Figure 9-1 Diagram of various types of neurons. (Redrawn from Martin S, Kessler M: *Neurologic interventions for physical therapy,* ed 2, St Louis, 2007, Saunders, p 9; Lundy-Ekman L: *Neuroscience fundamentals for rehabilitation,* ed 3, St Louis, 2007, Saunders, p 437; Gartner LP, Hiatt JL: *Color textbook of histology,* ed 2, Philadelphia, 2001, WB Saunders, p 187.)

to either make it easier or more difficult to generate an action potential. An axon can generate up to 1000 action potentials per second.

Myelin is a lipid and protein substance that covers axons and increases the speed of nerve impulse conduction. In the central nervous system (CNS), myelin is produced by glial cells called *oligodendrocytes;* in the peripheral nervous system (PNS), myelin is produced by Schwann cells. How fast impulses can be conducted depends on whether the nerve is myelinated or unmyelinated and on the diameter of the nerve fiber. The larger the diameter of the nerve, the faster the conduction of the action potential. The thicker the myelin surrounding the axon, the greater the conduction of the action potential.

Glia

Glia provide guidance, support, nutrition, and protection to the neurons and can be thought of as the connective tissue of the nervous system. Neurons do not survive in tissue cultures unless glial cells are present. Metabolically, they assist in regulating the concentration of sodium and potassium ions in the intracellular space; these ions affect the performance of the nerve cell and are active in repairing damage. Glial cells retain the ability to divide throughout the life of the individual. Injury to the CNS typically triggers glial cell proliferation as a means of repair. Normally, there are approximately 10 glial cells to every neuron, but because glia are smaller than neurons, they account for only half the volume of nervous tissue.

There are three types of glial cells: (1) macroglia, which include astrocytes and oligodendrocytes; (2) microglia; and (3) ependymal cells. The largest glial cell, the astrocytes, provide a vascular link via footlike projections between blood vessels, the brain, and the spinal cord. In the brain, protoplasmic astrocytes are part of the blood-brain barrier, which regulates the influx of vital nutrients and keeps out harmful substances. The "foot processes" surround the outside of capillary endothelial cells (Figure 9-2) and may assist

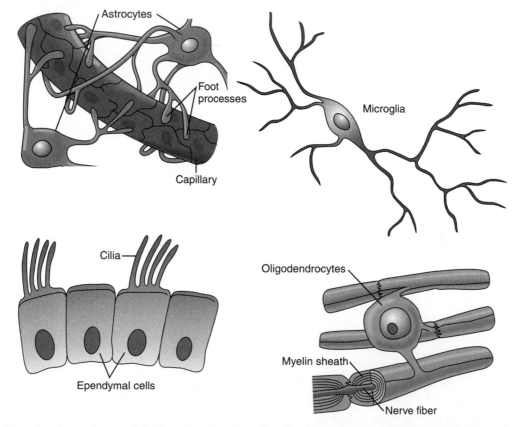

Figure 9-2 The four types of neuroglial cells: astrocytes, microglia, oligodendrocytes, and ependymal cells. (From Copstead LEC, Banasik JL: *Pathophysiology: biological and behavioral perspectives*, ed 2, Philadelphia, 2000, WB Saunders, p 987.)

in the formation and maintenance of the blood-brain barrier. In preterm infants, this barrier has not been formed. Therefore, foreign matter such as meconium, the first stool, may be deposited in brain structures and cause movement dysfunction.[3]

Astrocytes are involved in signaling neurons across an opening known as a gap junction. The signaling can occur from the neuron to the astrocyte or the astrocyte to the neuron. Astrocytes appear to play a key role in electrolyte homeostasis and regulating neurotransmitter release.[4] This bidirectional signaling is supported by the diffusion of Ca^{2+}. Astrocyte excitability seems to be based on the levels of intracellular calcium.

Astrocytes are also present in the spinal cord. They lend structural support to the nervous system and may eliminate interference or cross-talk in nerve cell transmission. Following injury, astrocytes and microglia clean up debris. Fibrous astrocytes fill in the space left by an injury and produce a glial scar, which can actually interfere with healing by blocking reestablishment of synaptic connections.

Microglia are derived from mesenchyme and can be found scattered throughout the CNS (see Figure 9-2). As the major scavenger cells (macrophages), they migrate to any area of injury to remove cellular debris, regardless of whether the spinal cord or brain is damaged. These small cells develop late in the fetal period after the CNS has been supplied by blood vessels.

Oligodendrocytes produce the myelin that covers the neural processes of the CNS (see Figure 9-2). The large number of this type of glial cell is a hallmark of the increasing evolutionary complexity of the nervous system.

Central Nervous System

The brain, brain stem, and spinal cord are collectively referred to as the CNS. The brain consists of two cerebral hemispheres, or cortices, the *brain stem* and the *cerebellum*. Each hemisphere of the cortex is divided into five lobes–frontal, parietal, temporal, occipital, and limbic–which are responsible for different body functions (Table 9-1). The areas that are directly related to processing sensory and motor information or coordinating movement are known as primary and association sensory (or motor) areas (Figure 9-3 and Table 9-2).

The concept that each side of the brain is specialized to perform certain functions has been widely accepted. Although the two cerebral hemispheres appear to be mirror images of each other, gross anatomical differences have been demonstrated by Geschwind and Levitsky.[5] Research has established that the processing and production of language are localized in the left hemisphere and spatial abilities are localized in the right (Table 9-3). The differences are likely to be related

---

Table 9-1

Functions of the Lobes of the Cortex of the Brain

Lobe	Structure	Function
Frontal	Primary motor cortex	Voluntary controlled movements
	Premotor area	Control of trunk and girdle muscles; anticipatory postural adjustments
	Supplementary area	Initiation of movement; orientation of eyes and head; bilateral, sequential movement
	Broca area in left hemisphere	Motor programming of speech
	Same are in right hemisphere	Nonverbal communication
Temporal	Primary auditory cortex	Discriminates loudness and pitch of sounds
	Wernicke area	Hears and comprehends spoken language; intelligence
Parietal	Primary somatosensory cortex	Discriminates texture, shape, and size of objects
	Primary vestibular cortex	Distinguishes head movements and head positions
Occipital	Primary visual cortex	Differentiates intensity of light, shape, size, and location of objects
Limbic	Anterior temporal lobe and inferior frontal lobe	Emotion, motivation, processing of memory; motivational drive to learn

Data from Lundy-Ekman L: *Neuroscience: fundamentals for rehabilitation*, ed 3, St Louis, 2007, Saunders.

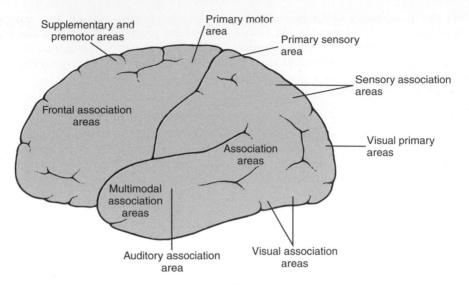

Figure 9-3 Primary and association sensory and motor areas of the brain.

to handedness because 95% of the population is left hemisphere, or right side, dominant.[6] The asymmetry of the two hemispheres is present even in infants.

The nervous system is somatotopically organized to relay signals throughout the body. Somatotopic arrangement of neurons in pathways allows for the localization of somatosensory stimulation. These topographic maps allow specialized axons from one part of the body to be in proximity to axons carrying related signals from adjacent parts of the body. This is true in both the motor and sensory cortices, where the parts of the body are represented. The size of the part is directly related to the functional importance of the part. For example, the sensory homunculus seen in Figure 9-4 depicts a caricature of a human being with oversized lips and thumb. The same type of organizational relationship is present

Table 9-2

Association Areas of the Brain

Association Area	Location	Function
Frontal	Prefrontal area	Goal-oriented behavior; self-awareness; elaboration of thought
Temporal	Temporal lobe	Recognition of faces or objects
Parietal	Posterior parietal lobe in right hemisphere	Attention to both sides of the body
	Posterior parietal lobe in left hemisphere	Attention to right side of the body
Parietooccipitotemporal	Junction of parietal, temporal, and occipital lobes	Interpretive meaning from sensory signals; sensory integration, problem solving, understanding spatial relationships
Limbic	Anterior temporal and inferior frontal lobes	Emotion, motivation, processing of memory

Data from Purves D, Augustine GJ, Fitzpatrick LC, et al: *Neuroscience,* Sunderland, Mass, 1997, Sinauer Associates.

Table 9-3

Behaviors Attributed to the Left and Right Hemispheres of the Brain

Behavior	Left Hemisphere	Right Hemisphere
Cognitive style	Processing information in a sequential, linear manner Observing and analyzing details	Processing information in a simultaneous, holistic, or gestalt manner Grasping overall organization or pattern
Perception/ cognition	Processing and producing language	Processing nonverbal stimuli (environmental sounds, speech intonations, complex shapes, designs) Visual-spatial perception Drawing inferences, synthesizing information
Academic skills	Reading: sound-symbol relationships, word recognition, reading comprehension Performing mathematical calculations	Mathematical reasoning and judgment Alignment of numerals in calculations
Motor	Sequencing movements Performing movements and gestures to command	Sustaining a movement or posture
Emotions	Expression of positive emotions	Expression of negative emotions Perception of emotion

From O'Sullivan SB, Schmitz TJ: *Physical rehabilitation: assessment and treatment*, ed 4, Philadelphia, 2001, FA Davis, p 536.

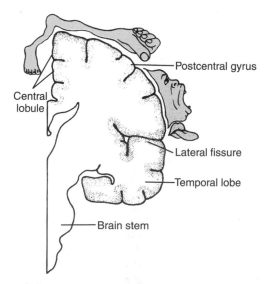

Figure 9-4 Sensory homunculus.

in the visual cortex as a visuotopic map and in the auditory cortex as a tonotopic map. This type of mapping occurs at every level of the nervous system.

The thalamus and the hypothalamus (Figure 9-5) lie deep within the cortex. All sensory systems, except for the olfactory, relay information through the thalamus to the cortex. Information from the basal ganglia and the cerebellum is also processed in the thalamus. Association nuclei integrate touch and visual information, in addition to processing emotional and memory information. Nonspecific nuclei are important for regulating consciousness, arousal, and attention.[7] The hypothalamus, named because of its anatomical relationship just inferior to the thalamus, is responsible for maintaining homeostasis. The hypothalamus integrates behavior and visceral functions by controlling eating, reproduction, and diurnal rhythms (see Chapter 11).

The *basal ganglia* are another group of nuclei found at the base of the cerebrum. This subcortical structure is in reality a group of structures composed of the caudate, putamen, globus pallidus, substantia nigra, and subthalamic nuclei. The basal ganglia regulate posture, muscle tone, and force production and are involved in cognitive functions related to movement. These related functions include motivation, memory for location of objects, changing behavior based on task demands, and awareness of body position in space.[8] Recent research suggests that the basal ganglia contributes to the neural networks that promote optimal motor and cognitive control. The basal ganglia uses the brain's reward system

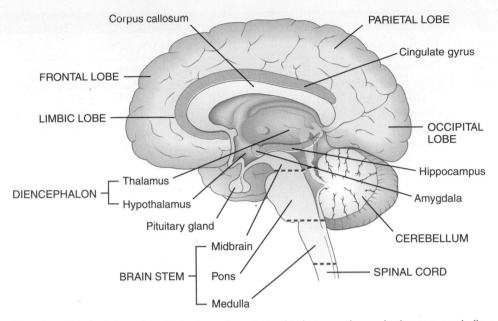

Figure 9-5 Schematic midsagittal view of the brain shows the relationship between the cerebral cortex, cerebellum, spinal cord, and brain stem and the subcortical structures important to functional movement.

to facilitate learning action sequences by trial and error learning.[9] When basal ganglia function is compromised because of a loss of the neurotransmitter dopamine, as happens in Parkinson disease, planning and programming of movement is impaired.

The *limbic system* is very complex. It consists of many interconnected structures, including the amygdala, hippocampus, and cingulate gyrus (see Figure 9-5). Other areas of the cortex and the thalamus are involved in addition to the hypothalamus. The limbic system regulates visceral and hormonal functions, such as eating, drinking, and reproduction. The role of the limbic system in memory is discussed at the end of this chapter.

The *cerebellum* is also made up of two hemispheres connected by a vermis. The cerebellum is involved in the initiation and timing of movements and in monitoring postural tone. By receiving sensory input from the vestibular, auditory, and visual systems, as well as from the spinal cord, it compares actual with anticipated motor performance, thereby functioning as a comparator. The cerebellum receives input from the cerebral cortex via nuclei in the pons, part of the brain stem. The cerebellum influences nuclei in the thalamus and brain stem to control movement, and its circuits are modified during motor learning. The cerebellum is all about timing, the timing of motor actions and the perceptual processing, which requires exact representation of temporal information.[10] "Studies on voluntary movements indicate that the

cerebellum is responsible for motor learning that consists of the development of new input-output associations.[11]"

The brain stem represents a transition between the brain and the spinal cord (see Figure 9-5). Its structures include the midbrain, pons, and medulla moving from the brain above to the spinal cord below. Reflex centers for visual, auditory, and tactile responses are found in the midbrain. The red nucleus, located in the brain stem, receives information from the cerebellum and the cerebral cortex and connects to the spinal cord via the rubrospinal tract. Activity in this tract contributes to upper limb flexion.

The *pons* assists the medulla in regulating the rate of breathing. Reflex centers in the pons assist with orientation of the head in response to auditory and vestibular stimulation. Postural muscle activity is controlled partially by tracts arising from vestibular nuclei located at the junction of the pons and medulla and connecting to the spinal cord.

The *medulla* houses nuclei that control and coordinate cardiovascular responses, breathing, and swallowing. The medulla contributes to the control of eye and head movements, which may be observed when head turning in an infant results in extension of the face arm (the arm toward which the face is turned) and flexion of the skull arm. This asymmetrical tonic neck reflex (ATNR) requires circuits in the medulla.[7] The eyes also turn toward the extended arm.

Loosely arranged groups of neurons within the core of the brain stem are responsible for keeping us alert to novel stimuli or for picking up information pertinent to movement safety. This group of neurons is called the *reticular activating system.* This system regulates the level of consciousness and the daily cycle of arousal, which includes periods of sleep and waking. Consciousness is governed by the reticular activating system, its ascending system that projects to the cortex, thalamus, and the basal forebrain (anterior to the hypothalamus). These latter structures constitute the cerebral part of the consciousness system.[7]

The brain stem, specifically the reticular activating system (RAS), produces generalized arousal and integrates all sensory information and cortical input. A part of the reticular formation contains autonomic nuclei, which interact with the parasympathetic and sympathetic portions of the autonomic nervous system to assist regulation of functions critical for life. Another part of the RAS regulates the flow of information regarding pain, level of awareness, and somatic motor activity. The brain stem acts to filter sensory input, such as pain, to the cortex.

The spinal cord is made up of groups of axons, called *tracts,* that ascend or descend within the spinal cord and relay input to and from CNS structures. Ascending tracts carry sensory information, and descending tracts direct movement. The two primary ascending tracts are the dorsal column and the anterolateral tract. The dorsal or posterior columns carry information about position sense (proprioception), two-point discrimination, deep touch, and vibration. The anterolateral or spinothalamic tract carries pain and temperature sensations to the thalamus for awareness. Light touch and pressure are carried in the dorsal and ventral columns.

The major descending tract located within the spinal cord originates in the frontal lobe from the primary motor cortex, the premotor cortex, and the supplementary motor cortex (see Figure 9-5). This efferent or motor tract is the corticospinal tract. The descending corticospinal tract carries impulses from the cortex, cerebellum, and basal ganglia down the spinal tract that synapse on cell bodies of motor neurons to control distal muscle movement in the arms, fingers, legs, and feet. The corticospinal tract is essential for planning, initiating, and coordinating voluntary movement.

Two additional descending motor tracts are the reticulospinal and vestibulospinal tracts, which travel from the reticular formation and the vestibular nucleus, respectively, to the spinal cord. The reticular formation is involved in providing feedforward control of posture as it anticipates a change in body posture and acts to ready posture for movement such as in gait. The vestibular nucleus provides information about movements generated in response to sensory signals of a postural disturbance and is part of a feedback mechanism for postural control. Gross motor movements can be controlled by these two brain stem pathways, but the motor cortex connections to the alpha motor neuron via the corticospinal tract are necessary for fine, fractionated extremity movements.

Peripheral Nervous System

The cranial and peripheral nerves along with their accompanying nerve nuclei or ganglia are referred to as the peripheral nervous system. *Ganglia* are groups of neuron cell bodies outside the CNS. All 31 pairs of spinal nerves are part of the PNS and have sensory and motor components. The sensory or afferent part is discussed in depth in Chapter 10.

The *efferent (motor) peripheral system* can be divided into the somatic nervous system and the autonomic nervous system (ANS). The *somatic efferent system* conducts impulses to skeletal muscle; the *autonomic efferent system* conducts impulses to smooth muscle, cardiac muscle, and glands. Both the somatic and the autonomic systems produce muscular contractions and change the rate of those contractions, but only the autonomic system causes the secretion of hormones.

The ANS is primarily responsible for maintaining an internal balance of visceral functions related to the heart, smooth muscle, and glands. It consists of three divisions: sympathetic, parasympathetic, and enteric. The sympathetic and parasympathetic divisions use acetylcholine as a neurotransmitter at the preganglionic synapse, as diagrammed in Figure 9-6. The parasympathetic division also uses acetylcholine at postganglionic synapses, whereas the sympathetic division uses norepinephrine to transmit nerve impulses to effector organs. Some effects of ANS activity are outlined in Table 9-4.

The third division of the ANS is contained within the walls of the gastrointestinal (GI) tract and controls digestive function. Although the GI tract receives both sympathetic and parasympathetic input, because of the built-in neural network, it acts independently to some degree. The release of over a dozen neurotransmitters by different types of enteric neurons has been documented (see Chapter 11).[12]

COMMUNICATION WITHIN THE NERVOUS SYSTEM

The nervous system is connected via synapses. The axon of a neuron contacts the cell body or dendrite of another neuron to make a synapse. The axon is the output cell of the neuron, while dendrites are the input

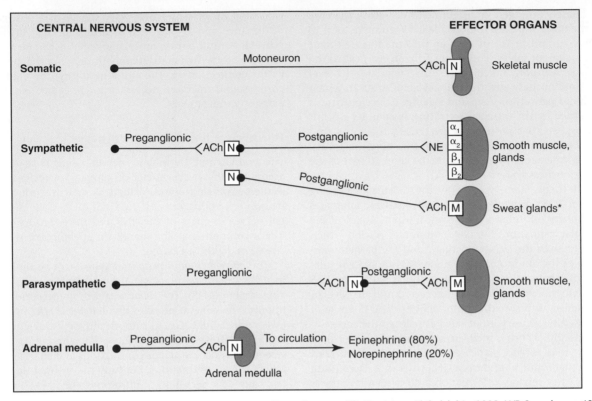

Figure 9-6 Organization of the autonomic nervous system. (From Costanzo LS: *Physiology*, Philadelphia, 1998, WB Saunders, p 40.)

cells of the neuron. As the system matures, more and more connections are made, both axonal and dendritic. A labyrinth of relay stations with an infinite number of ways to take in, disseminate, and combine information is formed (Figure 9-7). Dendritic spines are highly specialized subcellular structures that can change shape in a matter of seconds.[13] The increasing density and complexity of dendrites, the input cells, are a mark of advanced communication seen in phylogenetically higher animals. Dendritic branching increases the synaptic potential of the nervous system (Figure 9-8). Developmentally, branching occurs after initial pathways are formed with changes in spine morphology supporting changes in synaptic strength. The dynamic nature of change in dendritic spines provides a mechanism for correct information processing and storage in neural networks. Synaptic remodeling occurs throughout the life span in response to experience.[13,14]

Synapses

Neuron-to-neuron transmission of nerve impulses occurs at an interneuronal junction called a *synapse.* There are two basic types of synapses: chemical

and electrical. Electrical synapses, referred to as *gap junctions*, are instrumental in the development of the brain.[15] Their role will be discussed under life span changes. Only a few gap junctions were thought to be present in the adult human nervous system; however, functional electrical synapses have been shown to exist between GABAergic interneurons in the cortex of adult animals.[16] The human nervous system uses predominantly chemical synapses that are activated by substances called *neurotransmitters.*

More than 40 different chemical substances have been classified as neurotransmitters. A few of the best known are acetylcholine, norepinephrine, serotonin (5-HT), glutamate, gamma-aminobutyric acid (GABA), and dopamine. Dopamine, norepinephrine, and serotonin are slow-acting. Glutamate is a major excitatory neurotransmitter, and GABA is major inhibitory neurotransmitter; both are fast-acting. Transmission time for slow-acting neurotransmitters takes one tenth of a second to minutes compared with one-one thousandth of a second for fast-acting ones.[7] When an action potential reaches the end of an axon, it triggers the release of a neurotransmitter from synaptic vesicles. Sodium ions facilitate the depolarization of the presynaptic membrane, and calcium ions facilitate

Table **9-4**

Selected Effects of Autonomic Nervous System Activity

Organ	Effect of Sympathetic Stimulation	Effect of Parasympathetic Stimulation
Eye		
Pupil	Decrease dilation	Decrease constriction
Heart		
SA node	Increase heart rate	Decrease heart rate
Muscle	Increase rate and force	Decrease rate and force
Arterioles	Constriction	Dilation
Veins	Constriction	None
Lungs		
Bronchi	Dilation	Constriction
Gut		
Lumen	Decrease peristalsis	Increase peristalsis
Sphincter	Increase tone (usually)	Relax tone (usually)
Liver	Release glucose	Slight glucose synthesis
Kidney	Decrease output and renin secretion	None
Bladder	Relax detrusor muscle Contract trigone muscle	Contract detrusor muscle Relax trigone muscle
Glands		
Lacrimal	None/slight secretion	Copious secretion
Sweat	Copious sweat	Sweaty palms of hands
Basal metabolism	Increase	None

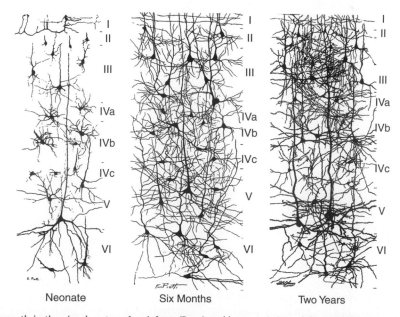

Neonate   Six Months   Two Years

Figure 9-7 Dendritic growth in the visual cortex of an infant. (Reprinted by permission of the publisher from Conel JL: *The postnatal development of the human cerebral cortex*, vol I-VIII, Cambridge, Mass, 1975, Harvard University Press (originally published in 1939).)

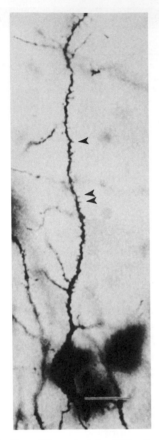

Figure 9-8 Portion of the apical dendritic of a pyramidal neuron illustrating dendritic spines. Golgi-Cox stain, human cerebral cortex; bar represents 20 g. (From Burt AM: *Textbook of neuroanatomy*, Philadelphia, 1993, WB Saunders, p 40.)

the release of the neurotransmitter. The transmitter diffuses across the space between the two neurons and binds to receptors on the postsynaptic neuron membrane.

Neurons can synapse on other neurons called *interneurons,* or they can synapse on muscle or glands. Interneurons are a major source of synaptic input to motor neurons. Interneurons are the links between motor neurons that form functional networks. Interneurons in the spinal cord receive sensory input that provides reflexive coordination between muscle groups. In addition, signals received from interneurons can facilitate or inhibit the firing of motor neurons.

Cortical Connections

Communication within the nervous system takes place via one of three ways: by association fibers, by commissural fibers, and by projection fibers. *Association areas* are cortical areas responsible for horizontally linking different parts of the cortex. The parietal, temporal, and occipital association areas are involved in perception. The sensory association cortex (see Figure 9-3) is responsible for interfacing sensory information from the three lobes to perceive and to attach meaning to sensory input, such as identifying shapes by touch. The thalamus and other nuclei in the brain stem relay sensory information to association areas for perceptual judgments. The prefrontal and the limbic association areas are concerned with movement and motivation, respectively (see Table 9-3).

Information is communicated not only within the hemispheres but also between the right and left hemispheres. A large group of nerve fibers, called the *corpus callosum,* transmits information between similar areas of the two sides of the brain (see Figure 9-5). For example, the anterior part of the corpus callosum transmits from the anterior cortex of one side to the anterior cortex of the opposite side.

Information is also shared vertically, up and down the neural axis, by tracts and nuclei that connect the cortex and the spinal cord. Afferent fibers bring sensory input into the spinal cord via the posterior root and connect with or continue as ascending tracts that carry information to various parts of the brain. Efferent fibers carry out commands from the motor cortex and prefrontal cortex, which travel in descending tracts to the anterior horn of the spinal cord.

ADAPTATION OF THE NERVOUS SYSTEM

Neural Plasticity

Neural plasticity is the ability of the nervous system to change. While it has always been hypothesized that the nervous system could adapt throughout life, there is now ample evidence that the adult brain maintains the ability for reorganization or plasticity.[17-19] Traditionally, it was always thought that plasticity was limited to when the nervous system was developing. *Critical periods* are times when neurons compete for synaptic sites. Activity-dependent changes in neural circuitry usually occur during a restricted time in development or critical period, when the organism is sensitive to the effects of experience. The concept of plasticity includes the ability of the nervous system to make structural changes in response to internal and external demands. Learning and behavior appear to modulate neurogenesis throughout life. Plastic changes can also include the ability of the neurons to change their function and the amount and type of neurotransmitter they produce.[20] The changes in structure and function of the building blocks of the nervous system are prime examples of nervous system plasticity.

After birth, the nervous system continues to mature. Although most of the 100 billion neurons are already formed at birth, neurons continue to make connections with other structures through dendritic branching and by remodeling other connections. Neuronal projections compete for synaptic sites during critical periods.[7] Persistent changes in spine morphology are seen when synaptic strength increases.[13] Neurons that fire together, wire together. The size of the spine is correlated with the strength of the synapse it forms.[14] Postnatal experience plays a major role in further inducing developmental changes by strengthening the pattern of synaptic connections of the system. Development and experience interact to produce change. Some types of mental retardation and cognitive disorders have been linked to spine density abnormalities (Figure 9-9).[13]

Experience is critical to development. Two types of neural plasticity have been described in the literature.[21] Unfortunately, the names given to them are confusing. One is experience-expectant, and the other is experience-dependent. In the course of typical prenatal and postnatal development, the infant is expected to be exposed to sufficient environmental stimuli at appropriate times. In fact, if the infant is not exposed to the proper quality and quantity of input, development will not proceed normally. This type of *experience-expectant* neural plasticity is exemplified in the sensory systems that are ready to function at birth but require experience with light and sound to complete maturation. Deprivation during critical time periods can result in the lack of expected development of vision and hearing.

Experience-dependent neural plasticity allows the nervous system to incorporate other types of information from environmental experiences that are relatively unpredictable and idiosyncratic. These experiences are unique to the individual and depend on the context in which development occurs, such as the physical, social, and cultural environment. Lebeer[22] refers to this as *ecological plasticity,* whereas Johnston[23] uses the term *activity-dependent plasticity.* Climate, social expectation, and child-rearing practices can alter movement experiences. What each child learns depends on the unique physical challenges encountered. Motor learning as part of motor development is an example of *experience-dependent neural plasticity.* Experiences of infants in different cultures may result in alterations in the acquisition of motor abilities. Similarly, not every child experiences the same exact words, but every child does learn language. *Activity-dependent plasticity* is what drives changes in synapses or neuronal circuits as a result of experience or learning.

Neuron Cell Death

Neuron cell death is an important occurrence in the development of the nervous system because the nervous system initially overproduces neurons. This overproduction ensures a sufficient number of neurons to complete the "wiring" of the organism and to support optimal function. Regressive phenomena take place at the end of neuron development and can result in cell loss as high as 70%.[24] Two regressive processes mold the developing nervous system. One is *apoptosis,* or programmed cell death, and the other is *axon pruning.* Apoptosis is a naturally occurring phenomenon within the nerve cell that is different from cell death that occurs secondary to injury or disease. The metabolic state of the extracellular environment appears to strongly influence this process. Those neurons deprived of trophic support, that is, those not nourished, degenerate and die. *Developmental apoptosis* is necessary for formation of normal neural networks. A major window of opportunity for programmed cell death ends around the time of birth. The trimming of extraneous axon connections, or *axon pruning,* occurs without harm to the cell of origin and allows for sculpting of the nervous system.

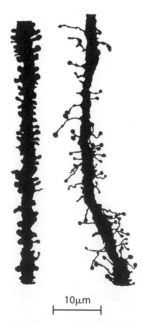

10μm

Figure 9-9 Dendritic spines from the brains of a normal 6-month-old child (*left*) and a severely cognitively impaired 10-month-old child (*right*). (From Purpura D: Dendritic spine "dysgenesis" and mental retardation, *Science* 186:1126-1128, 1974.)

Selective Neuronal Vulnerability

Plasticity is not always a positive occurrence. A defect in signaling or gene transcription can impair plasticity and affect learning and memory. Individuals with impaired plasticity would have cognitive deficits such as seen in Down syndrome. Excessive plasticity can lead to brain circuits that are unable to adapt to changes in connectivity. This type of plasticity has been linked to abnormalities in sensory system function and seizure generation. Lastly, plasticity that increases vulnerability to damage is demonstrated by the immature brain's inability to handle asphyxia.

Neurons are selectively vulnerable when synaptic connections are being assembled as during a critical period. Therefore, some periods of brain development afford more of a chance for damage to occur. For example, immature oligodendroglia that are positioned around the ventricles (periventricular) are particularly susceptible to damage from hypoxic ischemia.[25,26] Damage in this area is associated with spastic diplegia in premature infants.[27] Selective damage to the cortex and basal ganglia is associated with more severe motor problems involving the upper extremities more than the lower extremities. The molecular pathways that mediate these perinatal injuries are beginning to be unraveled.[25]

Neuroscience is only just beginning to understand the mechanisms of altered plasticity that occur after a developmental injury.[28] Some of the same processes that are crucial for establishing the appropriate connections within the developing nervous system may be appropriate to repair damage from injury, but others may be inappropriate. What is to prevent maladaptation by the nervous system? Giza and Prins[28] conclude that "young is not always better" in patients with developmental traumatic brain injury. The same statement can be made about the mature nervous system's response to injury, both of which are discussed below. Adaptive plasticity is defined as that which improves skill development or recovery from brain injury. Thus, the reorganization of circuits after neurological injury is also driven by activity-dependent plasticity as depicted in Figure 9-10. Plasticity is needed for learning to occur and for recovery of function following injury to the nervous system.

Cellular and molecular changes that occur with aging also render neurons vulnerable to damage.[29] Bartzokis[30] postulated that the same cortical regions (the frontal lobe and the hippocampus) that exhibit a protracted developmental course are vulnerable to degeneration later in life. Bartzokis[30] contends that the myelin breakdown in these regions is related to a decrement in the ability of the oligodendrocytes to continue to produce myelin in

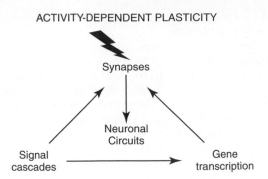

ACTIVITY-DEPENDENT PLASTICITY

Figure 9-10 Activity-dependent plasticity and refinement of synaptic connections are mediated through modulation of activity at synapses, which activate signaling cascades and gene transcription. Environmental sensory and behavioral conditions, drugs, toxins, nutritional disturbances, and genetic mutations affect the final formation of neuronal networks in the developing brain at multiple levels in this process. (From Johnson MV: Clinical disorders of brain plasticity, *Brain Dev* 26:73-80, 2004.)

the central nervous system. The last areas to myelinate appear to be the first to disconnect in Alzheimer disease and result in problems with new memory formation and higher cognitive functions. Mattson and Magnus[29] implicate the abnormal accumulation of proteins as the culprit in determining the age-related neuronal vulnerability in Parkinson, Alzheimer, and Huntington diseases. Oxidative stress is one major mechanism that can lead to damage and death of neurons. The most vulnerable neurons are large with myelinated axons that travel relatively long distances.

Response to Injury

The PNS retains the ability to regenerate, as evidenced by a return of muscle function after some types of peripheral nerve lesion. When peripheral nerve damage is severe enough to disrupt the myelin sheath and the axon, the axon will degenerate back to the node of Ranvier that is most proximal to the injury. This is called wallerian degeneration. After a time, the axon will regrow and try to reestablish contact. In a young healthy person, a peripheral nerve may grow a millimeter a day or an inch a month, given ideal circumstances.[7] The path of nerve growth can be followed by the Tinel sign (a tingling when the nerve is tapped) as the severed nerve grows and reestablishes contact with its receptor. In the most severe peripheral nerve injury, surgical intervention is required to reestablish the connection.

Adaptability within the CNS is functionally limited to reorganization because in most cases regeneration does not occur. Typically when a neuron dies, it is replaced by glial cells. When the brain is damaged by ischemia, some neurons die immediately, others are at risk of dying if blood supply is not reestablished. Neurons die via necrosis and apoptosis. The latter is programmed cell death that is triggered by an environmental event that sets in motion a cascade of events resulting in cell death. Additional neuron damage or death can occur because of excitotoxicity, during which time synaptic activity can contribute to ischemic injury. Excess secretion of the excitatory neurotransmitter glutamate can cause destruction and death of previously injured neurons. Adjacent neurons that are not directly injured may become inhibited from functioning. Blood flow changes can occur in areas remote from the original damage such that some areas of the cortex are less excitable.[31]

Recovery from neural injury involves resolution of edema, reperfusion of the damaged area, and mechanisms of neural plasticity. The initial inhibition of function is called *diaschisis*. Diaschisis is manifest by temporary blockage of function because of edema, shock, decreased blood flow, and underuse of glucose. Synaptic effectiveness is altered following neural injury. When local edema resolves, synaptic effectiveness improves. Denervation hypersensitivity also contributes to a decline in synaptic effectiveness. This happens when presynaptic neurons are destroyed, thereby depriving postsynaptic neurons of sufficient amounts of neurotransmitters. Through neural plasticity, new receptor sites are developed at the remaining synaptic terminals or some synapses become hypereffective by releasing more neurotransmitters than usual. There may also be reactive synaptogenesis when collateral sprouting occurs to reestablish synaptic sites on injured axons. There can also be *vicariation* of function when one area of the brain either cortically or subcortically takes over for a damaged area. While plasticity is usually thought of as a positive occurrence, it can also be maladaptive. Physical therapy interventions aimed at functional tasks such as the use of a treadmill for locomotor training take advantage of use-dependent cortical reorganization.[17,32]

SUMMARY OF STRUCTURE AND FUNCTION

Neurons are the means by which the nervous system communicates. All information is received by specialized receptors and transmitted along several distinct pathways to various regions of the brain, where it is interpreted, acted on, stored, or ignored. Structurally, neurons are produced to match their functions within the nervous system. Neurons increase their ability to communicate by the branching of dendrites and making of new synaptic connections. This branching can be very sophisticated and is related to the amount of information that can be processed. Complexity in dendrite formation is a mark of advanced evolution. As shown in Figure 9-9, fewer dendritic spines are seen in individuals with mental retardation.[33] The nervous system exhibits a great deal of plasticity throughout the life span. The brain is constantly changing and adapting to experience: those experiences that are expected and those that are unique to the individual. Scientists have shown that new neurons produced in the hippocampus are able to become fully functional. "While the vast majority of neurobiological models of memory have for a long time integrated synaptic plasticity as a fundamental mechanism for learning and memory formation, the addition of new neurons … suggests a new mechanism of plasticity.[19]" Research continues to analyze the structural and functional responses of the nervous system when it is damaged and to delineate the factors that influence a person's potential for recovery.

LIFE SPAN CHANGES

Prenatal Period

The CNS develops from specialized ectoderm at 3 weeks of gestation when the neural tube is formed. The brain is created from the cranial two thirds, and the spinal cord from the caudal one third, of the neural tube by the end of the fourth week of gestation—1 month before the mother feels the fetus move.[34] When this process is disturbed, severe brain and spinal cord anomalies may result, including anencephaly and myelomeningocele. During the fourth week of gestation, the embryo develops head and tail folds because of rapid growth of the cranial region and spinal cord. The head continues to enlarge during the succeeding weeks, with the brain being folded back onto itself. By 8 weeks, the head of the embryo is half the size of the body. At the end of the eighth week, the fetus looks definitely human and has completed the most critical period of CNS development.

Development of the nervous system is a complicated process. Via cytogenesis or cell production, the maximum number of neurons and glia are produced. Neurons of the spinal cord and brain stem are generated by the tenth week. The neurons of the forebrain, including the cerebral hemispheres, are produced by 20 weeks.[35] During histogenesis, or tissue formation, the structures of the brain and spinal cord are formed. Neurons move or migrate to their correct location within the nervous system, where they differentiate into different nerve cell types, form synaptic connections, and enlarge. Neuronal targets produce trophic substances that guide neuronal connections. Neuronal connections need to have the correct number of axons so that axons innervate the correct number of target cells.[6] Initially, there is polyneuronal innervation of prenatal muscle fibers compared with the 1:1 relationship seen in postnatal life.[7]

Nerve cell types are genetically determined. Therefore, the size and shape of the nerve cell, the pattern of axon or dendrite branching, and even the type of neurotransmitter a neuron will use are innately determined. The cerebral cortex begins as one layer only a few cells thick, known as the *germinal zone*.[36] Cell generation order and cell position in the cortex have an inside-out relationship because of the mechanism of cell migration. The cells formed earliest occupy the deepest layer of the cortex; the cells formed later occupy progressively more superficial layers.[35] These cells migrate using a system of guides, the radial glial fibers, which extend from the surface of the ventricles to the surface of the cortex. Structurally, the six layers of the cortex are completed during the last months of gestation and the first postnatal months of life.[36]

The first endocrine gland, the thyroid, develops at 24 days.[34] By the eleventh week, it begins to secrete thyroxin, a hormone necessary for proper brain growth. This hormone triggers the cessation of nerve cell proliferation and initiates nerve cell migration.[37] Without the thyroid hormone, axons are poorly myelinated and neurons do not completely branch. Too little hormone produces *cretinism*, a condition in which there is arrested mental and physical development.

Neuroglia form from the neuroepithelium as early as 3 weeks, although proliferation does not start until 18 weeks of gestation.[38] Microglia appear to be derived from mesenchymal cells late in the fetal period after blood vessels have established their connections. Glial tissue provides a kind of road map for migrating neurons within the brain.[39] The migration appears to be facilitated by some type of chemical affinity between neuronal and glial surfaces, at least in the cerebellum.[35]

Internal brain structures such as the thalamus and hypothalamus are present at 7 weeks of gestation. The internal structure of the spinal cord is achieved by 10 weeks. During the next 5 to 15 weeks, general structural features—sulci and gyri, cervical and lumbar enlargements of the spinal cord—are attained.[34] The 12 pairs of cranial nerves emerge during the fifth and sixth weeks of gestation.

In addition to giving rise to the neural tube, the neural plate gives rise to neural crest cells, which are the precursors of the PNS. The PNS begins as paired masses of neural crest cells, one on each side of the neural tube, that differentiate into the sensory ganglia of the spinal nerves. The neural crest cells in the brain region migrate to form sensory ganglia for cranial nerves V, VII, VIII, IX, and X.[34] Other structures also are produced from the neural crest cells: Schwann cells, meninges (the connective tissue covering of the brain), and many musculoskeletal components of the head.

Motor nerve fibers begin to appear in the spinal cord at the end of the fourth week of gestation, forming the spinal nerves. Next, the dorsal nerve root (consisting of sensory fibers) appears. It is made up of the axons of neural crest cells that have migrated to the dorsolateral part of the spinal cord, forming a spinal ganglion. The spinal nerves exit between the vertebrae, elongate, and grow into the limb buds, where they supply muscles that are differentiated from *mesenchyme*. The muscles innervated by segments of the spinal nerve are referred to as *myotomes*. Skin innervation occurs in the same segmental fashion, resulting in *dermatomes*.

Synapse formation occurs relatively late in the development of the nervous system, just before 6 to 7 weeks. Synapse formation is highly variable in pattern and distribution. The development of connections between the sensory neurons and the motor neurons is critical to laying the framework for spinal reflexes and for the pairing of sensory and motor information. A spinal reflex is the pairing of a sensory neuron and a motor neuron so that incoming stimuli produce a motor response. Once established, spinal reflexes are permanent[40] and considered "hard-wired." Reflexes can be monosynaptic or polysynaptic; that is, they can involve one or more than one synapse. The establishment of reflex connections provides the fetus and eventually the infant with survival reflexes, such as suck-swallow, rooting, and gag. Fetal movement begins in utero at about 6 to 7 weeks of gestation. Reflex movements in response to touch have been chronicled as early as 7 to 8 weeks of gestation. Reflex connections are established in utero in a cephalocaudal direction; arm withdrawal occurs earlier than leg withdrawal.

As another late-stage phenomenon of neural development, myelination starts after neuron formation (8 to 16 weeks of gestation) and overlaps with neuron migration (12 to 20 weeks of gestation). Myelination occurs first in those areas of the nervous system that will be used first. Myelin is initially laid down in the cervical part of the spinal medulla and in the cranial nerves related to sucking and swallowing, abilities needed for survival. The first axons to be myelinated are the anterior (motor) roots of the spinal cord at about 4 months of gestation. One month later, the posterior, or sensory, roots begin the process. Myelin is deposited as a sheath or covering in the spinal cord at the same time that functional connections (i.e., synapses) are being formed.[41] The vestibulocochlear system (cranial nerve VIII) is myelinated at the end of the fifth month of gestation[42] and is related to awareness of the head and body position in space.

Rapid periods of growth such as those seen in the fetal period are critical periods when the nervous system is most vulnerable to damage. The nervous system requires adequate nutrition for cell formation and myelination to occur.[43] For example, lipids in the form of fatty acids must be transported through the blood-brain barrier because there are no endogenous fats in the brain.[44] Birth occurs before CNS development is complete because the fetus outgrows the space, and the metabolic demand of the developing brain mass cannot be met by the mother's placenta.[45] Malnutrition or trauma can have dramatic effects on the developing system. A lack of nutrition results in a decrease in the number of synapses formed and in the amount of dendritic branching and myelination.[38]

Infancy and Early Childhood

At birth, the brain is one-fourth the weight of the adult brain, whereas the head is already 70% of its adult size. Critical periods for brain growth occur between 3 and 10 months and between 15 and 24 months of age.[24] Brain weight doubles by 6 months of age and is half the weight of the adult brain. Malnutrition during the first 2 years of life reduces the number of glial cells formed,[46] which may result in poorer vascular support for nervous

system function. The relationship of brain weight and brain growth is depicted in Figure 9-11. Children who are malnourished before 3 years of age reportedly have impaired motor ability.[47]

Brain metabolism changes with CNS maturation during infancy. Tracking glucose metabolism in the brain postnatally provides another means to document functional maturation. The pattern of activity, that is, where glucose is being used, corresponds to the areas of the brain that are maturing. In the newborn, the highest activity is found in the primary motor and sensory cortex, thalamus, brain stem, and midline of the cerebellum. By 2 to 3 months, increases in glucose use are evident in the parietal, temporal, and primary visual cortex; basal ganglia; and cerebellar hemispheres. The frontal cortex is the last area to demonstrate increased glucose use. The increase begins between 6 and 8 months, and by 8 to 12 months, use is widespread in the frontal lobes.[48] The increase in glucose use in the frontal lobes also corresponds to the expansion of dendritic branching and capillary networks in the frontal lobe.[49,50]

The cerebral metabolic rate of glucose use in infancy is 30% lower than in adulthood.[48] Figure 9-12 depicts the changes that occur in the metabolic rate of glucose use of the brain over time and compares the relative rate of use between children and adults. These changes over time partially mirror the time course for synaptogenesis. Synaptic proliferation occurs in the period between birth and 4 years of age. The typical 2-year-old has twice as many cerebral cortex synapses as an adult.[23] Between the ages of 2 and 3, the brain contains about 15,000

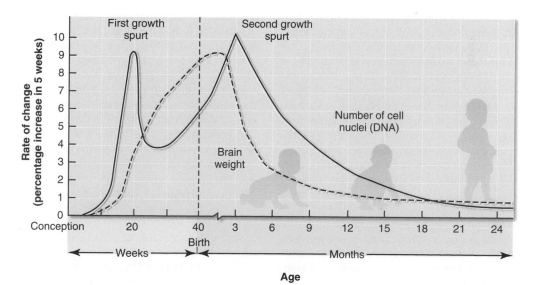

Figure 9-11 Relationship of brain weight *(dotted line)* and growth *(solid line)*. The DNA curve has two peaks: one reflecting neuron multiplication, and the other reflecting glial multiplication. (Data from Dobbing J: Undernutrition and the developing brain, *Am J Dis Child* 120:411-415, 1970.)

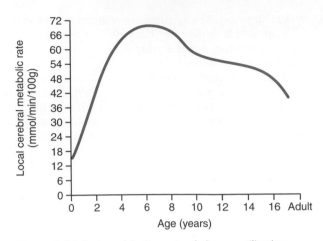

Figure 9-12 Brain metabolism rate of glucose utilization. (Adapted from Chugani HT: A critical period of brain development: studies of cerebral glucose utilization with PET, *Prev Med* 27:184-188, 1998.)

synapses per neuron. Pruning of excess synapses begins early in childhood, continues through adolescence and stabilizes during early adulthood.[51] The decline in rate of glucose use at adolescence is due to synaptic elimination that occurs in the cortex with a further diminishment of energy requirement to adulthood.[52]

Myelination of the PNS is largely complete at birth,[53] allowing the newborn immediate access to information about the environment through touch, motion, smell, and taste. The infant uses these sensory cues to carry out vital functions of eating, breathing, sleeping, and excreting. All cranial nerves (with the exception of the optic nerve) are completely myelinated at birth.

Although the PNS is ready to function at birth, myelination has only been occurring for 2 months in the brain (assuming that the infant is born at term, 40 weeks of gestation). Myelination in the CNS continues into young adulthood. The primary motor cortex develops ahead of the primary sensory cortex. The rates of myelination are related to when these areas reach adult levels of function.[54] Figure 9-13 shows when some major structures undergo myelination. "In general, … brain development progresses from posterior to anterior and from inferior to superior.[51]" The cerebellum and the brain stem myelinate before the cerebral hemispheres.[55] The midbrain and spinal cord are the most advanced portions at birth in terms of myelination, which may account for early descriptions of infants functioning only on a brain stem level. Early myelination of the brain stem supports the many vital functions controlled there and accounts for the fact that the newborn sleeps most of the time and is totally dependent on caregivers.

The first 2 months after birth are considered a period of CNS organization. During this time, the infant establishes physiological control of sleep and wakefulness as evidenced by the relationship between sleep states and electroencephalographic patterns, and by increasing the number and duration of periods of alertness. Social behavior begins around 2 months of age with the advent of the social smile. Circadian rhythm, or the 24-hour biological cycle, is established between 2 and 4 months of age without regard for night and day.[56] In other words, this is a time when infants can get their days and nights mixed up.

ANS changes occur during the first year of life as the newborn responds more via the sympathetic nervous system to ever-changing stressors such as light, gravity, and air. As internal body processes such as GI motility stabilize, behavioral responses gradually become more characteristic of the parasympathetic nervous system, which maintains the status quo or steady state.

Nerve conduction velocity increases over time in both skin and muscle fibers because of the change to saltatory conduction and the increase in nerve fiber diameter with age. Values for nerve conduction speed change remarkably quickly after birth. For example, ulnar nerve conduction in infants and young children increases from 30 to 50 m/sec from birth to 9 months of age and reaches adult values (60 m/sec) by 3 years of age.[57]

Brain structures are ready to support the development of function during the first year of life. The major efferent (motor) tract, the corticospinal tract, begins myelination 1 month before birth and completes the process by 1 year. The corticospinal tract in the newborn has not yet innervated the anterior horn, so during the first 6 months of life the infant demonstrates a Babinski sign.[7] Stroking the foot from the heel along the lateral border of the foot and then under the toes results in extension of the great toe. Although presence of this sign in individuals older than 6 months is indicative of corticospinal tract damage, in a young infant it is a sign of immaturity. There appears to be a correlation between late corticospinal tract development and late motor development.[58] Furthermore, the fact that the pattern of terminations of the corticospinal tract axons changes over the course of postnatal development is an example of activity dependent plasticity. The structure of the corticospinal axon terminals reflects sensory-motor cortex activity.[59] The sensory area of the brain catches up to the motor area by the age of 2. During the second year of life, the increasing speed and complexity of movement may be related to myelination. The process slows after 2 years and is mostly complete by 10 years of age.

The richness of the experiences that a child is exposed to during the first 3 years of life can be critical to cognitive development.[60] Brain growth during childhood is

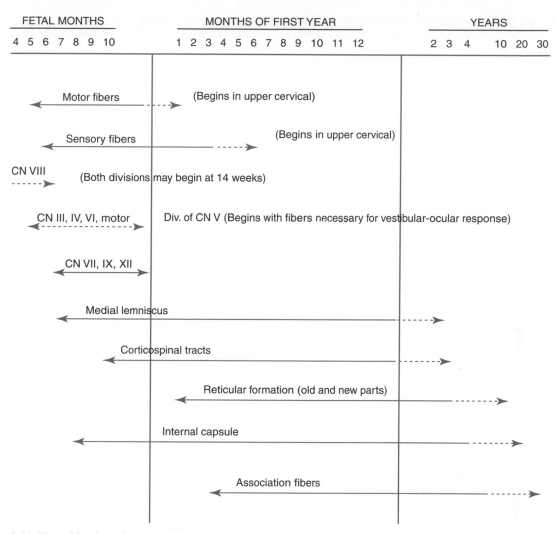

Figure 9-13 Timetable of myelination of selected nervous system structures. (Modified from Yakovlev PI, Lecours AR: The myelogenetic cycles of regional maturation of the brain. In Minkowski A, editor: *Regional development of the brain in early life,* Oxford, UK, 1967, Blackwell.)

thought to coincide with the stages of cognitive development as described by Piaget[61] and the development of language.[62] The infant's brain weight at 1 year is 60% of its adult weight, a gain of 10% in 6 months. During the next year, growth continues until 75% of adult brain weight is reached by age 2. The relationship of brain weight, age, and language acquisition is shown in Table 9-5. Myelination of structures that support speech development, such as the tectum, an integration center for auditory information, and the striatum, an integration center for language, occurs within the first year of life. Myelination of the striatum by 1 year of age coincides with the child's first spoken word. The pattern and density of dendritic branching have also been linked to language development, especially

the specialization of the left hemisphere as the language center in the majority of individuals.[62] A 2-year-old child can put together two-word combinations and by age 3 can speak in phrases and short sentences.

Childhood and Adolescence

Children develop fundamental skills such as jumping, throwing, catching, and balancing in early childhood (3 to 6 years). From 6 to 10 years of age, these skills become refined as ongoing myelination of the nervous system continues to increase the speed of conduction of nerve impulses and motor control becomes more automatic. The adolescent may continue to improve motor

Table 9-5

Relationship of Age, Brain Weight, and Language Acquisition

Age	Brain Weight (% of adult weight)	Language Level
Birth	25	Crying; no words
1 yr	60	Average age of first spoken word
18 mo to 2 yr	75	Two-word combinations
3 yr	80	Phrases and short sentences
6 yr	90	Five- to six-word sentences
Puberty	100	Abstract language concepts

skills with practice. The amount of change after adolescence is highly variable and depends more on practice, instruction, motivation, and innate ability.

To achieve its adult weight, the brain undergoes additional critical periods during growth spurts at 6 to 8 years, 10 to 12 years, and around 18 years of age. At 6 years of age, 90% of the adult brain weight is achieved, and the child is able to speak in five- to six-word sentences. Despite the fact that children exhibit a partially mature corticospinal tract between 6 and 9 years of age, the ability to conduct nervous impulses at adultlike speeds is not sufficient for proficient motor performance. A group of young school-age children could not perform a motor task as well as adults.[63] The corticospinal tract becomes morphologically mature by 10 years of age but not electrophysiologically mature until age 13.[63,64] In other words, the structure of the tract is adultlike in its connections and anatomical configuration before the tract is able to exhibit adult levels of neurotransmission.

Myelination continues during adolescence in the sensorimotor systems, including secondary cortical areas. The last areas to be myelinated are the association cortices in the frontal, parietal, and temporal lobes, along with other association fibers. At puberty, adult brain weight is attained, and abstract language concepts such as the use of complex clauses are demonstrated. Dendritic branching in the areas of the cortex involved with speech and language reaches adult levels of complexity between 12 to 16 years of age.[62] Additionally, low-frequency electroencephalographic rhythms change to adult high-frequency rhythms by 10 to 13 years of age.[65] The process of myelination of association areas continues through adulthood.[30]

The brain directs other body systems to change at puberty via hormonal influences. These changes include, but are not limited to, development of the secondary sex characteristics, changes in body composition, and the onset of menses (see Chapter 11).

Adulthood

Myelination continues into adulthood in those areas responsible for integrating information for purposeful action, the association areas of the brain. Myelination peaks about 50 years of age.[55] The majority of individuals between the ages of 20 and 29 years are at the peak of their ability to perform physically. Those involved in sports, such as recent Olympic competitors, are even younger. Despite the continued myelination of association areas, the nervous system begins to decline in adulthood. Brain weight and volume decline linearly with age in the average population.[66] Beginning at age 20, brain weight declines,[66] the cortex thins,[67] and the number of glial cells changes depending on type. Astrocytes and microglia increase, and oligodendrocytes decrease.[68] How much decline is necessary before functional abilities are affected is not known. We do know that age-related changes in the nervous system have far-reaching effects on all systems of the body.

"Age-related decrease in brain weight and dimension is very closely associated with deterioration of myelin.[69]" Any significant loss of neurons would be expected to cause an increase in glial cells.[70] While some have reported a decrease in glial cells in connection with the destruction of the myelin sheaths, others report that the number of glial cells does not increase in normal aging.[71] More importantly, it is thought that structural changes in several types of glial cells may have a greater effect on neuron function if, over time, such changes interfere with the transport of vital nutrients from the surrounding blood supply to the neuron.[72]

CNS changes related to aging are not the same for every part of the brain. Aging affects the frontal and temporal lobes more than the parietal lobes.[73] Positron emission tomography scans show decreased brain glucose metabolism in both of these areas in older individuals compared with young adults.[74,75] Previous reports of neuron loss from other areas of the cortex, such as the primary motor and sensory areas of the cortex, have not been substantiated by further research. Subcortical areas such as the thalamus, striatum, and locus ceruleus are more likely to lose neurons with aging.[76] Computed tomography scans confirm that atrophy of the brain occurs with aging.[77] In addition, there is ventricular enlargement. Cerebral volume declines by 11% in relation to cranial volume between the ages of 20 and 30.[78] A greater decline in brain volume has been reported in women than in men beginning in their 40s. Birge[79] reported on research findings in women that the loss primarily affects the hippocampus (in the temporal lobe) and parietal lobe. A total of about 15% of brain weight and volume is lost throughout the life span, beginning in middle adulthood.[80] The amount of these decreases is moderated by overall good health and varies according to the area of the brain studied. There is considerable interindividual variability in the patterns of brain changes.[81]

The hippocampus, a part of the limbic system associated with memory, has been reported to show a 30% decrease in neurons beginning after the age of 30.[82] This is due to the loss of pyramidal cells, which play an important role in memory and learning.[83] As stated earlier, research has shown that new neurons are produced in the hippocampus in adulthood.[19] In fact, exercise has been found to regulate adult hippocampal neurogenesis.[84]

In contrast to a litany of decreases in large populations of cells, the absence of significant age-related neuron cell loss has been documented in some discrete brain structures. The basal ganglia, which implement movement programs, maintain stability during adulthood.[72] Some brain stem nuclei show little or no neuron loss as a result of aging.[85] The dentate nucleus in the cerebellum and the nucleus basalis in the forebrain have not been shown to lose neurons.[86] The latter is responsible for the majority of cholinergic input for the cerebral cortex.

In the adult, nerve conduction velocity of peripheral nerves decreases.[87] The speed with which sensory nerves conduct impulses begins to decline after 30 years of age.[88] Motor nerve conduction velocity, according to Schaumburg and colleagues,[87] decreases by 1 m/sec per decade after 15 to 24 years of age. Therefore, sensory information continues to come into the nervous system, albeit more slowly.

The nervous system changes that result from aging begin at age 20. Brain weight and thickness of the cortex decline, whereas the number of glial cells increases. Whether the number of neurons increases, decreases, or stays the same with reduced neuron size is still being debated. Despite all of these occurrences, few overall changes in the structure of the brain and nervous system exceed 25% of the total area, except in disease states and only during the last few months of life.[89] The built-in redundancy of the nervous system by way of synaptic plasticity is such that even if neurons are lost in one place, other connections may be gained. Most areas of the brain stem that deal with vital functions are stable throughout adulthood and show minimal change with aging.

Older Adulthood

A major problem with identifying primary aging changes in the nervous system is that it is impossible to know with any degree of certainty if these are signs of preclinical pathology. The potential that both intrinsic and extrinsic environmental factors can produce changes with aging further compound the problem of identifying what are primary aging changes. Some degree of brain volume and neuron loss is probably inevitable, but it is not possible to state unequivocally what is "normal" or "typical" because universal or primary aging changes are difficult to separate from those that are harbingers of pathology. A cross-sectional comparison of a normal brain and an aging brain is shown in Figure 9-14.

Terry and colleagues[90] studied 51 brains from normal individuals aged 24 to 100 years and found that the overall total number of neurons, neuron density, and percentage of cell area occupied remained unchanged. A striking reduction in neuron size, however, was noted, along with a minor degree of neuronal loss when the entire cortex was considered. Large neurons in the frontal and temporal lobes shrank, whereas the number of smaller neurons increased.[90] Haug and associates[91] and Haug[92] concluded that the total number of neurons in the cortex does not change during the aging process and that the dominant age-related change is neuronal shrinkage. However, Pakkenberg and fellow researchers[71] found only a 10% change in number of total neurons in the brain from age 20 to 90 years.

Age-related decline in brain weight and volume is accompanied by neuronal atrophy, cell death, and ventricular enlargement. Resnick and colleagues[93] documented on average a 1.4 cm^3 increase in ventricular volume per year in healthy older adults. Gyral atrophy includes loss of gray and white matter, whereas white matter loss includes the loss of myelin. The volume of cerebrospinal fluid (CSF) remains constant until age 40, then increases with another rise after age 60.[86] Significant differences in brain volume are seen between young-old, middle-old, and oldest-old subjects.[94] Volume loss is seen to be minimal after age 65 with decline progressing at small constant rates from young-old to middle-old to oldest-old. The rate of loss is small and constant in the healthy older adults.

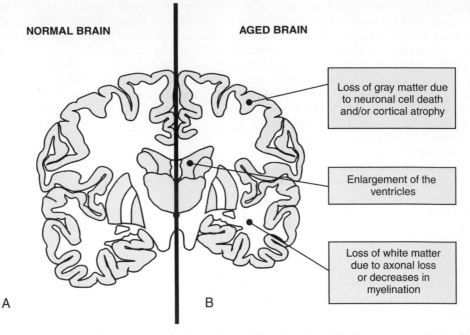

NORMAL BRAIN   **AGED BRAIN**

Loss of gray matter due to neuronal cell death and/or cortical atrophy

Enlargement of the ventricles

Loss of white matter due to axonal loss or decreases in myelination

A   B

Figure 9-14 Comparison of a normal and an aged brain. **A,** A normal hemisection of the human cortex. **B,** Aged human cortex. Researchers have observed several age-related gross anatomical changes, including a loss or atrophy of cortical neurons, a decrease in white matter (due to axonal or myelin loss), and an enlargement of the ventricles. (From Fox CM, Alder RN: Neural mechanisms of aging. In Cohen H, editor: *Neuroscience for rehabilitation*, ed 2, Philadelphia, 1999, Lippincott Williams & Wilkins, pp 401-418.)

Minor to moderate neuron loss and the loss of the ability of dendrites to produce new spines (sprouting) have been reported in many parts of the brain, but the link to a decline in function is far from apparent. Structural losses may be a result of an age-dependent decline in use because dendrites continue to grow into old age. Synaptic remodeling and growth also occur late in adulthood.[38] Synaptic plasticity can be assessed using positron emission tomography as a measure of cognitive reserve capacity. Dendritic complexity in older individuals who are cognitively intact supports the idea that the nervous system is still able to adapt well into the 70s.[70]

With the increased use of neuroimaging techniques such as magnetic resonance imaging (MRI) and positron emission tomography (PET), the longitudinal changes in aging brain function are becoming better elucidated. Volumetric imaging is one of the gold standards being used to understand the effects of increasing age on brain tissue. Specifically, voxel-based morphometry (VBM) has been used to localize loss in density of both gray and white matter. Good and colleagues[95] reported global loss of gray matter volume in older adults with a decline seen *primarily* in the parietal and frontal lobes. White matter loss was also seen, but the decline was

nonlinear and more prominent in the occipital and frontal regions. It appears that white matter loss is more accelerated in people in their 70s and 80s compared with people in their 50s and 60s. Resnick and associates[93] used MRI to longitudinally study the shrinking brain in adults aged 59 to 85 years at baseline. They found substantial declines in both gray and white matter.

White matter declines almost 30% with age.[96] It is the structure that declines the most with age. The commissures, major bundles of white matter that provide interhemispheric communication, are essential to human memory.[2] "The marked loss of myelinated nerve fibers with age could explain some of the cognitive decline seen in the elderly.[96]"

Minor changes in electroencephalographic patterns, such as a slowing of the alpha waves, have been reported with aging.[97] Additional evidence, however, suggests that no significant changes in pattern occur with age.[98] In fact, the temporal wave slowing, so often attributed to normal aging, has been linked to pathological brain changes.[99]

The cerebellum also shows age-related changes that could be associated with declines in posture, balance, and gait seen in the older adult. Although not proved to be cause and effect, the decrease in Purkinje cells and the fact that the cerebellum is highly myelinated seem to indicate a potential correlation.

Brain function as measured by glucose metabolism shows a 6% decline from ages 20 to 67 years.[100] Mielke and co-workers[101] have attributed "normal aging of the brain [to be] predominantly characterized by metabolic changes in the prefrontal cortex." The frontal lobes appear to be an area of the brain affected early and extensively by aging according to some researchers.[30] Indeed, studies of age-related memory loss show a decline with age that is related to the frontal lobe executive function abilities. Adults 60 years or older performed less well than young adults aged 20 to 40 on tasks that required orbitofrontal cortex function.[102] Itoh and colleagues[103] found that cerebral blood flow was preserved during aging even in the presence of brain atrophy, which progressed linearly. However, in a longitudinal study by Beason-Held and associates,[104] cerebral blood flow was shown to decrease with age in areas of the frontal, temporal, and occipital lobes. Structures such as the thalamus and caudate that border the lateral ventricles also showed a decrease in blood flow, which may reflect age-associated increases in ventricular volume.[93] Areas of the brain that showed an increase in blood flow included the hippocampus, cerebellum, and the prefrontal white matter. It has been postulated that these areas may represent preserved function in the brain relative to the global decline in blood flow seen with advanced age.[104]

The hippocampus exhibits a number of neurofibrillary tangles (NFTs) within the neuron cell body as a result of aging.[105] Although the incidence of NFTs increases with age in the healthy brain, an even greater incidence is seen in patients with dementia.[70] Neuritic or senile plaques and lipofuscin accumulation are additional cellular hallmarks of aging. A *senile plaque* is a thickened mass of degenerating *neurites* (small axons, some dendrites, astrocytes) with an *amyloid* (starchy glycoprotein) deposit in the center. Neuritic plaques occur as a result of pathological aging and are some of the earliest neuropathological hallmarks of Alzheimer disease (AD).[106]

The role of lipofuscin in normal aging and as a risk factor for AD has recently been studied and reviewed.[107,108] Lipofuscin, a byproduct of cell metabolism, is a pigment associated with aging. It accumulates in all cells of the brain. It also is deposited in other tissues of the body such as the heart. The amount of lipofuscin had previously been thought to roughly correlate to the degree of dementia in AD,[109] which has been linked to oxidative damage to neurons. Oxidative stress is a major theory of aging. Lipofuscin may be formed when there is incomplete degradation of lysosomes in mitochondria. So initially, lipofuscin may benefit the cell as a way to deal with degrading organelles. Extreme amounts of lipofuscin can negatively impact cell function and result in cell death. "Similarly, early in the development of AD, lipofuscin may be advantageous in delaying the development of AD-related pathology, but ultimately serve to synergize with other cellular factors to promote the development of AD pathology and AD dementia.[108]"

On a biochemical level, the loss of enzymes involved in neurotransmitter synthesis has been documented along with a moderate loss of receptor sites for certain neurotransmitters in both the CNS and the PNS.[110,111] A decline in motor system performance has been linked to a steady decrease in dopamine uptake sites because of an age-related loss of axons in basal ganglia pathways.[112] Loss of serotonin receptors in the cortex has been postulated to predispose older individuals to depression and cognitive impairment.[111] Cholinergic function declines in patients with AD; therefore, deficits in cholinergic function are also related to cognitive impairment. Specifically, the muscarinic type of cholinergic receptors decreases by 50% to 60% in the caudate, putamen, hippocampus, and frontal cortex between the ages of 4 and 93 years.[113] The declines in the serotonergic and cholinergic systems may play a role in cognitive decline associated with pathological aging.

Modest declines in dopamine content of the basal ganglia have been measured after midlife.[113] This 25% loss is in sharp contrast to the losses exhibited with severe lesions involving the basal ganglia or in Parkinson disease. The age-related alterations in the basal ganglia resemble those that occur in Parkinson disease, but the cell dropout is not as severe. Despite the similarity of brain cell degeneration, the causes for the changes are likely to be different.[114]

Aging changes in the ANS can be linked to changes in the sensitivity of sympathetic receptors to circulating neurotransmitters. *Aging* has been described as a hyperadrenergic state because of the more intense cardiac and vascular sympathetic responses seen in older adults.[115] In a review by Seals and Esler,[116] an age-related increase in total body sympathetic nervous system activity was reaffirmed. This increase is region specific and includes the gut, skeletal muscle,[116] heart, and liver[117] as targets but not the kidneys. Less epinephrine is released from the adrenal medulla in older adults at rest and in response to stress.[117] No consistent age-related changes in norepinephrine have been documented.[111]

Peripherally, over age 60, the loss of motor neurons and myelinated anterior root fibers contributes significantly to the gradual loss of muscle mass and strength seen with aging.[118] Decreased awareness of touch and vibration are two documented peripheral changes that occur by the age of 70.[119] Sensory changes are discussed more thoroughly in Chapter 10. The concept of "use it or lose it" cannot be overlooked when assessing the competence of any body system to adapt over time. It is especially true for the nervous system. As we age, lifestyles and habits formed early in life will be what motivate, inspire, and provide an impetus to move. If exercise, fitness, and health are valued and the individual stays physically fit and actively participates in life, how will the outcome differ?

FUNCTIONAL IMPLICATIONS

Two aspects of nervous system function—reaction time and cognition—are used to illustrate the relationship between nervous system development and acquisition of function. Reaction time is a measure of nervous system efficiency during movement. *Cognition* is that function of our brain that enables interaction with the environment. It is a complex brain function, whereas *reaction time* is a simple function. Both aspects of nervous system function—cognition and reaction time—change over time.

Reaction Time

The batter sees the ball, swings, and hits the ball. *Reaction time* is defined as the amount of time between presentation of a stimulus and the motor response. As would be expected, the reaction time of children is slower than that of adults.[120] Reaction time improves as the child develops more complex skills such as catching and hitting. Physical maturation affects information processing speed in 9 and 10 year olds, with early maturers being faster than late maturers.[120] Processing speed relative to cognitive tasks also increases in childhood with significant gain seen between 9 and 10 years and 11 and 12 years.[121] Reaction time peaks in young adulthood and then declines; it is slowed 15% to 30% in older persons.[68]

A simple response time (SRT) test measures reaction speed when only one response is required from a stimulus, such as hitting a key when a light flashes. Fast test responses are reported for subjects in their 20s, with the greatest consistency of response seen in subjects in their 30s. Responses on SRT tests slow with age.[122] A 20% increase in reaction time is seen in 60-year-old subjects compared with 20-year-old subjects.[123] Slowing reaction time or psychomotor speed has been recognized as a universal behavioral change in aging.[124]

Reaction time consists of three parts: (1) sensory transmission of input, (2) motor execution time, and (3) central processing.[125] The latter component makes up 80% of the total reaction time. Reaction time requires attention because attention is a prerequisite for sensory information to get into working memory, a concept that is discussed under cognition. Investigators using electromyography separate premotor time from motor time. *Premotor time* is the time between the stimulus and electromyographic activity and reflects the neural component of reaction time. Premotor time represents components 1 and 3. *Motor time* is defined as the time between the electromyographic activity and the movement and therefore reflects the muscular component of reaction time.

Both premotor and motor times are related to chronological age. Premotor time (the neural component) is slower in all older individuals regardless of task. Motor time (the motor component) depends more on the type of task, especially the amount of muscular force required. Simple tasks such as hand movement show more age-related effects on the premotor time[126]; jumping[127] and movement against resistance[128] show more age-related effects on the motor time. The more complicated the task, the more likely it is to be influenced by age-related change. In general, the more complicated the decision or task, the bigger is the difference seen in the reaction time of young and older adults.[129]

Complex or choice reaction time studies involve a choice between two responses. Light and Spirduso[130] confirmed that as the task becomes more complex, reaction time increases with the increasing age of the individual. In a complex task such as trying to recover balance, an individual's risk of falling increases with age. After the age of 60, reaction time variability increases relative to that of younger individuals. When Fozard and colleagues[131] compared simple and choice reaction times in a group of men and women ranging in age from 20 to 90 years; however, they found only slight slowing of simple reaction time but more dramatic slowing in choice reaction time.

Central and peripheral factors contribute to the slowing of reaction time. Laufer and Schweitz[132] reported that only 4% of the change in reaction time in aging individuals can be accounted for by the decrease in motor nerve conduction velocity, and 10% can be accounted for by the decrease in sensory nerve conduction velocity. The greater contribution to slowing comes from the central factors or premotor components. These premotor components include stimulus identification and processing, response selection, and response programming. Older subjects process sensory information for an aiming task, similar to younger subjects but at a lower speed.[133] Slowness is related to changes in neural pathways in the brain and brain stem that integrate sensory and motor information.[134]

Health and exercise may modify age-related changes in reaction time.[135] When the level of physical activity of the individual is considered, active older subjects have been found to have faster reaction times than sedentary older subjects.[136] Also, variability within older subjects increases such that on a day-to-day basis, responses are not as consistent as they are in younger individuals. The rate of slowing depends a great deal on the task.[137] Thus results involving reaction time in the elderly must be regarded cautiously.

Fitness training has positive benefits on both peripheral and central aspects of reaction time. Response times are faster for those individuals who had engaged in exercise for long periods of their lives. Those who exercised performed better than those who did not exercise on reasoning and working memory tasks. Training improved the performance of older adults engaged in multiple tasks. These improvements were retained for several months.[138] The aging brain generates new neurons in response to physical exercise, and it is thought that learning selectively enhances synaptogenesis well into adulthood.[84] The researchers postulated that physical activity enhanced the vascular response of the brain and that the neural component reflected learning.

Attention, Learning, and Memory

Cognition is the process of knowing and the application of that knowledge is intelligence. Cognitive processes include selective attention, learning, and memory. The ability to change the structure of the nervous system in response to experience is the basis for learning and memory.[139] Executive functions performed by the brain involve goal-directed, conscious decision-making and strategy selection. These functions require attention to select features on which to make decisions, to resolve conflicts, and to plan new actions.

Self-Control

Executive or focal attention is related to a person's ability to assess the many conflicting details of the environment and self and then make choices that influence cognitive and emotional function. Posner and Rothbart[140] posited that the ability to attend develops during the first year of life and is initially demonstrated by the infant's self-regulation of her own distress. Infants can consistently self-calm at 3 to 4 months when their attention is distracted. Posner and Rothbart[140] further hypothesized that the mechanism used by infants to cope with feelings of distress, or self-regulate, is transferred and applied to the control of cognition during later infancy and childhood.

The development of self-control begins in infancy with the regulation of distress and may involve interaction between areas in the frontal lobe, specifically the cingulate and the amygdala. For example, an 18-month-old shows context-sensitive learning when visually attending to her surroundings. Spatial locations are learned when the frontal areas of the brain develop a functional visual field. Self-control is needed for attention, and attention is needed for learning. Executive attention undergoes a dramatic change around 30 months of age. Patterns of response change, with older children becoming more accurate. Casey and co-workers[141] showed a significant correlation between the ability to perform tasks that relied on attentional control and the size of the right anterior cingulate in children aged 5.3 to 16 years. Further refinement of the attentional system occurs in adulthood. The development of self-control progresses slowly in early life, continues throughout adolescence, and becomes mutable during adulthood.[140]

Memory

The developmental psychologist Piaget[61] attributed the origin of intelligence to the pairing of sensory and motor experiences. He viewed cognitive development as necessary for memory development. The nervous system controls cognition by processing thought and memory. According to Guyton and Hall,[12] a thought reflects a pattern of stimulation of the cortex, thalamus, limbic system, and reticular formation of the brain stem. Physiologically, memories are produced by changes in the ability of one neuron to transmit to another neuron across a synapse, producing a "memory trace." Movement of energy leaves a residue by which use of the pathway can be assessed; think of a thermogram in which greater intensity of the color denotes warmth and increased blood flow. Memories can be considered immediate, short term, or long term depending on their duration. Immediate memories last for only a few seconds or a few minutes. Short-term memories can last for days or weeks but will eventually be lost if they are not converted to long-term memory. Long-term memory can be recalled years later and is thought to result from structural changes at the level of the synapses that influence signal conduction (Lynch, 1998).[142]

Types of Memory

There are two types of memory: implicit and explicit. *Implicit,* or procedural memory, relies on performance of procedural skills, which include forms of perceptual and motor learning that do not require verbal expression but are exhibited by alterations in task performance.

An example is matching shapes to a template. Researchers have shown that infants as young as 3 months remember a particular motor event. Rovee-Collier[143] experimented with connecting an infant's arm or leg to a mobile with a ribbon. The infant learned to move the mobile and even remembered which arm or leg to move after a short time had passed. Implicit memory is unconscious memory and is related to the cerebellum and striatum (caudate and putamen).[144,145]

Explicit, or declarative memory is the learning of facts and experiences that can be reported verbally, such as naming body parts, state capitals, or muscle origins and insertions. Explicit memory is conscious memory. It depends on structures in the medial part of the temporal lobe, including the hippocampus.[144,145] Because relative value is placed on this type of learning, the limbic system becomes involved. Declarative learning and memory allow for categorical aspects of higher cognitive and affective (emotional) processing such as abstract thought.

The development of memory occurs throughout life (Table 9-6). Before 6 months of age, there is no conscious memory, only a learned adaptive response. After 6 months of age, an infant learns object permanence, so she knows that an object does not disappear when it is out of sight. Conscious, explicit memory is demonstrated as early as 7 months, but recall of events is minimal until a child is about 3 years of age.

Conscious memory may be related to the linguistic ability of the child.

Between 5 and 7 years of age, the child begins to relate past and present memories and to reason more efficiently.[146] Children no longer just monitor perceptual information, such as size, shape, and color, but correlate perceptual information (e.g., "all round objects made of rubber bounce, whereas round stones do not"). They continue to pick up and reflect on relevant perceptual cues to solve increasingly complex problems or to perform tasks after the age of 6 or 7 years.[147] Around the age of 9 or 10 years, children begin to direct their thinking. They can evaluate, plan, and refine their own thinking about how best to solve a problem. Being able to think about thinking is called *metacognition,* a term that subsumes elaborate executive functions. The ability to think about remembering is called *metamemory.* We practice metacognition when encountering a patient with an undefined movement dysfunction and thinking of ways to approach the patient's problem. We practice metamemory when planning for a test by reviewing what one does and does not know.

With aging, there is a decrease in complex cognitive skills involving memory. As you may recall from Chapter 2, there are four types of long-term memory according to Tulving[148]: semantic memory, procedural memory, episodic memory, and perceptual representation memory. Nilsson,[149] reporting on the results

Table 9-6

Development of Memory

Type	Age	Neural Structures	Examples
Implicit (procedural)	First few months	Striatum (caudate and putamen); olivary-cerebellar complex	Procedural learning Conditioning
Preexplicit	Before 8 mo	Hippocampus and temporal lobe	Attention Recognition memory Novelty detection
Explicit (declarative)	Begins at 8-12 mo	Limbic and temporal lobe	Event sequence Novelty preference
Working	Begins at 8-12 mo; increases at 6-24 yr	Prefrontal lobes	Relate past events to present
Long term	Over life span	Hippocampus, basal ganglia, cerebellum, premotor cortex	Word meaning Motor behavior

Data from Nelson CA: The ontogeny of human memory: a cognitive neuroscience perspective, *Dev Psychol* 31:723-738, 1995; Purves D, Nelson CA: The nature of early memory, *Prev Med* 27:172-179, 1998; Augustine GJ, Fitzpatrick LC et al: *Neuroscience,* Sunderland, Mass, 1997, Sinauer Associates; Swanson HL: What develops in working memory? A life span perspective, *Dev Psychol* 35(4):986-1000, 1999.

of a large study in Sweden, states that there is a linear decline in episodic memory with age. Furthermore, there is a gender difference with women scoring higher than their male counterparts up to the age of 70. This same study reports a relatively constant performance in semantic and perceptual representation memory tasks with increasing age. Their study did not have any data on procedural memory performance, but they reported other data showing mixed results. As procedural memory is motor memory, the inconsistencies may be related to the tasks used to test this type of memory. If the tasks involve aspects of short-term memory, there might be a decline with age. If the task used in testing is purely procedural, it would only require activation of the primary motor cortex, which is relatively well preserved in older adults.[150]

Working memory is most affected by aging because information must not only be retained but also be manipulated or changed to be retrieved. New information can be registered and retrieved, but new information is forgotten more quickly. The speed with which information is processed slows with age and is a fundamental cause of age-related decline in memory.[151] This activity requires that information storage occurs at the same time as acquisition of new data, something that is difficult for the older learner. Older adults appear to have to redistribute resources from storage to allocation to keep up. A simple recall task without distraction showed no change in short-term memory with age in the Betula study.[149] However, others have reported that when older subjects had to process and store information simultaneously, there were significant age-related deficits.[152] Recently, Gazzaley and colleagues[153] looked at the effect of high memory load and distraction on older adults' ability to perform a delayed-recognition and recall task. Results showed that as the memory load increases, the older adult makes more errors in recognition. The frontal lobes are affected early by aging,[134] and the prefrontal cortex is involved with preserving memories in the face of distractions.[154] Changes in memory abilities need to be considered when giving verbal direction to older patients with movement dysfunction. Written instructions that parallel the verbal instructions are often critical to provide adequate carryover in a home program.

Intelligence

Cognition is functionally reflected in intelligence and development of executive function. "The development of the brain throughout infancy, childhood and adolescence is paralleled by the growth and maturation of the mind.[155]" Theory of mind refers to the ability of a person

to understand and reason. It implies that the person can appreciate how the desires and intentions of others are the same or different from her own. Children below the age of 4 do not demonstrate this ability. Looking at the development of executive function and its components will provide an overview of the changes that occurs in the brain over the life span.

Anderson's[156] model of executive function (Figure 9-15) identifies four aspects: attentional control, information processing, cognitive flexibility, and goal setting. Attentional control and information processing have already been discussed. Table 9-7 provides a broad general chronology of changes seen in all four aspects of executive function. Davidson and associates[157] looked at cognitive flexibility in children from 4 to 13 years of age. The ability to switch responses requires inhibition of previously learned responses and working memory. This ability begins to emerge between 3 and 4 years of age.[158] The child can handle more complicated tasks between 7 and 9 years, with gains continuing into early adolescence but not achieving adult levels.[157]

The frontal lobe is thought of as the seat of executive function. The frontal lobes are involved in planning and organization.[159] The frontal lobe is the last lobe of the brain to complete its development and is not fully mature in adolescence. Adolescence is a unique

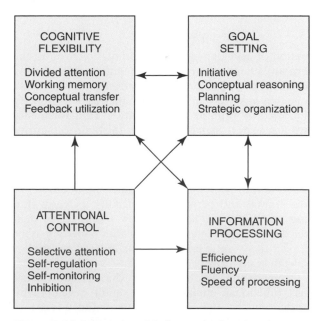

Figure 9-15 Proposed model of executive function. (From Anderson P: Assessment and development of executive function (EF) during childhood, *Child Neuropsychol* 8[2]:71-82, 2002.)

Table 9-7

Development of Executive Function

Attentional Control	Information Processing	Cognitive Flexibility	Goal Setting
By 12 months can inhibit certain behaviors			
By 3 years can inhibit "instinctive" behaviors	See an increase between 3 and 5 years	Between 3 and 4 years can switch response sets	4 year olds demonstrate simple planning abilities; can generate new concepts
Impulse control improves up to 6 years		Between 7 and 9 can handle more complicated tasks	Rapidly develop organizational skills between 7,
9 year olds can monitor and regulate own actions	Significant gains seen between 9 and 10 years	Gains continue through childhood	10,
Some increase in impulsivity seen at 11 years	Significant gains continue from 11-12 years	Gains continue into adolescence	and 11 years of age
	Minimal changes after 15 years	At age 13, still not at adult level	Some regression at 12-13 years, refinement and improvement during the rest of adolescence

Source: Anderson P: Assessment and development of executive function (EF) during childhood, *Child Neuropsychol* 8(2):71-82, 2002; Davidson MC, Amso D, Anderson LC, et al: Development of cognitive control and executive functions from 4 to 13 years: evidence from manipulations of memory, inhibition, and task switching, *Neuropsychologia* 44:2037-2078, 2006.

period of development. The prefrontal cortex and the limbic system undergo major reorganization during this time period. Axons in the prefrontal cortex are still myelinating.[160] Synaptic density increases in puberty followed by pruning after puberty.[161] Functional MRI studies seem to support that both the brain's cognitive appraisal system and its emotion processing systems develop in adolescence.[162,163] Structures that make up the limbic system such as the amygdala show greater activation in adolescents than adults. White matter in the frontal and parietal lobes steadily increases during childhood and adolescence,[164] whereas gray matter declines. Gray matter decline after puberty may be linked to synaptic pruning and is inversely related to overall brain growth.[55,164]

Remodeling of the cortex during adolescence has functional implications for adult development. "Environment and genetic programming interact to regulate synaptic organization during the critical period resulting in a mature cortex.[165]" Behaviorally, a teen's performance on tasks involving decision making, working memory, processing speed, and inhibitory control improves during adolescence.[166,167] These tasks represent different facets of executive function, which are the purview of the frontal cortex. Consistent improvement is correlated with pruning of synapses and myelination. Regulation of emotional behavior is thought to be related to integration of information from the cortex and the limbic system. Benes and associates[168] supported this explanation by documenting increased myelination of the involved structures.

A key factor in cognitive development is *working memory*. In working memory, information is manipulated. This action is supported by recruiting areas of the frontal cortex, specifically the dorsolateral prefrontal cortex (DLPFL) and the superior parietal cortex. The brain accumulates information about experiences in the external world and develops an internal world in the temporal and parietal association cortices.[155] The frontal association area manipulates thought models like images or scenarios to simulate what could happen in the real world. These thought models are shared with the cerebellum so that eventually thinking can be more automatic and less conscious.[155] Crone and associates[169] found that 8 to 12 year olds did not perform as well as 13 to 17 or 18 to 25 year olds on an object-working memory task. They concluded that increased recruitment of DL and PFC by adolescents resulted in their improved ability to work with object representations.

Adult executive function appears to depend on a set of interrelated cortical and cerebellar regions that are also involved in early motor skill acquisition. "The cerebellum and prefrontal cortex participate as critical parts of a neural circuit that is important when (1) a cognitive task is difficult as opposed to easy, (2) a cognitive task is new as opposed to familiar and practiced, (3) conditions of the cognitive task change, as opposed to when they remain stable and predictable, (4) a quick response is required, as opposed to longer response latencies being acceptable, and (5) one must concentrate instead of being able to operate on 'automatic pilot.'[170]" Ridler and co-workers[171] showed that the frontocerebellar system used for executive function, is anatomically related to systems associated with typical infant motor development. They looked at two groups of adults; one group had schizophrenia and the other were nonpsychotic. The group with earlier motor skill development had superior executive function while the group with delayed motor skill development had impaired executive function. If there is a common anatomical substrate for motor and executive function, then early motor behavior might be able to predict who might develop poor executive

function. However, it is more likely "adult executive systems emerge developmentally by integration of additional (prefrontal and lateral cerebellar) regions with a "core" or prototypic, frontal premotor-medial cerebellar circuit that has previously matured in support of early motor skills.[171]"

Horn and Donaldson[172] described two types of intellectual ability: fluid intelligence and crystallized intelligence (Figure 9-16). *Fluid intelligence* is the ability to form novel associations, to reason logically, and to solve problems. It can be measured by looking at reaction time and memory. Fluid intelligence peaks in the early 20s and declines throughout adulthood (see Figure 2-13. *Crystallized intelligence* is experiential learning, education, and stored information. It is the ability to use judgment to decide on a course of action. This type of intelligence incorporates a lifetime of decision-making and is postulated to improve with age.[172]

According to measures of intelligence, intellectual ability peaks between ages 20 and 30 and is maintained until at least 75 years of age.[115] Despite all we do know about the aging changes related to cognition or intelligence, we do not understand why some older individuals remain alert, sharp, and active participants in the world around them and others lose touch, disengage, or show signs of dementia. To date, there is insufficient research to relate loss of neurons from the nervous system to functional decline in cognitive function in healthy aging individuals. Intellectual changes seen in

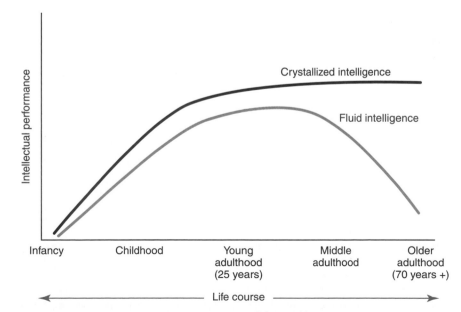

Figure 9-16 Comparison of age-related changes in fluid and crystallized intelligence.

later life that are considered "normal" include (1) slowing of reaction time or cognitive processing, (2) decline in fluid intelligence, and (3) impairment in some aspects of short-term memory.[99]

Exercise appears to mediate cognitive changes in the brain that occur from aging. Erickson and Kramer[173] support the premise that 6 months of moderate aerobic exercise can produce significant improvements in cognitive function in older adults. The effect of the exercise occurs in the area of executive function. In their review of studies, the ability to plan and coordinate a task was enhanced by an aerobic exercise program. Williamson and colleagues[174] also report a positive benefit of physical activity on cognitive function in a pilot study involving over 100 sedentary older adults aged 70 to 89 years.

The typical life span course of the nervous system can be perturbed anywhere along its developmental path. Two examples of disruption of the nervous system are fetal alcohol syndrome and Alzheimer disease. These examples provide a marked contrast to typical development in one case and a possible variant of aging in the other case.

Fetal Alcohol Syndrome

Fetal alcohol syndrome (FAS) causes significant learning and sensory deficits in children and is a leading cause of mental retardation in the western hemisphere.[175] Along with fetal alcohol effects (FAE), FAS has been described as a spectrum disorder. As such, the term spectrum disorder is recognized as an umbrella designation to encompass the full range of observed outcomes in individuals prenatally exposed to alcohol. The ingestion of alcohol during pregnancy can produce a myriad of physiological and behavioral abnormalities. Visuospatial functioning is impaired as is attention, verbal, and nonverbal learning. These deficits affect overall executive function or the ability to make decisions and solve problems. Behavioral manifestations can also include attention deficit/hyperactivity disorder. "FAS is the most common known cause of mental retardation and occurs more often than two other common birth defects (Down syndrome and spina bifida) combined.[176,177]" Fetal alcohol spectrum disorders (FASD) are a major public health problem.[178]

The incidence of FAS is 0.97 per 1000 births worldwide with different countries reporting widely varied estimates.[179] Reports vary country to country. Higher rates of FAS, on average 9 per 1000, are seen in certain populations such as Native Americans.[180] Prevalence has been reported as high as 7 per 1000 in one Italian province.[181] The problem is worse when trying to estimate the rate of prevalence of all FASDs. A prevalence as high as 1 in 100 live births has been reported.[175] Pregnant women continue to drink alcohol, with 13% reporting frequent or binge drinking.[182] Binge drinking is more detrimental to the fetus than chronic low levels of drinking because it takes the fetus days to detoxify what the mother's liver can dissipate in hours.[183]

Clinical Features

The classic presentation from which the term fetal alcohol syndrome was coined came from Jones and Smith in 1973.[184] The triad of signs that constitute FAS are facial dysmorphology, prenatal and postnatal growth disturbances, and central nervous system deficits including mental retardation. The facial features are shown in Figure 9-17 and consist of short palpebral fissures, short nose, an elongated midface, wide set eyes, thin upper lip, and a long, undefined philtrum (area between the nose and upper lip). Children with FAS show decreases in both weight and length/height, characteristically falling below the 10th percentile for age or gestational age.[185] A head circumference at or below the 10th percentile is part of the Institute of Medicine guidelines for diagnosing FAS.[186] IQ scores for children with FAS are usually between 40 and 80.[187] There can be wide individual differences with some children having an IQ within the average range in childhood after a diagnosis of FAS in infancy. It should be noted that FAS is a diagnosis of exclusion, as other disorders such as Williams, DeLange, and velocardiofacial share some of the same facial characteristics.[178]

FASD is the result of altered neural plasticity. Animal research supports the fact that alcohol disrupts the development of sensory circuits in the developing rat/ferret brain. Early on the development of functional

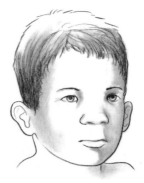

Figure 9-17 Characteristic facial features of a child with fetal alcohol syndrome. (From Ratliffe KT: *Clinical pediatric physical therapy*, St Louis, 1998, Mosby. p 331.)

maps of the sensory cortex and the visual cortex are disrupted by alcohol exposure. Later, the development of the frontal lobes, known to be involved in executive function, is negatively impacted by alcohol ingestion.

Adolescence

Blakemore and Choudhury[164] suggest that because puberty is a time when synaptic reorganization occurs, it may represent a critical or sensitive period for development of social cognition as well as executive functions. Social cognition is the knowledge of social rules, norms, or behaviors usually learned by observation of others. Adolescent alcohol abuse interferes with development of the frontal lobe and maturation of executive function. Figure 9-18 is a model of the effect that alcohol abuse has on adolescent and subsequent adult development. See the Clinical Implications Box 9-1 for further information regarding how alcohol can affect development across the life span.

Alzheimer Disease

Alzheimer disease (AD) is a progressive degenerative dementia that is the fourth leading cause of death in adults.[188] A major reason that memory loss is so feared by the elderly is because of the association between memory loss and AD. AD is characterized by a slow decline in memory, cognition, and functional abilities. "The transition from age-associated memory impairment (AAMI) to the dramatic loss of cognitive abilities accompanying Alzheimer's disease requires progressive development of neocortical pathology that results in neuron death.[189]" AAMI appears to be linked to alterations in neuronal spines and synapses that fall short of producing cell death.[189] A condition called mild cognitive impairment is thought to be an early sign of AD. This condition consists of a persistent mild loss of memory for recent events. People with mild cognitive impairment convert to having AD at a rate of 10% to 15% a year.[190]

Age and genetics are two risk factors for the development of AD. With increased age comes an increased risk of AD; the prevalence goes up with each decade. Aging contributes to an increased potential for neuronal injury. The production of free radicals in response to oxidative stress may play an early role in the pathophysiology of AD.[191] The presence of NFTs inside the neurons and of neuritic plaques outside the neurons is a hallmark of the neuropathology of AD. This involvement is most often seen in the temporal and parietal lobes with extension into the frontal region.[192] Pathological changes are seen in Figure 9-19. If neuronal repair is inadequate, as is supposed in AD, this defective response could lead to aberrations in the processing of beta-amyloid precursor proteins. Amyloid, an insoluble fibrous substance, makes up the core of the plaques. Tangles tend to form in cortical areas that have the least myelin and a greater degree of dendritic plasticity.[193] The genes associated with the amyloid precursor protein on chromosome 21

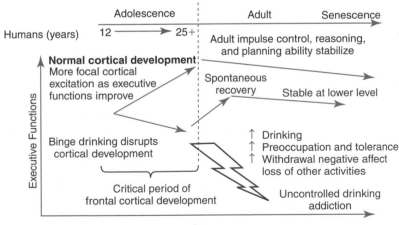

Figure 9-18 A schematic diagram of how adolescent alcohol abuse disrupts frontal cortical development and maturation of executive function. The upward narrowing arrow emphasizes the normal focusing of cortical excitation during cognitive tasks that occurs during the transition from adolescence to adulthood. The model suggests that interventions to reduce adolescent drinking will improve abilities and reduce addiction. (From Crews F, He J, Hodge C: Adolescent cortical development: a critical period of vulnerability for addition, *Pharmacol Biochem Behav* 86:189-199, 2007.)

CLINICAL IMPLICATIONS Box 9-1

Alcohol and Development

Use and abuse of alcohol take a huge toll on the health of individuals across the life span. Alcohol is a teratogen and therefore can cause birth defects if ingested during pregnancy. "Alcohol use disorders are the most prevalent substance use disorders in the United States.[199]" Alcohol abuse is a public health problem of gargantuan proportions. This clinical box highlights some of the issues related to alcohol use from a developmental perspective.[164,165,199-209]

Prenatal

- Fetal alcohol syndrome and fetal alcohol effects are part of the fetal alcohol spectrum of disorders.
- Prenatal exposure to alcohol puts the developing fetus at risk for developmental disabilities.
- Prenatal exposure puts the individual at risk for alcohol abuse later in life.
- Fetal alcohol spectrum disorders are totally preventable.

Infancy

- Babies can be exposed to alcohol when breast-fed.
- Contrary to popular belief, use of alcohol by a lactating mother decreases milk production and disrupts important hormones involved in supporting lactation.
- Prenatal and postnatal exposure to flavors and odors, including alcohol, can predispose to behaviors and preferences during infancy and childhood.

Childhood/Adolescence

- The onset of drinking occurs in middle school.
- Half of adolescents are active drinkers.
- Adolescents are less sensitive to the sedative effects of alcohol but more sensitive to the memory disruptions caused by alcohol ingestion.
- Being insensitive to the intoxicating effects of alcohol has been shown to predict later problems with

alcohol, as well as being a characteristic of persons at genetic risk for alcoholism.
- Binge drinking may lead to long-term changes in executive function because of the disruption of the neuromaturation of numerous brain regions, such as the hippocampus, prefrontal cortex, and the limbic system.
- Alcohol is involved in 1400 deaths and 50,000 injuries in college-age students.
- A college-age student's brain is still developing and at risk for further damage from over imbibing.

Adults

- Ten percent of pregnant women used alcohol, and 2% engaged in binge drinking according to a behavioral risk factor survey.
- More than half of the women of childbearing age did not use birth control and used alcohol, and 13% reported binge drinking.
- Prenatal alcohol use is one of the leading preventable causes of developmental disabilities.

Older Adults

- Alcohol misuse in older adults increases the likelihood of physical and mental problems.
- The National Institute on Alcohol Abuse and Alcoholism[176] recommends that persons over 65 years of age limit themselves to only one drink a day.
- Ten percent of older adults surveyed nationally reported being "binge drinkers," which is drinking five or more drinks on one occasion at least 12 times in the previous year.
- Alcohol use in the elderly is a public health issue.
- Hazardous drinking is a pattern of alcohol consumption that carries a risk of harmful consequences to the drinker or others.
- Harmful drinking is a pattern of drinking that causes physical or mental damage to the drinker's health but without being dependent.

---

and presenilin-1 and -2 are involved in only a small percentage of cases of AD. These patients have an earlier onset of AD, before the age of 60.

The brain areas involved in AD include the limbic, hippocampus, and cortical association areas. Arendt and colleagues,[193] Mattson and Magnus,[29] and Bartzokis[30]

have all related the increased vulnerability of those brain regions involved in AD with increased neuroplasticity. Loss of the long corticocortical projections in the association areas is most directly related to the dementia seen in AD.[189] The aggregation of tau proteins and beta-amyloid can precipitate a neuroinflammatory response

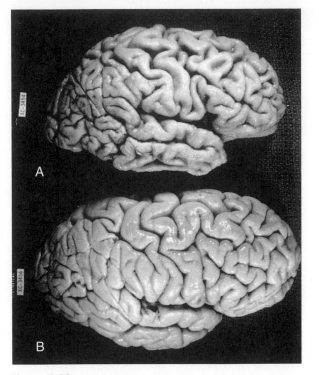

Figure 9-19 Pathological changes seen in Alzheimer disease. **A,** Alzheimer diseased brain shows reduced size, narrow gyri, and wide sulci in frontal and temporal lobes. **B,** Age- and sex-matched control. (From Damjanov I, Linder J, editors: *Anderson's pathology*, ed 10, St Louis, 1996, Mosby.)

that further contributes to eventual neuron death.[194] Senile plaques appear to be associated with a locally induced chronic inflammatory response. Microglia are activated early in AD pathology and this activation precedes the development of NFTs.[195] Accumulation of tau and amyloid proteins accentuates oxidative stress and in turn produces more reactive oxygen species that ultimately trigger apoptosis and neuron cell death. The neurotransmitter systems demonstrate impaired function in response to amyloid accumulation and NFTs by exhibiting decreased levels of serotonin, norepinephrine, dopamine, and glutamate.

Not all memory loss is pathological. In a study using a series of memory tasks, Carlesimo and colleagues[196] demonstrated quantitative and qualitative differences in memory loss between normal and pathological aging. They noted a progressive decline in episodic memory with age in all groups of normal aging individuals. The group with AD showed an even greater decline in the learning of a word list than

did the normal groups. This is "consistent with the view that a sort of continuum exists between memory changes resulting from normal aging and the memory impairment caused by AD.[196]" Two other aspects of memory showed specific deterioration in the AD group, whereas the performance of normally aging individuals remained stable. These aspects are episodic memory or word recall and semantic memory. It was hypothesized that these tasks required more attention and allocation of processing resources than individuals with AD possess. Lastly, procedural learning tasks were found to be unaffected by either aging or dementia. The neurological changes associated with normal aging are compared with those seen in AD in the Clinical Implications Box 9-2.

Females have an increased risk for developing AD. This may be due to the fact that women live longer than men or that, after menopause, the drop in estrogen negatively influences brain processes that increase the risk for developing AD.[197] Estrogen may protect against AD by improving cerebral blood flow, influencing neural transmission, and blunting the neurotoxic effects of beta-amyloid.[197,198] Even though results of hormone replacement therapy have been controversial, there may be a critical period when estrogen replacement alone may be beneficial for cognitive function in women. "Estrogen levels affect spine density on pyramidal neurons in the prefrontal cortex; these neurons may provide many of the same circuits implicated in AAMI.[189]" Therefore there appears to be an interaction between reproductive and neural senescence.

SUMMARY

When looking at the function of the nervous system, we must understand that it is constantly changing in response to environmental demands, both from within and from without. The degree of adaptation and accommodation varies from one person to another. Movement, language, and cognitive changes that occur across the life span are based on the interaction between the structure and function of the nervous system. How and why we move, talk, and think depend on the integrity of our nervous system. Our ability to learn and to adapt to the environment reflects the development of our unique nervous system characteristics across the life span. Our ability to perform the functions of the nervous system—thinking, talking, and reacting—continue as long as our system's reserves are maintained and not compromised by disease.

CLINICAL IMPLICATIONS Box 9-2

Alzheimer Disease: A Variation of Normal Aging?

Alzheimer disease (AD) is the most common form of progressive degenerative dementia. There are presently 4 million people with AD in the United States, and it is the fourth leading cause of death in adults.[188] Diagnosis is based on a history of progressive deterioration in at least two aspects of cognition, one of which is typically memory. If we live long enough, is dementia of the Alzheimer type inevitable? There are reports of increased risk in individuals over age 90.[210] However, there are differences between normal aging and AD; differences are seen in the areas of the brain that are involved and the structural and functional changes that occur.[79,106,111,192,196,211,212]

Normal Aging

- Changes in frontal cortex and subcortical areas.
- Diffuse amyloid B protein deposition; some neurofibrillary tangles (NFTs) in limbic structures, almost none in neocortical structures
- No language impairment
- No change in implicit memory or learning
- Word recall declines

- Semantic memory stable
- Older adults use list making as a memory strategy
- No consistent change in neurotransmitters
- Estrogen deficiency speeds aging effects on memory in women

Alzheimer Disease

- Changes in association areas in temporal, parietal, and frontal lobes
- Dense NFTs and neuritic plaques in all limbic structures; density related to severity of dementia
- Loss of word finding; inability to remember names; anomia; receptive aphasia
- Loss of ability to learn new information
- Word recall declines greater than normal
- Semantic memory declines
- Older adults use rehearsal as a memory strategy; external cues do not help
- Decreased activity in cholinergic neurons; norepinephrine and serotonin decreased in early onset
- Women have a two to three times greater prevalence

REFERENCES

1. Erikson EH: *Identity, youth, and crisis*, New York, 1968, WW Norton.
2. Zaidel DW: The case for a relationship between human memory, hippocampus and corpus callosum, *Biol Res* 28:51–57, 1995.
3. Volpe JJ: *Neurology of the newborn*, ed 3, Philadelphia, 1995, WB Saunders.
4. DeKeyser J, Mostert JP, Koch MW: Dysfunctional astrocytes as key players in the pathogenesis of central nervous system disorders, *J Neurol Sci* Oct 10, 2007 (Epub ahead of print).
5. Geschwind N, Levitsky W: Human brain: left-right asymmetries in temporal speech regions, *Science* 161:186–187, 1968.
6. Purves D, Augustine GJ, Fitzpatrick LC, et al: *Neuroscience*, Sunderland, Mass, 1997, Sinauer Associates.
7. Lundy-Ekman L: *Neuroscience: fundamentals for rehabilitation*, ed 3, St Louis, 2007, Saunders/Elsevier.
8. Alexander GE, Crutcher MD, DeLong MR: Basal ganglia-thalamocortical circuits: parallel substrates for motor, oculomotor, "prefrontal" and "limbic" functions, *Prog Brain Res* 85:119–146, 1990.
9. Graybiel AM: The basal ganglia: learning new tricks and loving it, *Curr Opin Neurobiol* 15:638–644, 2005.

10. Salman MS: The cerebellum: it's about time! But timing is not everything: new insights into the role of the cerebellum in timing motor and cognitive tasks, *J Child Neurol* 17(1):1–9, 2001.
11. Manzoni D: The cerebellum and sensorimotor coupling: looking at the problem from the perspective of vestibular reflexes, *Cerebellum* 6:24–37, 2007.
12. Guyton AC, Hall JE: *Textbook of medical physiology*, ed 11, Philadelphia, 2006, WB Saunders.
13. Carlisle HJ, Kennedy MB: Spine architecture and synaptic plasticity, *Trends Neurosci* 28(4):182–187, 2005.
14. Lippman J, Dunaevsky A: Dendritic spine morphogenesis and plasticity, *J Neurobiol* 64(1):47–57, 2005.
15. Sutor B, Hagerty T: Involvement of gap junctions in the development of the neocortex, *Biochim Biophys Acta* 1719(1–2):59–68, 2005.
16. Hestrin S, Galarreta M: Electrical synapses define networks of neocortical GABAergic neurons, *Trends Neurosci* 28(6):304–309, 2005.
17. Butefisch C: Plasticity in the human cerebral cortex: lessons from the normal brain and from stroke, *Neuroscientist* 10(2):163–173, 2004.
18. Doyon J, Benali H: Reorganization and plasticity in the adult brain during learning of motor skills, *Curr Opin Neurobiol* 15:161–167, 2005.

19. Bruel-Jungerman E, Rampon C, Laroche S: Adult hippocampal neurogenesis, synaptic plasticity and memory: facts and hypotheses, *Rev Neurosci* 18:93–114, 2007.

20. Woolf CJ, Slater MW: Neuronal plasticity: increasing the gain in pain, *Science* 288:1765–1768, 2000.

21. Black JE: How a child builds its brain: some lessons from animal studies of neural plasticity, *Prev Med* 27:168–171, 1998.

22. Lebeer J: How much brain does a mind need? Scientific, clinical and educational implication of ecological plasticity, *Dev Med Child Neurol* 40:352–357, 1998.

23. Johnston MV: Clinical disorders of brain plasticity, *Brain Dev* 26:73–80, 2004.

24. Rabinowicz T, De Courten-Myers G, McDonald-Comber Petetot J, et al: Human cortex development: estimates of neuronal numbers indicate major loss late in gestation, *J Neuropathol Exp Neurol* 55:320–328, 1996.

25. Johnston MV: Excitotoxicity in perinatal brain injury, *Brain Pathol* 15(3):234–240, 2005.

26. Johnston MV, Trescher WH, Ishida A, et al: Neurobiology of hypoxic-ischemic injury in the developing brain, *Pediatr Res* 49(6):735–741, 2001.

27. Volpe J: Brain injury in premature infant: neuropathology, clinical aspects, and pathogenesis, *Ment Retard Dev Disabil Res Rev* 3:3–12, 1997.

28. Giza CC, Prins ML: Is being plastic fantastic? Mechanisms of altered plasticity after developmental traumatic brain injury, *Dev Neurosci* 28(4–5):364–379, 2006.

29. Mattson MP, Magnus T: Ageing and neuronal vulnerability, *Nature* 7:278–294, 2006.

30. Bartzokis G: Age-related myelin breakdown: a developmental model of cognitive decline and Alzheimer's disease, *Neurobiol Aging* 25:5–18, 2004.

31. Landers M: Treatment-induced neuroplasticity following focal injury to the motor cortex, *Int J Rehabil Res* 27:1–5, 2004.

32. Taub E, Uswatte G, Elbert T: New treatments in neurorehabilitation founded on basic research, *Nat Rev Neurosci* 3(3):228–236, 2002.

33. Purpura D: Dendritic spine "dysgenesis" and mental retardation, *Science* 186:1126–1128, 1974.

34. Moore KL, Persaud TVN: *The developing human: clinically oriented embryology*, ed 7, Philadelphia, 2003, WB Saunders.

35. Evrard P, Minkowski A, editors: *Developmental neurobiology*, vol 12, New York, 1989, Raven Press.

36. Green E: Developmental neurology. In Stokes M, editor: *Neurological physiotherapy*, St Louis, 1998, Mosby, pp 215–228.

37. Ford DH, Cramer EB: Developing nervous system in relationship to thyroid hormone. In Grave GD, editor: *Thyroid hormones and brain development*, New York, 1977, Raven Press, pp 1–18.

38. Herschkowitz N: Brain development and nutrition. In Evrard P, Minkowski A, editors: *Developmental neurobiology*, vol 12, New York, 1989, Raven Press, pp 297–304.

39. Brittis PA, Sliver J: Exogenous glycosaminoglycans induce complete inversion of retinal ganglion cell bodies and their axons within the retinal neuroepithelium, *Proc Natl Acad Sci U S A* 91:7539–7542, 1994.

40. Sperry R: Growth of nerve circuits, *Sci Am* 201:5–68, 1959.

41. Martinez M: Biochemical changes during early myelination of the human brain. In Evrard P, Minkowski A, editors: *Developmental neurobiology*, vol 12, New York, 1989, Raven Press, pp 185–200.

42. Almli CR, Moore NM: Normal sequential behavior and physiological changes throughout the developmental arc. In Umphred DA, editor: *Neurological rehabilitation*, ed 3, St Louis, 1995, CV Mosby, pp 33–65.

43. Wiggins RC, Fuller G, Enna SJ: Undernutrition and the development of brain neurotransmitter systems, *Life Sci* 35:2085–2094, 1984.

44. Bourre JM: Developmental synthesis of myelin lipids: origin of fatty acids: specific role of nutrition. In Evrard P, Minkowski A, editors: *Developmental neurobiology*, vol 12, New York, 1989, Raven Press, pp 111–154.

45. Deacon D: Co-founder of the creative thinking association, *Caring* 21(5):20–22, 2002.

46. Dobbing J: Infant nutrition and later achievement, *Nutr Rev* 42:1–7, 1984.

47. Kretchmer N: Nutritional influences on neurological development: a contemplative essay. In Evrard P, Minkowski A, editors: *Developmental neurobiology*, vol 12, New York, 1989, Raven Press, pp 261–264.

48. Chugani HT: A critical period of brain development: studies of cerebral glucose utilization with PET, *Prev Med* 27:184–188, 1998.

49. Diemer K: Capillarisation and oxygen supply of the brain. In Lubbers DW, Luft EC, Thews G, et al, editors: *Oxygen transport in blood and tissue*, Stuttgart, Germany, 1968, Thieme, pp 118–123.

50. Schade JP, van Groenigen WB: Structural organization of the human cerebral cortex, *Acta Anat (Basel)* 47:74–111, 1961.

51. Gothelf D, Furfaro JA, Penniman LC, et al: The contribution of novel brain imaging techniques to understanding the neurobiology of mental retardation and developmental disabilities, *Ment Retard Dev Disabil Res Rev* 11:331–339, 2005.

52. Chugani HT: Development of regional brain glucose metabolism in relation to behavior and plasticity. In Dawson G, Fischer KW, editors: *Human behavior and the developing brain*, New York, 1994, Guilford, pp 153–175.

53. Bishop B, Craik RL: *Neural plasticity*, Washington, D.C., 1982, American Physical Therapy Association.

54. Bronson GW: Structure, status and characteristics of the nervous system at birth. In Stratton P, editor: *Psychobiology of the human newborn*, New York, 1982, Wiley, pp 99–118.

55. Sowell ER, Thompson PM, Toga AW: Mapping changes in the human cortex throughout the span of life, *Neuroscientist* 10(4):372–392, 2004.

56. Stratton P: Rhythmic functions in the newborn. In Stratton P, editor: *Psychobiology of the human newborn*, New York, 1982, J Wiley & Sons, pp 119–145.

57. Thomas JE, Lambert EH: Ulnar nerve conduction velocity and H-reflex in infants and children, *J Appl Physiol* 15:1–9, 1960.

58. Martin JH: The corticospinal system: from development to motor control, *Neuroscientist* 11(2):161–173, 2005.

59. Friel KM, Martin JH: Role of sensory-motor cortex activity in postnatal development of corticospinal axon terminals in the cat, *J Comp Neurol* 485(1):43–56, 2005.

60. Kotulak R: Inside the brain: revolutionary discoveries of how the mind works, *Prev Med* 27:246–247, 1998.

61. Piaget J: *Origins of intelligence*, New York, 1952, WW Norton.

62. Hallett T, Proctor A: Maturation of the central nervous system as related to communication and cognitive development, *Infant Young Child* 8:1–15, 1996.

63. Heinen F, Fietek UM, Berweck S, et al: Fast corticospinal system and motor performance in children: conduction precedes skill, *Pediatr Neurol* 19:217–221, 1998.

64. Nezu A, Kimura S, Uehara S, et al: Magnetic stimulation of motor cortex in children: maturity of corticospinal pathway and problem of clinical application, *Brain Dev* 19:176–180, 1997.

65. Valadian I, Porter D: *Physical growth and development from conception to maturity*, Boston, 1977, Little, Brown.

66. Duara R, London ED, Rapoport SI: Changes in structure and energy metabolism of the aging brain. In Finch CE, Schneider EL, editors: *Handbook of the biology of aging*, New York, 1985, Van Nostrand Reinhold, pp 595–616.

67. Magnotta VA, Andreasen NC, Schultz SK, et al: Quantitative in vivo measurement of gyrification in the human brain: changes associated with aging, *Cereb Cortex* 9:151–160, 1999.

68. Willott JF: *Neurogerontology*, New York, 1999, Springer.

69. Patten C, Craik RL: Sensorimotor changes and adaptation in the older adult. In Guccione AA, editor: *Geriatric physical therapy*, ed 2, St Louis, 2000, Mosby, pp 78–109.

70. Mrak RE, Griffin ST, Graham DI: Aging-associated changes in human brain, *J Neuropathol Exp Neurol* 56:1269–1275, 1997.

71. Pakkenberg B, Pelvig D, Marner L, et al: Aging and the human neocortex, *Exp Gerontol* 38:95–99, 2003.

72. Whitbourne SK: *The aging individual: physical and psychological perspectives*, New York, 1996, Springer.

73. Jack CR Jr, Petersen RC, Xu YC, et al: Medial temporal atrophy on MRI in normal aging and very mild Alzheimer's disease, *Neurology* 49:786–794, 1997.

74. DeSanti S, de Leon MJ, Convit A, et al: Age-related changes in brain: II. Positron emission tomography of frontal and temporal lobe glucose metabolism in normal subjects, *Psychiatr Q* 66:357–370, 1995.

75. Eberling JL, Nordahl TE, Kusubov N, et al: Reduced temporal lobe glucose metabolism in aging, *J Neuroimaging* 5:178–182, 1995.

76. Kemper TL: Neuroanatomical and neuropathological changes during aging and dementia. In Albert ML, Knoefel JE, editors: *Clinical neurology of aging*, New York, 1994, Oxford University Press, pp 3–67.

77. Stafford JL, Albert MS, Naeser MA, et al: Age-related differences in computed tomographic scan measurements, *Arch Neurol* 45:409–415, 1988.

78. Yamamura H, Ito M, Kubota K, et al: Brain atrophy during aging: a quantitative study with computed tomography, *J Gerontol* 35:492–498, 1980.

79. Birge SJ: Hormones and the aging brain, *Geriatrics* 53(Suppl 1):S28–S30, 1998.

80. Double KL, et al: Topography of brain atrophy during normal aging and Alzheimer's disease, *Neurobiol Aging* 17:513–521, 1996.

81. Whitbourne SK, editor: *Gerontology: an interdisciplinary perspective*, New York, 1999, Oxford University Press.

82. Mouritzen Dam A: The density of neurons in the human hippocampus, *Neuropathol Appl Neurobiol* 5:249–264, 1979.

83. Fox CM, Adler RN: Neural mechanism of aging. In Cohen H, editor: *Neuroscience for rehabilitation*, ed 2, Philadelphia, 1999, Lippincott Williams & Wilkins, pp 401–418.

84. Fabel K, Kempermann G: Physical activity and the regulation of neurogenesis in the adult and aging brain, *Neuromolecular Med* 10(2):59–66, 2008.

85. Konigsmark BW, Murphy EA: Neuronal population in the human brain, *Nature* 228:1335–1336, 1970.

86. Bondareff W: Brain & Central Nervous System. In Birren JE, editor: *Encyclopedia of gerontology*, ed 2, vol 1, Boston, 2007, Academic Press, pp 187–190.

87. Schaumburg HH, Spencer PS, Ochoa J: The aging human peripheral nervous system. In Katzman R, Terry RD, editors: *The neurology of aging*, Philadelphia, 1983, FA Davis, pp 111–122.

88. Buchtal F, Rosenfalck A, Behse F: Sensory potentials of normal and diseased nerves. In Dyck PJ, Thomas PK, Griffin JW, et al, editors: *Peripheral neuropathy*, ed 2, Philadelphia, 1984, WB Saunders, pp 442–464.

89. Cotman CW, Holets VR: Structural changes at synapses with age: plasticity and regeneration. In Finch CE, Schneider EL, editors: *Handbook of the biology of aging*, New York, 1985, Van Nostrand Reinhold, pp 617–644.

90. Terry RD, De Teresa R, Hansen LA: Neocortical cell counts in normal human adult aging, *Ann Neurol* 21:530–539, 1987.

91. Haug J, Kuhl S, Mecke E, et al: The significance of morphometric procedures in the investigation of age changes in cytoarchitectonic structures of human brain, *J Hirnforsch* 25:353–374, 1984.

92. Haug J: Are neurons of the human cerebral cortex really lost during aging? A morphometric examination. In Traber J, Gispen WH, editors: *Senile dementia of the Alzheimer type*, New York, 1985, Springer-Verlag, pp 150–163.

93. Resnick SM, Pham DL, Kraut MA, et al: Longitudinal magnetic resonance imaging studies of older adults: a shrinking brain, *J Neurosci* 23(8):3295–3301, 2003.

94. Mueller EA, Moore MM, Kerr DC, et al: Brain volume preserved in healthy elderly through the eleventh decade, *Neurology* 51:1555–1562, 1998.

95. Good CD, Johnsrude IS, Ashburner J, et al: A voxel-based morphometric study of ageing in 465 normal adult human brains, *Neuroimage* 14:21–36, 2001.

96. Marner L, Nyengaard JR, Tang Y, et al: Marked loss of myelinated nerve fibers in the human brain with age, *J Comp Neurol* 462:144–152, 2003.

97. Friedlander WJ: Electroencephalographic alpha rate in adults as a function of age, *Geriatrics* 13:29–31, 1958.

98. Shigeta M, Julin P, Almkvist O, et al: EEG in successful aging: a 5-year follow-up study from the eighth to the ninth decade of life, *Electroencephalogr Clin Neurophysiol* 95:77–83, 1995.

99. Keefover RW: Aging and cognition, *Neurol Clin* 16:625–648, 1998.

100. Petit-Taboue MC, Landeau B, Desson JF, et al: Effects of healthy aging on regional cerebral metabolic rate of glucose assessed with statistical parametric mapping, *Neuroimage* 7:176–184, 1998.

101. Mielke R, Kessler J, Szelies B, et al: Normal and pathological aging: findings of positron-emission-tomography, *J Neural Transm* 105:821–837, 1998.

102. Resnick SM, Driscoll I, Lamar M: Vulnerability of the orbitofrontal cortex to age-associated structural and functional brain changes, *Ann N Y Acad Sci* 1121:562–575, 2007.

103. Itoh M, Hatazawa J, Miyazawa, et al: Stability of cerebral blood flow and oxygen metabolism during normal aging, *Gerontology* 36(1):43–48, 1990.

104. Beason-Held LL, Kraut MA, Resnick SM: I. Longitudinal changes in aging brain function, *Neurobiol Aging* 29:483–496, 2006.

105. Bell MA, Ball MJ: Neuritic plaques and vessels of visual cortex in aging and Alzheimer's dementia, *Neurobiol Aging* 11:359–370, 1990.

106. Haroutunian V, Perl DP, Purohit DP, et al: Regional distribution of neuritic plaques in the nondemented elderly and subjects with very mild Alzheimer disease, *Arch Neurol* 55:1185–1191, 1998.

107. Keller JN, Dimayuga E, Chen Q, et al: Autophagy, proteasomes, lipofuscin, and oxidative stress in the aging brain, *Int J Biochem Cell Biol* 36:2376–2391, 2004.

108. Keller JN: Age-related neuropathology, cognitive decline, and Alzheimer's disease, *Ageing Res Rev* 5:1–13, 2006.

109. Brody H, Vijayashanker N: Anatomical changes in the nervous system. In Finch CE, Hay-Flick L, editors: *Handbook of biology and aging*, New York, 1977, Van Nostrand Reinhold, pp 241–256.

110. Rogers J, Bloom FE: Neurotransmitter metabolism and function in the aging nervous system. In Finch CE, Schneider EL, editors: *Handbook of the biology of aging*, New York, 1985, Van Nostrand Reinhold, pp 645–691.

111. Strong R: Neurochemical changes in the aging human brain: implications for behavioral impairment and neuro-degenerative disease, *Geriatrics* 53(Suppl 1):S9–S12, 1998.

112. Volkow ND, Gur RC, Wang GJ, et al: Association between decline in brain dopamine activity with age and cognitive and motor impairment in healthy individuals, *Am J Psychiatry* 155:344–349, 1998.

113. DeKosky ST, Palmer AM: Neurochemistry of aging. In Albert ML, Knoefel JE, editors: *Clinical neurology of aging*, ed 2, New York, 1994, Oxford University Press, pp 79–101.

114. Hubble JP: Aging and the basal ganglia, *Neurol Clin* 16:649–657, 1998.

115. Katzman R, Terry RD: Normal aging of the nervous system. In Katzman R, Terry RD, editors: *The neurology of aging*, Philadelphia, 1983, FA Davis, pp 15–50.

116. Seals DR, Esler MD: Human ageing and sympathoadrenal system, *J Physiol* 528:407–417, 2000.

117. Esler M, Lambert G, Kaye D, et al: Influence of ageing on the sympathetic nervous system and adrenal medulla at rest and during stress, *Biogerontology* 3:45–49, 2002.

118. Lexell J: Evidence for nervous system degeneration with advancing age, *J Nutr* 127:1011S–1013S, 1997.

119. Potvin AR, Syndulko K, Tourtellote WW, et al: Human neurologic function and the aging process, *J Am Geriatr Soc* 28:1–9, 1980.

120. Eaton WO, Ritchot KIM: Physical maturation and information-processing speed in middle childhood, *Dev Psychol* 31:967–972, 1995.

121. Kail R: Sources of age differences in speed of processing, *Child Dev* 57:969–987, 1986.

122. Birren JE, Fisher LM: Aging and speed of behavior: possible consequences for psychological functioning, *Annu Rev Psychol* 110:1571–1576, 1995.

123. Birren JE, Woods AM, Williams MV: Speed of behavior as an indicator of age changes and the integrity of the nervous system. In Hoffmeister F, Muller C, editors: *Brain function in old age*, New York, 1979, Springer-Verlag, pp 10–44.

124. Kail RV, Salthouse TA: Processing speed as a mental capacity, *Acta Psychol (Basel)* 86:199–225, 1994.

125. Schaie KW, Willis SL, editors: *Adult development and aging*, ed 4, New York, 1996, Harper Collins.

126. Welford AT: Between bodily changes and performance; some possible reasons for slowing with age, *Exp Aging Res* 10:73–88, 1984.

127. Onishi N: Changes of the jumping reaction time in relation to age, *J Sci Labour* 42:5–16, 1966.

128. Singleton WT: The change of movement timing with age, *Br J Psychol* 45:166–172, 1954.

129. Spirduso WW: *Physical dimensions of aging*, Champaign, Ill, 1995, Human Kinetics.

130. Light KE, Spirduso WW: Effects of adult aging on the movement complexity factor of response programming, *J Gerontol* 45:P107–P109, 1990.

131. Fozard JL, Vercruyssen M, Reynolds SL, et al: Age differences and changes in reaction time: the Baltimore longitudinal study of aging, *J Gerontol B Psychol Sci Soc Sci* 49:179–189, 1994.

132. Laufer AC, Schweitz B: Neuromuscular response tests as predictors of sensory-motor performance in aging individuals, *Am J Phys Med* 47:250–263, 1968.

133. Chaput S, Proteau L: Aging and motor control, *J Gerontol B Psychol Sci Soc Sci* 51:P346–P355, 1996.

134. Woodruff-Pak DS: *The neuropsychology of aging*, Malden, Mass, 1997, Blackwell.

135. Emery CF, Huppert FA, Schein RL: Relationships among age, exercise, health, and cognitive function in a British sample, *Gerontologist* 35:378–385, 1995.

136. Spirduso WW: Physical fitness, aging and psychomotor speed: a review, *J Gerontol* 35:850–865, 1980.

137. Stine-Morrow EAL, Soederberg-Miller LM: Basic cognitive processes. In Cavanaugh JC, Whitbourne SK, editors: *Gerontology:an interdisciplinary perspective*, New York, 1982, Oxford University Press, pp 186–212.

138. Churchill JD, Galvez R, Colcombe S, et al: Exercise, experience and the aging brain, *Neurobiol Aging* 23:941–955, 2002.

139. Bertoni-Freddari C, Fattoretti P, Paoloni R, et al: Synaptic structural dynamics and aging, *Gerontology* 42:170–180, 1996.

140. Posner MI, Rothbart MK: Attention, self-regulation and consciousness, *Philos Trans R Soc Lond B Biol Sci* 353:1915–1927, 1998.

141. Casey BJ, Trainor R, Giedd J, et al: The role of the anterior cingulate in automatic and controlled processes: a developmental neuroanatomical study, *Dev Psychobiol* 3:61–69, 1997.

142. Lynch G: Memory and the brain: unexpected chemistries and a new pharmacology, *Neurobiol Learn Mem* 70:82–100, 1998.

143. Rovee-Collier C: Learning and memory in children. In Osofsky JD, editor: *Handbook of infant development*, ed 2, New York, 1987, J Wiley & Sons, pp 98–148.

144. Nelson CA: The ontogeny of human memory: a cognitive neuroscience perspective, *Dev Psychol* 31:723–738, 1995.

145. Nelson CA: The nature of early memory, *Prev Med* 27:172–179, 1998.

146. Mussen PH, Conger JJ, Kagan J, editors: *Child development and personality*, ed 4, New York, 1974, Harper & Row.

147. Paris SC, Lindauer BK: The development of cognitive skills during childhood. In Wolman BB, editor: *Handbook of developmental psychology*, Englewood Cliffs, NJ, 1982, Prentice-Hall, pp 333–349.

148. Tulving E: Organization of memory: Quo vadis? In Gazaniga MS, editor: *The cognitive neuroscience*, Cambridge, Mass, 1995, MIT Press, pp 839–847.

149. Nilsson LG: Memory function in normal aging, *Acta Neurol Scand Suppl* 179:7–13, 2003.

150. Raz N, Briggs SD, Marks W, et al: Age-related deficits in generation and manipulation of mental images: the role of the dorsolateral prefrontal cortex, *Psychol Aging* 14:436–444, 1999.

151. Luszcz MA, Bryan J: Toward understanding age-related memory loss in late adulthood, *Gerontology* 45:2–9, 1999.

152. Backman L, Small B, Wahlin A: Aging and memory: cognitive and biological processes. In Birren JE, Schaie KW, editors: *Handbook of psychology of aging*, ed 5, New York, 2001, Academic Press, pp 349–377.

153. Gazzaley A, Sheridan MA, Cooney JW, et al: Age-related deficits in component processes of working memory, *Neuropsychology* 21(5):532–539, 2007.

154. Sakai K, Rowe JB, Passingham RE: Active maintenance in prefrontal area 46 creates distractor-resistant memory, *Nat Neurosci* 5:479–485, 2002.

155. Ito M: Nurturing the brain as an emerging research field involving child neurology, *Brain Dev* 26:429–433, 2004.

156. Anderson P: Assessment and development of executive function (EF) during childhood, *Child Neuropsychol* 8(2):71–82, 2002.

157. Davidson MC, Amso D, Anderson LC, et al: Development of cognitive control and executive functions from 4 to 13 years: evidence from manipulations of memory, inhibition, and task switching, *Neuropsychologia* 44:2037–2078, 2006.

158. Espy K: The shape school: assessing executive function in preschool children, *Dev Neuropsychol* 13:495–499, 1997.

159. Fuster JM: Frontal lobe and cognitive development, *J Neurocytol* 31:373–385, 2002.

160. Yakovlev PI, Lecours AR: The myelogenetic cycles of regional maturation of the brain. In Minkowski A, editor: *Regional development of the brain in early life*, Oxford, UK, 1967, Blackwell.

161. Huttenlocher PR, Dabholkar AS: Regional differences in synaptogenesis in human cerebral cortex, *J Comp Neurol* 387(2):167–178, 1997.

162. Monk CS, McClure EB, Nelson EE, et al: Adolescent immaturity in attention-related brain engagement to emotional facial expressions, *Neuroimage* 20:420–428, 2003.

163. Paus T: Mapping brain maturation and cognitive development during adolescence, *Trends Cogn Sci* 9(2):60–68, 2005.

164. Blakemore SJ, Choudhury S: Development of the adolescent brain: implications for executive function and social cognition, *J Child Psychol Psychiatry* 47(3/4):296–312, 2006.

165. Crews F, He J, Hodge C: Adolescent cortical development: a critical period of vulnerability for addition, *Pharmacol Biochem Behav* 86:189–199, 2007.

166. Luciana M, Conklin HM, Hooper CJ, et al: The development of nonverbal working memory and executive control processes in adolescents, *Child Dev* 76(3):697–712, 2005.

167. Luna B, Garver KE, Urban TA, et al: Maturation of cognitive processes from late childhood to adulthood, *Child Dev* 75(5):1357–1372, 2004.

168. Benes FM, Turtle M, Khan Y, et al: Myelination of a key relay zone in the hippocampal formation occurs in the human brain during childhood, adolescence, and adulthood, *Arch Gen Psychiatry* 51(6):477–484, 1994.

169. Crone EA, Wendelken C, Donohue S, et al: Neurocognitive development of the ability to manipulate information in working memory, *Proc Natl Acad Sci U S A* 103:9315–9320, 2006.

170. Diamond A: Close interrelation of motor development and cognitive development and of the cerebellum and prefrontal cortex, *Child Dev* 71(1):44–56, 2000.

171. Ridler K, Veijola JM, Tanskanen P, et al: Fronto-cerebellar systems are associated with infant motor and adult executive functions in healthy adults but not in schizophrenia, *Proc Natl Acad Sci U S A* 103(42):15651–15665, 2006.

172. Horn JL, Donaldson G: Cognitive development in adulthood. In Brim OG, Kagan J, editors: *Constancy and change in human development*, Cambridge, Mass, 1980, Harvard University Press, pp 445–529.

173. Erickson KI, Kramer AF: Aerobic exercise effects on cognitive and neural plasticity in older adults, *Br J Sports Med* 43:22–24, 2009.

174. Williamson JD, Espeland M, Kritchevsky SB, et al: Changes in cognitive function in a randomized trial of physical activity: results of the lifestyle interventions and independence for elders pilot study, *J Gerontol A Biol Sci Med Sci* 64(6):688–694, 2009.

175. Sampson PD, Streissguth AP, Bookstein FL, et al: Incidence of fetal alcohol syndrome and prevalence of alcohol-related neurodevelopmental disorder, *Teratology* 56:317–326, 1997.

176. National Institute on Alcohol Abuse and Alcoholism (NIAAA): *Seventh special report to the U.S. Congress on alcohol and health*, Washington D.C., 1990, US Government Printing Office.

177. Rasmussen C: Executive functioning and working memory in fetal alcohol spectrum disorder, *Alcohol Clin Exp Res* 29(8):1359–1367, 2005.

178. Riley EP, McGee CL: Fetal alcohol disorder: an overview with emphasis on changes in brain and behavior, *Exp Biol Med* 30:357–365, 2005.

179. Abel EL: An update on incidence of FAS: FAS is not an equal opportunity birth defect, *Neurotoxicol Teratol* 17:437–443, 1995.

180. May PA, Gossage JP: Epidemiology of alcohol consumption among American Indians living in four reservations and in nearby border towns, *Drug Alcohol Depend* 63:S100, 2001.

181. May PA, Fiorentino D, Gossage JP, et al: Epidemiology of FASD in a province in Italy: prevalence and characteristics of children in a random sample of schools, *Alcohol Clin Exp Res* 30(9):1562–1575, 2006.

182. Tsai J, Floyd RL, Green PP, et al: Patterns and average volume of alcohol use among women of childbearing age, *Matern Child Health J* 11(5):437–445, 2007.

183. Ratliffe KT: *Clinical pediatric physical therapy*, St Louis, 1998, Mosby.

184. Jones KL, Smith SW: Recognition of the fetal alcohol syndrome in early infancy, *Lancet* 2:999–1001, 1973.

185. Sokol RJ, Clarren SK: Guidelines for the use of terminology describing the impact of prenatal alcohol on offspring, *Alcohol Clin Exp Res* 13:597–598, 1989.

186. Hoyme HE, May PA, Kalberg W, et al: A practical clinical approach to diagnosis of fetal alcohol spectrum disorders: clarification of the 1996 Institute of Medicine criteria, *Pediatrics* 115:39–47, 2005.

187. Niccols A: Fetal alcohol syndrome and the developing socio-emotional brain, *Brain Cogn* 65(1):135–142, 2007.

188. Fuller KS: Degenerative diseases of the central nervous system. In Goodman CG, Boissonnault WG, editors: *Pathology: implications for the physical therapist*, Philadelphia, 1998, WB Saunders, pp 723–747.

189. Morrison JH, Hof PR: Life and death of neurons in the aging cerebral cortex, *Int Rev Neurobiol* 81:41–57, 2007.

190. Fuller KS, Winkler PA, Corboy JR: Degenerative diseases of the central nervous system. In Goodman CG, Boissonnault WG, editors: *Pathology: implications for the physical therapist*, ed 3, Philadelphia, 2009, WB Saunders, pp 1402–1448.

191. Polidori MC, Griffiths HR, Mariani E, et al: Hallmarks of protein oxidative damage in neurodegenerative diseases: focus on Alzheimer's disease, *Amino Acids* 32:553–559, 2007.

192. Davis KL: Alzheimer's disease: seeking new ways to preserve brain function, *Geriatrics* 54:42–47, 1999.

193. Arendt T, Bruckner MK, Gert HJ, et al: Cortical distribution of neurofibrillary tangles in Alzheimer's disease matches the pattern of neurons that retain their capacity of plastic remodeling in the adult brain, *Neuroscience* 83:991–1002, 1998.

194. Eikelenboom P, Veerhuis R, Scheper W, et al: The significance of neuroinflammation in understanding Alzheimer's disease, *J Neural Transm* 113:1685–1695, 2006.

195. Arends YM, Duyckaerts C, Rozemuller JM, et al: Microglia, amyloid and dementia in Alzheimer's disease. A correlative study, *Neurobiol Aging* 21:39–47, 2000.

196. Carlesimo GA, Mauri M, Graceffa A, et al: Memory performances in young, elderly, and very old healthy individuals versus patients with Alzheimer's disease: evidence for discontinuity between normal and pathological aging, *J Clin Exp Neuropsychol* 20:14–29, 1998.

197. Candore G, Balistreri CR, Grimaldi MP, et al: Age-related inflammatory diseases: role of genetics and gender in the pathophysiology of Alzheimer's disease, *Ann N Y Acad Sci* 1089:472–486, 2006.

198. Genazzani AR, Pluchino N, Luisi S, et al: Estrogen, cognition and female ageing, *Hum Reprod Update* 13(2):175–187, 2007.

199. Fisher CB, Lerner RM, editors: *Encyclopedia of applied developmental science*, vol 1, Thousand Oaks, Calif, 2005, Sage Publications.

200. Alati R, Al Mamum A, Williams GM, et al: In utero alcohol exposure and prediction of alcohol disorders in early adulthood: a birth cohort study, *Arch Gen Psychiatry* 63:1009–1016, 2006.

201. CDC: *Alcohol use and pregnancy* (website): http://www.cdc.gov/ncddd/factsheets/FAS_alcoholuse.pdf. Accessed November 10, 2007.

202. Babor TG, Higgins-Biddle JC: *Brief intervention for hazardous and harmful drinking. A manual for use in primary care*, Geneva, Switzerland, 2001, Department of Mental Health and Substance Dependence, World Health Organization.

203. Centers for Disease Control: *Alcohol consumption among women who are pregnant or who might become pregnant - United States, 2002* (website): http://www.cdc.gov/mmwr/preview/mmwrhtml/mm5350a4.htm. Accessed November 10, 2007.

204. Culberson JW: Alcohol use in the elderly: beyond the CAGE part 1 of 2: prevalence and patterns of problem drinking, *Geriatrics* 61(10):23–27, 2006.

205. Mennella JA: Regulation of milk intake after exposure to alcohol in mothers' milk, *Alcohol Clin Exp Res* 25:590–593, 2001.

206. Mennella JA, Pepino MY, Teff KL: Acute alcohol consumption disrupts the hormonal milieu of lactating women, *J Clin Endocrinol Metab* 90:1979–1985, 2005.

207. Molina JC, Spear NE, Spear LP, et al: The International Society for Developmental Psychobiology 39th annual meeting symposium: Alcohol and Development: Beyond Fetal Alcohol Syndrome, *Dev Psychobiol* 49(3):227–242, 2007.

208. Schuckit MA: Low level of response to alcohol as a predictor of future alcoholism, *Am J Psychiatry* 151:184–189, 1994.

209. Substance Abuse and Mental Health Services Administration (Office of Applied Studies). Results from the 2001 National Household Survey on Drug Abuse: vol 1. Summary of National Findings. (NHSDA Series H-17, DHHS Publication No. SMA 02-3758) Rockville, Md: Department of Health and Human Services, 2002.

210. Ritchie K, Kildea D: Is senile dementia "age-related" or "ageing-related"? Evidence from meta-analysis of dementia prevalence in the oldest old, *Lancet* 346: 931–934, 1995.

211. Haroutunian V, Purohit DP, Perl DP, et al: Neurofibrillary tangles in nondemented elderly subjects and very mild Alzheimer disease, *Arch Neurol* 56:713–718, 1999.

212. McDougall GJ: Predictors of the use of memory improvement strategies by older adults, *Rehabil Nurs* 21:202–209, 1996.

CHAPTER 10

Sensory System Changes

OBJECTIVES

After studying this chapter, the reader will be able to:

1. Discuss the role of sensation in perception and movement.

2. Describe age-related sensory system changes across the life span.
3. Correlate sensory system changes with function across the life span.

Our senses provide the only means of communicating with and about the world around us. The psychologist J. J. Gibson[1] introduced the concept of *affordance* to describe the complementary effect of the environment on the developing organism. Sensation affords interaction between the infant and the environment, as well as interaction between the environment and the infant in such a manner that both are changed. The environment includes the biophysical and sociocultural surroundings that affect movement outcome (Figure 10-1). These surroundings can also encompass people and objects. No wonder Piaget[2] described the origins of intelligence as the sensorimotor period. An infant's initial foray into the world is guided by sensations that are paired with movement to initiate communication, motor control, and intelligence.

Because the sensory system is part of the nervous system, sensory and motor systems have a common goal—movement production. The role of sensory input in the development and control of posture and movement is well documented.[3-7] Initially, sensory input is paired with motor output, resulting in reflexes such as flexor withdrawal and positive support. Infants learn to maintain their posture and balance in response to sensory input with the development of *postural reactions* that automatically occur to maintain the alignment of the head and trunk in response to a weight shift; these include protective extension of the extremities, righting, and equilibrium reactions of the head and trunk. Automatic postural reactions in response to anteroposterior body sway (postural sway) are governed by somatosensory, vestibular, and visual input (see Chapter 12).

Sensory input aids the process of learning movement by providing feedback for movement accuracy, such as in reaching for or rolling toward a desired object. Once movement is learned, sensation may not be as necessary for the movement to occur. When movement becomes more automatic, however, sensation becomes an anticipatory signal to move; for example, gathering your things when you hear the bell ring at the end of class or changing your walk to a run when you think you may miss your bus. The way a movement feels can be recalled when playing a once-forgotten piano piece or riding a bicycle. Once you learn, you do not forget how, although execution may be impaired through nervous or muscular system deficits.

Sensory systems are important to functional movement. The majority of what we know about the senses comes from research with animals and infants. We also need to understand the age-related changes in sensory function across the life span, including the importance of state and stimulus novelty. The normally expected changes in sensory awareness with age are just beginning to be distinguished from pathological changes, and our knowledge of the functional implication of age-related sensory deficits for movement is still preliminary.

CHARACTERISTICS OF SENSORY SYSTEMS

Sensation entails the reception of afferent stimuli from both the internal milieu of the body and the external world. To receive input, the body must be sufficiently aroused. The state of arousal that an infant experiences will determine the level of responsivity to sensory stimuli. A patient in a coma may respond only to painful stimuli. With recovery, sensory awareness grows. Reception of sensory stimuli does not always imply

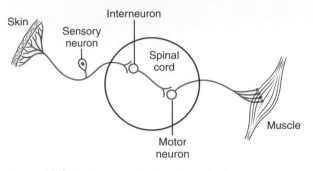

Figure 10-1 Environmental factors that affect movement outcome.

that the sensation reaches conscious awareness. Each sensory system has its own unique set of receptors and pathways it travels to reach conscious awareness.

The senses monitor internal processes related to vital functions such as breathing, eating, sleeping, and excreting, as well as producing arousal in the form of general alerting, sexual responses, and fight-or-flight reactions. The arousal functions are choreographed by various subsystems of the nervous system (central, peripheral, and autonomic) in concert with the brain stem reticular activating, hypothalamic, and limbic systems. The interpretation of sensory stimuli is often determined by the state of the autonomic nervous system. Think of how slowly you respond to the alarm clock in the morning when you have an 8 o'clock class. Your parasympathetic system predominates during vegetative functions such as sleep, but you animatedly respond to cold water when showering, a sympathetic response to a brief cold stimulus.

Sensory input comes in via special receptors, is conveyed by nerve fibers, and is disseminated to appropriate regions of the central nervous system (CNS). For example, your eye picks up a moving image and relays the information to the brain, which identifies a hummingbird. In the meantime, your eye muscles track the bird's movements while you safely continue your forward progression on the nature path. Different sensory receptors have sent a variety of messages to the brain that have been interpreted and have resulted in an adaptive response to allow you to enjoy a pleasurable activity while continuing a motor task. Some pathways relay information from only one type of sensory receptor such as mechanoreceptors; others carry information about pain and temperature. All sensory systems have the ability to transform one type of energy (the stimulus) into an electrical signal, code for specific qualities of the stimulus, be represented topographically on many levels of the nervous system, integrate information between

one or more sensory systems, and participate in motor responses both in a preparatory and reactive manner.

The Senses

Somatic Senses

Touch, temperature, pain, and awareness of joint position (proprioception) are conveyed by mechanoreceptors, thermoreceptors, and nociceptors. Touch and proprioception contribute to the development of body scheme and awareness of our relationship to the outside world. Touch defines the limits of the body and provides information about people and objects in the environment. Temperature detection ensures survival and efficient physiological function of the body. Pain protects the body from too much pressure, as from sitting too long in one position, and from overexposure to the sun, snow, or chemicals. Somatic receptors convey pressure, vibration, temperature, pain, and some proprioceptive information about the body.

Free nerve endings are found in the skin, muscle, joints, and viscera. These nociceptors convey noxious stimuli. As such, they can respond to mechanical, thermal, and chemical stimuli, either on the skin or internally at the periosteum, arterial walls, and joint surfaces. Thermoreception also occurs by activating free, unencapsulated nerve endings. Thermoreceptors detect hot and cold by responding to changes in their own metabolic rate relative to actual temperature changes in the ambient air. Extremes of hot or cold can be detected as pain through the stimulation of pain receptors in addition to the temperature receptors.

The majority of *mechanoreceptors* are encapsulated and include *pacinian corpuscles, Meissner corpuscles, Merkel disks,* and *Ruffini endings.* Pacinian corpuscles respond to tissue vibration and rapid changes in the mechanical state of the tissues.[8] They are found in the skin and joints. Meissner corpuscles are sensitive to light touch and vibration, whereas Merkel disks respond to pressure. The latter receptor is found in hairy skin, and the former two receptors are found primarily in hairless skin. Ruffini endings convey stretch of the skin and of joints.

Muscle spindles and Golgi tendon organs are examples of mechanoreceptors but are also classified as proprioceptors. Proprioceptive receptors detect the position of body parts in space and are found in the vestibular part of the ear as well as in muscles, tendons, and joints. Muscle spindles are stretch-sensitive and provide information about muscle length and velocity of contraction. The awareness of joint movement or kinesthesia along with joint position sense make up the functions collectively referred to as "proprioception.[9]"

Joint position receptors relay knowledge of joint angulation, especially at end ranges. More than half of the innervation to a muscle conveys information to and from the muscle spindles, the body's primary source of proprioceptive information.[10] The muscle spindle provides sensory feedback during reflexive and voluntary movement.

The Golgi tendon organ, located in the muscle tendon, detects tension generated by the contraction or stretch of that muscle and safeguards the muscle from overwork by inhibiting or stopping the muscle from contracting. Articular receptors in the joint capsule and ligaments also provide proprioceptive information. The pacinian corpuscles respond to mechanical stimulation during movement, whereas Ruffini endings become active when the joint is at the extremes of its movement. However, the loss of joint receptors because of surgery or anesthesia does not seem to impair motion detection.[11-13] Various cutaneous sensory receptors are shown in Figure 10-2.

Vestibular Sense

The ear is a special part of our anatomy that is crucial to motion sense as well as the sense of hearing. It is, therefore, important to understand its various parts and how they work (Figure 10-3). The vestibular system relays input about the body's relationship to gravity, head position, and head movement. Although it is

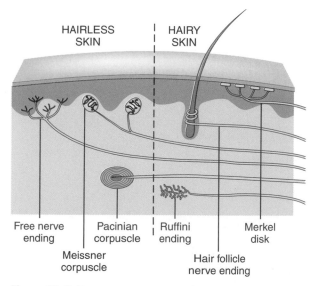

Figure 10-2 Cutaneous receptors include the free nerve ending, Meissner corpuscle, and pacinian corpuscle found in hairless skin and the Ruffini ending and Merkel disk in hairy skin. (From Lundy-Ekman L: *Neuroscience fundamentals for rehabilitation*, ed 3, Philadelphia, 2007, WB Saunders, p 107.)

considered part of proprioception in some regards, it is discussed separately because of its intimate relationship to movement. Vestibular receptors in the inner ear provide information about head position and head movement in space. Vestibular information is used to update postural tone and equilibrium and to ensure gaze stability during head movements.[14] Gaze stability allows the eyes to fix on an image even though the head is moving. The vestibular system resolves intersensory conflicts about balance. If the proprioceptors think the body is not moving and the eyes think the body is moving, the input of the vestibular system decides what the real situation is and relays information to appropriate motor centers.

The vestibular receptors are located within the membranous labyrinth of the inner ear. The labyrinth is made up of three fluid-filled semicircular ducts and the utricle and saccule (Figure 10-4). The vestibular receptors are specialized hair cells located in the ampullae of the semicircular ducts and the maculae of the saccule and utricle (Figure 10-5). The semicircular ducts respond to angular head movement. The saccule and utricle detect gravity; the utricle also monitors the position of the head when one is upright, and the saccule monitors it when one is lying down. Both respond to linear acceleration from the deflection of the hair cells. The three semicircular ducts are oriented at right angles to each other and respond to angular acceleration. When these paired structures are stimulated, the hair cells (receptors) are deformed (bent). They transmit electrical signals via the vestibular part of cranial nerve VIII to the vestibular ganglion and on to the vestibular nuclei in the medulla and vestibulocerebellum. These relay nuclei also communicate with the cervical spinal cord, oculomotor system, cerebellum, vestibular nuclei of the other side of the body, brain stem reticular formation, thalamus, and hypothalamus. Although the vestibular system exerts an influence on all other sensory systems,[14,15] it exerts more influence on the motor systems by contributing to postural tone. Postural tone is sufficient tone in postural muscles to sustain a posture.

Special Senses

Vision, hearing, taste, and smell are considered the traditional special senses and are subserved by specific cranial nerves. Specialized receptors found in the eye, ear, tongue, and nose are specifically and uniquely designed to sense light, sound, taste, and odors. The distance receptors—vision and hearing—have been the most thoroughly studied.

Vision is the most complex special sense. The sharpness of vision (acuity) and the ability to focus on near and far objects (accommodation) are functions of the

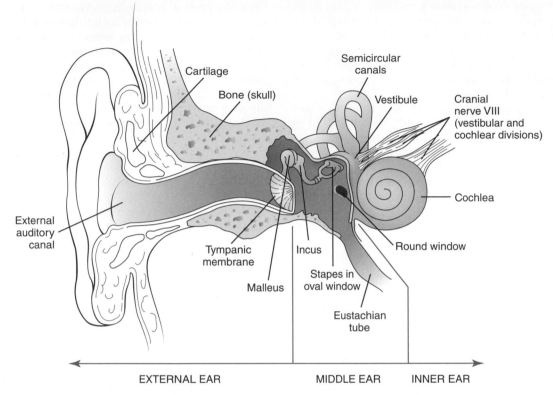

Figure 10-3 Anatomy of the ear. (Redrawn from Applegate E: *The anatomy and physiology learning system*, ed 2, Philadelphia, 2000, WB Saunders, p 194.)

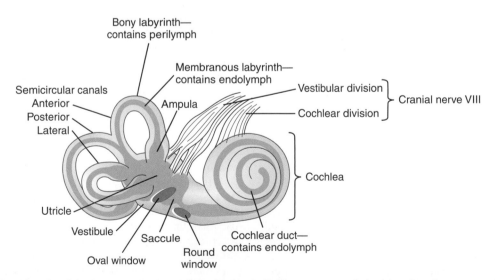

Figure 10-4 Labyrinths of the inner ear. (Redrawn from Applegate E: *The anatomy and physiology learning system*, ed 2, Philadelphia, 2000, WB Saunders, p 195.)

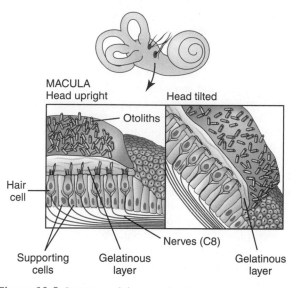

MACULA
Head upright
Head tilted
Otoliths
Hair cell
Supporting cells
Gelatinous layer
Nerves (C8)
Gelatinous layer

Figure 10-5 Structure of the macula. (Redrawn from Applegate E: *The anatomy and physiology learning system,* ed 2, Philadelphia, 2000, WB Saunders, p 198.)

structure of the eye. The eye is the organ of sight, but the photoreceptors are the rods and cones within the retina of the eye. A very small area of the retina called the macula is capable of detailed and acute vision. The center of this small area, the fovea, consists of only cones. Cranial nerves II, III, IV, and VI are involved in vision. Visual recognition of objects and the interpretation of their meaning involve the occipital cortex and the limbic system.

Hearing is possible because sound waves are transformed into vibration in the ear. Sound is captured by the external ear and funneled to the eardrum, or tympanic membrane. Three small bones form the ossicular chain (the malleus, incus, and stapes) and transmit sound vibration to the cochlea in the inner ear (see Figure 10-3). Remember that the cochlea is embedded in the temporal bone or bony labyrinth and is a set of fluid-filled coiled tubes. The sound wave travels along the basilar (bottom) membrane of the cochlear duct like a ripple of water on a pond. The hair cells of the organ of Corti lying on the basilar membrane receive the vibration and generate nerve impulses in the auditory division of cranial nerve VIII. The signals are conveyed via complex connections in the brain stem to the cerebral cortex, where sound is perceived and the meaning can be interpreted.

Taste and smell are involved in the vital functions of eating and smelling and are considered near and far receptors, respectively. These receptors are the only ones that are continually being replaced. Substances in the mouth enter taste pores and interact with the membranes of the taste receptors (buds). The chemical stimulus is transduced into taste sensation. Taste buds are found in special skin structures called *papillae,* which are innervated by branches of cranial nerves VII, IX, and X. Three distinct types of papillae are present in humans and located on different parts of the tongue, soft palate, and epiglottis.

Smell is the most primitive special sense. It has a direct connection to the limbic, or emotional, system as well as to the cortex. The olfactory receptor is a remarkably simple structure found in the olfactory mucosa. Olfactory hairs, or cilia, project into the mucus, react to odors, and stimulate the olfactory cells. As a bipolar neuron, the olfactory receptor is the actual cell body of the sensory neuron. The receptor can be replaced if damaged. Its axon forms cranial nerve I.

Perception and Integration Sensory input plays a major role in perceptual development. When meaning is attached to sensory information, sensation becomes perception. Detection, awareness, and localization of sensory information are components of perception. The ability to discriminate comes before discrimination of sensory information. Sensory information is shared between senses to provide for the identification and manipulation of objects and people within the environment.

Sensory integration is the ability to use sensory information to move efficiently. *Integration* means a putting together of many sensory inputs for the purpose of adapting to the task at hand. Integration enhances adaptation by making an individual's response more effective. An individual who has difficulty processing any of the many sensory inputs might exhibit difficulty in planning or executing certain tasks. Perceptual abilities and sensory integration develop over time and reflect the increasing adaptation of the individual to the environment and the tasks encountered within the environment.

There are three types of sensory integration. *Intrasensory* integration occurs when information is shared within the same sensory system. Input from both eyes provides for the perception of depth. *Intersensory* integration occurs when two different sensory systems combine to impart a richer understanding than could be provided by only one sensory dimension. For example, touch and proprioception combine to provide a sense of body scheme. The last type, *sensorimotor* integration, involves the interaction of sensory and motor systems, as with the combining of vision and movement to draw or write. The combination of head turning, looking, and hearing to localize an auditory cue is another example. The linking of movement awareness and language results in the establishment of directionality or the ability of the child to use spatial cues. Others have called this *spatial cognition*.

The role of *sensation* in perceptual organization was defined by Ayres[15] as being able to make use of sensory information. A later definition explains that the sensory information from within the body and from the environment is processed to allow the individual to move effectively within the environment.[16] Sensory integration is an adaptive phenomenon that takes place within the context of a specific task and environment. It is one thing to maneuver a wheelchair through an obstacle course and quite another to walk on the deck of a rolling ship in a storm.

Cortical and subcortical structures participate in sensory integration. Association cortices, the thalamus, and the brain stem reticular system can process, amplify or dampen, and direct sensory information to other areas of the brain. The thalamus relays the sensory stimulus to the cortex and to the appropriate association areas to plan a response. Recognition and interpretation of the stimulus occur in the primary sensory cortex, such as the realization that you have been touched and the quality of that touch (gentle or rough). The touch is further interpreted in the higher association areas as emotionally pleasing or dangerous. In an open system, interconnected structures regulate and organize sensory input into a conceptual whole to allow us to identify shapes by touch. This ability is called *stereognosis*. Perceptual abilities and sensory integration develop over time and reflect the increasing adaptation of the individual to the environment.

LIFE SPAN CHANGES

Prenatal Period

The senses of touch, smell, and taste are ready to function at birth, as evidenced by the complete myelination of their respective neural pathways. The vestibular, visual, and auditory senses are capable of some level of function at birth but require additional time and environmental experience to complete myelination and maturation of central pathways. The sensory systems develop in utero in the following order: touch, vestibular, smell, hearing, vision, taste, and proprioception.

Somatic Senses

The fetus develops the ability to respond to touch around the mouth as early as 7½ weeks of gestation.[17] The earliest response to touch is avoidance, or turning away. By 17 weeks, cutaneous sensation spreads to the entire body with the exception of the top and back of the head; these areas are subjected to the most sensory input during delivery.

Proprioceptive receptors are well developed by midfetal life.[18] Tapping, stretching, or even a change in amniotic fluid pressure can cause a response in the fetus.[19] Muscle spindles are known to differentiate between 11 and 12 weeks.[20] The Golgi tendon organ does not differentiate until 16 weeks of gestation. Pacinian corpuscles are found in the distal parts of limbs at 20 weeks of gestation but are immature.

Sensory nerve endings capable of carrying pain are present throughout the body of the fetus by 20 weeks of gestation. However, the fetus is not aware of the pain because the pathway from the spinal cord to the cortex is incomplete. This pathway connects to the thalamus by 24 to 26 weeks of gestation, making cortical perception of pain possible.[21] The nociceptive system is completely myelinated by 37 weeks of gestation.[22] Knowing that preterm infants feel pain makes it imperative that pain management strategies be implemented in this population.

Vestibular Sense

The vestibular apparatus begins as a thickening of ectoderm, or placode, in the primitive ear early in the fourth week of gestation. A *placode* is a common precursor of most sensory organs. The semicircular canals, utricle, and saccule are completely formed at 9½ weeks of gestation.[23] The fetus moves constantly in utero, and the vestibular apparatus provides information about that movement. The fetus shows a generalized body response to changes in body position, including the ability to right the head. Movement in utero has been linked to later movement competence.[24] Neural connections link the labyrinths and the oculomotor nuclei in the brain stem between 12 to 24 weeks of gestation, which will be important for establishing gaze stability and spatial orientation. This is the first sensory system to be myelinated and the first to function. However, although it is structurally complete at birth, maturation continues to assist the child to develop postural control, movement, and balance.[25]

Special Senses

Vision The eyes also develop during the fourth week of gestation from a placode that forms a vesicle. The optic vesicle folds in onto itself to produce a two-layered optic cup, from which the retina is derived. The neural cells of the retina differentiate into 10 layers containing photoreceptors (the rods and cones), cell bodies of bipolar neurons, and ganglion cells. Because of the infolding, the photoreceptors are adjacent to the pigment layer. Therefore, light must pass through the retina to reach the receptors.

Neurons in the occipital cortex are organized into their adult layers during the second half of gestation,[26] so they are ready to receive input after birth. Myelination begins at the optic chiasm around 13 weeks of gestation, and the rods and cones differentiate at 16 weeks. Light perception is possible in utero[27]; the fetus exhibits reflexive eye blinking at 6 months of gestation. Thalamic connections begin to myelinate before term and continue until the fifth postnatal month of life. The thalamic connections, those to the lateral geniculate nucleus, are crucial to the development of more sophisticated visual perceptual abilities. Central visual pathways develop postnatally, even though the neurons that constitute these pathways are formed prenatally.

Hearing The ectoderm of the otic placode forms both the membranous labyrinth of the vestibular system and the structures of the inner ear—the cochlear duct and the organ of Corti—during the fourth week of gestation. The hair cells differentiate by 16 weeks of gestation.[27] The remaining structures of the ear, including ligaments and muscles, come from the branchial arches. Hearing in utero is possible as early as 24 weeks of gestation and is consistently present after 28 weeks of gestation.[28]

Taste The tongue is developed from the mandibular arch at 26 to 31 days of gestation. Formation is completed by the 37th day; the various types of taste buds reach maturity by 13 weeks of gestation.[26] Ingestion of amniotic fluid in utero is thought to contribute to the development of the primitive gut and to the regulation of amniotic fluid volume. Taste is functional in utero in the last third of the pregnancy. The amniotic fluid is rich in chemicals such as sugars, salts, acids, and lactate that can be "tasted" by the fetus.[29] Steiner[30] reports that infants born at 6 to 7 months of gestation can detect citric acid.

Smell The olfactory placode also forms during the fourth week of gestation. It is the earliest distance receptor to develop. The fifth cranial nerve innervates the walls of the nose at 5 weeks; the olfactory organ (bulb) is well developed by the fifth and sixth months of gestation. The unmyelinated nerve fibers of cranial nerve I are the olfactory nerve. It is these fibers that end in the olfactory bulb. Olfactory discrimination is possible in preterm infants beyond 29 weeks of gestation.[18]

Infancy and Early Childhood

All sensory systems are capable of functioning at birth because the peripheral nervous system is completely myelinated. However, complete maturation of sensory pathways occurs after birth. Physiological changes occur after birth in all sensory systems, as evidenced by an increase in nerve conduction velocity (time to conduct) with myelination, redistribution of axon branching, and increased synaptic efficacy. Functional changes are apparent as the infant interacts more meaningfully with the world.

State and Novelty

Behavioral state and novelty of stimulus play a role in the infant's level of interest in sensory information. A sleeping or overstimulated infant is not able to react to a new stimulus. On the other hand, a quietly alert infant looking at a mobile will generally become attentive to a new toy. Sensory awareness requires that the infant be sufficiently aroused. The concept of state was first described by Prechtl[31] as levels of alertness ranging from sleep to crying. The quiet alert state has been deemed the most appropriate for testing an infant's responses to sensory stimulation. Studies show that an infant's state will affect the level of reflex and motor responsiveness.[32] The ability of the infant to change states smoothly is also an indication of the degree to which the CNS is organized.

Many studies of visual preference in infants have pinpointed the role of novelty in gaining attention and producing motor behavior. The behavior may be looking, reaching, vocalizing, or even quieting, but the common denominator is that the infant responds to a certain level of stimulus novelty. For example, when an infant is shown two pictures, the infant typically attends to the new picture. From the earliest moment that the infant is quietly alert, there is the ability to perceive sensory stimuli and to demonstrate preferences. Novelty and complexity guide infants' exploratory behavior.[33] Learning and adaptation occur much earlier than was once believed. Perceptual abilities once reserved as the province of the older child are consistently being documented in infants. Sensory perception, that is, the ability to attach meaning to sensory information, occurs from the beginning of extrauterine life.

Self-Perception

Infants develop a sense of self as young as 2 to 3 months. Hand-to-mouth and hand-to-face behavior is typical in an infant. This cutaneous self-stimulation does not trigger any of the typically observed rooting responses when an external object contacts the same facial location. Rochat and Hespos[34] suggest that the infant can distinguish between self-touch and touch of another person. The self-stimulation would involve proprioceptive stimulation from self-movement as well as touch. When touching their own face, infants experience a unique sensorimotor event that potentially identifies their body as a differentiated body. Rochat categorizes infants' self-exploration of their own bodies as visual-proprioceptive calibration: "infants appear fascinated by the simultaneous experience of seeing and feeling the limbs of their own body moving through space.[35]" Three-month-old infants begin to show systematic visual and proprioceptive self-exploration.[36]

During the second year of life, the child develops a sense of "me." Before that time, the infant may distinguish her own image from another infant's image in a mirror but still does not have a real sense of herself and only herself. In an experiment where a Post-it note is stuck to a child's forehead and the child looks in the mirror and removes the Post-it, the concept of me is thought to exist. This action occurs by age 2 but the development of the child's sense of self continues until 4 to 5 years of age, according to Rochat.[37] The reader is referred to his description of levels of self-awareness.

Somatic Senses

Touch The perception of touch and pain is crucial to the newborn's survival. Although the defensive movements to light touch seen in utero fade by birth, the newborn reflexively moves to clear the nose and mouth of any object that obstructs the airway. The first responses to touch are generalized diffuse responses, such as random arm and leg movements. Information from touch is initially used by the infant to locate food. Within a few days after birth, head turning in response to touching the mouth is precisely related to the part of the mouth touched. Although touch and pain are not completely differentiated in the full-term newborn, pain sensitivity has been shown to increase over the first 4 days of life.[38]

Early tactile input plays a role in parent-infant attachment, stress-coping mechanisms, sociability, and cognitive development. The use of tactile input to recognize differences develops gradually; a 1-month-old infant is able to distinguish between pacifier shapes.[39] Prechtl[40] reports a refinement in the receptive field for touch-mediated reflex responses such as flexor withdrawal. Touch to any part of the leg of a newborn results in a reflexive withdrawal. Gradually, the receptive field becomes limited to the sole of the foot.

Touch sensation can be localized generally at 7 to 9 months; specific localization is demonstrated by 12 to 16 months of age.[18] General localization is exhibited by the infant's moving the extremity; specific localization involves the infant's touching or looking at the area touched. A toddler can touch the place where she was touched and will either rub the area or push away the

stimulus. The spot also will be noticed visually, which supports the possibility that intersensory association occurs between touch and vision.

The ability to use touch to identify objects is called *haptic perception*.[1] *Haptic* means "able to lay hold of" and is appropriate because the majority of information about objects comes from manipulation. Nine-month-old infants have been found to possess this ability, as determined by manual exploration.[41] When visual information is combined with touch, infants as young as 6 months can pick out toys that were touched previously without being seen.[42]

Temperature The newborn must regulate its own body temperature at birth and is sensitive to the temperature of the ambient air. Responses to changes in air temperature are often seen in common body postures assumed by the infant. Infants who are too warm may appear to be "sunbathing," decrease their calorie intake, sleep, and show peripheral vasodilation. Sweating and panting responses mature later. Conversely, the infant will wake and move about if too cool. Discrimination of hot and cold is possible early on and is characterized by more reactivity to cold. Respiratory changes, limb movement, and state changes have been documented for temperatures varying as little as 5° to 6°.

Pain Pain receptors are equally prevalent in infants and adults,[21] with pain sensitivity appearing to increase in the first month of life.[43] Puchalski and Hummel[44] reviewed development of the nociception and stressed the fact that infants remember pain. Newborn infants and preterm infants may experience pain more acutely because descending inhibition is not present developmentally.[45,46] Studies of infant circumcision[47] show that physiological changes in response to the procedure occur and that preterm infants display behavioral and physiological changes in response to painful stimuli.[48] Pain is the fifth vital sign and as such should be assessed. Evidence suggests that there may be long-term consequences of not treating pain in infants,[45] which may include diminished social control, poor adaptive behavior, and impulsivity. Altered responses to pain, both hyperresponses and hyporesponses, have been reported. In the case of extremely preterm infants, plasticity of the brain can result in negative consequences, as hyperinnervation may result from repeated painful procedures.[44]

Proprioception Proprioception is the foundation for purposeful movements such as imitation, reaching, and locomotion. It is used for action very early after birth, when the tactile and vestibular systems are functioning.

The fact that newborn infants imitate mouth opening and tongue protrusion is interpreted as a pairing of visual and proprioceptive input.[49] In the same way a child handles objects to gain haptic perception, infants move to gain proprioceptive information. Self-perception in the infant appears to depend on touch and proprioception.[50] Research has shown that reaching behavior in 5-month-olds depends more on the infant's motor ability and proprioception than on visual control; no difference is seen between reaching in the dark and reaching in the light.[51] Vision becomes more important as the system matures, as evidenced by more successful reaching with vision in the 7-month-old.[52,53]

Achieving and maintaining an upright posture depend on the infant's ability to interpret and respond to information about body sway, which comes from vestibular, visual, and proprioceptive input. Multiple studies have shown that infants use vision proprioceptively in sitting and standing to maintain stable postures.[54-57] When proprioceptive and vestibular input indicated that the body was stable and visual input indicated movement, the majority of subjects made compensatory movements.

Vestibular Sense

The vestibular system defines the body's relationship to gravity and is completely myelinated at birth. Many of the infant's earliest activities are related to achieving and maintaining stable postures against gravity. Preterm infants were initially found to have delayed vestibular responses to movement,[58] especially preterm infants, who are also small for gestational age. This delay in responding is due to immaturity, not pathology,[59] and is related to the difficulty preterm infants have in maintaining alert wakefulness. When alert and awake, even preterm infants can demonstrate vestibular responses.[60] Newborn infants' vestibular function was found to be better when tested in a supine position than in a prone position. It has been postulated that this positional difference in physiological function may contribute to the protective effect of the supine position in preventing sudden infant death syndrome.[61]

The first postnatal vestibular ocular reflex (VOR) demonstrated by the infant is called the *Doll eye phenomenon*. When a typical newborn is held in dorsal suspension and the head is moved horizontally, the eyes appear to move in the opposite direction of the head motion. This eye movement corresponds to the slow component of nystagmus. Persistence of the Doll eye phenomenon after the first 2 weeks of life indicates serious brain damage. A normal VOR should be present by 2 months of age[62] and consists of both the slow and fast component of nystagmus being present. Nystagmus is an alternating sequence of fast and slow horizontal eye movements normally seen in response to a series of rotatory movements of the head. The form and amount of nystagmus normally present in infants change between birth and the first year of life.[63]

The vestibular system provides a functional connection with the visual system by related eye movements to head movements. Saccadic movements of the eye are quick movements, which bring the image onto the fovea of the eye. As the saccadic system matures, the eyes can then demonstrate the fast component of nystagmus, a jerking back to central gaze. Optokinetic nystagmus is nystagmus that results from viewing a rotating drum stimulus. Infants as young as 3 to 6 months of age can demonstrate optokinetic nystagmus. A VOR can also generate eye movements to compensate for head motion to maintain a stable retinal image. The saccadic system responsible for the fast component of nystagmus continues to mature up to the age of 2.[25,62] A lack of VOR responses at 10 months of age is abnormal.[25,64]

Vestibular sensitivity increases from birth to a peak between 6 and 12 months of age. After this peak, there is a decline to 2½ years and a more gradual decline to puberty. Infants are more sensitive to vestibular input, and that oversensitivity may explain their relative unsteadiness. The slow maturation of vestibular sensitivity is a result of changes in synaptic strength and connectivity in the brain stem and higher centers.[60] Maturation of the vestibular system contributes to postural control and general motor development through its contributions to developmental reflexes, such as the Moro and head righting (see Chapter 12).

Special Senses

Vision Newborns were always thought to have relatively poor, if any, visual abilities at birth. However, as technology for testing has become more sophisticated, so has the understanding of the infant's visual system. Newborns have pattern preference and can maintain attention if a stimulus is novel enough or resembles a face. To obtain visual alerting behavior, newborns need to be approached from the side because they are unable to maintain their heads in the midline until 4 months of age. Visual acuity at birth appears to be about 20/800,[65] and steadily increases with age. Some authors report that adult levels of vision (20/20) are achieved as early as 1 year,[43] but others use 3 years as the age at which adult resolution is possible.[65]

The infant sees initially in black and white. As the cones (the color receptors) mature over the first several months, color vision develops. Two month olds see the colors red and yellow, and full-color vision is present by 4 months.

Smooth tracking abilities begin by 2 months of age[66] and progress over an ever-widening arc as the infant matures and head control is achieved. Smooth pursuit is the ability to track a target smoothly without jerking. Myelination of the pathway that subserves smooth pursuit is complete at 5 months.[67] Accommodation is possible at 2 months but improves to adult levels by 6 months. Depth and size perception begin to develop with the ability to use the two eyes together to converge or diverge on near and far objects. This may be aided by the development of head control in the prone position as the infant practices looking down at her hands or up at toys.

Vision provides vital information for balance and head control: "perceptual sensitivity to visual information improves rapidly during the first few months after birth."[68] Head control contributes to the ability of the infant to visually fix on objects. Conversely, visual fixation contributes to postural stability of the head and neck. Visual information is used to control posture even before infants can sit. Optical flow is detected peripherally by infants and used as a cue to make a compensatory response. "Optical flow refers to the perceived motion of the visual field that results from an individual's own movement through the environment.[69]"

Binocular vision depends on adequate alignment of the eyes. Most infants demonstrate good visual alignment between 3 and 6 months of age. Shimojo and colleagues[70] postulate that the change in binocular function seen at 3 months is related to the separation of the afferent input from the two eyes into columns within the visual cortex. These bands of cells are known as *ocular dominance columns*. If the input from each eye is the same, the columns will be the same size. Two-year olds-exhibit adultlike binocular vision. Table 10-1 provides a list of changes in visual development along with changes in visual motor behavior.

Table **10-1**		

Visual Development First Two Years of Life

Age	Visual Development	Visual-Motor Behavior
Newborn	Focal distance 7-10 in 20/800 acuity	Hands fisted Doll eye Tracks toy to midline Prefers black and white
1 mo	Focal distance ≥ 1-3 ft Frontal visual fields mature	Tracks 180 degrees Prefers face to object Tracks horizontally
2 mo	Accommodation develops Depth and size perception developing Dichromatic (red and yellow)	Unilateral hand regard Asymmetrical tonic neck reflex Hands open, manipulates red ring, swipes
3 mo	Head turning with eyes Binocular vision begins Improved visual attention	Strong visual inspection of hands at midline Mouths objects
4 mo	Sees in full color Well-developed binocular vision Accommodates over wide range of distances	Bilateral reach at midline Hits and shakes objects Instinctive grasp Holds one cube
5 mo	Vision directs grasp and manipulation	Turns head to follow vanishing object Raking; holds two cubes
6 mo	Adult accommodation 20/40 acuity	Tracks objects in all directions Transfers at midline Palmar grasp

Table 10-1—cont'd

Visual Development First Two Years of Life

Age	Visual Development	Visual-Motor Behavior
7 mo		Transfers hand to hand
		Radial palmar grasp
8 mo	Macula more mature	Anticipates future position of objects in motion
		Reaches for hidden objects
9 mo		Radial digital grasp
10 mo		Recognizes object by seeing only part of it
		Inferior pincer grasp (9-12 mo)
12 mo	20/20 acuity	Follows rapidly moving objects
		Visually monitors hand play
		Neat pincer grasp
2 yr	Adult binocular vision	

Hearing At birth, the infant physiologically responds to sound by changing respiratory patterns or heart rate. Sensory thresholds are slightly higher than those of adults.[71] Behaviorally, the infant may demonstrate facial grimacing, eye blinking, and crying at loud noises. The auditory system is completely myelinated 1 month after birth. By 3 months of age, head turning to localize sound is well established. In the appropriate state of wakefulness, a newborn may exhibit eye or head turning to sound. New sounds will produce searching behavior in infants older than 4 months and will encourage the infant to babble in vocal play. Vocal imitation follows, with words being produced by the first year. Locke[72] suggests that the infant's orientation to the voices and location of people speaking may be an important precursor to the development of spoken language.

The 2-year-old develops listening skills, which refine the production of speech and facilitate the rapid acquisition of language. Speech is learned by successive approximations of the correct sound. Basic auditory listening skills are mastered by 3 years of age.[18] Data from auditory-evoked potentials document adult latency values by the age of 4 years, indicating the early postnatal maturation of the auditory system.[73]

Ear infections that result in increased fluid in the ear are a common problem in infants and preschoolers. Because fluid in the middle ear can produce a conductive hearing loss, these infections are now treated aggressively. Previously, many children with a chronic ear infection showed delayed development of language.

Dynamic balance problems and delays in gross motor development have been reported in children with chronic ear infections.[74]

Taste and Smell These two chemical senses are significant to the newborn. Although obviously linked to feeding, these senses are also involved in parent-infant communication, control of respiration, and cognition.[43] Taste may assist in modulating oral intake, as well as in coordinating breathing and eating. Smell may be related to infant attention, although this has not been adequately studied. Infants may use smell to identify familiar features of the environment, including people, before the visual system is effective in performing this function. A 5-day-old newborn can selectively orient to her mother's breast pad based on odor.[75] Both taste and smell are functional at birth and quickly become connected to feeding reflexes. Infants discriminate between all four primary taste sensations but prefer to ingest sweet things.

Childhood and Adolescence

Sensory changes continue during childhood and adolescence. It is during childhood that the integration of sensation and movement occurs. The perceptual process, although evident in early development, is further refined by the child's increased ability to attend to more than one characteristic of a stimulus, to attach meaning to sensory stimuli, and to plan a motor response. Cognitive and language development is of paramount importance in developing and verbalizing spatial and directional concepts that build on the increased awareness of self and the surroundings.

Somatic Senses

The somatic senses of touch and proprioception continue to be refined in childhood. Two-point discrimination is possible by 4 years of age.[76] Children can usually identify familiar objects by touch at 5 years of age. Knowledge of where the body is in space and the sequence of movements that must be planned to perform a motor task is based on appropriate interpretation of tactile and proprioceptive input. The ability to motor plan, or praxis, emerges during childhood. Tactile and proprioceptive sensation also refine the changing adolescent's body scheme and the affective view of the body.

The coupling of movement and perception is a central process in perceptual development. Bigelow[77] identified how children use proprioceptive information in visual self-recognition. Children recognized moving images of themselves sooner than they did static pictures, which supports the belief that children move their bodies purposefully to gain proprioceptive information. Thelen[78] believed that individuals perceive in order to move and move in order to perceive. Rochat[37] thinks that the highest level of self-awareness is achieved around the age of 5. This belief is supported by the ability of children to develop representations of objects and people in their mind between the ages of 4 and 5. Infants begin with no awareness of self and as children are able to develop a meta-level of self-awareness by age 5. For a thorough discussion of all five levels, the student is referred to Rochet's article where he describes a self-discovery paradigm using a Post-it note and looking in the mirror.[37]

Kinesthetic acuity improves with age. *Kinesthetic acuity* is the ability to proprioceptively discriminate differences in location, distance, weight, force, speed, and acceleration of movement. For example, an individual can distinguish objects by weight when held in the hand while blindfolded. Based on research using the Kinesthetic Acuity Test (KAT), Elliot and associates[79] reported that performance in children improves from age 5 through 12 and sometimes beyond. Livesey and Parks[80] and Livesey and Intilli[81] have now used the KAT with preschool children and have documented that kinesthetic sense can be tested in children as young as 3 years of age. In the 1995 study, they found that kinesthetic sense improves with age and that boys performed better than girls. However, when visual-spatial cues were reduced in the follow-up 1996 study, the gender differences were no longer present. Kinesthetic acuity improves more quickly than kinesthetic memory. Memory for movement is *kinesthetic memory*. Examples of movement tasks performed from memory are a dance routine and the sequence of step-hopping that occurs in skipping. Adult levels of kinesthetic acuity are achieved by 8 years of age, whereas kinesthetic memory maturity is not usually achieved until age 12.[82]

Vestibular Sense

Vestibular responses change greatly between preadolescence and adulthood.[59] The most striking maturational changes occur in preschool children.[25] Vestibular sensitivity declines from 2½ years to puberty. Before 3 years of age, infants and children engage in repetitive self-stimulation, such as rocking in a rocking chair or spinning themselves around, but this is not a pervasive activity. This period of vestibular stimulation begins around 6 to 8 months of age and coincides with a peaking of vestibular sensitivity. With increasing maturation, these behaviors decline. Children have a stronger response to vestibular stimulation than adults, who respond less intensely as the system matures. Although maturation of vestibular nystagmus is thought to be completed between 10 and 14 years of age,[59] vestibular function relative to postural control in standing does not reach adult levels even at the age of 15.[4] See Chapter 12 for a further discussion of sensory organization in postural control.

Special Senses

Vision   Many aspects of visual perception develop in childhood. The child shows refinement of size constancy: the ability to recognize that objects remain the same size even if the distance of the viewer from the object changes. The ability to separate the figure from the background, or *figure-ground perception,* improves with age. By 8 years of age, most children are as good as adults in performing this perceptual task.[83]

Visual perception related to object identification, movement, and task performance seems to follow the same trend. By 5 years of age, children demonstrate *visual closure,* or the ability to discern a shape when seeing only part of it. Between 5 and 10 years of age, children accurately track moving objects, such as a softball.[84] Perceptual judgments regarding the size of various objects at different distances become mature at the age of 11 years.[85] Adult levels of depth perception are achieved at 12 years of age.

Spatial Awareness   *Spatial awareness* is the internalization of our own location in space and object localization. The teacher stands in front of the students with the blackboard behind her. *Space perception* is the ability to perceive direction or distance. Combining visual information with proprioception allows the child to recognize the location and orientation of objects within the environment. By age 3 to 4 years, most children have conceptualized the spatial dichotomies of over/under, top/bottom, front/back, and in/out. The sequence of acquisition of these spatial directions is vertical to horizontal, then diagonal or oblique.[83] Knowledge of the spatial environment is necessary to construct effective motor programs. Objects are first related to the child and later related to other objects. Space perception and spatial awareness are needed for successful execution of a motor program when accommodating to changing environmental demands.

Most 5-year-old children know the right side of the body from the left side. This concept of *laterality* is a conscious internal awareness of the two sides of the body. However, it is not until children are 8 years of age that they consistently and accurately answer questions about right-left discrimination.[82] It is also at this age that children can begin to relay information in directional terms such as "the playground is on the right."

Directionality, the motor expression of laterality and spatial awareness, develops between 6 and 12 years of age.[86] Directionality is initially demonstrated at 6 years when the child mirrors and imitates movement. At 7 years of age, the child uses the body as a directional reference: "The ball is in front of me." Next, the child can reference objects objectively, such as, "The water fountain is on the left." By 10 years of age, the child can identify the right and left of the person opposite her. She will no longer mirror movements but will move the right arm when the other person moves the right arm. At 12 years of age, the child can use a natural frame of reference so that she can describe that the sun sets in the west.

Adulthood and Aging

Sensory abilities present in adolescence continue to guide motor activities. Information from different sensory systems continue to be combined during adulthood. This *intersensory integration* allows the adult mover to use visual and auditory cues to provide increased perception of the task at hand. Many combinations of sensory inputs are possible. The response time in a motor task can be shortened when a person attends to a combination of sensory inputs rather than to a single sensory input.[87] Despite the development of intersensory associations and the maintenance of a steady functional state of sensory receptors up to middle age, a decline in sensory function does begin in adulthood and progresses with advanced age. Peripheral and central changes are documented in many of the sensory systems, although these changes are not always directly related to a decline in function, nor are they universal.

Somatic Senses

Some older adults show a diminished ability to detect touch, vibration, proprioception, temperature, and pain.[88] Structural changes in skin such as loss of dermal thickness, decline in nutrient transfer, and loss of collagen and elastin fibers contribute to a decline in the functions of the skin. Physiologically, the growth rate, healing response, sensory perception, and thermoregulation of the skin decline.[89]

The skin receptors responsible for the perception of pressure and light touch, *pacinian* and *Meissner corpuscles,* decline in number with age.[90,91] By the ninth decade, they are only one third of their original density. Both of these receptors also undergo morphological or structural changes. Verillo[92] attributed decreased vibrotactile sensitivity with age to structural changes in the pacinian corpuscle pathways. Meissner corpuscles change relative to whether we have performed physical labor. With manual labor, the corpuscles become winding and large; without manual labor, they develop neurofibrillary networks. Regardless of the structural changes, older adults can lose up to 90% of these receptors. *Merkel disks,* another type of pressure receptor, appear to be unchanged.[93,94] With the loss of pressure and light touch receptors, valuable feedback about the environment is decreased, and balance responses may be impaired.

Tactile acuity declines with age. Touch thresholds in the fingers of older adults were found to be elevated 2½ times over younger adults.[95] Spatial acuity as tested by two-point discrimination has been found to be impaired with age. Stevens and colleagues[96] documented a lower ability to detect gap discrimination on five body areas (plantar and dorsal surfaces of the forefoot, volar forearm, and upper and lower surfaces of the forefinger) in older adults compared with young adults. The rate of deterioration of spatial acuity is slower in the proximal parts of the body compared with the distal parts.[97] However, the upper and lower surfaces of the fingertips and feet show identical declines in tactile acuity so that it is incorrect to attribute this effect of aging to wear and tear.[98]

One of the most common sensory losses documented in older adults is the loss of vibratory sensation. The decline in the pacinian and Meissner corpuscles correlates with impairments in detecting vibration seen in older adults. Awareness of vibration begins to decline at 50 years of age,[99] with the lower extremities more affected than the upper extremities.[100] Perry[101] studied vibration perception on the plantar surface of older and younger adults using monofilaments. Older adults were less sensitive at all sites tested compared with young adults. Vibration perception thresholds were found to double in the early 70s. Clinically it is important to include vibratory testing of the lower extremity in older adults when screening for sensory impairments because losses may be related to impaired balance. See Table 10-2 for a summary of the age-related changes in cutaneous somatosensation.

Joint position sense (JPS) definitely declines with age,[102] especially in the lower extremities. Distal joints are more affected than proximal joints with the differences possibly being related to weight bearing. A decrease in JPS has been documented in the big toe and in the ankle in weight bearing and nonweight bearing.[103,104] However, in the knee the decrease was present in partial weight bearing but not in weight bearing.[105] In an older study, women exhibited an age-related decline in proprioception and static joint position sensation of the knee.[106] The more recent studies have looked at dynamic movement, which may explain the differences in the results. Subjects using a visual analog scale also reported an age-related decline in position sense of the knee.[107] No difference in hip JPS in older subjects compared with younger ones was reported in a study by Pickard and colleagues.[108] Functionally, the decline in proprioception in the lower extremities has tremendous implications for compromising balance in older adults.

Compromised thermoregulation can predispose older adults to hypothermia or heat stroke. Control of body temperature regulation by the hypothalamus is altered significantly with age. The ability of the sympathetic nervous system to cause vasoconstriction and impede heat loss is impaired. As a result, mild hypothermia occurs in a large number of older adults in cooler rooms, which is why older people accommodate by more often wearing sweaters, coats, and hats. Thermoregulatory deficiency is also a result of a decline in temperature perception.[109]

Effects of aging on pain perception have become clearer over the last several years. Gibson and Farrell[110] provide a substantial review of age differences in the nociceptive system. The threshold at which pain is

Table 10-2

Age-Related Changes in Somatosensation

Function	Receptor	Nature of Change
Touch/Pressure	Fewer free nerve endings ↓ number of pacinian corpuscles ↓ concentration of Meissner corpuscles	Significant increase in thresholds after age 40 years Lower thresholds in fingers than toes Light touch thresholds significantly increase in hands and feet Men are generally less sensitive than women
Vibration	↓ number of pacinian corpuscles ↓ concentration of Meissner corpuscles	Diminished vibration threshold Lower extremities more affected than upper extremities Greatest decline after 80 years
Proprioception (passive joint position)	↓ number of intrafusal fibers in the spindle ↓ in all joint receptor types	Decreased joint position sense in the big toe and ankle Thresholds for lower extremity joints twice as great after 50 years of age than before 40 years
Kinesthesia (active joint motion)	Alterations in distal sensory axons	Few age-related changes generally if minimal memory involved Age-related changes increase with greater memory demands

Data from Shaffer SW, Harrison AL: Aging of the somatosensory system: a translational perspective, *Phys Ther* 87:193-207, 2007; Williams HG: Aging and eye-hand coordination. In Bard C, Fleury J, Hay L, editors: *Development of eye-hand coordination*, Columbia, SC, 1990, University of South Carolina Press, p 352.

perceived provides an early warning system for the body to avoid injury. Based on substantial support from the literature, Gibson and Farrell[110] conclude that pain thresholds increase with age when certain stimulus factors are present. The stimuli that show an increased threshold tend to be brief, be small in spatial extent, and involve peripheral or visceral sites. These occasions would put the older person at risk for injury. Because it takes more stimuli for pain to register, the person can sustain an injury before pain is identified.[110] The function of the myelinated fibers that subserve pain are changed secondary to aging, leaving the perception of pain and temperature to be conducted by slower unmyelinated fibers.[111] Sensitivity of age-injured tissue may become maladaptive if the hyperalgesia does not resolve during the healing process. Additional age-related changes in somatosensation are listed in Table 10-3.

Vestibular Sense

Dizziness and vertigo are common disturbances in persons older than 50 years. Structures of the vestibular system such as the hair cells undergo degeneration.[112] A 20% to 40% reduction in hair cells has been reported

in the saccule and utricle and in the semicircular canals. Neuronal loss has been documented in parts of the vestibular nuclear complex that receive input from the semicircular canals.[113] Neural changes in the vestibular nerve are evident in older adults and may begin as early as 40 years of age. By 75 years, the number of myelinated vestibular nerve fibers declines almost 40%.[114] The older individual may exhibit dysequilibrium from age-related changes in the peripheral or central vestibular system. There is an increased gain in the vestibular-ocular reflex (VOR) in older adults, which can result in the person perceiving movement of the environment when the head is moved.[115] The nervous system compensates for age-related deterioration of the vestibular system as evidenced by not all older adults exhibiting vestibular disorders. However, dizziness and vestibular dysfunction may manifest themselves when the nervous system is no longer able to compensate.[116]

Presbystasis is the age-related decline in equilibrium or dynamic balance seen when no other pathology is noted.[117] Reliance on vestibular input alone may result in loss of balance and even falls in the older adult.[118,119] Healthy older adults without general sensory deficits do

Table **10-3**	

Age-Related Changes in Vision

Function	Nature of Change
General	Decreased transparency of lens
	Decreased amount of light reaching the eye
	Decrease in number of macular neurons by almost half from 20 to 80 years
Visual acuity	Usually retained throughout life; slight decrease from 20 to 50 years
	More rapid decrease from 60 to 80 years; need more light to detect objects
Light adaptation	Sharp decline in ability to quickly adapt from dark to light environments after 40 years; dramatic decrease after 60 years
Contrast sensitivity	Three times as much contrast needed by older individuals as younger ones to perceive a coarsely structured target
Dark adaptation	Little or no change from 20 to 40 years
	Significant increase in time to adapt after 70; an 80-year-old requires 40+ minutes
Depth perception	Little or no changes to 60+ years
	Accelerated decrease from 60 to 75 years
Visual information processing	Older individuals are one-third slower than younger ones
	Significant decrease in peripheral and central information between 50 and 60 years

Modified from Williams HG: Aging and eye-hand coordination. In Bard C, Fleury J, Hay L, editors: *Development of eye-hand coordination*, Columbia, SC, 1990, University of South Carolina Press, p 350.

not exhibit as much of an increase in postural sway as do older adults who show sensory deficits. The latter group is more likely to experience falls.[3,120,121] Postural sway is described in Chapter 12.

Special Senses

Vision Visual acuity increases in the 20s and 30s, remains stable in the 40s and 50s, and then declines.[122] The most rapid decrease in acuity occurs between 60 and 80 years of age. By 85, there is an 80% loss from the acuity level present at 40 years of age.[123] Structural changes in the optical part of the eye contribute to these age-related changes in function. The cornea and lens thicken, the lens curvature decreases, and a yellowish pigment accumulates. Aging changes in the lens protein may be a result of oxidative damage.[109] Table 10-3 lists some age-related changes in vision.

Central vision can be impaired by cataracts, a decrease in the transparency of the lens. The increase in lens density is due to accumulation of pigments. Cataracts begin to form in everyone older than 30 years,[124] and a little over 17% of those older than 40 have at least one cataract.[89] The rate of progression, however, is different for every individual. Most cataracts develop bilaterally in those older than 50 years and are present to some degree in all 70 year olds.[125] Fully developed cataracts are documented in one-third of persons 80 years old.[124] Visual acuity of 20/50 or worse is an indication for surgical removal. Those with diabetes have a higher incidence of cataracts than do the rest of the population.

Color discrimination in the green-blue end of the spectrum becomes more difficult as the lens of the eye yellows with aging. Pupil size declines with age, allowing less light into the eye. By 60 years of age, retinal illumination is reduced by one third, and the older adult is less able to detect low levels of light. Because of the lens changes, light may be scattered over more of the retinal surface, resulting in glare. Glare introduces extraneous light into the eye and may be particularly troublesome for older adults. Because of retinal sensitivity loss, the elder's eyes are overstimulated by oncoming headlights or sudden flashes of light.

Contrast sensitivity and dark adaptation decline with age. Contrast sensitivity loss causes a loss of depth perception, which can be especially dangerous when going up or down stairs. Adaptation to dim light decreases with age, which can be hazardous when entering a darkened house or a less well illuminated room. A teenager needs only 6 to 7 minutes to adapt to darkness, but an 80-year-old may need more than 40 minutes.[126] These changes are related to a decline in the number of receptors and a decreased regeneration capacity of photoreceptor pigment.[93]

Presbyopia is the diminished ability to focus clearly at normal reading distances. One contributing cause is the thickening of the lens due to continued growth of lens fibers.[124] The ciliary muscle normally acts to change the curvature of the lens to focus the image. With aging, the ciliary muscles become less able to adequately accommodate to distance changes; those over 40 often complain, "My arms are not long enough to read the print of the newspaper." Accommodation difficulties may also impair the older person's ability to read the speedometer in the car because of a decreased ability to change the lens size when switching from far to near vision. Corrective lenses such as bifocals or trifocals become necessary. By the age of 60, when the lens can no longer accommodate, presbyopia exists.

Hearing *Presbycusis,* an age-related decline in hearing acuity, is due to a loss of sensory cells in the inner ear or, more specifically, the organ of Corti. Structural changes that contribute to age-related hearing loss include degeneration of the hair cells at the base of the cochlea, degeneration of nerve cells in the spiral ganglia, atrophy of associated vascular and connective tissue, and loss of neurons in the cortical auditory centers.[93] Because the loss typically occurs at the base of the structure, hearing is initially impaired for high-frequency tones such as the whistle of a tea kettle or a doorbell. Speech perception is preserved because speech is heard at lower sound frequencies. This type of hearing loss is associated with aging and can begin as early as 30 years of age and progress until 80.

Presbycusis is more than a simple hearing loss of pure tones. It also involves speech processing and discrimination. Although speech perception is preserved, the ability to discriminate or recognize what is being said decreases. The loss of discrimination is greater than would be expected from the hearing loss alone. Seventy-five percent of adults older than 70 years will exhibit hearing loss of this type. The environment and heredity can contribute to the onset of presbycusis, so it is important to know the risk factors. Noise exposure, smoking, ototoxic medications, hypertension, and family history have been identified by Gates and Mills[127] in their review of presbycusis as risk factors.

Taste and Smell Taste and smell are intimately linked to the perception of the flavor of food. Age-related deficits can lead to poor appetite and lower food intake in older adults.[128] A diminished sensitivity of taste and smell can be expected in adults approximately 60 years of age. The thresholds for detecting tastes and smells increase with aging, with losses occurring more quickly after the age of 70. Loss of taste bud function is documented[129] and has been related to changes in taste cell membranes rather than to an actual loss of taste buds.[130] Pressure detection on the tongue is the only parameter that declines with age.[131]

The loss of smell is greater than that of taste.[128] In an earlier review, Schiffman[132] noted that there is a modest loss of taste in normal healthy aging. Smell identification declines progressively with age.[133] Identification of tastes declines with age. Memory distortion, changes, or both in the social and emotional context in which eating occurs may also contribute to a decreased perception of the flavor and appeal of food for older adults. Poor appetite can cause a decline in energy and activity and ultimately lead to a decline in overall function.

Functional Implications

Impairment of any one sensory system during early development can lead to difficulty in function. Hearing loss affects the development of motor skills and balance.[134] Because the eighth cranial nerve subserves both hearing and motion sense, it stands to reason that if one part is damaged, the other portion may also be damaged. Many children with hearing impairments have poor vestibular function, resulting in balance deficits.[135] Some children with primarily vestibular deficits are unsafe without protective headgear.

The effects of deficits in tactile, vestibular, and proprioceptive systems on sensory integration are also well documented.[14] Deficits are linked to poor body scheme, self-image, difficulty in motor planning, or sequencing movement and balance. Sensory information is used to learn movement. The ability to process sensory information and thus integrate it with movement in a planned and organized manner is important for motor coordination.

The effects of visual deficits on the developmental course were documented by Jan and colleagues.[136] Visually impaired children must substitute auditory cues to direct movement; because so many movements are visually guided, their acquisition of motor milestones is delayed. Children with crossed eyes, or strabismus, may have difficulty in developing head control or midline reaching. The earlier that the visual alignment deficits are detected and corrected, the better off children are in terms of upper extremity control. The ability to prevent or detect visual deficits earlier may decrease the concomitant activity and participation limitations.

A decline in function of any one sensory system because of aging can have serious functional implications. For example, presbyopia makes it more difficult for the older adults to read dials on the stove or to do needle work. A decline in depth perception can contribute to an increased potential for falling while going up or down stairs. Presbycusis may isolate an elder from a lively conversation or decrease awareness of a warning siren while driving the automobile with the radio turned on. Food preparation and mealtime may be less enjoyable because of age-related changes in smell and taste abilities. Changes in somatosensation in the lower extremities and motion sense may contribute to an increased likelihood of falling or an increased fear of falling, which can lead to hypoactivity. Any or all of the potential sensory changes with aging can curtail an individual's range of movement by increasing dependence on compensatory devices or strategies.

Because vision is so important to development across the life span, two conditions that affect vision, amblyopia and macular degeneration, are discussed in detail. One occurs early in development and is potentially reversible, whereas the other occurs at the end of the life span. Both are examples of sensory changes that can have significant functional implications. An important life skill that can be impeded by either of these conditions is driving. It is our most relied-on means of mobility and is prized as a reward by the adolescent, deemed almost as a right of passage. Adults depend on driving to get to and from jobs, appointments, shopping, and leisure activities. Driving becomes a significant quality-of-life issue as individuals reach older age and strive to maintain independence.

Amblyopia

Amblyopia is derived from the Greek word for "blunt or dull sight." The loss of sight can occur in childhood. The brain depends on receiving simultaneous clear focused images from both eyes for the visual pathways to develop properly.[137] Because of difficulty in producing a single image when looking with both eyes, the person with amblyopia elects to see with only one eye to see one image. The lazy eye, if deprived of visual input for sufficient time, will lose sight, and the child will become functionally blind because of a lack of visual cortex development. This problem may be associated with an eye that is deviated in any direction–in, out, up, or down–a condition known as strabismus. However, strabismus is not necessarily a cause of amblyopia. In addition, the use of only one eye may not be apparent unless screening is conducted.

In 2002, the American Academy of Pediatrics (AAP) issued a statement regarding the use of photoscreening, a vision screening technique, as a method of identification of children with visual problems.[138] The AAP reaffirmed this position in August 2008. All children should be screened for risk factors associated with amblyopia. The prevalence of amblyopia is thought to be 1% to 4%.[139] However, almost 80% of children in preschool *never* get screened.[140] With only 21% of children being screened, there is a very real possibility that a lot of children with visual problems are not being identified. The difficult to screen population such as the very young and developmentally delayed are at even greater risk for not being screened for preventable visual loss or treatable visual conditions. The AAP[138] recommends use of a photoscreening method that would facilitate screening in all children. Salcido and colleagues[141] found photoscreening more efficient than traditional screening in a group of 3- and 4-year-old children. A U.S. preventive task force[142] recommended that photoscreening was able to identify amblyogenic factors, such as significant refractory error, strabismus, and media opacities but not amblyopia.

Amblyopia, or lazy eye, is a deficit of visual acuity initially not thought to be correctable with glasses. Traditionally, treatment of amblyopia consisted of occlusion or patching of the eye with corrective lenses being used as an adjunctive treatment. As the ability to detect and assess refractive errors in children with amblyopia improved, the effect of correction of these errors were studied.[143] Evidence now appears to demonstrate that refractive correction can benefit children with amblyopia and refractive errors if the correction is used earlier in treatment, not just as an adjunct to occlusion.[144] In those children with refractive errors and amblyopia, one-fourth to one-third of the children treated first with corrective lenses did not require occlusion therapy.[145] It is recommended, however, that those children who do not improve with corrective lenses should proceed to occlusion therapy.

Childhood amblyopia is also the leading cause of loss of vision in one eye in adults.[139] The potential for loss of vision occurs during critical periods in the postnatal development of the visual system. Maturation of the visual system is activity dependent; that is, the eye must be exposed to sensory stimulation to complete its development (Clinical Implications Box 10-1: Amblyopia: A Preventable Loss of Vision).

Macular Degeneration

The macula is the part of the eye where the most acute vision occurs because it contains the fovea, the central focusing point of the optic system. Age-related maculopathy is more likely to be seen after age 50.[146] With aging, vascular and nutritional changes can affect the function of the macula. Age-related macular degeneration (AMD) is the late stage of age-related maculopathy and has a prevalence of 15% in adults over the age of 85.[147] Macular degeneration is the most common cause of irreversible loss of eyesight late in life.[148]

Clinically, the early stage of AMD is marked by the presence of *drusen,* which are extracellular deposits and

CLINICAL IMPLICATIONS Box 10-1
Amblyopia: A Preventable Loss of Vision

Deprivation of visual input during a critical period can lead to a permanent visual deficit. There are three critical periods for visual acuity: during development from early gestation through 3 to 5 years of age; during a period of deprivation, possible from the first few months to 7 to 8 years of age[168]; and during the recovery period from the time of deprivation into adulthood.[169] Many motor and sensory conditions can lead to amblyopia, including strabismus, myopia, astigmatism, cataract, and refractive differences between the two eyes.

Prevention Focuses

- Screening for risk factors associated with amblyopia should be performed as early as possible and on a regular basis during childhood.[138]
- Screening of all children 3 to 4 years of age for amblyopia and strabismus[138,142]; despite a prevalence of 1% to 4%,[139] most children are not screened.[140]
- Use of photoscreening is supported by the American Academy of Pediatrics[138] with further research into its cost effectiveness and efficacy.
- Regardless of the type of testing, evaluators need to be competent in the application and interpretation of the tests.[138]

pigment abnormalities in the retinal pigment epithelium. There are two types of AMD: a "wet" type and a "dry" type. The exudative or wet type is less common than the dry type.[148] The dry type is also referred to as *geographic atrophy.* It is responsible for a large number of cases of moderate visual loss in older adults. There is no treatment for this type. The wet type of AMD is caused by the leakage of newly formed blood vessels that have grown into the eye. Severe vision loss can occur because of these new blood vessels, pigment epithelial detachment, and disciform scarring. However, if the wet type is detected early, it can be treated by laser therapy or with medications.[148] There are 200,000 new cases of this exudative type of AMD diagnosed annually in the United States.[148] AMD pathogenesis has been linked to oxidative damage of the retinal pigment epithelium. There is evidence that the intraocular inflammation seen in AMD may be caused by an immune response.[149] The link between oxidation-induced events and the onset and progression of AMD may also be supported by the fact that dietary supplement and antioxidants have been used to reduce the risk of severe visual loss.[150,151]

Macular degeneration begins differently in every person. Some common symptoms include a gradual loss of the ability to see objects clearly, distorted vision, a gradual loss of clear color vision, and a dark or empty area in the center of vision. These symptoms are not unique to AMD but do indicate the need to seek professional assessment. The Amsler grid is an early detection chart that may be used independently, alerting the clinician to changes in vision that should be assessed by an optometrist (Figure 10-6). While the Amsler grid has been the

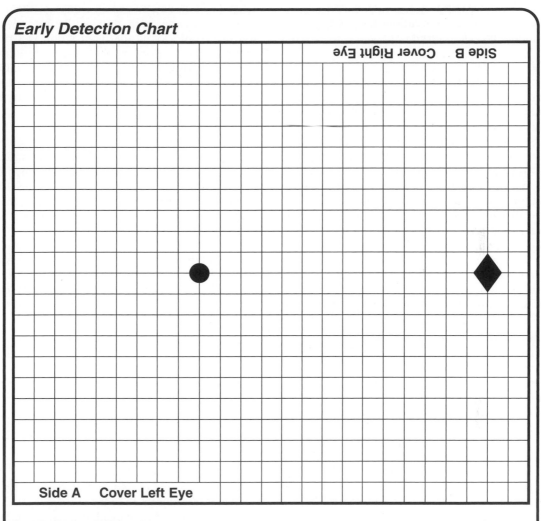

Early Detection Chart

Side B   Cover Right Eye

Side A   **Cover Left Eye**

Directions for using the chart:
1. Wear your reading glasses or bifocals and have good lighting on card. Hold card facing you so you can read side A. Cover your left eye.
2. Hold card at arm's length and stare only at small dot while bringing chart toward your eye.
3. Pull the card toward you until the large "♦" disappears from view. The lines should look straight and black.
4. If lines appear wavy, grey or fuzzy, draw on top of them and show chart to your optometrist.

5. Turn card upside down to read side B. Close your right eye and follow steps 2, 3 and 4.

Be sure to call your optometrist immediately if you notice a change, or if you don't understand how to use the chart. This screening test does not replace a thorough eye examination by your optometrist.

 American Optometric Association
243 North Lindbergh Blvd., St. Louis, MO 63141

Figure 10-6 Amsler grid: early detection chart. (From the American Optometric Association.)

most frequently recommended method for monitoring vision in those at risk, new technology that involves a computer-based program to detect distortions has been found to be more sensitive.[152] There is no way to restore central vision once it is lost, but peripheral vision is not damaged and low vision aids can be helpful. It is important to be aware of risk factors and potential prevention strategies (Clinical Implications Box 10-2: Macular Degeneration: Who Is at Risk?).

Driving

Retention of the ability to drive in older adulthood is a significant quality-of-life issue. In one study, a group of older adults who chose to stop driving reported experiencing loneliness and isolation as consequences.[153] Depression is a common finding in older men who cease driving.[154] Healthy older adult drivers drive more slowly, which could reflect their insight into their own limitations.[155] Although some report driving skills are preserved in healthy older persons,[156] others have documented that older healthy drivers make fewer steering corrections and eye-movement excursions than do younger drivers.[157] Three categories of age-related changes can affect driving: sensory, cognitive, and motor function. These are found in Table 10-4.

Driving is a very visual task. Decline in visual acuity, contrast sensitivity, visual attention, and useful field of view are frequently mentioned as reasons for impaired performance of motor vehicle operational skills.[124,157,158] A decline in function of any part of the visual system, whether peripheral (as in the eye with changes in lens accommodation) or central (as with processing of sensory information), results in the modification of motor behavior. A decline of visual acuity to 20/50 or less means restriction from driving. Ragland, Satariano, and MacLeod[159] found that poor vision was the most common reason given by older adults for limiting or stopping driving. The implications of visual difficulties for the ability of the individual to drive (especially at night), to be mobile on uneven terrain, or to be in unfamiliar environments are vast.

Useful field of view (UVOF) is defined as "the area of the visual field that is functional for an observer at a given time and for a given task.[65]" The useful field of view becomes smaller in older adults when distractions are present, making visual search less efficient. Cross and colleagues[160] report that a greater than 35% reduction in UVOF is significantly associated with an increased rate of motor vehicle collisions (MVCs) in a three-state cohort of older drivers. This same study found that there was no association between visual acuity and contrast sensitivity in older adults and MVC involvement. Furthermore, the presence of cataracts or glaucoma was not associated with an increased rate

---

CLINICAL IMPLICATIONS Box 10-2

Macular Degeneration: Who is at Risk?

Age-related macular degeneration (AMD) is the leading cause of legal blindness among older adults in the United States and Europe.[148] Unfortunately, few of the many potential risk factors are modifiable. Increased public awareness of AMD as a common cause of irreversible loss of eyesight in older adults may promote further research into the prevention of blindness.

Risk Factors
- *Age:* Women 75 years old or older are twice as likely to develop early AMD and have a seven times greater incidence of later AMD.[170]
- *Race:* Blacks have a lower prevalence rate than whites.[171]
- *Heredity:* A positive family history (parent or sibling with AMD) is a strong predictor; Myers[172] found 100% concordance among identical twins with AMD.
- *Environment:* Cigarette smoking increases the risk[173]; Hammond and colleagues[174] found an inverse

relationship between cigarette smoking and macular pigment density; light exposure data are inconclusive, but it has been difficult to study lifetime effects of light exposure.

Potential Prevention Strategies
- Wear sunglasses, coated to "filter out" ultraviolet light, at all times when in the sun.
- Increase intake of carotenoids (sources of vitamin A), which have been found to have a protective effect against AMD.[175] The consumption of foods rich in carotenoids, such as corn and spinach, promoted the elevation of macular pigment density.[176]
- Have regular vision assessments.
- Use an Amsler grid as a means to detect early AMD in those at risk and to recognize progression if already diagnosed (see Figure 10-6).
- Use a computer-based program to detect visual distortions.[152]
- Take a good multivitamin.

Table 10-4

Age-Related Physiological Changes That May Affect Driving

Type of Change	Examples
Sensory changes	Presbycusis (hearing loss)
	Visual decrements in static visual acuity
	Acuity under low illumination
	Resistance to glare
	Contrast sensitivity (static and dynamic)
	Visual fields
	Depth perception
Cognitive changes	Distraction by irrelevant stimuli
	Memory retrieval impairment
	Decline in spatial orientation
	Decreased visual searching
	Decreased visuomotor integration
Psychomotor changes	Slowed speed of behavior
	Decreased reaction time
	Declines* in:
	Strength
	Range of motion
	Trunk and neck mobility
	Proprioception

*The contribution of age-related changes versus deconditioning and diseases remains unclear. From Reuben DR: Driving. In Duthie EH Jr, Katz PR: *Practice of geriatrics*, ed 3, Philadelphia, 1998, WB Saunders, p 58.

of MVCs. Cross and associates[160] recommend that an evidence-based battery of vision tests needs to be developed to screen for high-risk drivers.

Cognitive impairments, especially those related to Alzheimer disease, are associated with an increased risk in driving.[124] Individuals with Alzheimer disease can be easily distracted, not remember where they are going, and may even have a greater decrease in visual-spatial processing and orientation. Drivers with Alzheimer disease tend to drive faster than do older adults without Alzheimer disease.[155] In a study of more than 14,000 adults aged 70 or older, Anstey and colleagues[161] reported that cognitive function and perceived self-health were stronger predictors of whether an older adult would cease driving than sensory function and medical conditions. Older adults with poor memory, slow processing speed, or poor self-rated health had a higher probability of driving cessation within a subsequent 5-year period. In a survey of older adults with dementia, 54% of participants ceased driving because of increasing cognitive deficits.[162] Family encouragement and physician input were also factors in the decision-making process.

Perceptual-motor performance declines as evidenced by a decrease in reaction time. This may be related to difficulty sustaining attention or managing divided attention for the many visually related driving tasks. The impact of the loss of mobility, both real and perceived, can substantially affect an individual's self-image.

Safety is always a concern for older adults. As individuals live longer, there will be greater numbers of geriatric drivers. Remaining independent requires the ability to get to and from the physician's office, grocery store, and friends' and relatives' homes. Maintaining independence by being able to come and go whenever the need arises is important to the average elder. Older drivers are less likely to drive under compromising visual conditions, such as at night or in inclement weather. Are older drivers safe? Older drivers have a crash rate per vehicle mile of travel similar to young drivers.[160] They are more likely to be fatally injured when involved in a vehicular crash.[163] Difficulty with seeing instrument panels, dealing with glare and haze, and judging vehicle speed have also been reported by older drivers.[164] Because so many problems are related to visually related driving tasks, some states have initiated the use of state-mandated tests of visual acuity in 70-year-old drivers. The testing has been associated with lower fatal crash rates.[165] However, as previously discussed, testing visual acuity without testing UVOF may not be sufficient to identify at risk drivers. The UVOF test assesses visual attention and processing speed.[160]

Fatality rates over the last decade are showing a downward trend from previous reports.[166] Some of this decline may be related to gender differences in the self-regulation and cessation of driving. Gender differences are seen in the crash risk, rate and types of crashes, driving patterns, self-regulation, and cessation of driving. As might be expected, both older men and women are likely to have more serious injuries secondary to comorbidities and frailty. Although older women have been found to be safer drivers than older men, older women cease driving at an earlier age than older men.[167] Women may stop driving for different reasons than men, such as lack of confidence, fear of crime, or cost to operate a motor vehicle. Because women are safer drivers, it would make sense to keep them driving as a way to ensure they will have mobility as they age and require less caregiving. Rehabilitation therapists can play a vital role in enhancing the mobility of older drivers.

SUMMARY

Sensory input plays an important role in the learning and refinement of movement. The integration of multiple sensory input and the association-coordination of sensory and motor information form the basis for cognition and perception. Sensory input from the external environment initiates the activity that shapes synaptic connections. The autonomic nervous system and the reticular system act as gatekeepers, determining which sensory information reaches consciousness and which is dampened. The thalamus is a central relay station that directs the flow of sensory information to association cortices. All sensory systems have similar characteristics: transduction and coding, representation, and integration at all levels of the nervous system. Sensory systems develop early in utero to be ready to function at birth. Some, such as vision and hearing, must have additional input to completely develop the neural pathway. Sensory abilities change with age; deficits in any sensory system, whether from congenital absence, trauma, or decline with age, can result in functional impairment of movement. Presbystasis, presbyopia, and presbycusis are all seen in older adults but not to the same degree in all individuals. Age-related changes in the sensory systems, therefore, are neither uniform nor universal.

REFERENCES

1. Gibson JJ: *The senses as perceptual systems*, Boston, 1966, Houghton-Mifflin.
2. Piaget J: *Origins of intelligence*, New York, 1952, International University Press.
3. Lord SR, Ward JA, Williams P, et al: Physiological factors associated with falls in older community-dwelling women, *J Am Geriatr Soc* 42:1110–1117, 1994.
4. Hirabayashi S, Iwasaki Y: Developmental perspective of sensory organization on postural control, *Brain Dev* 17(2):111–113, 1995.
5. Nougier V, Bard C, Fleury M, et al: Contribution of central and peripheral vision to the regulation of stance: developmental aspects, *J Exp Child Psychol* 68:202–215, 1998.
6. Shumway-Cook A, Woollacott MH: *Motor control: theory and practical applications*, ed 2, Baltimore, 2007, Williams & Wilkins.
7. Ferber-Viart C, Ionescu E, Morlet T, et al: Balance in healthy individuals assessed with Equitest: maturation and normative data for children and young adults, *Int J Pediatr Otorhinolaryngol* 71:1041–1046, 2007.
8. Guyton AC, Hall JE: *Textbook of medical physiology*, ed 11, Philadelphia, 2006, WB Saunders.
9. Shaffer SW, Harrrison AL: Aging of the somatosensory system: a translational perspective, *Phys Ther* 87:193–207, 2007.
10. Boyd IA: The isolated mammalian muscle spindle. In Evarts EV, Wise SP, Bousfield D, editors: *The motor system in neurobiology*, New York, 1985, Elsevier, pp 154–167.
11. Cuomo F, Birdzell MG, Zukerman JD: The effect of degenerative arthritis and prosthetic arthroplasty on shoulder proprioception, *J Shoulder Elbow Surg* 14:345–348, 2005.
12. Khabie V, Schwartz MC, Rokito AS, et al: The effect of intra-articular anesthesia and elastic bandage on elbow proprioception, *J Shoulder Elbow Surg* 7:501–504, 1998.
13. Nallegowda M, Singh U, Bhan S, et al: Balance and gait in total hip replacement: a pilot study, *Am J Phys Med Rehabil* 82:669–677, 2003.
14. Fisher AG, Murray EA, Bundy AC, editors: *Sensory integration: theory and practice*, Philadelphia, 1991, FA Davis.
15. Ayres AJ: *Sensory integration and learning disorders*, Los Angeles, 1972, Western Psychological Services.
16. Ayres AJ: *Sensory integration and praxis tests*, Los Angeles, 1989, Western Psychological Services.
17. Hooker D: *The prenatal origin of behavior*, Lawrence, Kan, 1952, University of Kansas Press.
18. Lowrey GH: *Growth and development of children*, ed 8, Chicago, 1986, Year Book.
19. Windle WF: *Physiology of the fetus*, Philadelphia, 1940, WB Saunders.
20. Wyke B: The neurological basis of movement: a developmental review. In Holt KS, editor: *Movement and child development*, Philadelphia, 1975, JB Lippincott, pp 19–33.
21. Anand KJ, Hickey PR: Pain and its effect in the human neonate and fetus, *N Engl J Med* 31:1321–1329, 1987.
22. Gilles FH, Leviton A, Dooling EC: *The developing human: growth and epidemiologic neuropathology*, Boston, 1983, John Wright.
23. Humphrey T: The embryologic differentiation of the vestibular nuclei in man correlated with functional development. In *International Symposium on Vestibular and Oculomotor Problems*, Tokyo, 1965, p 51.
24. Milani-Comparetti A: The neurophysiological and clinical implications of studies on fetal motor behavior, *Semin Perinatol* 5:183–189, 1981.
25. Ornitz EM, Atwell CW, Walter DO, et al: The maturation of vestibular nystagmus in infancy and childhood, *Acta Otolaryngol* 88:244–256, 1979.
26. Meisami E, Timiras PS: *Handbook of human growth and developmental biology, vol I, part B*, Boca Raton, Fla, 1988, CRC Press.
27. Almli CR, Mohr NM: Normal sequential behavioral and physiological change throughout the developmental arc. In Umphred DA, editor: *Neurological rehabilitation*, ed 3, St Louis, 1995, Mosby, pp 33–65.
28. Birnholz JC, Benacerraf BR: The development of human fetal hearing, *Science* 222:516–518, 1983.
29. Beauchamp GK, Cowart BJ, Schmidt HJ: Development of chemosensory sensitivity and preference. In Getchell TV, Doty RL, Bartoshuk LM, editors: *Smell and taste in health and disease*, New York, 1991, Raven Press, pp 405–416.

30. Steiner JE: Human facial expression in response to taste and smell stimulation, *Adv Child Dev* 13:257–295, 1979.
31. Prechtl HFR: Behavioral states of the newborn infant (a review), *Brain Res* 76:185–212, 1974.
32. Smith SL, Gossman M, Canan BC: Selected primitive reflexes in children with cerebral palsy: consistency of response, *Phys Ther* 62:1115–1120, 1982.
33. Sahoo SK: Novelty and complexity in human infants' exploratory behavior, *Percept Mot Skills* 86:698, 1998.
34. Rochat P, Hespos SJ: Differential rooting response by neonates: evidence for an early sense of self, *Early Dev Parent* 6:105–112, 1997.
35. Rochat P: Self-perception and action in infancy, *Exp Brain Res* 123:102–109, 1998.
36. Rochat P, Morgan R: Spatial determinants in the perception of self-produced leg movements by 3–5 month-old infants, *Dev Psychol* 31:626–636, 1995.
37. Rochat P: Five levels of self-awareness as they unfold early in life, *Conscious Cogn* 12:717–731, 2003.
38. Kaye H, Lipsitt L: Relationship of electro to actual threshold to basal skin conductance, *Child Dev* 35:1307–1312, 1964.
39. Meltzoff AN, Borton R: Intermodal matching by human neonates, *Nature* 282:403–404, 1979.
40. Prechtl HFR: The directed head turning response and allied movements of the human baby, *Behavior* 13:212–242, 1958.
41. Gottfried AW, Rose SA: Tactile recognition in infants, *Child Dev* 51:69–74, 1980.
42. Rose SA: From hand to eye: findings and issues in infant cross-modal transfer. In Lewkowicz DJ, Lickliter R, editors: *The development of intersensory perception*, Hillsdale, NJ, 1994, Erlbaum, pp 265–284.
43. Salapatek P, Cohen L: *Handbook of infant perception: from sensation to perception*, New York, 1987, Academic Press.
44. Puchalski M, Hummel P: The reality of neonatal pain, *Adv Neonatal Care* 2(5):233–247, 2002.
45. Fitzgerald M, Walker SM: Infant pain management: a developmental neurobiological approach, *Nat Clin Pract Neurol* 5(1):35–50, 2009.
46. Simons SHP, Tibboel D: Pain perception development and maturation, *Semin Fetal Neonatal Med* 11:227–231, 2006.
47. Gunnar M, Fisch R, Korsvik S, et al: The effects of circumcision on serum cortisol and behavior, *Psychoneuroendocrinology* 6:269–275, 1981.
48. Craig KD, Whitfield MF, Grunau RVE, et al: Pain in the preterm neonate: behavioral and physiological indices, *Pain* 52:238–299, 1993.
49. Meltzoff AN, Moore MK: Imitation of facial and manual gestures by human neonates, *Science* 198:75–78, 1977.
50. Morgan R, Rochat P: Intermodal calibration of the body in early infancy, *Ecol Psychol* 9:1–24, 1997.
51. Sugden DA: The development of proprioceptive control. In Whiting HTA, Wade MG, editors: *Themes in motor development*, Boston, 1986, Nijhoff, pp 21–39.
52. Lasky RE: The effect of visual feedback of the hand on the reaching and retrieval behaviour of young infants, *Child Dev* 48:112–117, 1977.
53. Von Hofsten C: Development of visually directed reaching: the approach phase, *J Hum Mov Stud* 5:160–178, 1979.
54. Butterworth GE, Ciccheti D: Visual calibration of posture in normal and motor retarded Down's syndrome infants, *Perception* 7:513–525, 1978.
55. Butterworth GE, Hicks L: Visual proprioception and postural stability in infants: a developmental study, *Perception* 6:255–262, 1977.
56. Lee DN, Aaronson E: Visual proprioceptive control of standing in infants, *Percept Psychophys* 15:529–532, 1974.
57. Sundermier L, Woollacott MH: The influence of vision on the automatic postural muscle responses of newly standing and newly walking infants, *Exp Brain Res* 120:537–540, 1998.
58. Eviatar L, Eviatar A, Naaray I: Maturation of neurovestibular responses in infants, *Dev Med Child Neurol* 16:435–446, 1974.
59. Ornitz EM: Normal and pathological maturation of vestibular function in the human child. In Romand R, editor: *Development of auditory and vestibular systems*, New York, 1983, Academic Press, pp 479–536.
60. Eliot L: *What's going on in there? How the brain and mind work the first five years of life*, New York, 1999, Bantam.
61. Marmur R, Sabo E, Carmeli E, et al: Optokinetic nystagmus as related to neonatal position, *J Child Neurol* 22(9):1108–1110, 2007.
62. Weissman BM, DiScenna AO, Leigh RJ: Maturation of the vestibulo-ocular reflex in normal infants during the first 2 months of life, *Neurology* 39:534–538, 1989.
63. Eviatar L, Eviatar A: The normal nystagmic response of infants to caloric and perrotatory stimulation, *Laryngoscope* 89:1036–1044, 1979.
64. Fife TD, Tusa RJ, Furman JM, et al: Assessment: vestibular testing techniques in adults and children: report of the therapeutics and technology assessment subcommittee of the American Academy of Neurology, *Neurology* 55(10):1431–1441, 2000.
65. Coren S, Ward LM, Enns JT: *Sensation and perception*, ed 5, Fort Worth, Tex, 1999, Harcourt.
66. Aslin RN: Development of smooth pursuit in human infants. In Fisher DF, Monty RA, Senders JW, editors: *Eye movements: cognition and visual perception*, Hillsdale, NJ, 1981, Erlbaum, pp 31–51.
67. Nandi R, Luxon LM: Development and assessment of the vestibular system, *Int J Audiol* 47:566–577, 2008.
68. Bertenthal BI, Rose JL, Bai DL: Perception-action coupling in the development of visual control of posture, *J Exp Psych* 23:1631–1643, 1997.
69. Kandel ER, Schwartz JH, Jessell TM: *Principles of neural science*, ed 4, New York, 2000, McGraw-Hill.
70. Shimojo SJ, Bauer J, O'Connell KM, et al: Pre-stereoptic binocular vision in infants, *Vision Res* 26:501–510, 1986.
71. Werner LA, Marean GC: *Human auditory development*, Boulder, Colo, 1996, Westview Press.
72. Locke J: A theory of neurolinguistic development, *Brain Lang* 58:265–326, 1997.
73. Allison T, Hume AL, Wood CC, et al: Developmental and aging changes in somatosensory, auditory and visual evoked potentials, *Electroencephalogr Clin Neurophysiol* 58:14–24, 1984.

74. Cohen H, Friedman EM, Lai D, et al: Balance in children with otitis media with effusion, *Int J Pediatr Otorhinolaryngol* 42:107–115, 1997.

75. MacFarlane A: Olfaction in the development of social preferences in the human neonate, *Ciba Found Symp* 33:103–113, 1975.

76. Hermann RP, Novak CB, Mackinnon SE: Establishing normal values of moving two-point discrimination in children and adolescents, *Dev Med Child Neurol* 38:255–261, 1996.

77. Bigelow A: The correspondence between self and image movement as a cue to self-recognition for young children, *J Genet Psychol* 139:11–26, 1981.

78. Thelen E: Motor development: a new synthesis, *Am Psychol* 50:79–95, 1995.

79. Elliot JM, Connolly KJ, Doyle AJR: Development of kinaesthetic sensitivity and motor performance in children, *Dev Med Child Neurol* 30:80–92, 1988.

80. Livesey DJ, Parks NA: Testing kinaesthetic acuity in preschool children, *Aust J Psychol* 47(3):160–163, 1995.

81. Livesey DJ, Intili D: A gender difference in visual-spatial ability in 4-year-old children: effects on performance of a kinesthetic acuity task, *J Exp Child Psychol* 63:436–446, 1996.

82. Gabbard CP: *Lifelong motor development*, ed 3, Dubuque, Iowa, 2000, Brown and Benchmark.

83. Williams HG: *Perceptual and motor development*, Englewood Cliffs, NJ, 1983, Prentice Hall.

84. Haywood KM: Eye movements during coincidence-anticipation performance, *J Mot Behav* 9:313–318, 1977.

85. Collins JK: Distance perception as a function of age, *Aust J Psychol* 28:109–113, 1976.

86. Long AB, Looft WR: Development of directionality in children: ages six through twelve, *Dev Psychol* 6:375–380, 1972.

87. Nickerson RS: Intersensory facilitation of reaction time, *Psychol Rev* 80:489–509, 1973.

88. Kenshalo DR: Age changes in touch, vibration, temperature, kinesthesis, and pain sensitivity. In Birren JE, Schaie KW, editors: *Handbook of psychology of aging*, New York, 1977, Van Nostrand Reinhold, pp 562–579.

89. Duthie EH, Katz PR, Malone ML: *Practice of geriatrics*, ed 4, Philadelphia, 2007, WB Saunders.

90. Cauna N, Mannan G: The structure of human digital pacinian corpuscles (corpus cula lamellosa) and its functional significance, *J Anat* 92:1–20, 1958.

91. Iwasaki T, Goto N, Goto J, et al: The aging of human Meissner's corpuscles as evidenced by parallel sectioning, *Okajimas Folia Anat Jpn* 79:185–189, 2003.

92. Verillo RT: Change in vibrotactile thresholds as a function of age, *Sens Processes* 3:49–59, 1979.

93. Meisami E: Aging of the sensory systems. In Timiras PS, editor: *Physiological basis of aging and geriatrics*, ed 2, Boca Raton, Fla, 1994, CRC Press, pp 115–132.

94. Weisenberger JM: Touch and proprioception. In Birren JE, editor: *Encyclopedia of gerontology*, ed 2, San Diego, 1996, Academic Press, pp 591–603.

95. Bruce MF: The relation of tactile threshold to histology in the fingers of elderly people, *J Neurol Neurosurg Psychiatry* 43:730–734, 1980.

96. Stevens JC, Alvarez-Reeves M, Dipietro L, et al: Decline of tactile acuity in ageing: a study of body site, blood flow, and lifetime habits of smoking and physical activity, *Somatosens Mot Res* 20:271–279, 2003.

97. Stevens JC, Choo KK: Spatial acuity of the body surface over the life span, *Somatosens Mot Res* 13:153–166, 1996.

98. Wickremaratchi MM, Llewelyn JG: Effects of ageing on touch, *Postgrad Med J* 82:301–304, 2006.

99. Steiness I: Vibratory perception in normal subjects, *Acta Med Scand* 158:315–325, 1957.

100. Merchut MT, Toleikis SC: Aging and quantitative sensory thresholds, *Electromyogr Clin Neurophysiol* 30:293–297, 1990.

101. Perry SD: Evaluation of age-related plantar-surface insensitivity and onset age of advanced insensitivity in older adults using vibratory and touch sensation test, *Neurosci Lett* 392:62–127, 2006.

102. Skinner HB, Barrack RL, Cook SD: Age-related decline in proprioception, *Clin Orthop Relat Res* 184:208–211, 1984.

103. Kokmen E, Bossemeyer RW Jr, Williams WJ: Quantitative evaluation of joint motion sensation in an aging population, *J Gerontol* 33:62–67, 1978.

104. Verschueren SM, Brumagne S, Swinnen SP, et al: The effect of aging on dynamic position sense at the ankle, *Behav Brain Res* 136:593–603, 2002.

105. Bullock-Saxton JE, Wong WJ, Hogan N: The influence of age on weight-bearing joint reposition sense of the knee, *Exp Brain Res* 136:400–406, 2001.

106. Kaplan FS, Nixon JE, Reitz M, et al: Age-related changes in proprioception and sensation of joint position, *Acta Orthop Scand* 56:72–74, 1985.

107. Barrett DS, Cobb AG, Bently G: Joint proprioception in normal, osteoarthritic and replaced knees, *J Bone Joint Surg* 73B:53–56, 1991.

108. Pickard CM, Sullivan PE, Allison GT, et al: Is there a difference in hip joint position sense between young and older groups? *J Gerontol A Biol Sci Med Sci* 58:631–635, 2003.

109. Timiras PS: *Physiological basis of aging and geriatrics*, Boca Raton, Fla, 1994, CRC Press.

110. Gibson SJ, Farrell M: A review of age differences in the neurophysiology of nociception and the perceptual experience of pain, *Clin J Pain* 20(4):227–239, 2004.

111. Tucker MA: Age associated changes in pain threshold measured by transcutaneous neuronal electrical stimulation, *Age Ageing* 18:241–246, 1989.

112. Ochs A, Newberry J, Lenhardt M, et al: Neural and vestibular aging associated with falls. In Birren JE, Schaie KW, editors: *Handbook of the psychology of aging*, ed 2, New York, 1985, Van Nostrand Reinhold, pp 378–399.

113. Lopez I, Honrubia V, Baloh RW: Aging and the vestibular nucleus, *J Vestib Res* 7:77–85, 1997.

114. Bergstrom B: Morphology of the vestibular nerve: III. Analysis of the myelinated vestibular nerve fibers in man at various ages, *Acta Otolaryngol* 76:331–338, 1973.

115. Paige GD: Senescence of human visual-vestibular interactions. I. Vestibular-ocular reflex and adaptive plasticity with aging, *J Vestib Res* 2:133–151, 1992.

116. Matheson AJ, Darlington CL, Smith PF: Dizziness in the elderly and age-related degeneration of the vestibular system, *N Z J Psychol* 28(1):10–16, 1999.

117. Kennedy R, Clemis JD: The geriatric auditory and vestibular system, *Otolaryngol Clin North Am* 23:1075–1082, 1990.

118. Wolfson L, Whipple R, Derby CA, et al: A dynamic posturography study of balance in healthy elderly, *Neurology* 42:2069–2075, 1992.

119. Sturnieks DL, St George R, Lord SR: Balance disorders in the elderly, *Neurophysiol Clin* 38(6):467–478, 2008.

120. Duncan G, Wilson JA, MacLennen WJ, et al: Clinical correlates of sway in elderly people living at home, *Gerontology* 38:160–166, 1992.

121. Ring C, Nayak USL, Isaacs B: The effect of visual deprivation and proprioceptive change on postural sway in healthy adults, *J Am Geriatr Soc* 37:745–749, 1989.

122. Pitts DG: Visual function as a function of age, *J Am Optom Assoc* 53:117–124, 1982.

123. Weale RA: Senile changes in visual acuity, *Trans Ophthalmol Soc UK* 95:36–38, 1975.

124. Duthie EH, Katz PR: *Practice of geriatrics*, ed 3, Philadelphia, 1998, WB Saunders.

125. Cleary BL: Age-related changes in the special senses. In Matteson MA, McConnell ES, Linton AD, editors: *Gerontological nursing*, ed 2, Philadelphia, 1997, WB Saunders, pp 385–405.

126. Williams HG: Aging and eye-hand coordination. In Bard C, Fleury M, Hay L, editors: *Development of eye-hand coordination*, Columbia, SC, 1990, University of South Carolina Press, pp 327–357.

127. Gates GA, Mills JH: Presbycusis, *Lancet* 366:1111–1120, 2005.

128. Schiffman SS, Graham BG: Taste and smell perception affect appetite and immunity in the elderly, *Eur J Clin Nutr* 54(Suppl 3):S54–S63, 2000.

129. Miller IJ: Human taste bud density across adult age groups, *J Gerontol A Biol Sci Med Sci* 43:26–30, 1988.

130. Mistretta CM: Aging effects on anatomy and neurophysiology of taste and smell, *Gerodontology* 3:131–136, 1984.

131. Weiffenbach JM, Bartoshuk LM: Taste and smell, *Clin Geriatr Med* 8:543–555, 1992.

132. Schiffman SS: Effects of aging on the human taste system, *Ann N Y Acad Sci* 1170: 725–729, 2009.

133. Ship J: The influence of aging on oral health and consequences for taste and smell, *Physiol Behav* 66:209–215, 1999.

134. Horak FB, Shumway-Cook A, Crowe TK, et al: Vestibular function and motor proficiency of children with impaired hearing or with learning disability and motor impairments, *Dev Med Child Neurol* 30:64–79, 1988.

135. Rine RM, Cornwall G, Gan K, et al: Evidence of progressive delay of motor development in children with sensorineural hearing loss and concurrent vestibular dysfunction, *Percept Mot Skills* 90:1101–1112, 2000.

136. Jan JE, Sykanda A, Groenveld M: Habilitation and rehabilitation of visually impaired and blind children, *Pediatrician* 17:202–207, 1990.

137. American Academy of Pediatrics: Committee on Practice and Ambulatory Medicine: Eye examination and vision screening in infants, children, and young adults, *Pediatrics* 98:153–157, 1996.

138. American Academy of Pediatrics: Committee on Practice and Ambulatory Medicine: Use of photoscreening for children's vision screening, *Pediatrics* 109:524–525, 2002.

139. Simmons K: Preschool vision screening: rationale, methodology and outcome, *Surg Ophthalmol* 41:3–30, 1996.

140. Castanes MS: Major review: the underutilization of vision screening (for amblyopia, optical anomalies and strabismus) among preschool age children, *Binocul Vis Strabismus Q* 18(4):217–232, 2003.

141. Salcido AA, Bradley J, Donahue SP: Predictive value of photoscreening and traditional screening of preschool children, *J AAPOS* 9(2):114–120, 2005.

142. US Preventive Services Task Force: *Guide to clinical preventive services*, ed 2, Alexandria, Va, 1996, International Medical Publishing.

143. Moseley MJ, Neufield M, McCarry B, et al: Remediation of refractive amblyopia by optical correction alone, *Ophthalmic Physiol Opt* 22:296–299, 2002.

144. Moseley MJ, Fielder AR, Stewart CE: The optical treatment of amblyopia, *Optom Vis Sci* 86(6):1–5, 2009.

145. Stewart CE, Moseley MJ, Fielder AR, et al: Refractive adaptation in amblyopia: quantification of effect and implications for practice, *Br J Ophthalmol* 88:1552–1556, 2004.

146. Kliffen M, van der Schaft TL, Mooy CM, et al: Morphologic changes in age-related maculopathy, *Microsc Res Tech* 36:106–112, 1997.

147. Patten C, Craik RL: Sensorimotor changes and adaptation in the older adult. In Guccione AA, editor: *Geriatric physical therapy*, ed 2, Philadelphia, 2000, WB Saunders, pp 78–109.

148. Kaufman SR: Developments in age-related macular degeneration: diagnosis and treatment, *Geriatrics* 64(3):16–19, 2009.

149. Nussenblatt RB, Liu B, Li Z: Age-related macular degeneration: an immunologically driven disease, *Curr Opin Invest Drugs* 10(5):434–442, 2009.

150. Chong EW, Kreis AJ, Wong TY, et al: Dietary omega 3 fatty acid and fish intake in the primary prevention of age-related macular degeneration: a systematic review and meta-analysis, *Arch Ophthalmol* 126(6):826–833, 2008.

151. Age-Related Eye Disease Study Research Group: A randomized, placebo-controlled, clinical trial of high-dose supplementation with vitamins C and E, beta carotene, and zinc for age-related macular degeneration and vision loss: AREDS report no. 8, *Arch Ophthalmol* 119(10):1417–1436, 2001.

152. Trevino R, Kynn MG: Macular function surveillance revisited, *Optometry* 79(7):397–403, 2008.

153. Johnson JE: Urban older adults and the forfeiture of a driver's license, *J Gerontol Nurs* 25:12–18, 1998.

154. Ragland DR, Satariano WA, MacLeod KE: Driving cessation and increased depressive symptoms, *J Gerontol A Biol Sci Med Sci* 60(3):399–403, 2005.

155. Fitten LF, Perryman KM, Wilkinson CJ, et al: Alzheimer and vascular dementia and driving: a prospective road and laboratory study, *JAMA* 273:1360–1365, 1995.

156. Carr D, Jackson WJ, Madden DJ, et al: The effect of age on driving skills, *J Am Geriatr Soc* 40:567–573, 1992.

157. Perryman KM, Fitten LJ: Effects of normal aging on the performance of motor-vehicle operational skills, *J Geriatr Psychiatry Neurol* 9:136–141, 1996.

158. Owsley C, McGwin G Jr: Vision impairment and driving, *Surv Ophthalmol* 43:535–550, 1999.

159. Ragland DR, Satariano WA, MacLeod KE: Reasons given by older people for limitation or avoidance of driving, *Gerontologist* 44:237–244, 2004.

160. Cross JM, McGwin G, Rubin GS, et al: Visual and medical risk factors for motor vehicle collision involvement among older drivers, *Br J Ophthalmol* 93:400–404, 2009.

161. Anstey KJ, Windsor TD, Luszcz MA, et al: Predicting driving cessation over 5 years in older adults: psychological well-being and cognitive competence are stronger predictors than physical health, *J Am Geriatr Soc* 54:121–126, 2006.

162. Croston J, Meuser TM, Berg-Weger M, et al: Driving retirement in older adults with dementia, *Top Geriatr Rehabil* 25(2):154–162, 2009.

163. Insurance Institute for Highway Safety: Status report: special issue, *Older Drivers* 36:1–7, 2001.

164. Scialfa CT, Thomas DM: Age differences in same-different judgments as a function of multidimensional similarity, *J Gerontol* 49:P173–P178, 1994.

165. Levy DT, Vernick JS, Howard KA: Relationship between driver's license renewal policies and fatal crashes involving drivers 70 years or older, *JAMA* 274:1026–1030, 1995.

166. Eberhard JW, Mitchell CGB: Recent changes in driver licensing rates, fatality rates, and mobility options for older men and women in the United States and Great Britain, *Top Geriatr Rehabil* 25(2):88–98, 2009.

167. Morgan CM, Winter SM, Classen S, et al: Literature review on older adult gender differences for driving self-regulation and cessation, *Top Geriatr Rehabil* 25(2):99–117, 2009.

168. Lewis TL, Mauer D: Effects of early pattern deprivation on visual development, *Optom Vis Sci* 86:1–7, 2009.

169. Daw NW: Critical periods and amblyopia, *Arch Ophthalmol* 116:502–505, 1998.

170. Klein R, Klein BE, Jensen SC, et al: The five-year incidence and progression of age-related maculopathy: the Beaver Dam eye study, *Ophthalmology* 104:7–21, 1997.

171. Ryskulova A, Turczn K, Makuc DM, et al: Self-reported age-related eye diseases and visual impairment in the United States: results of the 2002 national health interview study, *Am J Pub Health* 98(3):454–461, 2008.

172. Myers SM: A twin study on age-related macular degeneration, *Trans Am Ophthalmol Soc* 92:775–844, 1994.

173. Klein R, Knudtson MD, Cruickshanks KJ, et al: Further observations on the association between smoking and the long-term incidence and progression of age-related macular degeneration: the Beaver Dam eye study, *Arch Ophthalmol* 126(1):115–121, 2008.

174. Hammond BR Jr, Wooten BR, Snodderly DM: Cigarette smoking and retinal carotenoids: implications for age-related macular degeneration, *Vision Res* 36:3003–3009, 1996.

175. Berger JW, Fine SL, Maguire MG: *Age-related macular degeneration*, St Louis, 1999, Mosby.

176. Hammond BR Jr, Johnson EF, Russell RM, et al: Dietary modification of human macular pigment density, *Invest Ophthalmol Vis Sci* 38:1795–1801, 1997.

CHAPTER 11

Vital Functions

OBJECTIVES

After studying this chapter, the reader will be able to:

1. Describe vital human functions.
2. Define homeostasis.
3. Describe the role of the endocrine system in vital functions.
4. Discuss changes in vital functions across the life span.

We define vital functions as those functions necessary for survival. In humans, vital functions are breathing, sleeping, eating, and eliminating. All of these functions involve multiple systems of the body. And these systems interact to produce functions that support our ability to explore the environment and to experience life. Homeostasis also is important to vital functions because it is the process that keeps the internal environment constant or in balance. Homeostasis of the vital functions allow individuals to participate fully in all life roles such as play, work, and leisure.

The four vital functions—breathing, sleeping, eating, and eliminating—can be broken down into six processes: ventilation-respiration, sleep-wakefulness, ingestion, digestion, absorption, and excretion. All processes must occur for life to be sustained.

These processes and functions are cyclical. Each process has a rhythm or occurs in a cycle. Breathing brings air in and lets carbon dioxide out; wakefulness and sleep occur in patterns that generally correspond to day and night; food and water are ingested and wastes are eliminated. Circadian rhythms (from *circa*, which means "about," and *dies*, which means "day") are innately directed rhythms that occur every 24 hours. These rhythms affect all aspects of human physiology. Easily recognizable rhythms include the sleep-wake cycle and the cyclical release of hormones. Biologically, the cycles of change seen in these vital functions make it easier to adapt to different environments.

The cyclical nature of the vital functions provides a clue to their control and a way to explain behavior. Hormonal control of cyclical vital functions is mediated by the autonomic nervous system and the endocrine system, which together maintain the body's internal homeostasis. The circadian timing system is a neural system composed of a biological clock with input and output pathways. The central nervous system site of the biological clock in humans is found in the anterior hypothalamus.[1,2]

The hypothalamus and its related structures oversee the vegetative functions of the brain such as body temperature, thirst and satiation centers, and osmolality of body fluids. These functions are vital to the maintenance of homeostasis and represent basic physiological needs. The human species has a need to drink and to take in salt, to maintain body temperature, to eat, to reproduce, and to respond to stress.[3] These basic physiological drives ensure the survival of the species.

The control of vegetative functions is therefore closely related to behavior. In addition to its major role in controlling vegetative and endocrine functions of the body, the hypothalamus controls many aspects of emotional behavior. Because the hypothalamus is a major part of the limbic system, it is not surprising that our emotional state can and does affect basic bodily functions. Homeostasis is disrupted by our thoughts, emotion, and stress, which are manifested in physiological changes in vegetative functions, as anyone nervously waiting for an important interview can attest. The hypothalamus directs its actions through the endocrine and autonomic nervous systems. The latter is discussed in Chapter 9, and the endocrine system is discussed here.

ENDOCRINE SYSTEM

The endocrine system consists of a collection of glands that manufacture and secrete hormones into the bloodstream. These chemical messengers affect various cells of the body and regulate many aspects of physiological function. The endocrine system plays a role in the rate of growth, basal metabolic rate, stress responses, and reproduction. The endocrine system is second only to the nervous system in terms of its ability to act as a major communication system. It is composed of the pituitary gland, thyroid, parathyroid, adrenal cortex, adrenal medulla, islet cells of the pancreas, secretory cells in the intestines, and the gonads. The hypothalamus is also considered part of the endocrine system because it releases hormones that control the activity of the pituitary gland.

The hypothalamus monitors physiological set points for almost every internal body function. For example, there are set point values for body temperature, blood glucose levels, blood pressure, and salt concentration in the blood. If these values are under or over the normal range, sensing mechanisms relay information to the hypothalamus or subsystems under its control, and steps are taken to correct the error. Negative feedback is the most common way in which values are corrected. Set points for regulated variables can be changed or reset. Set points can be changed by external or internal stimuli. Some set points, such as body temperature, display a circadian rhythm; body temperature is higher during the day than during the night.

Homeostatic Control Mechanisms

Reflexes control some endocrine functions. A stimulus is received that is interpreted as an error by an integrating center. The integrating center stimulates an effector, which is typically a muscle or a gland, which in turn produces a response that corrects the error, reestablishing homeostasis. The muscle may act to change blood flow to an area to prevent heat loss. The hypothalamus relays commands to the autonomic nervous system to activate heat-gain or heat-loss mechanisms. When an increase in blood sugar is detected, insulin is secreted by the pancreas. The level of glucose in the blood declines, and insulin secretion ceases. Negative feedback systems are corrective by nature. An error must be detected for the system to be engaged.

Another way in which homeostasis is controlled by the endocrine system is by local responses. Local homeostatic responses occur within the tissues. For example, skin is damaged by a puncture. The damaged cells in the area release chemicals that assist in preventing further injury. Chemical messengers are used in reflex and local homeostatic responses. There are many categories of chemical messengers. An example of a chemical messenger is human growth factor; there are at least 50 growth factors, so they represent a family of chemical messengers.[4]

Circadian rhythms provide an anticipatory facet to homeostasis. These rhythms are internally driven by hormones and entrained by external factors. One of the strongest of these cues is the duration of light and dark. Even in the absence of cues, however, the rhythms run free; that is, they maintain the cycle. A biological rhythm is an example of a feedforward system that operates without detectors.

Endocrine Changes Across the Life Span

Hormones, their roles in growth and development, and the effects of aging associated with the body's responses and changes are found in Table 11-1.

Prenatal

The endocrine system develops in stages in utero after the second month of gestation. The first endocrine gland to develop is the thyroid gland, at 24 days of gestation.[5] Thyroid hormone plays a major role in the development of the brain and nervous system. The pituitary forms at 4 weeks and is composed of ectoderm from two different sources, which explains why there are two different tissue types (glandular and neural) composing the gland. The function of these tissues contributes to the maximum rate of growth in height of the fetus seen around the fourth month of gestation.[6] The fetal adrenal gland produces steroids that influence the maturation of the liver, epithelium of the digestive tract, and the lungs.[7]

Fetal growth is primarily nutrition dependent and therefore reliant on the mother's nutritional intake and the integrity of the placenta. Neither the sex hormones or growth hormone play a role in fetal growth. The placenta is an endocrine gland that supplies the developing fetus with peptide hormones, neurohormones, and steroids. The placenta converts steroids produced by the fetus' adrenal gland to biologically active steroids such as estrogens. The placenta secretes substances autonomously without being regulated by fetal or maternal signals.[8] Placental insufficiency and poor maternal nutrition are causes of intrauterine growth retardation.[9]

Table **11-1**		

Hormonal Actions During Growth and Aging

Hormone	Influence on Growth	Effects of Aging
Aldosterone	Secretion increases	Levels decline Adaptive response fails

Cortisol	High concentrations inhibit growth
	Prolonged secretion can cause
	   breakdown of bone and inhibit
	   secretion of growth hormone
	Catabolizes protein
		Levels maintained

Epinephrine		Unchanged in young–old Increased in oldest–old
Estrogen	Increases GH at puberty Stimulates closure of epiphyses	Secretion declines, then ceases Increased risk of fractures
Glucagon		Secretion maintains or increases
Growth hormone (GH)	Major postnatal growth stimulus Highest secretion in adolescence	Secretion declines
Insulin	Stimulates fetal growth	Decreased sensitivity
Norepinephrine		Secretion increases
Testosterone	Increases GH at puberty Stimulates eventual closure of epiphyses	Secretion declines

Thyroid hormones	Prenatally needed for central nervous
	   system development
	Needed for GH secretion in childhood
	   and adolescence
		Secretion declines
		Decreased target cell response

Vasopressin (antidiuretic
   hormone)
		Increased sensitivity
		Decreased adaptive response with
		   change in posture
		Decreased target cell response

Data from Davis PJ, Davis FB, Leinung MC: Endocrine disorders. In Duthie EH, Katz PR, Malone ML, editors: *Practice of geriatrics*, ed 4, Philadelphia, 2007, WB Saunders, pp 645-664; Goodman CC: The endocrine and metabolic systems. In Goodman CC, Fuller KS, editors: *Pathology: implications for the physical therapist*, ed 2, Philadelphia, 2009, WB Saunders, pp 453-518; Norwak FV, Mooradian AD: Endocrine function and dysfunction. In Birren JE, editor: *Encyclopedia of gerontology*, ed 2, San Diego, 2007, Academic Press, pp 480-494; Purushothaman R, Morley JE: Endocrinology in the aged. In Gass GH, Kaplan HM, editors: *Handbook of endocrinology*, ed 2, Boca Raton, Fla, 1996, CRC Press, pp 241-260.

Infancy Through Adolescence

Growth hormone is the main impetus for postnatal growth.[8] Whereas it has no effect on fetal growth, growth hormone exerts a profound effect on cell proliferation in target tissues. Too much growth hormone can produce gigantism; too little, dwarfism. Secretion of human growth hormone controls the rate of growth and development. It sustains the normal rate of protein synthesis in the body and is needed for cartilage cell proliferation at the epiphyseal plates of bone.

Growth hormone works indirectly on cell division by influencing the liver to secrete insulin-like growth factor I. This growth factor in turn stimulates protein synthesis and impedes protein degradation. Insulin-like growth factor II is also a growth hormone, which plays a role in postnatal growth, but its exact function is unclear. A peak level of insulin-like growth factor is seen in adolescence. Growth hormone and insulin-like growth factor I levels are low during the day, but 1 to 2 hours after falling asleep, large amounts are secreted.

The amount of growth hormone produced at night can represent 20% to 40% of the day's total output.

Thyroid and parathyroid hormones are important to the growth of bones, teeth, and the brain. Insufficient thyroid hormone results in retardation of bone growth. And the brain does not develop properly in utero without the thyroid hormone. After birth, the effects of a deficit are apparent in sluggish thought processes or jitteriness resulting from excessive production. The amount of thyroid hormone secreted declines slightly from birth to puberty and then increases for an adolescent growth spurt. Parathyroid hormone is involved in maintaining calcium homeostasis by acting at three sites: the bones, the gastrointestinal (GI) tract, and the kidneys. This involvement continues throughout the life span. The thyroid hormones have an effect on dental development, so it is not surprising to find that skeletal maturity and dental maturity are usually correlated.

The earliest signs of puberty—the acquisition of axillary and pubic hair—are a result of increased secretion of androgens by the adrenal gland. The adrenal gland is directed to secrete androgens by corticotropin released from the pituitary. The adrenal androgens also play a major part in directing the course of the adolescent growth spurt in both sexes. The remaining changes that occur during puberty are the result of increased activity within the hypothalamic anterior pituitary system.

The hypothalamus produces increased amounts of gonadotropin-releasing hormone just before puberty. During childhood, only low levels of gonadotropin-releasing hormone, pituitary gonadotropins, and estrogen or testosterone are secreted. Gonadotropin-releasing hormone is released in rhythmic bursts during the night at 2-hour intervals, causing nocturnal release of gonadotropins, which in turn stimulate the cells of the ovary or testicle to secrete estrogen or testosterone. Testosterone and the adrenal androgens produce greater growth of muscle in the male. Female growth for the most part is dependent on the androgens of the adrenal cortex alone.[6]

The rise in estrogen triggers menarche, the first menstrual period. On average, the onset of menarche in the United States is 12 years.[10] The advent of the first period is a late-stage phenomenon of puberty occurring after development of the breast and pubic hair and growth spurt. The onset of menses may be associated with the age-related change in body composition and body mass, such as the attainment of 17% body fat and a weight of 103 to 109 pounds.[11] This may explain the lack of onset of menarche or the cessation of menses in female athletes with low body fat and body mass. Rising estrogen levels also cause the epiphyses to close, thus terminating skeletal growth. Because girls go through puberty earlier than do boys, they attain peak height earlier and develop secondary sex characteristics sooner than do boys.

Testosterone is critical to the attainment of sexual maturity in males. Spermatogenesis begins at puberty under the direction of testosterone. It has negative-feedback effects on the hypothalamus and anterior pituitary. Testosterone also induces changes in the male reproductive organs and development of the secondary sex characteristics and sex drive. Testosterone stimulates growth during puberty through its effect on growth hormone secretion. It also causes the eventual closure of the epiphyses. Testosterone, unlike estrogen, has a strong anabolic effect on protein synthesis that can also account for the increased muscle mass of men compared with women. Anabolic steroids are synthetic agents that are converted into testosterone by the body. Some male and female athletes use anabolic steroids to build body mass and strength, but these drugs are potentially very dangerous and can have serious side effects such as liver damage.

Adulthood

During adulthood, our hormones are integrally associated with our normal physiological response to stress. The hypothalamus and anterior pituitary coordinate the release of corticotropin, which stimulates the adrenal cortex to secrete cortisol. The activity of the sympathetic nervous system is also increased during stress. The familiar fight-or-flight reaction is accompanied by an increased secretion of epinephrine, additionally readying the body for physical activity and for coping with new situations. The secretion of most other hormones also is affected by stress. Prolonged stress has been linked to increased susceptibility to disease by depressing the immune system.

Older Adulthood

As the body ages, it is less resilient to environmental stress. It becomes more difficult to maintain the status quo or homeostasis. There are four patterns of change in endocrine function during normal aging. The first pattern is related to endocrine gland failure, which is exemplified by the ovary during menopause. The second pattern of change is associated with a decrease in sensitivity of target organs. Examples include the age-related decline in peripheral tissue response to insulin and the progressive resistance of the renal system to the effects of antidiuretic hormone or vasopressin. The third pattern is seen in the failure of an expected adaptive response, such as an insufficiency in the expected normal increase in blood pressure on standing from a supine or seated position caused by a lack of renin. The final pattern is marked by an increased sensitivity within the endocrine system as seen when there is a more aggressive response to an increase in antidiuretic hormone in older adults for a given level of osmolality. Older individuals tend to retain fluid more easily.

Menopause Menopause is part of normal aging for a woman. On average, the menstrual cycles become less regular around the age of 50. The cessation of those cycles is known as *menopause.* Many changes occur during menopause. The failure of the ovaries to produce estrogen affects the genitourinary tract, the skeletal system, and body composition. A woman may experience an increased need to urinate and some urethral irritability. Loss of minerals from the bone puts a woman at risk for osteoporosis (see Chapter 6). Loss of estrogen also increases a woman's risk for cardiovascular disease.

Physiological changes associated with menopause include thinning of the walls of the vagina and decreased lubrication, vasomotor changes leading to hot flashes or flushes, less immediate responses to sexual arousal, and fewer contractions during orgasm. There is a discernible decrease in function of the endocrine system in females at three levels. The decline at the organ level, the ovary, and effects of decline in circulating hormone levels have been briefly described. Last, target organs, the estrogen receptors in the body, also are affected. The breasts lose connective tissue, the skin becomes thin, and sweat glands and hair follicles become dry and less resilient due to the loss of estrogen.[12]

As the population ages, health maintenance in postmenopausal women will be a huge concern of all health care providers. Screening for conditions related to loss of estrogen such as osteoporosis, coronary artery disease, and breast and colorectal cancer are extremely important. Symptoms of menopause need to be managed on an individual basis taking into consideration each woman's unique health and family history. A recent review of recommendations for health maintenance in this population can be found in an article by Rao and colleagues.[13]

Andropause Men undergo less dramatic changes relative to a reduction in circulating testosterone levels. However, there is a steady decline in testosterone from the age of 60.[14] The decline in the amount of testosterone in the circulation does not indicate a decrease in potency. Sperm continue to be produced but in smaller quantities. The decline in sperm production appears to be linked to connective tissue changes around the inside of the seminiferous tubules. This decline begins in the 40s and 50s, with a decrease in motility noted after the age of 50.

Androgen deficiency and erectile dysfunction are two separate clinical entities.[15] The decline in testosterone with age does cause the libido to diminish but does not cause impotence. Impotence is typically related to vascular disease and present in half of men over the age of 70.[16] The fact that the amount of gonadotropins in the serum increases with age supports the likelihood that the testes are less responsive to their effects. The term *androgen decline in the aging male* (ADAM) is a clinical entity with the symptoms mimicking the age-related loss of testosterone. There are no consistent criteria for diagnosing ADAM. The prevalence of ADAM in men with erectile dysfunction is high but may be related to the presence of additional pathology.[15] Additional studies are needed to clarify aging effects from effects from pathology. At present, there are hormonal changes in men with age, which may be as universal as menopause is in women. Testosterone replacement therapy for age-related decline is not warranted based on the present data.[17]

LIFE SPAN CHANGES OF VITAL FUNCTIONS

Ventilation-Respiration

Oxygen is needed by the body to convert organic carbon compounds into usable energy. Oxygen, however, cannot be stored in the body. The cardiovascular, pulmonary, musculoskeletal, and nervous systems work together to take in oxygen and to expel carbon dioxide in the act of *ventilation. Respiration,* the process of gas exchange, occurs at the cellular level within the alveoli. Ventilation and respiration involve the lungs, heart, thorax, diaphragm, central nervous system breathing centers, and central and peripheral chemoreceptors.

Control Mechanisms

Control of ventilation is achieved by two interacting systems, each with a specific purpose and affected by different stimuli. One system is neural and the other is chemical. Both systems are automatic but can be overridden by the need to talk, swallow, or perform other desired tasks such as swimming underwater. The neural and chemical systems act on the muscular contraction of the diaphragm and intercostal muscles that are involved in the inspiratory phase of ventilation. During quiet breathing, expiration is usually passive. During forceful expiration, as in a cough, the abdominal muscles are activated.

Neural System At least three brain stem centers coordinate the rhythmic ventilatory cycle and maintain the depth of ventilation. These sites are located in the medulla and the pons of the brain stem. The first site consists of several nuclei in the medulla. The inspiratory neurons provide the stimulus to fire the muscles of breathing. Voluntary control of breathing occurs through the corticospinal tract. The group of neurons in the medulla sends out repetitive bursts of inspiratory signals. The bursts of firing are cyclical and alternate with quiet periods. One center in the pons modulates the output of the medullary inspiratory neurons, which can regulate the depth of ventilation. The other center in the pons is active in the transition between inspiration and expiration. If this area of the pons is damaged, apneustic breathing occurs, which is characterized by long inspiratory gasps.

Chemical System The chemical system regulates alveolar ventilation and monitors the blood gases. The central and peripheral chemoreceptors primarily control ventilation at rest. Central chemoreceptors located in the medulla respond to the composition of the extracellular fluid of the brain—specifically to the hydrogen ion concentration in that fluid. Although hydrogen ions cannot pass through the blood-brain barrier, carbon dioxide in the extracellular fluid reacts with water to form hydrogen ions. Therefore a rise in arterial PCO_2 causes an increase in hydrogen ion concentration and, consequently, an increase in ventilation. The neurons in the medullary inspiratory area are also very sensitive to chemicals, such as morphine and barbiturates, and can become so depressed that ventilation ceases.

Ventilation can be stimulated reflexively by a large decrease in arterial PO_2. This mechanism uses the peripheral chemoreceptors: the aortic and carotid bodies. The chemoreceptors are directly influenced by the oxygen content of circulating arterial blood. A decrease in oxygen content excites the receptors to cause an increase in depth and rate of breathing. Peripheral receptors provide an accessory mechanism for controlling breathing activity. It is the central receptors, however, that account for approximately 70% of the increased ventilation due to chemical changes.

Breathing patterns can also be modified by sensory input from the lungs and chest wall, as in the case of a person who hyperventilates. By increasing the depth and rapidity of inspiration, alveolar and arterial carbon dioxide levels decrease and arterial oxygen levels increase. Swimmers may hyperventilate to increase the length of time they can hold their breath. Another example of altered breathing occurs when a person blows off too much carbon dioxide too quickly. The delay in the detection of the change in blood chemistry by the ventilatory centers causes periodic breathing,

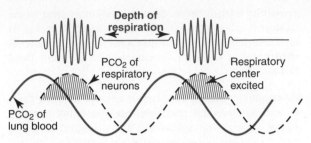

Figure 11-1 Cheyne-Stokes breathing showing the changing PCO_2 in the pulmonary blood *(solid line)* and the delayed changes in PCO_2 of the fluids of the respiratory center *(dashed line)*. (From Guyton AC, Hall JE: *Textbook of medical physiology*, ed 11, Philadelphia, 2006, WB Saunders.)

or Cheyne-Stokes breathing (Figure 11-1). This type of breathing is seen in patients with brain damage or chronic or severe cardiac failure.

Function Across the Life Span

Prenatal The lungs develop early during gestation, but it is not until a pulmonary blood supply is established and adequate amounts of surfactant are produced that the lungs become capable of efficient gas exchange. The heart, although not a part of the pulmonary system per se, is needed to perfuse the lungs with blood to allow gas exchange to take place. For the fetus to receive an adequate supply of oxygen through the placenta, the fetal heart must pump a large volume of blood.

Although ventilation cannot occur during fetal life, respiratory movements do occur in utero. Respiratory movements are possible at the end of the first trimester, but because the amniotic fluid is very thick, the fetus "breathes" only a small amount. Fetal breathing movements, however, are a vital factor in the development of normal lungs.[18] Fox and colleagues[19] note that fetal breathing ceases for up to 1 hour after maternal ingestion of alcohol, which may be related to the developmental problems seen as a result of fetal alcohol syndrome.

The pattern of fetal breathing is used to diagnose labor and to predict the outcome of preterm delivery.[5] Breathing movements in utero appear to condition the respiratory muscles and may produce a pressure gradient between the lungs and the amniotic fluid. At birth, the lungs are half-filled with fluid, so the first breath is possible only if the fluid is cleared from the lungs. This process is assisted by compression of the thorax during vaginal delivery.

Infancy and Childhood The newborn infant must breath through its nose because the tongue takes up all of the space in the oral cavity. Babies efficiently use nasal breathing to bypass the impenetrable oral cavity. This anatomical arrangement provides a protective feature for the infant because breathing is not yet coordinated with sucking and swallowing. However, when a baby has a cold, it is difficult to shift to breathing through the mouth, as occurs in older children and adults.

The depth and rate of ventilation change in relationship to the activity or work to be performed. The diaphragm is the major muscle of inspiration until around 5 to 7 years of age, after which the thoracic muscles play a larger role. According to Adkins,[20] four components–the diaphragm, chest, neck accessory, and abdominal muscles–may contribute to breathing. Usually the adult breathing pattern consists of an equal combination of diaphragm and chest movements (two diaphragm, two chest). Pathological changes in the musculoskeletal and cardiovascular systems can have a significant effect on the breathing pattern, as in scoliosis, spinal cord injury, or congenital heart defect. The relationship among work capacity, ventilation, and oxygen consumption is the same for a child as for an adult.

Older Adulthood   With normal aging, functional changes are seen in the volume of air moved, the rate of the airflow, and the amount of oxygen exchanged. Although the overall total lung volume remains constant, individual lung volumes change (for specific examples, see Chapter 8). Total lung capacity remains the same because the stiffness of the chest wall is balanced by the loss of elastic recoil of the lungs. Arterial oxygen tension (PaO_2) is the measure most often used of the amount of oxygen in the blood. There is a 4-mm Hg drop in PaO_2 per decade.[21] This decline has been attributed to increasing variability in ventilation-perfusion matching in different parts of the lung and premature airway closure. In addition, the amount of hemoglobin available for oxygen transport diminishes with age.[22] Despite these documented age-related changes in the cardiovascular and pulmonary systems, pulmonary function can be improved with a program of moderately intense exercise training.[23]

Sleep-Wakefulness

Sleeping is a large part of our lives, but the exact benefits or purposes of sleep continue to be studied and elucidated. On the surface sleep appears to be a passive process, but in reality it is actually quite an active period for building memories. Sleep is a basic physiological drive like hunger or thirst. For most of us, sleep is a rhythmic, predictable process that occurs at night. It has always been said that a good night's sleep repairs the mind and the body. Anyone who has had

difficulty sleeping knows the far-reaching effects of a lack of sleep. Research links sleep to time needed to allow the nervous system to reorganize and to promote memory and learning. Sleep has been associated with memory consolidation and offline learning in children and adults.[24,25] Most of us have had the experience of going to bed trying to solve a problem and awaking in the morning to find the solution.

The sleep-wakefulness cycle consists of periods of sleep lasting from 6 to 10 hours and periods of wakefulness lasting from 14 to 18 hours a day. Timing of sleep and wakefulness is largely determined by internal factors, part of the so-called biological clock, and external factors such as the light in the environment. Physiologically, sleep is a state of unconsciousness from which a person can be aroused.[4] Human beings alternate between three states: wakefulness, nonrapid eye movement (NREM) sleep, and rapid eye movement (REM) sleep.

Wakefulness is associated with an increase in most physiological parameters from sleep levels; further increases in blood pressure and rate of breathing are associated with sympathetic nervous system activation. When we are awake, the brain wave pattern seen on an electroencephalogram is desynchronized (Figure 11-2).

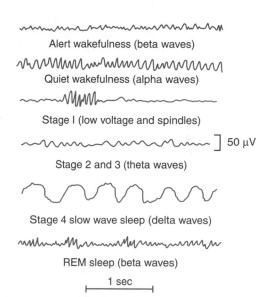

Alert wakefulness (beta waves)

Quiet wakefulness (alpha waves)

Stage I (low voltage and spindles)

] 50 µV

Stage 2 and 3 (theta waves)

Stage 4 slow wave sleep (delta waves)

REM sleep (beta waves)

|— 1 sec —|

Figure 11-2 Progressive change in the characteristics of the brain waves during different stages of wakefulness and sleep. Stages of slow wave sleep and corresponding electroencephalographic patterns. Stage 1: Very light sleep, low-voltage synchronized waves with sleep spindles. Stages 2 and 3: Light sleep characterized by low-voltage theta waves. Stage 4: Deep sleep characterized by high-voltage delta waves. (From Guyton AC, Hall JE: *Textbook of medical physiology*, ed 11, Philadelphia, 2006, WB Saunders.)

An alpha rhythm is most likely to be recorded in an awake, relaxed adult whose eyes are closed. When attention is directed toward an external stimulus, the alpha rhythm is replaced by a beta rhythm. Arousal is the lowest level of attention. Once aroused, alertness is possible. When we are able to avoid distractions, it is termed *directed attention*. We can be so focused on a task that even a novel stimulus does not produce an orienting response.

There are two types of sleep: NREM sleep and REM sleep. Each involves the brain, lungs, heart, and specific brain stem centers. NREM sleep is the initial phase of sleep and has four stages. Stage 1 is the lightest sleep, and stages 2, 3, and 4 are increasingly deeper. Each successive stage of NREM sleep exhibits a slower frequency and higher amplitude brain wave than the previous stage. The last two stages of NREM sleep are also known as *slow wave sleep* (SWS) because of their unique slow wave sleep pattern on electroencephalography. NREM sleep occurs when decreased activity in the reticular activating system in the brain stem causes the brain waves to slow down. SWS is associated with a 10% to 30% decrease in blood pressure, rate of ventilation, and basal metabolic rate.[4] Declarative memory is consolidated during SWS.[24] Consolidation is the process of interaction between the cortex and the hippocampus coordinated by the fluctuations seen in this stage of sleep.[26] All four stages of NREM sleep and REM sleep exhibit characteristic physiological functions and are further distinguished by different brain wave patterns (see Figure 11-2).

REM sleep occurs when the brain waves do not slow down but the person is asleep and exhibits rapid eye movements and muscle atonia. These incongruent characteristics explain why REM sleep is also called *paradoxical sleep*. Dreaming occurs in REM sleep, but the muscle atonia prevents us from acting out the dreams. An irregular heart rate and breathing rate and increased brain metabolism are characteristics of paradoxical sleep. Periods of paradoxical, or REM, sleep are interspersed between periods of NREM sleep and are characterized by low-voltage, asynchronous brain waves.

Sleep begins with stage 1 of NREM sleep and progresses to stage 4 in approximately 30 to 40 minutes. The cycle then reverses itself by going from stage 4 back to stage 1. At this point, the sleeper experiences an episode of REM sleep. Each period of REM sleep in adults can last from 5 to 40 minutes and usually happens every 90 minutes of sleep. Depending on how long we sleep, we may experience four or five episodes of REM sleep. When awakened while in REM sleep, we can recall our dreams. The relative amount of NREM and REM sleep does change over the course of a night's sleep. Early in the night, SWS (stages 3 and 4 of NREM sleep) prevail, whereas stage 2 of NREM and REM sleep are dominant in the last half of the night.[27]

Control Mechanisms

At least three endogenous pattern generators are responsible for the sleep-wake cycle. These centers are located in the brain stem. One group known as the *raphe nuclei* secretes serotonin, a major neurotransmitter associated with sleep. Stimulation of the raphe nuclei causes sleep. Another collection of cells called the *locus ceruleus*, secrete norepinephrine. According to one theory, activity in the neurons that secrete serotonin and norepinephrine is greater during wakefulness while cholinergic neurons are dominant during REM sleep. In this model, NREM sleep is an intermediate state. The third group of generators involved in sleep is located in the hypothalamus and is the site of the biological clock in humans. These areas produce sleep and arousal. Sleep, then, is attributed to an active inhibitory process.[4]

Melatonin is produced by the pineal gland and is secreted in a diurnal cycle. More melatonin is produced at night than during the day. Sleep onset occurs with the onset of melatonin secretion. Melatonin production is controlled by the suprachiasmatic nucleus in the hypothalamus. The timing of its secretion is capable of causing phase shifts in the sleep-wakefulness cycle. Light coming in through the retina can affect the suprachiasmatic nucleus. When environmental stimuli adjust the function of the suprachiasmatic nucleus and other rhythm-generating systems of the brain, it is called *entrainment*.

A less well-defined group of cells, the reticular activating system, is responsible for arousing the cortex. If the reticular activating system is not inhibited by the sleep centers, the reticular nuclei spontaneously become active and continue to be aroused by the positive feedback from the cortex and the peripheral nervous system. Serotonin adjusts the body's general arousal level. Levels are high when alert, low in NREM sleep, and lowest in REM sleep. When the reticular activating system tires or is inhibited, sleep occurs. Research continues on isolating additional transmitter substances and sleep factors. Although the first human gene that controls the sleep cycle has been discovered,[28] there continues to be no complete explanation for the reciprocal, cyclical operation of the sleep-wake cycle.

Function Across the Life Span

Prenatal Milani-Comparetti[29] noted that the fetus had alternating periods of sleep and wakefulness at 29 weeks of gestation. Rosen and coresearchers[30] distinguished

REM, NREM, and wakefulness electroencephalographic patterns in the fetus during labor. Sleep in the fetus appears to be important in the continued development of the nervous system.[31] It is thought that sleep induces early development of central sensory processing centers to prepare them to receive input at birth. This is supported by the early myelination of these areas and the importance of experience or activity dependent maturation of the sensory systems during postnatal development.

Infancy Preterm infants exhibit *ultradian rhythms,* which are rhythms with period lengths of less than 24 hours. This lack of circadian rhythm may reflect the effect of infant care schedules.[2] A term newborn's 4-hour sleep-wake cycle appears to be related to cyclical variation in gastrointestinal physiology and can be altered by changing the infant's feeding schedule. Newborns may spend as much as 16 hours sleeping each day. Half of that sleep will be REM sleep, which supports its speculated role in nervous system organization. A stable circadian rhythm is established between the second and fourth months after birth. Very little melatonin is produced until 3 months of age.[32] At that time, wakefulness is recognized as a stable state necessary for the infant to learn about the environment. Sleep reflects the infant's capability for self-regulation.[33] Gradually, the naps between wakeful periods at night lengthen until the infant sleeps through the night, at about 28 weeks after birth. The 3-month-old spends only 40% of sleeping time in REM sleep.[34] By 3 years of age, the child's amount of REM sleep constitutes 20% to 25% of the total sleep time, the same percentage as an adult.[35] This appears to be the result of functional maturation of the inhibitory systems active during REM sleep.

An infant's sleep begins with REM sleep and progresses to NREM, whereas an adult's sleep begins with NREM sleep. The quality of sleep within a state, changes in electroencephalographic activity, and percentage of time spent in different stages of sleep and wakefulness change during the first 2 years of life. Infants do not exhibit SWS at birth. It develops by 2 to 6 months of age.[35] Infants and children spend more time in slow wave sleep than adults.[24] Gomez and colleagues[36] found that 15-month-old infants who napped had better recall. NREM sleep is especially enhanced during early childhood and has been linked to an increase in protein synthesis and release of growth hormone. The ability of the nervous system to inhibit REM sleep, thus allowing more NREM sleep, may also be a result of central nervous system maturation.[37] Others have postulated a two process model to account for sleep-wake regulation. In this model, sleep is regulated by a circadian process that generates 24-hour cycles of behavior and a homeostatic process that reflects the amount of proper sleep and wakefulness.[35]

State Sleep-wake states have traditionally been used to classify newborn behavior. Prechtl[38] first identified six behavioral states in newborns ranging from sleeping to crying. These states are taken into consideration when testing newborns. The six states are found in Table 11-2. Prechtl's states are related to physiology and are used to assess the newborn's ability to adjust to the extrauterine environment.

Sudden Infant Death Unfortunately, sleep in infants is also linked to sudden death. Sudden infant death syndrome, or SIDS, is defined as the sudden death of an infant for no apparent reason due to a cessation of breathing. SIDS is the third leading cause of death in the first year of life and together with congenital malformations and disorders related to prematurity and low birth weight accounts for 43% of all infant deaths.[39] When SIDS was shown to be related to sleeping in a prone position, the American Academy of Pediatrics recommended that infants sleep in positions other than prone. A "Back to Sleep" program was launched in 1994. Preventive programs have decreased the incidence of SIDS by more than 50%.[40] The incidence of SIDS is higher in prematurely born infants and those with a low birth weight. A study found that a disproportionate number of cases of SIDS, more than 20%, occur in child care settings.[41] This finding was explained by a lack of instruction of caregivers regarding sleeping posture. Despite the fact that only 20% or less of infants sleep on their backs,

Table **11-2**	
Infant Behavioral States	
Prechtl	**Infant State**
Deep sleep, regular breathing, eyes closed	1
Active rapid eye movement sleep, irregular breathing, eyes closed but movement can be detected	2
Drowsy, eyes open or closed, variable activity level	3
Quiet alert, focused attention, minimal motor activity	4
Active awake, eyes open, considerable motor activity	5
Crying, jerky motor movements	6

Data from Prechtl H: *The neurological examination of the full-term newborn infant,* ed 2, Philadelphia, 1977, JB Lippincott.

CLINICAL IMPLICATIONS Box 11-1

Sudden Infant Death Syndrome

Sudden infant death syndrome (SIDS) is the most common cause of death in infants under a year of age with an incidence of 0.54/1000 live births.[99] The peak occurrence is between 2 and 4 months of age with 90% of deaths happening before 6 months of age.[40] According to the Triple Risk Model of Filiano and Kinney,[100] three factors converge to act on a vulnerable infant to cause SIDS. These factors are (1) underlying vulnerability of the infant; (2) critical period in development of homeostatic control between birth and 6 months; and (3) an external stressor such as the prone sleep posture. Immaturity of autonomic control of the cardiorespiratory system, failure of an arousal response, or abnormal serotonin function in the brain stem have all been postulated to be possible causal agents in SIDS.

Fifty to 75% of infants with SIDS have abnormalities in the brain stem system that supports respiration, sleep, and arousal. "The serotonergic system is considered to be critical for the modulation and integration of diverse homeostatic functions."[101] Prenatal exposure to alcohol and smoke via maternal use may impair the development of the serotonin-mediated homeostatic systems in the brain stem.[102] This impairment could make the infant vulnerable to exogenous stressors during a critical developmental period.

Premature infants have a fourfold increased risk of SIDS.[40] At one time it was thought that apnea was a predecessor of SIDS but that has not been borne out by research. Therefore, use of an apnea monitor is not recommended as a strategy to reduce SIDS.[103] In a study of more than 20,000 infants, Kato and associates[104] found that infants who subsequently died from SIDS had fewer occurrences of spontaneous arousal.

The following risk factors for SIDS have been compiled from multiple sources[101,103,105]:
- Extrinsic risk factors
  - Sleeping prone
  - Sharing a bed
  - Air pollution
  - Soft bedding
  - Bed clothes that cover the head
  - Too many clothes
- Intrinsic risk factors
  - Male (2:1)
  - Black or Native American
  - Prematurity
  - Perinatal smoke exposure
  - Parental smoking, alcohol ingestion, drug use
  - Socioeconomic disadvantage
- Risk reduction and intervention
  - Back to sleep
  - Use a firm mattress
  - Do not smoke during pregnancy
  - Use a pacifier at nap times and bedtime
  - Share a room but not a bed
  - Reinforce back to sleep at secondary care sites and with secondary caregivers
  - Tummy time

30% to 50% of infants with SIDS are found in a prone position.[42,43] See the Clinical Implications Box 11-1 for more information on SIDS.

Childhood Children require sleep for learning. Backhaus and associates[44] studied the ability of 9- to 12-year-old children to remember word pairs relative to immediate and post-learning sleep. Both conditions resulted in a significant gain in the number of pairs recalled. School performance and sleep or lack of sleep have been studied in school-age children. Processing skills may be sensitive to long-term sleep loss or deprivation.[45] African American (AA) children and children of lower socioeconomic status (SES) may be more vulnerable to effects of disturbed sleep.[46] Cognitive performance of AA children in the study was more negatively affected by sleeping less and having a more variable schedule of sleeping and waking than the European

American children. Both groups performed similarly when they experienced a more consistent sleep schedule. However, when children with a higher SES experienced sleep disruptions, they were able to perform better cognitively than children with lower SES.

Adolescence and Adulthood Adolescents need about 10 hours of sleep a day, but many fall short of achieving the recommended amount. Loss of sleep has been shown to interfere with daytime functioning.[47] Before puberty, the adolescent is an effective sleeper. However, after the onset of puberty, the adolescent's sleep and waking behavior changes. Levels of melatonin decline just before puberty.[48] The adolescent stays up later but still has to get up early for school, and that dichotomy results in sleep deprivation.[49] By the age of 16, the average amount of sleep has dropped from 10 hours in middle childhood to less than 8 hours.[50]

Sleep also affects creativity, emotional regulation, and memory in the adolescent. Wagner and associates[51] studied the process of sleep-dependent creative insight in young adults using a math task. The subjects were able to solve the task faster after a night of sleep. Emotional regulation may also be affected by sleep. Emotion can modulate memory processing. Experiences associated with and triggered by strong emotions tend to produce stronger memories. One just has to think of special events in one's life to remember an experience. The neuroanatomical areas involved in emotion appear to also be involved in REM sleep.[52] Wagner and colleagues[53] demonstrated that emotional memories could be retrieved 4 years after an experiment involving exposure to emotionally arousing material if a short 3-hour period of sleep ensued after the exposure.

An adult generally spends about 8 hours sleeping, but there are great variations in adults' sleep needs. Some require as little as 5 hours, whereas others would prefer 10 hours for peak function. On average, a young adult sleeps 7 hours a night.[54] An adult spends 75% of the time in NREM sleep and 25% in REM sleep. Decrements in the deeper stages of NREM sleep are commonly seen in early adulthood. By midlife, the amount of SWS an adult gets has declined.[24] Backhaus and associates[55] demonstrated that subjects between 48 and 55 years of age had a decreased ability to consolidate declarative memories that correlated with decreased SWS. Work, family, and social demands can diminish total sleep time over the next several decades.

Older Adulthood   As we age, the length of time spent in deep, SWS (stage 3 and 4) sleep decreases; the quality of the sleep decreases; and the amount and relative proportion of REM to NREM sleep decreases (Figure 11-3). Older adults take longer to fall asleep, wake up more frequently, and wake up earlier. Daily average sleep time has been reported to be 7 hours, the same as young adults.[56] Daytime napping often occurs as a means to maintain an adequate amount of total sleep time. Sleep efficiency as measured by the relative percentage of time spent in bed sleeping declines from 90% in young adults to 75% in older adults.[57] The decline in sleep efficiency in the elderly has continued to be shown in a recent meta-analysis of sleep parameters across age groups.[58] The changes appear to be related to a decrease in both homeostatic drive for sleep and the strength of the circadian signal for early morning sleep.[59] Melatonin levels decline with advanced age, which also alters the sleep-wake cycle. Despite the fact that the need for sleep does not decline with age, the older adult's ability to maintain a sleep state is impaired. The inability to stay asleep at night results in daytime sleepiness.

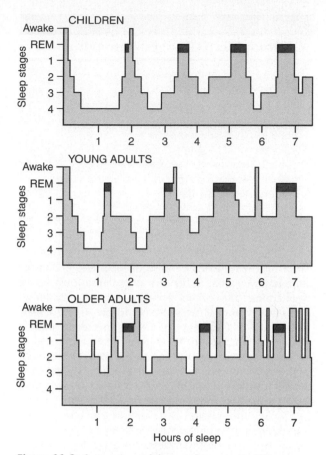

Figure 11-3 Comparison of sleep cycles across the life span. Note the dramatic changes in rapid eye movement sleep in the early years. As we get older, it takes us longer to fall asleep, and we have less deep sleep, more awakenings, and less rapid eye movement sleep. (Redrawn from Kales A, Kales JD: Sleep disorders: recent findings in the diagnosis and treatment of disturbed sleep, *N Engl J Med* 290:(9)487-499, 1974.)

Circadian rhythms begin to shift with age. As we grow older, there is an advancement of the sleep phase, meaning that we become sleepy earlier in the evening. After 6 to 8 hours of sleep, we may awake even though it may be 4 or 5 AM. In addition, older adults may have other poor sleep habits such as remaining in bed when unable to sleep, which, when combined with the phase advancement, can lead to a decline in total nocturnal sleep time. The typical changes in sleep that occur with aging are found in Box 11-1.

The likelihood of experiencing temporary cessation of breathing during sleep, or sleep apnea, increases with age. *Sleep-disordered breathing may result from many anatomical or physiological changes in the structures and function of the breathing system.* When adequate airflow

Box 11-1

Common Sleep Changes with Aging

Decrease in actual time asleep
Difficulty falling asleep
Advance of the normal circadian phase: early to sleep, early awake
Reduction in slow wave sleep
Reduction in REM sleep
Reduced threshold for arousal
Frequent arousal resulting in fragmented sleep
Napping during the day

Adapted from Wolkove N, Elkholy O, Baltzan M, et al: Sleep and aging: 1. Sleep disorders commonly found in older people, *CMAJ* 176(9):1299-1304, 2007.

cannot be maintained because of recurrent periods of complete or partial upper airway collapse, obstructive sleep apnea (OSA) occurs. Apnea is defined as "a period of cessation (or near cessation) of airflow lasting at least 10 seconds."[60] Prevalence of OSA is greater in middle age men than women. Nine percent of women 30 to 60 years of age have OSA compared with 24% of men in the same age group. A study in community-dwelling older adults found 24% of people 65 years or older had five or more apnea episodes per hour of sleep, and 62% had 10 or more episodes per hour.[61] Research has shown that the quality of sleep in persons over 50 years of age can be improved by relying less on medication as a sleep aid, spending less time in bed when awake, and increasing exposure to bright light in the evening.[54]

Studies have indicated that changes in sleep patterns are not purely associated with age but rather with the level of activity that an individual is involved with on a daily basis. Older adults who exercise, such as walking or swimming, for at least 30 minutes per day or spend greater than 50% of their day involved in functional activities have been shown to sleep for 6- to 7-hour periods without experiencing difficulty falling or staying asleep.[62] Increased daytime activity and exercise, along with proper hydration and nutrition, and stress reduction, such as through biofeedback, meditation, and humor, have been shown to be effective in relieving the older adult's feelings of impaired nocturnal sleep.[62]

Deep sleep cycles are crucial for repair and healing for all age groups. It is during this time that all hormonal substances and their substrates needed for the efficient functioning of the neuroendocrine system are produced.[63] It has been demonstrated that submaximal activity and exercise level stimulate the production of interleukin 1, a powerful component of immune system functioning. Interleukin 1 induces deep/slow wave sleep, suppresses REM sleep, and stimulates the production of growth hormone. Sleep patterns change in response to infections; therefore, sleep can be considered a specific healing mechanism vital for the maintenance of health at all ages. For an excellent review of the interconnection between the immune system and sleep, the reader is referred to Imeri and Opp.[64]

Ingestion and Digestion

Eating involves taking in food to provide needed nutritional substrates that foster growth, maturation, and repair of all the body's systems (consult a basic nutrition text for the specific nutritional requirements for each system). Eating, a pleasurable experience for some people, is seen by others as merely something that must be done to keep the body fueled for movement. The initial act of ingesting food or taking in liquid continues in the acts of digestion, absorption, and elimination. Digestion and elimination are crucial to the smooth running of the human body and the maintenance of the internal chemical balance needed for homeostasis. The digestive and excretory systems function together to process all nutrients, except oxygen. The useful components of ingested food and liquids are extracted during the process of digestion and absorption. Waste products are removed and excreted via the GI or the genitourinary tract during elimination.

The act of eating is a skeletal motor activity that demands close coordination with breathing. Eating also requires neuromuscular coordination for mastication (chewing) and deglutition (swallowing), as well as the use of sensory input for motivation and feedback. The process of ingestion involves the mouth, teeth, tongue, pharynx, and esophagus. The process of digestion and absorption also requires the stomach, intestines, salivary glands, pancreas, liver, and gallbladder. The digestive tract consists of a hollow tube that begins at the mouth and ends at the anus. From the midesophagus to the anus, its wall contains two layers of smooth muscle cells: the inner layer is circular and can produce sphincterlike contractions, and the outer layer is longitudinal and can shorten the digestive tract when contracted.

There are three phases of swallowing: the oral phase, the pharyngeal phase, and the esophageal phase. Before swallowing, food is taken into the mouth and changed into a manageable bolus. During the oral phase, the bolus is moved to the back of the pharynx by the tongue. In the second stage, the bolus moves past the throat arches to begin the swallow. The epiglottis folds over the trachea to direct the bolus into the esophagus. Lastly, the bolus is transported down the esophagus by a peristaltic wave toward the stomach (Figure 11-4).

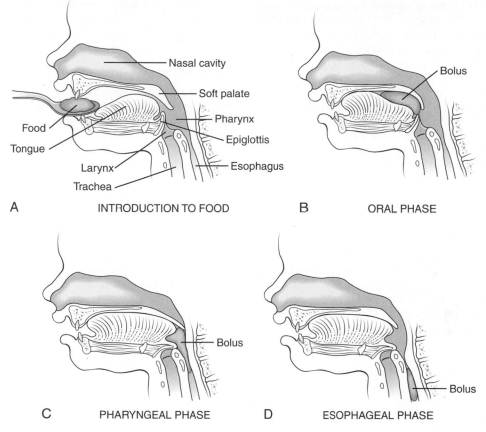

A   INTRODUCTION TO FOOD   B   ORAL PHASE

C   PHARYNGEAL PHASE   D   ESOPHAGEAL PHASE

Figure 11-4 Three phases of swallowing. **A,** Introduction of food. **B,** Oral phase. **C,** Pharyngeal phase. **D,** Esophageal phase. (Adapted from Batshaw ML: *Children with disabilities,* ed 4, Baltimore, 1997, Brookes, 1997, p 622.)

Control Mechanisms

The phases of swallowing are controlled by a complex reflex that allows sequential control of multiple muscles. After the food is chewed, the body of the tongue presses against the roof of the mouth and, in a wavelike motion, propels the food into the pharynx. As the food travels farther back in the pharynx, the epiglottis folds over to close the glottis, preventing food from going into the trachea. Touch receptors in the pharynx elicit the swallow, a series of peristaltic waves, which propels the food into the esophagus. All of this occurs within seconds and is controlled by an area in the brain stem. The control of the phases of swallowing comes from the coordination of "brain stem and cortical central pathways, and the enteric nervous systems of the esophagus that control the smooth muscle segments.[65]"

The esophagus has two sphincters: the upper and lower. The esophageal phase of swallowing is marked by the relaxation of the upper sphincter. The size of the bolus dictates the amount the diameter of the upper sphincter increases. In the esophagus, the food is further conducted to the stomach by peristalsis. The lower esophageal sphincter opens at the end of the peristaltic wave to allow food into the stomach. The pharynx and the upper third of the esophagus are made up of skeletal muscle that is innervated by the glossopharyngeal (cranial nerve IX) and vagus (cranial nerve X) nerves. The remaining two-thirds of the esophagus is made up of smooth muscle that is controlled by the myenteric plexus via the vagus nerve; thus, there is a backup system for food to reach the stomach even if the swallowing reflex is paralyzed. The lower sphincter relaxes to allow food into the stomach and then closes. When the lower sphincter is inefficient, gastric contents can reflux into the esophagus, resulting in gastroesophageal reflux (GER). GER can be a common problem in children with neurological impairments because of poor neuromuscular control.[66]

Although the reflex explanation for chewing and swallowing is documented, there has also been shown to be a functional connection between sucking and swallowing, and swallowing and respiration. Broussard and Altshchuler's[67] study of the timing of swallowing and respiration provided evidence that groups of pre-motor neurons function as pattern generators to initiate the repetitive rhythmic muscle activity seen in swallowing. Recently, Barlow[68] reviewed the current findings on the differential maturation of central pattern generators for feeding and respiration. It is known that the function of these groups of neurons that support the rhythmicity of feeding can be modified by sensory input. The development of motility of the oral, pharyngeal, and esophageal structures occurs in infancy and early childhood. It can be influenced by dietary and postural habits in addition to neuromuscular maturation.

The regulation and control of digestion take place within the GI tract itself. GI reflexes cause changes in muscle wall contractility and the secretion of digestive enzymes. Two major nerve plexuses control these reflexes: the myenteric plexus and the submucosal plexus. Together, they are called the enteric nervous system. The myenteric plexus lies within the intestinal wall between the two muscular layers. It controls the motor activity of the wall and the sphincters that separate the parts of the digestive tract and is needed for effective peristalsis. The submucosal plexus controls the local segmental responses, such as secretion, absorption, and contraction. Endocrine cells scattered in the epithelial walls of the stomach and small intestine secrete the hormones that control the digestive system. Contractility of the wall of the digestive system is determined by the internal concentration of calcium ions in the smooth muscle cells of the lining.[69] Receptors for the two plexuses, along with the parasympathetic and sympathetic innervation, provide the neural support for the GI reflexes, which respond to the following conditions: stretch of the wall, concentration of the chyme, acidity of the chyme, and presence of specific organic digestive byproducts.[4] Secretions within the GI tract are therefore under hormonal, central, and local nervous system control.

Control of the GI tract can be divided into three phases: cephalic, gastric, and intestinal. These phases are named for where the initial stimulus occurs, not for where the reflex occurs. The first phase begins even before the food reaches the stomach, when the sight, smell, taste, and texture of the food and the emotional state of the person eating trigger the secretion of pepsinogen, the precursor of pepsin, an enzyme that digests protein. Next, gastrin is released in response to local vagal reflexes, which stimulates gastric acid secretion. The amount of acid secreted by the stomach is balanced by the absorptive and digestive abilities of the small intestines. Finally, secretin, cholecystokinin, and glucose-dependent insulinotropic peptide are secreted during the intestinal phase. The three phases occur in temporal order only at the beginning of a meal. Thereafter, the reflexes may occur simultaneously during ingestion and absorption.

Structural Changes Across the Life Span

The structures that support ventilation/respiration, ingestion, digestion, and absorption grow over the course of the life span. These structural changes support the function of these three processes. For example, an infant goes from using one tube for both breathing and eating to using two tubes: the trachea for breathing and the esophagus for eating. The relationship between structure and function becomes apparent when examining the oropharyngeal and digestive systems. The oropharyngeal anatomy of the newborn is significantly different from that of an adult. The infant's lower jaw is retracted and smaller (Figure 11-5). The oral cavity is small, with the tongue occupying all of the space and being in proximity to the roof and floor. The chubby-cheeked appearance of the newborn is due to the presence of fat pads. These pads make sucking easier.

Up until 3 to 4 months, the child's epiglottis and soft palate are approximated. The larynx is elevated and in proximity to the base of the tongue. With growth, the posterior part of the tongue will descend with the larynx to become a segment of the front wall of the pharynx. The oral cavity enlarges with growth, and the elongation of the neck and pharynx changes the relationship of the tongue, larynx, and epiglottis.

The digestive system also begins in a more elevated location in the infant than the adult. The ends of the esophagus are two vertebral levels higher in the infant than in the adult. The capacity of the stomach increases from 30 mL at birth to 90 mL approximately 2 weeks later. At 1 year, the capacity increases further to 500 mL and finally to 1500 mL in adulthood.[6] The digestive system descends with growth like the respiratory system.

Length of the small intestines increases from infancy to puberty. Also because of the size of the infant pelvis, only a small amount of the intestines extend into the pelvis. In the adult, the majority of the small intestine and even some of the stomach may be in the pelvic region. Structurally, the wall of the intestines is thin and only with age develops the musculature needed for peristalsis. "Villi continue to form in the small intestine until puberty."[6]

Five percent of the infant's body weight is due to the relatively large size of the liver, an organ of digestion. The liver has many important functions during intrauterine life, one of which is producing many types of blood cells. At adulthood, the liver will take up only 2.5% of the body's weight.

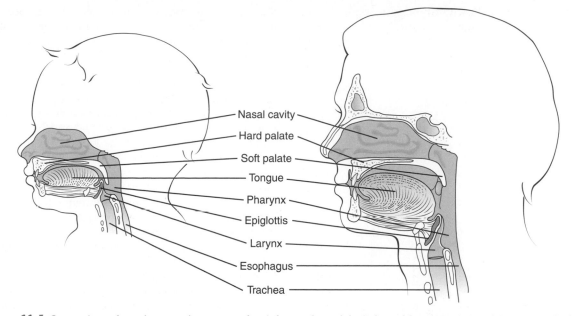

Figure 11-5 Comparison of oropharyngeal anatomy of an infant and an adult. (Adapted from Morris SE, Klein MD: *Pre-feeding skills*, Tucson, 1987, Therapy Skill Builders, p 8.)

Function Across the Life Span

Prenatal The earliest oral reflex in utero is the gag reflex, which is present at 17 weeks of gestation. Other oral reflexes, such as rooting and suck-swallow, are present by 28 weeks of gestation. The fetus has been shown to suck its thumb as well as to take in amniotic fluid. The oral reflexes are elicited by touch or pressure and can be considered survival reflexes because their purpose is to obtain nutrition and to protect the fetus from swallowing unwanted material.

The gut starts to develop around 4 weeks of gestation, the myenteric plexus at around 8 to 9 weeks, followed a few weeks later by the submucosal plexus.[70] Buchan and colleagues[71] demonstrated the presence of regulatory gut peptides or hormones as early as 8 to 10 weeks after conception. These protein complexes regulate the activity of the digestive system. Aynsley-Green[72] documented a large number of gut hormones and metabolites in the fetal and maternal circulations at 18 to 21 weeks of gestation and postulated that these circulating peptides facilitate the development of the fetal lung and GI tract. By the fifth month of gestation, the fetus shows peristaltic movements within the GI tract, and the liver is secreting bile. GI tract function approaches that of a normal newborn by 6 to 7 months of gestation.[4] Meconium, from the unabsorbed amniotic fluid and excretory byproducts, is continually formed and excreted in small amounts.

All of these developments appear necessary to prepare the fetus to independently seek, find, and assimilate food efficiently after birth.

Infancy Through Childhood The fetus uses glucose, which is primarily obtained from the mother's blood. Once the umbilical cord is cut, the infant must regulate her own blood glucose level. Because the infant has a very limited amount of stored glucose, the supply is quickly depleted. Because the infant's liver is not functionally adequate at birth, stored fats and proteins must be used as energy sources until feeding can begin.

The introduction of food produces changes in the digestive system and endocrine system that allow efficient use of food. Levels of blood glucose and plasma insulin increase after the first enteral or by-mouth feeding. Within days, the secretion of digestive hormones has fostered growth of the gastric mucosa. Their secretion also fosters the development of gastric motility and secretion, pancreatic endocrine function, and liver metabolism. Typically, term infants have low acid output initially, which becomes normal within several days.[73] Regulation of postnatal nutritional adaptation is schematically represented in Figure 11-6.

Human milk is the optimal nutritional source of calcium during the first year of life.[74] Human milk also contributes trophic factors that aid digestive system maturation and immunoglobulins that reduce the risk of infection.[75] Evidence has been found that prolactin

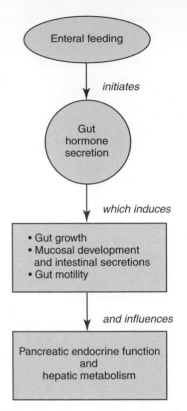

Figure 11-6 Hypothesis to explain regulation of postnatal nutritional adaptation. (Redrawn from Aynsley-Green A: Metabolic and endocrine interrelations in the human fetus and neonate, *Am J Clin Nutr* 41:399-417, 1985.)

in maternal milk helps regulate the newborn's immune system, lending further support to the benefits of breast-feeding.[76] The need for calcium to promote bone growth and metabolism in infants has led manufacturers of infant formulas to increase the concentration of calcium in their formulas to match the levels received in human milk.

Proteins in human milk influence the newborn's gut immune system.[77] The gut of the newborn needs to be colonized by specific gut flora. The maternal environment plays a role in the development and maturation of the infant's gut. Babies born by cesarean section had different gut bacteria than those born vaginally.[78] An infant's GI tract is sterile at birth. The GI tract becomes populated by bacteria during the birth process. Penders and associates[79] noted that infants born vaginally at term and who were only breast-fed had the most beneficial gut microbiota.

Ingestion   Ingesting food progresses from being reflexive at birth to being voluntary at 2 to 5 months of age. At this time, a voluntary sucking pattern is established

that allows the tongue to stroke the food source. In the process of obtaining food, the tongue's shape is modified. This change also prepares the tongue for articulating specific speech sounds and is an example of feeding as preparation for speech. As oral control improves, the lips can close around a spoon to remove food and the infant learns to drink liquids from a cup. Again, this oral motor skill carries over into the ability to produce closed mouth sounds such as "*p*," "*b*," and "*m*."

The elevated position of the larynx and the space occupied by the tongue allow the infant to breathe while feeding. Liquid flows down either side of the epiglottis and the uvula that are in contact while swallowing. Thus the airway is protected anatomically during swallowing. When the one-tube system of eating and breathing is replaced with the adult two-tube system, the valving at the epiglottis is needed to protect the airway during swallowing.

Between 5 and 8 months of age, oral motor behavior shifts from sucking to chewing. This transition is supported by growth changes in the skull and mandible, peripheral afferent input, neural maturation, and motor learning. The pharynx has elongated, and the larynx has descended providing more space in the oral cavity. The soft palate is no longer in contact with the epiglottis. The infant is maintaining an erect sitting posture for a short period of time. For further discussion of oral motor development, the reader is referred to Morris and Klein[80] and Delaney and Arvedson.[81]

The infant is ready to transition to spoon feeding and for the introduction of solid food around the age of 6 months. The infant is no longer able to obtain sufficient amounts of iron from human or formula milk. The digestive system seems unprepared for solid food until 4 to 6 months. The kidney also requires at least 4 months to mature to the point of being able to handle the higher osmolar load of solid foods. Adequate nutrition in the form of solid food allows infants to triple their birth weight by 1 year of age and quadruple it by age 2. Foods should be introduced one at a time to detect potential allergies.[82]

Dental Development   Dental development begins during gestation and continues through adolescence. The tooth buds of the deciduous or baby teeth form at 6 weeks of gestation. Some tooth buds of permanent teeth are formed before birth, whereas others are not developed until after birth. Healthy teeth are important to our nutrition, general health, and appearance. The timing of tooth eruption varies greatly among infants, although there is a set sequence. The average infant's first tooth appears at about 6 months; the remainder of the 20 baby teeth are in place by 2½ years of age. Typically, the first permanent tooth erupts at 6 years, with the third molars or wisdom teeth appearing last at 17 years. The replacement of the baby teeth by the 32 permanent ones is gradual and can span up to 11 years. Dental age can supplement bone age as a way to estimate skeletal maturity.

Digestion/Absorption Digestion begins in the mouth, where the food is chewed and first exposed to saliva. In the absence of food, the mouth is kept moist by saliva. Salivation is triggered by chemoreceptors. The salivary glands are the most productive exocrine glands in the body given their size. After swallowing, digestion continues in the stomach, where chyme is produced. Chyme is partially digested food that is acidified by adding gastric acid. The amount of acid secreted into the stomach increases relative to the protein content of the meal. The final stage of digestion occurs in the small intestine, where food is maximally digested and absorbed. The pancreas and gallbladder supply organically specific digestive enzymes and bile to aid this process. The small intestine absorbs the nutrients, so that by the time material reaches the large intestine, the volume has been significantly reduced. Waste is stored temporarily until its bulk is sufficient for it to be moved on to the last segment of the GI tract, the rectum, where, after distention, defecation is initiated.

Motility in the small intestines initially takes place by segmentation that involves a stationary contraction and relaxation of segments of the intestinal wall. During this process, there is ongoing division and subdivision of the intestinal contents, allowing the mixing of the chyme. This mixing brings the chyme into contact with the intestinal wall. Motility is affected by the enteric nervous system, hormones, and our emotional state. After most of the meal is absorbed, segmentation is replaced by peristalsis. Peristalsis is a contraction of a segment of the digestive tract that moves undigested content to the large intestines. Slower contractions of the smooth muscle wall of the large intestine mean that content remains for a longer period of time until sufficient bulk is achieved. Mass movements occur three or four times a day in the large intestines. These intense contractions occur generally after a meal and spread to the rectum. If the time is not right for defecation, we inhibit the relaxation of the external sphincter, and reverse peristalsis sends the fecal mass back to the colon.

Older Adulthood

Dentition Good oral hygiene and a regular schedule of preventive care will help us keep our teeth for our entire life span. However, oral tissues undergo substantial changes with age. Teeth can be lost because of deterioration in periodontal structures such as the gums, bones of the jaw, and membranes around the teeth. In the past, many older adults did not take proper care of their teeth, which resulted in tooth loss. Today, more older adults are retaining their teeth into advanced age.[83,84] Shay[83] states that one third of those over 65 years have no teeth. Ninety percent of those without teeth wear dentures. Although dentures can provide a more positive self-image, they may be a source of discomfort so there may continue to be nutritional concerns for the older adult. Oral health and oropharyngeal function can be maintained throughout an individual's life by using preventive dentistry.[83]

Digestion/Absorption Physiological changes in the digestive system related to aging are less obvious than in other systems. There are minor changes in all phases of digestion, but they appear to have a relatively small impact on function. A decrease in the amount of saliva produced was once thought to be a normal consequence of aging. Indeed, dry mouth is a common complaint by older adults, but it is not a normal change of aging.[83] Rather, it is a common side effect of medication. Saliva is important for taste and maintenance of oral health. Although the amount of saliva produced by the parotid gland does not decline with age, there are conflicting reports about declines in the output from other salivary glands. Older adults need to chew their food more to achieve the desired degree of maceration before swallowing. The sequence of swallowing, especially the oral and pharyngeal phases, takes longer in the older adult but again with no apparent functional consequences unless the person has a neuromuscular disease.

Many community-dwelling older adults have a calorie intake below the recommended dietary allowance. Protein is less easily digested because of a decline in gastric acid production, an approximate 25% loss by the age of 60.[85] Daily protein requirements for an older person are 0.8 g/kg of body weight.[86] Carbohydrates are also not as well metabolized as one ages. Aging individuals have an increase in fasting glucose concentration. There is also a decrease in insulin sensitivity with aging. The interplay of these two occurrences explains the abnormal glucose metabolism demonstrated by older adults.[87] Blood glucose levels may rise to the point at which the older adult develops diabetes, but this is not a normal consequence of aging. Adult-onset diabetes is a disease related to genetics and obesity.

Despite some structural changes in the villi of the small intestines with age, absorption remains functional for macronutrients such as fat, protein, sodium, and potassium. The aging GI tract is less efficient in absorbing vitamin B_{12}, vitamin D, and calcium.[88] Vitamin B_{12} deficiency can cause memory impairment, dementia, and balance and gait problems.[86] A recent review states that the lack of absorption of vitamin B_{12} may only be seen in older adults who do not have sufficient stomach acid to access the B_{12}.[89] Vitamin D and calcium are important for bone integrity. Alterations in calcium absorption in the intestine are related to bone loss and osteoporosis (see Chapter 6). Calcium supplements are commonly prescribed. There also appears to be a significant vitamin D inadequacy in this population.[90] New recommended dietary allowances have been proposed for vitamin D.[91] Nutrition requirements in the aging population continue to be updated as new research becomes available.

Fat is digested within the small intestines through the action of bile secreted by the liver. The liver shows definite anatomical changes with age, but because of its large margin of safety, none of these structural changes affects the production and secretion of bile; therefore, intestinal function, with regard to the digestion of fat, remains essentially unchanged. However, on a microscopic level there is a decrease in smooth endoplasmic reticulum (ER) and fewer mitochondria. Because the liver plays a pivotal role in the metabolism of many drugs, the decrease in the ER causes a marked decline in the first phase of drug metabolism.[92] Older men are more affected by this decline than older women. During the first phase of drug metabolism, the original compound is transformed by some chemical process such as hydrolysis or reduction. Aging appears to have less of an effect on the second phase of drug metabolism.[89] During the second phase of drug metabolism, the original compound or the resultant product of phase I metabolism is conjugated. Conjugation involves coupling the original compound or the resultant product of phase 1 metabolism with some endogenous substance.

Elimination

The fourth vital function is elimination. Elimination includes defecation of solid waste, which is an extension of digestion, and micturition, which is the excretion of liquid waste from the urinary system.

Defecation

Control Mechanisms Spinal level reflexes coordinate contraction of the colon and rectum to expel feces. These autonomic reflexes are mediated by the parasympathetic system and involve sacral cord segments S2-S4. These segments may be spared in a patient with an incomplete spinal cord lesion, allowing bowel control. The exit route for feces, the anus, is usually kept closed by contraction of the internal anal sphincter. This sphincter is made of smooth muscle, whereas the external anal sphincter is made of skeletal muscle and thus is under voluntary control. Mass movement

of fecal material distends the rectal wall and initiates the defecation reflex. The defecation reflex consists of contraction of the rectum and external anal sphincter, relaxation of the internal sphincter, and increased peristalsis in the colon. After sufficient pressure builds up, the external sphincter reflexively relaxes and allows the stool to be passed.

Childhood Children are usually ready to control defecation around the age of 2 years, but the age is highly variable. The following cues are helpful to determine a child's readiness to be toilet trained: regular bowel movements, the ability to sit alone well, the ability to recognize the need for a bowel movement, and the desire to cooperate with an adult, as seen when releasing an object on request. Guidelines for assessing toilet training readiness by the American Academy of Pediatrics recommend a child-oriented approach.[93]

Older Adulthood Despite what television commercials imply about an older adult's need for laxatives, there is no evidence for decreased motility in the large intestine. Autonomic nervous system responses to stress can aggravate GI function by decreasing salivary and gastric secretions. Other factors, such as decreased physical activity, decreased fluid or fiber intake, and living alone, often lead to, or compound, functional constipation. Unsound dietary practice, including decreased caloric and water intake, in addition to habitual use of laxatives, is far more likely to create constipation than any structural or physiological age-related change.

The Valsalva maneuver assists defecation but can be dangerous in older individuals with cardiovascular disease, especially if they are constipated. Along with the rise in abdominal pressure from bearing down, intrathoracic pressure rises, causing a rise in blood pressure and a decrease in the venous return to the heart.

Fecal continence requires good sphincter control. Although there is some evidence that sclerosis of the internal anal sphincter occurs with age, the majority of individuals with fecal incontinence do not demonstrate the associated decline in anal canal pressure. Rather, these individuals are likely to have some type of neurological disease.

Micturition

The process of micturition is far more complex than defecation. The urinary system is made up of two kidneys, two ureters, a bladder, and a urethra. The kidneys have been described as 1 million functional units held together by connective tissue. Normal function depends on circulatory, endocrine, and nervous system interaction. The kidneys are the filtering system for the body, and they produce urine as the byproduct of filtering the plasma. The purpose of the kidneys is to maintain water and electrolyte balance within the body and to regulate plasma concentration. Homeostasis of our internal environment is achieved via the multiple processes of filtration, absorption, and secretion.

Structural changes occur over the first year of life as the kidneys become fully functional. Their growth corresponds to that of the body as a whole during this period of development as evidenced by the organs' weight doubling in 6 months and tripling by the end of the first year.[6] Renal tubules continue to form, and glomeruli enlarge. Most importantly, the epithelial layer of cells in the capsule of the glomeruli changes from being cuboidal to flat, allowing better filtration after the first year. As with many structures in the body, work demand induces a change in the size of the kidneys.

The bladder is located in the abdominal cavity during infancy and moves into the pelvis only as that structure expands. The characteristic pyramidal shape of the bladder is achieved by the age of 6 years, at which time the bladder occupies its adult position. The ureters lengthen to accommodate the gradual change in position.[6] As with defecation, micturition depends on the physical control of sphincters, which is achieved somewhere between 18 and 24 months of age.

Control Mechanisms Arterial blood pressure is controlled by the kidney. Too much fluid causes the pressure to rise, too little fluid causes the pressure to drop. The two determinants of arterial blood pressure are the volume of renal output and the amount of salt and water in the system. The kidneys control renal output by changing the extracellular fluid volume. An increase in extracellular fluid increases blood volume and ultimately cardiac output, which increases arterial pressure. This increase in arterial pressure is accomplished by controlling the amount of salt in the system, which is the main determinant of the amount of extracellular fluid.

As part of the endocrine system, the kidneys have an additional means of controlling arterial pressure. The renin-angiotensin system is a more powerful and complex mechanism than the one previously described. After a drop in blood pressure, the kidneys release renin, which enzymatically causes the release of angiotensin I. Within seconds, angiotensin I is converted by an enzyme in the lungs to angiotensin II. The latter produces systemic vasoconstriction and decreased excretion of salt and water by the kidney. Angiotensin can secondarily cause fluid retention by stimulating the adrenal gland to secrete aldosterone. The renin-angiotensin system maintains normal arterial blood pressure despite wide fluctuations in salt intake. The system takes about 20 minutes to become fully active.

Function Across the Life Span

Prenatal The human embryo develops three different sets of kidneys from mesoderm.[5] The first set is rudimentary and nonfunctional. The second set does function for a short time in utero but is replaced by a third and final set of permanent kidneys, which develop in the early part of the fifth week of gestation and are capable of producing urine 6 weeks later. The collecting tubules and ducts are of endodermal origin, as is the urinary bladder. Urine formation continues throughout fetal life and makes up a large part of the amniotic fluid. Because the placenta removes the waste products from the fetus, the kidneys do not need to function until after birth. However, because the mature fetus swallows amniotic fluid daily that is absorbed by the fetal intestines, the fetal kidneys do play a role in regulating amniotic fluid volume. The permanent kidneys ascend to their adult position around the ninth week of gestation.[5]

Infancy Through Childhood The infant's kidney function is adequate but immature for the first few weeks of life. The rate of fluid intake and output in the infant is seven times that of the adult. The infant cannot readily adjust to large changes in fluid loads; any undue loss of water and solutes from fever, vomiting, and diarrhea can be life threatening. Renal function changes rapidly in response to increased blood flow at birth and steadily increasing metabolic demands. By 4 months of age, the kidneys have developed sufficiently to manage solid foods that create a higher osmolar demand than milk.[94] Renal function improves greatly by 6 months; mature function of sphincters is possible between 18 months and 2 years of age. The kidneys enlarge after birth due to hypertrophy of the nephrons. In infants and children, the bladder occupies space within the abdomen. At 6 years, the bladder is still not fully contained in the pelvis; only after puberty is the bladder considered a pelvic organ.

Maturation of bladder function occurs by 4 years of age.[95] During infancy, the bladder wall responds to a small amount of urine, contracting to expel its contents. Expulsion is automatic. From 18 months to 2½ years of age, the child develops an awareness of having to void and can retain urine for short periods before voiding. The daily urine volume gradually increases, and as a child gains control over the diaphragm and the abdominal and perineal muscles, she learns to initiate voiding. Bladder control continues to improve as she retains larger volumes of urine for longer periods. Mature bladder control is finally achieved between 2½ and 4½ years of age. A child may first sleep through the night dry when the bladder can retain about 10 to 12 oz (300 to 360 mL) of urine. This is not quite double the amount normally voided during the day. There are gender differences in toileting. A boy's ability to gain bladder control appears to be related to maturation of sleep cycles, that is, being able to wake up in time to void.[96] More boys are prone to nocturnal enuresis (bedwetting).[97] The fact that boys take longer to train than girls, by about 6 months, may be related to their anatomy and need to adopt a separate posture for elimination. Although bowel maturation precedes bladder maturation, bladder control is attained about 6 months before bowel control in toddlers. Brazelton and colleagues[96] reported that most toddlers are completely trained at 2 to 3 years of age.

Toilet training can be a stressful time for both toddler and parents. Enuresis and encopresis do not occur in the majority of children, but the loss of bladder and bowel control can be disturbing to the child and parent. Encopresis is fecal incontinence. Seeking the advice of the pediatrician in these cases is always a good idea.

The kidneys contribute to homeostasis by expelling waste products in the form of urine and by regulating the balance of fluid and electrolytes in the body. One measure of kidney function and health status is how quickly certain substances, such as creatinine, are cleared from the body. Normal creatinine clearance averages 124 mL/min in men. The kidneys also secrete substances that are part of the hormonal system, including erythropoietin, renin, and active forms of vitamin D.[4] Renin is synthesized and stored in the kidneys and is important in the control of blood pressure.

Older Adulthood   Renal function declines with age; older adults have 40% of normal adult capacity to clear creatinine from the body.[98] Gross anatomical changes occur, with loss of nephrons and renal mass and thickening of membranes. Physiologically, the surface area for filtration decreases. Renal blood flow decreases with age, as does the glomerular filtration rate. The endocrine functions of the kidneys also change with age. The amount of renin declines, which may be why the ability to conserve salt and water diminishes with age. A decrease in erythropoietin, the hormone secreted by the kidney to stimulate red blood cell production, may contribute to anemia. The ability to concentrate urine is lessened, and the diurnal rhythm of urine production is lost because of age-related changes in the renal tubules. These tubular changes may significantly affect the ability of older adults to benefit from medication. An adult dose may have an adverse rather than a beneficial effect because of the lower excretion rate in an individual.

The smooth muscular wall and elastic tissue of the bladder are replaced by noncontractile connective tissue as a result of aging. The person older than 65 years will experience the need to void earlier due to a reduction in the amount the bladder can store. Recognition of the need to void may occur closer to the bladder's capacity, failing to provide sufficient warning and necessitating a dash to the restroom. Weakening of the bladder and pelvic floor muscles prevents its complete emptying and may lead to *stress incontinence,* defined as a loss of urine associated with laughing, coughing, or lifting. Stress incontinence is primarily a problem of reduced urethral resistance. *Urge incontinence* is often related to prostate disease. The loss of self-esteem related to bladder dysfunction in the older adult is significant. Additional types of urinary incontinence are listed in Table 11-3.

Table 11-3

Types of Urinary Incontinence and Associated Symptoms and Etiologies

Type of Urinary Incontinence	Common Symptoms	Common Causes
Stress	Leakage with physical activities that increase abdominal pressure	Sphincteric dysfunction Urethral hypermobility Radical prostatectomy
Urge	Urgency, frequency, nocturia, urine leakage before reaching toilet	Detrusor overactivity Neurological disorder Spinal cord injury
Overflow	Frequent small-volume leaks often not associated with activity	Detrusor failure Neurological disorders Spinal cord injury
Functional	Leakage symptoms are variable	Mobility impairment Cognitive impairment
Mixed	Leakage symptoms are variable	Cause is variable

From Griebling TL: Urinary incontinence in the elderly, *Clin Geriatr Med* 25:445-457, 2009.

CLINICAL IMPLICATIONS Box 11-2

Urinary Incontinence and Age

Urinary incontinence (UI) is a common condition, but it should not be viewed as an inevitable consequence of aging. Urinary incontinence is an involuntary loss of urine. Twenty-five percent to 30% of all adults will experience UI at some time in their lives. However, the incidence and prevalence of UI are higher in older adults than in younger adults.[106] There are several types of UI seen in older adults, which are listed in Table 11-3. The most common types of urinary incontinence are designated as stress and urge incontinence. Increased intra-abdominal pressure is associated with stress incontinence, which may be caused by sneering, laughing, or physical activity. Urge incontinence is linked to detrusor contractions and instability, and it is manifested by an abrupt, overwhelming need to void.

Urinary incontinence is a social and a hygiene problem, which has tremendous impact on a person's health-related quality of life. UI has been linked to depression and functional disability. Older adults with UI are at greater risk for falls than those older adults who do not have UI.[107] Both men and women exhibit urinary incontinence, but women appear to be twice as likely to be affected. This may be related to the added stress of pregnancy on the efficacy of the pelvic floor muscles and to the loss of estrogen at menopause. For more information, the reader is referred to Griebling,[106] DuBeau,[108] or Pauls.[109]

Urinary incontinence:
- Is a prevalent and costly health condition
- Significantly affects quality of life
- Affects both women and men
- Is not a natural consequence of aging
- Is more likely to be experienced by the oldest-old

Risk factors:
- Increased age
- Higher than normal body mass index
- Presence of chronic disease, such as diabetes or chronic obstructive pulmonary disease
- History of having had a hysterectomy

Prevention and intervention:
- Bladder training
- Timed voiding
- Kegel exercises
- Pelvic floor muscle exercises
- Use of anticipatory contraction of pelvic muscles before change of position, such as sit to stand

The prevalence of urinary incontinence has been estimated at 15% to 30% in women. The prevalence is less in men. Many older women seem to expect some degree of incontinence to occur as a result of aging. Therefore, it is important to teach Kegel exercises to prevent stress incontinence. Urinary incontinence is not, however, inevitable (Clinical Implications Box 11-2: Urinary Incontinence and Age).

SUMMARY

All of the vital functions depend on an adequate blood supply to deliver the necessary nutrients to the organs involved. The skeletal system provides the frame on which the muscles of mastication, ventilation, digestion, and elimination work. The autonomic nervous system and the endocrine system play a significant role in maintaining homeostasis. Ventilation-respiration and sleep/wakefulness and ingestion are cyclical activities that conform to neural control mechanisms based on oscillations. Developmentally, intrinsic pacemakers for these repetitive functions buy time until other structures and the systems they serve mature. Vital functions that do not appear to have such neural control, such as digestion, absorption, and elimination, do exhibit cyclical function and require precise neural coordination demonstrated by the GI nervous system, which has as many neurons as the spinal cord. The ability to maintain a fixed level of performance allows each of us to adapt to a fluctuating environment.

The environment can and does influence the adaptation of vital functions to changing internal and external demands. Humans are motivated to preserve life and to satisfy the basic drives for air, food, and water. Possibly because these functions are vital, the age-related changes in them do not often result in significant or life-threatening effects. No one system of the body works entirely without the other. If one system malfunctions, it will affect all the others, in some way, at some time, and eventually lead to either adaptation or failure.

REFERENCES

1. Moore RY: A clock for all ages, *Science* 284:2102–2103, 1999.
2. Rivkees SA: Developing circadian rhythmicity: basic and clinical aspects, *Pediatr Endocrinol* 44:467–487, 1997.
3. Iverson S, Iverson L, Saper CB: The autonomic nervous system and the hypothalamus. In Kandel ER, Schwartz JH, Jessell TM, editors: *Principles of neuroscience*, ed 4, New York, 2000, McGraw-Hill, pp 960–981.
4. Guyton AC, Hall JE: *Textbook of medical physiology*, ed 11, Philadelphia, 2006, WB Saunders.
5. Moore KL, Persaud TVN: *Before we are born: essentials of embryology and birth defects*, Philadelphia, 2003, WB Saunders.
6. Sinclair D, Dangerfield P: *Human growth after birth*, ed 6, New York, 1998, Oxford University Press.
7. Carlson BM: *Human embryology and developmental biology*, ed 4, Philadelphia, 2009, Mosby Elsevier.
8. Johnson LR, editor: *Essential medical physiology*, ed 3, San Diego, 2003, Academic Press.
9. Cetin I, Alvino G: Intrauterine growth restriction: implications for placental metabolism and transport. A review, *Placenta* 30(Suppl A):S77–S82, 2009.
10. Anderson SE, Dallal GE, Must A: Relative weight and race influence on average age at menarche: results from two nationally representative surveys of US girls studied 25 years apart, *Pediatrics* 111(4 pt 1):844–850, 2003.
11. Santrock JW: *Child development*, ed 4, New York, 1998, McGraw-Hill.
12. Smith M: Gynecologic disorders. In Duthie EH, Katz PR, editors: *Practice of geriatrics*, Philadelphia, 1998, WB Saunders, pp 524–534.
13. Rao SS, Singh M, Parkar M, et al: Health maintenance for postmenopausal women, *Am Fam Physician* 78(5):583–591, 593–594, 2008.
14. Harman SM, Metter EJ, Tobin JD, et al: Longitudinal effects of aging on serum total and free testosterone levels in healthy men. Baltimore longitudinal study of aging, *J Clin Endocrinol Metab* 86:724–731, 2001.
15. Kohler TS, Kim J, Feia K, et al: Prevalence of androgen deficiency in men with erectile dysfunction, *Urology* 71:693–697, 2008.
16. Purushothaman R, Morley JE: Endocrinology in the aged. In Gass GH, Kaplan HM, editors: *Handbook of endocrinology*, ed 2, Boca Raton, Fla, 1996, CRC Press, pp 241–260.
17. Davis PJ, Davis FB, Leinung MC: Endocrine disorders. In Duthie EH, Katz PR, Malone ML, editors: *Practice of geriatrics*, ed 4, Philadelphia, 2007, Saunders Elsevier, pp 445–664.
18. Goldstein RB: Ultrasound evaluation of the fetal thorax. In Callen PW, editor: *Ultrasonography in obstetrics and gynecology*, ed 3, Philadelphia, 1994, WB Saunders, pp 426–455.
19. Fox HE, Steinbrecher M, Pessel D, et al: Maternal ethanol ingestion and the occurrence of human fetal breathing movements, *Am J Obstet Gynecol* 132:354–358, 1978.
20. Adkins HV: Improvement of breathing ability in children with respiratory muscle paralysis, *Phys Ther* 48:577–581, 1968.
21. Crapo RO, Jensen RL, Berlin SL: PaO_2 in healthy subjects at 1500 m altitude are well predicted by meta-analysis, *Chest* 100:96S, 1991.
22. Nilsson-Ehle H, Jagenburg RJ, Landahl S, et al: Decline of blood hemoglobin in the aged: a longitudinal study of an urban Swedish population from age 70–81, *Br J Haematol* 71:437–442, 1989.
23. Deley G, Kervio G, Van Hoecke J, et al: Effects of a one-year exercise training program in adults over 70 years old: a study with a control group, *Aging Clin Exp Res* 19(4):310–315, 2007.
24. Rasch B, Born J: Reactivation and consolidation of memory during sleep, *Curr Dir Psychol Sci* 17(3):188–192, 2008.
25. Fischer S, Wilhelm I, Born J: Developmental differences in sleep's role for implicit off-line learning: comparing children with adults, *J Cogn Neurosci* 19(2):214–227, 2007.
26. McClelland JL, McNaughton BL, O'Reilly RC: Why there are complementary learning systems in the hippocampus and neocortex: insights from the successes and failures of connectionist models of learning and memory, *Psychol Rev* 102:419–457, 1995.
27. Walker MP: The role of sleep in cognition and emotion, *Ann N Y Acad Sci* 1156:168–197, 2009.
28. Chicurel M: Mutant gene speeds up the human clock, *Science* 291:226–227, 2001.
29. Milani-Comparetti A: The neurophysiological and clinical implications of studies on fetal motor behavior, *Semin Perinatol* 5:183–189, 1981.
30. Rosen MG, Scibetta JJ, Chik L, et al: An approach to the study of brain damage: the principles of fetal EEG, *Am J Obstet Gynecol* 115:37–47, 1973.
31. Peirano P, Algarin C, Uauy R: Sleep-wake states and their regulatory mechanisms throughout early human development, *J Pediatr* 143(Suppl 4):S70–S79, 2003.
32. Waldhauser F, Ehrhart B, Forster E: Clinical aspects of the melatonin action: impact of development, aging and puberty, involvement of melatonin in psychiatric disease and importance of neuroimmunoendocrine interactions, *Experientia* 49:671–681, 1993.
33. Novosad C, Freudigman K, Thoman EB: Sleep patterns in newborns and temperament at eight months: a preliminary study, *J Dev Behav Pediatr* 20:99–105, 1999.
34. Coons S, Guilleminault C: Development of consolidated sleep and wakeful periods in relation to the day/night cycle in infancy, *Dev Med Child Neurol* 26:169–176, 1984.
35. Markov D, Goldman M: Normal sleep and circadian rhythms: neurobiologic mechanisms underlying sleep and wakefulness, *Psychiatr Clin North Am* 29:841–853, 2006.
36. Gomez RL, Bootzin RR, Nadel L: Naps promote abstraction in language-learning infants, *Psychol Sci* 17:670–674, 2006.
37. Challamel MBJ: Development of sleep and wakefulness. In Meisami E, Timiras PS, editors: *Handbook of human growth and developmental biology, vol I, part B*, Boca Raton, Fla, 1988, CRC Press, pp 269–284.

38. Prechtl H: *The neurological examination of the full-term newborn infant*, ed 2, Philadelphia, 1977, JB Lippincott.

39. Kung HC, Hoyert DL, Xu JQ, et al: *E-stat deaths: preliminary data for 2005 health E-stats*, Hyattsville, Md, 2007, US Department of Health and Human Services, CDC.

40. Moon RY, Horne RSC, Hauck FR: Sudden infant death syndrome, *Lancet* 370:1578–1587, 2007.

41. Moon RY, Patel KM, Shaefer SJ: Sudden infant death syndrome in child care settings, *Pediatrics* 106(2 pt 1):295–300, 2000.

42. Corwin MJ, Lesko SM, Heeren T, et al: Secular changes in sleep position during infancy: 1995–1998, *Pediatrics* 111:52–60, 2003.

43. Mitchell EA, Bajanowski T, Brinkmann B, et al: Prone sleeping position increases the risk of SIDS in the day more than at night, *Acta Paediatr* 97:584–589, 2008.

44. Backhaus J, Hoeckesfeld R, Born J, et al: Immediate as well as delayed post learning sleep but not wakefulness enhances declarative memory consolidation in children, *Neurobiol Learn Mem* 89:76–80, 2008.

45. Dahl RE: Sleep, learning, and the developing brain: early-to-bed as a healthy and wise choice for school-aged children: comment on Fallone, et al, *Sleep* 28:1498–1499, 2005.

46. Buckhalt JA, El-Sheikh M, Keller P: Children's sleep and cognitive functioning: race and socioeconomic status as moderators of effects, *Child Dev* 78(1):213–231, 2007.

47. Wolfson AR, Carskadon MA: Sleep schedules and daytime functioning in adolescents, *Child Dev* 69:875–887, 1998.

48. Cavallo A: Melatonin and human puberty: current perspectives, *J Pineal Res* 15:115–121, 1993.

49. Keenan SA: Normal human sleep, *Respir Care Clin N Am* 5:319–331, 1999.

50. Allen R: Social factors associated with the amount of school week sleep lag for seniors in an early starting suburban high school, *Sleep Res* 21:114–119, 1992.

51. Wagner U, Gais S, Halder H, et al: Sleep inspires insight, *Nature* 427:352–355, 2004.

52. Nishida M, Pearsall J, Buckner RL, et al: REM sleep, prefrontal theta, and the consolidation of human emotional memory, *Cereb Cortex* 19(5):1158–1166, 2009.

53. Wagner U, Hallschmid M, Rasch BH, et al: Brief sleep after learning keeps emotional memories alive for years, *Biol Psychiatry* 60:788–790, 2006.

54. Neikrug AB, Ancoli-Isreal S: Sleep disorders in the older adult: a mini-review, *Gerontology* 181–189, 2009.

55. Backhaus J, Born J, Hoeckesfeld R, et al: Midlife decline in declarative memory consolidation is correlated with a decline in slow wave sleep, *Learn Mem* 14:336–341, 2007.

56. Foley D, Ancoli-Israel S, Britz P, et al: Sleep disturbances and chronic disease in older adults: results of the 2003 National Sleep Foundation Sleep in America Survey, *J Psychosom Res* 56:497–502, 2004.

57. Bundlie SR: Sleep imaging, *Geriatrics* 53(Suppl 1):541–543, 1998.

58. Ohayon MM, Carskadon MA, Guilleminault C, et al: Meta-analysis of quantitative sleep parameters from childhood to old age in healthy individuals: developing normative sleep values across the human life span, *Sleep* 27(7):1255–1277, 2004.

59. Dijk DF, Duffy JF, Riel E, et al: Ageing and the circadian and homeostatic regulation of human sleep during forced desynchrony of rest, melatonin and temperature rhythms, *J Physiol* 516(pt 2):611–627, 1999.

60. Norman D, Loredo JS: Obstructive sleep apnea in older adults, *Clin Geriatr Med* 24:151–165, 2008.

61. Ancoli-Israel S, Kripke DF, Mauber MR, et al: Sleep disordered breathing in community-dwelling elderly, *Sleep* 14:486–495, 1991.

62. Guilleminault C: Sleep and sleep disorders in the elderly. In Cassel S, Walsh B, editors: *Geriatric medicine*, New York, 1994, Springer-Verlag, pp 342–351.

63. Sapolsky RM, Krey LC, McEwen BS: The neuroendo-crinology of stress and aging: the glucocorticoid cascade hypothesis, *Endocr Rev* 17:284–289, 1996.

64. Imeri L, Opp MR: How (and why) the immune system makes us sleep, *Nat Rev* 10:199–210, 2009.

65. Miller AF: The neurobiology of swallowing and dysphagia, *Dev Dis Res Rev* 14:77–86, 2008.

66. Altaf MA, Sood MR: The nervous system and gastrointestinal function, *Dev Dis Res Rev* 14:87–95, 2008.

67. Broussard DL, Altshchuler SM: Central integration of swallow and airway-protective reflexes, *Am J Med* 108(Suppl 4a):62S–67S, 2000.

68. Barlow SM: Oral and respiratory control for preterm feeding, *Curr Opin Otolaryngol Head Neck Surg* 17(3):179–186, 2009.

69. Hirst GDS: A calcium window to the gut, *Nature* 399:16–17, 1999.

70. Wallace AS, Burns AJ: Development of the enteric nervous system, smooth muscle and interstitial cells of Cajal in the human gastrointestinal tract, *Cell Tissue Res* 319:367–382, 2005.

71. Buchan AMF, Bryant MG, Polak JM, et al: Development of regulatory peptides in the human fetal intestine. In Bloom SR, Polak JM, editors: *Gut hormones*, London, 1981, Churchill Livingstone, pp 119–126.

72. Aynsley-Green A: Metabolic and endocrine interrelations in the human fetus and neonate, *Am J Clin Nutr* 41:399–417, 1985.

73. Marciano T, Wershil BK: The ontogeny and developmental physiology of gastric acid secretion, *Curr Gastroenterol Rep* 9:479–481, 2007.

74. American Academy of Pediatrics: Breastfeeding and the use of human milk, *Pediatrics* 115:496–506, 2005.

75. Werk LN, Alpert JJ: Solid feeding guidelines, *Lancet* 352:1569–1570, 1998.

76. Ellis LA, Mastro AM, Picciano MF: Do milk-borne cytokines and hormones influence neonatal immune cell function? *J Nutr* 127:985S–988S, 1997.

77. Xanthou M: Immune protection of human milk, *Biol Neonat* 74:121–133, 1998.

78. Adlerberth I, Lindberg E, Aberg N, et al: Reduced enterobacterial and increased staphylococcal colonization of the infantile bowel: an effect of hygienic lifestyle? *Pediatr Res* 59:96–101, 2006.

79. Penders J, Thijs C, VInk C, et al: Factors influencing the composition of the intestinal microbiota in early infancy, *Pediatrics* 118:511–521, 2006.

80. Morris SE, Klein MD: *Pre-feeding skills*, ed 2, Austin, Tex, 2000, Pro-Ed.

81. Delaney AL, Arvedson JC: Development of swallowing and feeding: prenatal through first year of life, *Dev Dis Res Rev* 14:105–117, 2008.

82. Samour PQ, King K: *Handbook of pediatric nutrition*, Sudbury, UK, 2006, Jones and Bartlett.

83. Shay K: Dental and oral disorders. In Duthie EH, Katz PR, Malone ML, editors: *Practice of geriatrics*, ed 4, Philadelphia, 2007, Saunders Elsevier, pp 547–561.

84. Ship JA: The influence of aging on oral health and consequences for taste and smell, *Physiol Behav* 66:209–215, 1999.

85. Whitbourne SK: *The aging individual: physical and psychological perspectives*, New York, 1996, Springer.

86. Abbasi A: Nutrition. In Duthie EH, Katz PR, editors: *Practice of geriatrics*, Philadelphia, 1998, WB Saunders, pp 145–158.

87. Scheen AJ: Diabetes mellitus in the elderly: insulin resistance and/or impaired insulin secretion? *Diabetes Metab* 31(special issue 2):5S27–5S34, 2005.

88. Russell RM: The aging process as a modifier of metabolism, *Am J Clin Nutr* 72 (Suppl 2):529S–532S, 2000.

89. Bhutto A, Morley JE: The clinical significance of gastrointestinal changes with aging, *Curr Opin Clin Nutr Metab Care* 11:651–660, 2008.

90. Hansen KE, Binkley N: Osteoporosis. In Duthy EH, Katz PR, Malone ML, editors: *Practice of geriatrics*, ed 4, Philadelphia, 2007, Saunders Elsevier, pp 231–243.

91. Hollis BW: Circulating 25-hydroxyvitamin D levels indicative of vitamin D sufficiency: implications for establishing a new effective dietary intake recommendation for vitamin D, *J Nutr* 135:317–322, 2005.

92. Cotreau MM, von Moltke LL, Greenblatt DJ: The influence of age and sex on the clearance of cytochrome P450 3A substrates, *Clin Pharmacokinet* 44:33–60, 2005.

93. American Academy of Pediatrics: Toilet training guidelines: parents - the role of the parents in toilet training, *Pediatrics* 103(6 pt 2):1362–1363, 1999.

94. Hendricks KM, Badruddin SH: Weaning recommendations: the scientific basis, *Nutr Rev* 50:125–133, 1992.

95. Berk LB, Friman PC: Epidemiologic aspects of toilet training, *Clin Pediatr (Bologna)* 29:278–281, 1990.

96. Brazelton TB, Christophersen ER, Frauman AC, et al: Instruction, timelines, and medical influences affecting toilet training, *Pediatrics* 103(6 pt 2):1353–1358, 1999.

97. Howe AC, Walker CE: Behavioral management of toilet training, enuresis, and encopresis, *Pediatr Clin North Am* 39:413–432, 1992.

98. Rowe JW, Andres RA, Tobin JD, et al: The effect of age on creatinine clearance in man, *J Gerontol* 31:155–163, 1976.

99. Mathews TJ, MacDorman MF: Infant mortality statistics from the 2003 period linked birth/infant death data set, *Natl Vital Stat Rep* 54(16):1–29, 2006.

100. Filiano JJ, Kinney HC: A perspective on neuropathologic findings in victims of the sudden infant death syndrome: the triple-risk model, *Biol Neonat* 65(3–4):194–197, 1994.

101. Kinney HC, Thach BT: The sudden infant death syndrome, *N Engl J Med* 361:795–805, 2009.

102. Kinney HC: Brainstem mechanisms underlying the sudden infant death syndrome: evidence from human pathologic studies, *Dev Psychobiol* 51:223–233, 2009.

103. American Academy of Pediatrics Task Force on Sudden Infant Death Syndrome: The changing concept of sudden infant death syndrome: diagnostic coding shifts, controversies regarding the sleeping environment, and new variables to consider in reducing risk, *Pediatrics* 116:1245–1255, 2005.

104. Kato I, Franco P, Groswasser J, et al: Incomplete arousal processes in infants who were victims of sudden death, *Am J Respir Crit Care Med* 168:1298–1303, 2003.

105. Rakesh S, Fifer WP, Myers MM: Identifying infants at risk for sudden infant death syndrome, *Curr Opin Pediatr* 19(2):145–149, 2007.

106. Griebling TL: Urinary incontinence in the elderly, *Clin Geriatr Med* 25:445–457, 2009.

107. Morris V, Wagg A: Lower urinary tract symptoms, incontinence and falls in elderly people: time for an intervention study, *Int J Clin Pract* 61:320–323, 2007.

108. DuBeau CE: Beyond the bladder: management of urinary incontinence in older women, *Clin Obstet Gynecol* 50(3):720–734, 2007.

109. Pauls J: Urinary incontinence and impairment of the pelvic floor in the older adult. In Guiccione AA, editor: *Geriatric physical therapy*, ed 2, St Louis, 2000, Mosby, pp 340–350.

CHAPTER 12

Posture and Balance

OBJECTIVES

After studying this chapter, the reader will be able to:

1. Define posture, balance, righting, and equilibrium.
2. Discuss the theoretical approaches to the study of posture and balance.
3. Differentiate between static and dynamic balance and between reactive and anticipatory postural control.
4. Describe posture and balance across the life span.

*P*osture is defined as the attitude or position of the body.[1] As such, being in a prone position and in a sitting position are both postures. When talking about someone's posture, most of us think of the alignment of body segments with respect to each other as well as with respect to the outside world. Posture has three functions. First, posture functions to maintain alignment of the body's segments in any position: supine, prone, sitting, quadruped, and standing. Second, posture can function to anticipate change to allow the body to engage in voluntary, goal-directed movements. When reaching or stepping, the body may make postural adjustments before, during, and after a movement. Third, posture may function to react to unexpected perturbations or disturbances in balance. This last function requires quick adaptation. Thus, posture is more than just maintaining a position of the body such as standing. Posture is active, whether it is sustaining an existing posture or moving from one posture to another.

Posture is determined and maintained by coordination of the various muscles that move the limbs, by proprioception, and by the sense of *balance*. Control of posture is balance. The term *postural control* is often used by physical therapists to describe balance; in this chapter, it is synonymous with balance. The goal of the postural control system is to attain a stable vertical posture of the head and trunk against the force of gravity. When this is accomplished, a base is provided for adequate reaching, sitting, standing, and walking.[2]

MODELS OF POSTURAL ORGANIZATION

Posture is organized at two different levels.[3] The first level is that of the body scheme. The body scheme includes posture as a reference to gravity, its anatomical relationships, and the concept of support. The postural body scheme represents the body's structures such as the head, trunk, and feet and the sensory receptors that provide information about gravity and the external environment.

The second level organizes postural control on the basis of the information from the representational level to form postural networks. The internal representation of the body segments involved in a posture makes up the representational level. The ways in which the various segments of the body relate to one another and how the relationships change based on sensory information are also represented within the *postural networks*. Posture is represented as a whole entity rather than as just its component parts.

Postural networks are formed during development. For example, as a child experiences sitting, postural muscles are activated. The large numbers of muscle combinations that are initially available are eventually narrowed to those combinations that are most functional. The process of selection forms networks and is illustrated in Figure 3-7. The neural basis for the development of these postural networks is discussed in Chapter 3.

Assaiante and Amblard[4] proposed an ontogenetic model for the sensorimotor organization of balance control. Their model is based on two functional principles. One principle assumes that the organization of balance depends on which frame of reference is used by the body. The two possible frames of reference are the support surface and gravity. If the support surface is the frame of reference, balance control is organized in an ascending direction from the feet to the head (as seen in a quiet standing posture) or from the hip to the head (as seen in locomotion). If the vertical line of gravity is the frame of reference, balance control is organized in a descending direction from head to feet. A second functional principle is that children learn to control increasing degrees of freedom during a movement. The linkage between the head and trunk can be "en bloc" or articulated. When the head and trunk are en bloc, they move as a unit so that the head is stable on the trunk. When the linkage between the head and neck is articulated, the head is stable in space.

The model of Assaiante and Amblard[4] is based on typical, natural movement activities of children when balance is not disturbed. Four periods of development of postural control have been identified across the life span (Figure 12-1). In the figure, the direction of the organization is listed across the top along with the organization of the head and trunk linkage. From birth to the achievement of upright stance, a cephalocaudal or descending type of organization is predominant. Control appears first in the muscles of the neck, then in the trunk, and finally in the legs. The second period lasts from the achievement of upright bipedal posture up to 6 years of age.

During this second period, control is ascending from the support surface, that is, from the feet during standing or ascending from the hips up during locomotion.

At age 7, there is a return to a descending organization with an articulated linkage between the head and trunk. This is not a return to the original condition found in the first period but rather a progression to establishment of head stabilization in space strategy (HSSS). HSSS is a basic means of organizing descending temporal control of balance. By being able to master the degrees of freedom allowed by the neck joint, the child improves the accuracy of the visual and vestibular messages received relative to balance or postural control. The final period of postural development adds a measure of selectivity to the articulated operation of the head and trunk unit. This selective control of the degrees of freedom is presumed to be task dependent. The fourth period is present in adulthood.

TYPES OF POSTURAL CONTROL

There are four types of postural control: static, reactive, anticipatory, and adaptive. *Static postural control* ensures stability by maintaining the body's center of mass (COM) within its base of support (BOS). All of the forces acting on the body are balanced when the COM is within its limits of stability; that is, within the

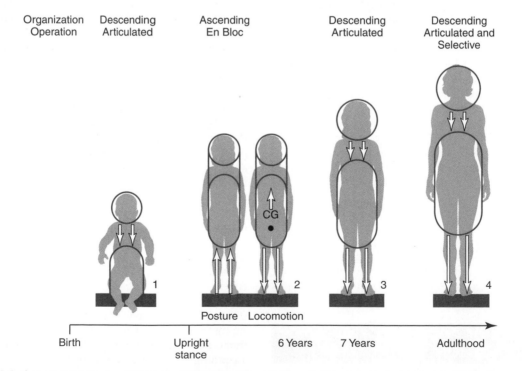

Figure 12-1 Ontogenetic scheme of the organization of posturokinetic activities. (Adapted and reprinted from *Human movement science*, vol 14, 1995, pp 13-43; Assaiante C, Amblard B: An ontogenetic model of the sensorimotor organization of balance control in humans, p 13, 1995, with permission from Elsevier Science.)

boundaries of the BOS. When static posture is controlled, we are said to have good static balance in a particular position. Although balance in quiet standing is considered static, there is movement occurring during quiet standing. Static posture is also termed *steady-state posture,* exemplified when we gently sway over our ankles. The area circumscribed by the sway represents a cone of stability (Figure 12-2). The cone represents the limits of stability for that posture.

Reactive postural control governs the unexpected movement of the COM within or outside the BOS. Various balance responses are possible given the speed of the displacement and whether the displacement results in the COM exceeding the BOS. Righting or equilibrium reactions are produced in response to weight shifts within

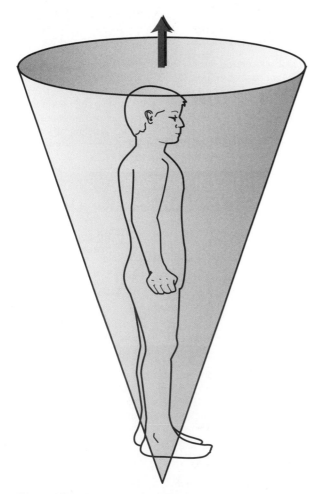

Figure 12-2 Cone of stability. (From Martin ST, Kessler M: *Neurologic intervention for physical therapist assistants,* Philadelphia, 2000, WB Saunders, p 37.)

the BOS. When the COM moves out of the BOS, as in a slip or fall, additional automatic postural responses occur. An unexpected perturbation on a force platform is an example of reactive postural control or balance. In this case, the movement of the platform shifts the person's COM resulting in the need for a postural adjustment.

Postural adjustments made before a movement are classified as *anticipatory.* We typically make such postural adjustments before reaching, lifting, and stepping. Anticipatory postural adjustments require that the nervous system feed information forward to postural muscles to prepare for the movement to follow. Think of being a water skier in the water, waiting for the first pull of the rope. You may hear the acceleration of the boat before you feel the pull, but you had better be ready to successfully achieve your goal of being lifted to an upright position. When you prepare to lift a box of heavy books, you expect the load and you prepare your posture accordingly. Experience is important in acquiring *anticipatory postural control.*

Lastly, *adaptive postural control* is demonstrated when we modify a motor response because of a change in environmental conditions or task demands. Most individuals change their speed and step width when walking on slippery ground. Aspects of cognition, such as attention, motivation, and intention, influence anticipatory and adaptive postural control. When attention is directed away from the balance task, it may be more difficult to adapt.

Postural control is the process by which the central nervous system, sensory system, and musculoskeletal system produce muscular strategies to regulate the relationship between the COM and BOS.[5] Stability involves the use of two mechanisms. The first involves development of torques at the joints of the supporting leg or legs and trunk to control COM motion without changing the base of support. More recently this strategy has been identified as a feet-in-place strategy. The second mechanism involves stepping or grasping movements of the limbs to alter the BOS when a person's balance is disturbed. This is a change in support strategy. If the source of the destabilization is recognized, it can be anticipated. Sensory information about the body's orientation and motion is also needed and may not be available ahead of an unexpected disturbance in balance. In that case, the sensory information of the instability can either be fed forward or fed back for postural correction. The way in which the postural system may operate is shown in Figure 12-3.

There are three types of perturbations possible: physiological, mechanical, and informational. Physiological events can disrupt the operation of the nervous system

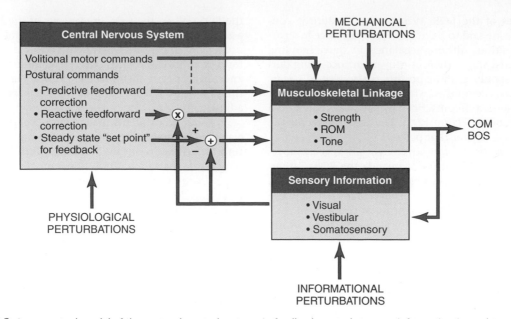

Figure 12-3 A conceptual model of the postural control system. In feedback control, sensory information is used to continuously update the corrective changes to the center of mass (COM) or base of support (BOS). In feedforward control, preprogrammed stabilizing reactions are released, either predictively (anticipatory postural adjustments) or in reaction to sensory information pertaining to the state of instability (triggered postural reactions). Mechanical perturbations involve changes in the forces acting on the body (due to movement of the body or interaction with the environment). Informational perturbations pertain to transient changes in the nature of the orientational information available from the environment. Physiological perturbations refer to transient internal events that disrupt the operation of the neural control system. *ROM,* range of motion. (Adapted from Maki BE, McIlroy WE: Postural control in the older adult, *Clin Geriatr Med* 12(4):635-658, 1996.)

control by changing the set point and blocking incoming sensory information. Examples of mechanical disturbances of balance are changes in the forces acting on the body, such as a push or shove, slip, or trip. Another example could come from a change in range of motion at the ankle that could change the available BOS in standing. A change in the ambient light, as when walking into a dark room, is an example of an informational perturbation. Changes in sensory information coming in from the environment can affect the set point or reactive balance.

COMPONENTS OF A POSTURAL CONTROL SYSTEM

During the 1990s, posture came to be recognized as a complex interaction of biological, mechanical, and movement components. A conceptual model of the systems involved in postural control is depicted in Figure 12-4. Seven components have been identified: limits of stability, sensory organization, eye-head stabilization, the musculoskeletal system, motor coordination, predictive central set, and environmental adaptation.

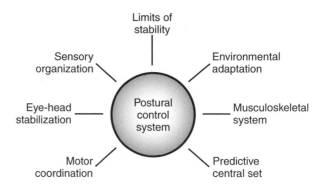

Figure 12-4 Components of normal postural control. (Adapted from Duncan P: *Balance. proceedings of the APTA forum*, Alexandria, Va, 1990, American Physical Therapy Association, with permission of the American Physical Therapy Association.)

Limits of Stability

Every posture has a BOS. The BOS is that area of the body in contact with the support surface. The perimeter of the BOS is the typical limit of stability. When the mass of the body is maintained within the limits of the

BOS, the posture is maintained. Developmental postures such as sitting, quadruped, and standing all have a different BOS. Keeping the COM of body within the BOS constitutes balance. During quiet stance, as the body sways, the limits of stability depend on the interaction of the position and velocity of movement of the COM. We are more likely to lose balance if the velocity of the COM is high and at the limits of the BOS. The body perceives changes in the COM in a posture by detecting amplitude of center of pressure (COP) motion. The COP is the point of application of the ground reaction force. In standing, there would be a COP under each foot. Feel how the COP changes as you shift weight forward and back while standing.

Sensory Organization

The visual, vestibular, and somatosensory systems provide the body with information about movement and cue postural responses. The maturation of the sensory systems and their relative contribution to balance have been extensively studied with some conflicting findings. Some of these conflicts may be related to the way balance is studied, whether static or dynamic balance is assessed, and to the maturation of sensorimotor control. Regardless of these differences, sensory input appears to be needed for the development of postural control.

Vision is very important for the development of head control. Newborns are sensitive to the flow of visual information and can even make postural adjustments in response to this information.[6] Input from the visual system is mapped to neck movement initially and then to trunk movement as head and trunk control is established. The production of spatial maps of the position of various body parts appears to be linked to muscular action. The linking of posture at the neck to vision forms before somatosensation is mapped to neck muscles.[7] Most everyone agrees that vision is the dominant sensory system for the first 3 years of life and that infants rely on vision for postural control in the acquisition of walking.

Vestibular information is also mapped to neck muscles at the same time as somatosensation is mapped. Eventually, mapping is done of combinations of sensory input such as visual-vestibular information.[8] This bimodal mapping allows for comparisons to be made between previous and present postures. The mapping of sensory information from each individual sense proceeds from the neck to the trunk and on to the lower extremities.[7] Information from vision acts as feedback when the body moves and as an anticipatory cue in a feedforward manner before movement. As the child learns to make use of somatosensory information from the lower extremities, somatosensory input emerges as the primary sensory input on which postural response decisions are made.

Somatosensation is the combined input from touch and proprioception. Adults use somatosensation as their primary source for postural response. When there is a sensory conflict, the vestibular system acts as a tiebreaker in making the postural response decision. If somatosensation says you are moving and vision says you are not, the vestibular input should be able to resolve the conflict to maintain balance. However, vestibular function relative to standing postural control does not reach adult levels, even at the age of 15, according to Hirabayashi and Iwasaki.[9]

Eye-Head Stabilization

The head carries two of the most influential sensory receptors for posture and balance: the eyes and labyrinths. These two sensory systems provide ongoing sensory input about the movement of the surroundings and head, respectively. The eyes and labyrinths provide orientation of the head in space. The eyes must be able to maintain a stable visual image even when the head is moving, and the eyes have to be able to move with the head as the body moves. The labyrinths relay information about head movement to ocular nuclei and about position, allowing the mover to differentiate between *egocentric* (head relative to the body) and *exocentric* (head relative to objects in the environment) motion. Lateral flexion of the head is an egocentric motion. The movement of the head in space while walking or riding in an elevator is an example of exocentric motion.

The HSSS involves an anticipatory stabilization of the head in space before body movement. A child first displays this strategy at 3 years of age while walking on level ground.[10] By maintaining the angular position of the head with regard to the spatial environment, vestibular inputs can be better interpreted. The HSS strategy appears to be mature in 7 year olds.[4] Older adults have been shown to adopt this strategy when faced with distorted or incongruent somatosensory and visual information.[11]

Musculoskeletal System

The body is a mechanically linked structure that supports posture and provides a postural response. The viscoelastic properties of the muscles, joints, tendons, and ligaments can act as inherent constraints to posture and movement. The flexibility of body segments such as the neck, thorax, pelvis, hip, knee, and ankle contribute to attaining and maintaining a posture or making a postural response. Each body segment has mass and grows at a different rate. Each way in which a joint can move represents a degree of freedom. Because the body has so many individual joints and muscles with many possible ways in which to move, certain muscles work together in synergies to control the degrees of freedom.

Normal muscle tone is needed to sustain a posture and to support normal movement. *Muscle tone* has been defined as the resting tension in the muscle[12] and the stiffness in the muscle as it resists being lengthened.[13] Muscle tone is determined by assessing the resistance felt during passive movement of a limb. Resistance is due mainly to the viscoelastic properties of the muscle. On activating the stretch reflex, the muscle proprioceptors, the muscle spindles, and Golgi tendon organs contribute to muscle tone or stiffness. The background level of activity in antigravity muscles during stance is described as postural tone by Shumway-Cook and Woollacott.[7] Others also describe patterns of muscular tension in groups of muscles as postural tone.[14] Together, the viscoelastic properties of muscle, the spindles, Golgi tendon organs, and descending motor commands regulate muscle tone.

Motor Coordination

Motor coordination is the ability to coordinate muscle activation in a sequence that preserves posture. The use of muscle synergies in postural reactions and sway strategies in standing are examples of this coordination and are described in the upcoming section on neural control. Determination of the muscles to be used in a synergy is based on the task to be done and the environment in which the task takes place.

Strength and muscle tone are prerequisites for movement against gravity and motor coordination. Head and trunk control require sufficient strength to extend the head, neck, and trunk against gravity in prone; to flex the head, neck, and trunk against gravity in supine; and to laterally flex the head, neck, and trunk against gravity in side-lying.

Predictive Central Set

Predictive central set can best be thought of as postural readiness. This ability to anticipate the need for a change in posture is part of anticipatory postural control. Recognizing the consequence of a movement would allow an individual to prepare for the movement. Think of how you prepare for the act of catching a ball. Sensation and cognition are used as anticipatory cues before movement. Anticipatory postural adjustments serve three purposes.[3] One purpose is to keep postural disturbance to a minimum. A second purpose is to prepare for movement as initiating gait. A third purpose is to assist a movement in terms of force or velocity such as throwing a ball. It appears that an internal representation of the dynamics of movements is built up during development that allows for anticipatory postural control to guide movement under similar task conditions.

Environmental Adaptation

Postural responses are made in reaction to internally and externally perceived needs. Movement performance is changed when we encounter ice on a sidewalk. A young child may change the manner in which stairs are descended based on perception of safety. Developmentally, the sensorimotor system of an infant must adapt to gravity. The nervous system generates movement solutions to the problems the infant encounters during the attainment of an upright erect posture. The sensory systems also signal the need for automatic postural reactions to preserve posture. With development of postural networks, anticipatory postural control develops and is used to preserve posture (see Chapter 4). Adaptive postural control allows changes to be made to movement performance in response to internally or externally perceived needs.

NEURAL BASIS FOR POSTURAL CONTROL AND BALANCE

There are two ways to view the neural basis of postural control. One is the traditional reflex and hierarchical model of postural control already discussed in Chapter 4. The development of postural control does appear to follow a hierarchy and to proceed in a cephalocaudal sequence. Head control is developed before trunk control. Once an erect posture is achieved, however, it is more beneficial to use a systems approach to analyzing postural control.

Hierarchical Model

Postural Reflexes

Reflexes and reactions help to restore stability before the activation of voluntary systems. As described in Chapter 4 the hierarchical view of motor control attributes certain reflexes and reactions to specific levels of the nervous system. Cervicospinal and vestibulospinal reflexes assist in maintaining postural stability. Vestibular responses are used primarily to stabilize the head in space. Therefore, the brain stem is involved in postural control. It coordinates information from the spinal cord, cerebellum, cerebrum, and special senses. "Brainstem nuclei act reflexively to stimuli and in response to commands issued by other motor centers.[15]" The reticular formation within the brain stem contributes to postural tone by balancing activation of flexor and extensor muscles to allow us to express these reflexes. Posture and proximal movement emanate from brain stem centers.[12]

Automatic Postural Adjustments

The act of bringing or moving body segments into alignment with one another has traditionally been referred to as *righting* the head or the body. Righting means to bring the body into "normal" alignment. For humans, normal alignment is considered erect bipedal stance. Newborn infants cannot stand up by themselves or balance. During the first year of life, infants acquire righting and balance abilities that enable them to move from a lying to standing position and to balance in the transitional postures they might assume while rising: sitting, quadruped, and kneeling. Righting functions enable an individual to move from one stable posture, such as lying supine, to another stable posture, such as lying prone. The essence of righting is movement from one stable posture to another while seeking a more upright posture. When we can stand without assistance, we move out of the period of infancy and enter childhood. Thus the postural function of rising is so important to our development that it has been used as a marker of transition to childhood.

Postural reactions are the basis of voluntary movement in a reflex/hierarchical model of postural control. The postural reactions of protective extension, head- and trunk-righting, and equilibrium responses are seen as providing a basis for posture/balance, locomotion, and prehension. These postural reactions occur in response to changes in the body's orientation to gravity and in the pattern of weight distribution within the BOS. Automatic postural reactions maintain or regain balance and make it safe to move voluntarily. There are three kinds of automatic postural reactions: protective, righting, and equilibrium.

The earliest *protective reactions* are seen in response to quick lowering of the body toward a support surface. A protective reaction is an extremity response to a quick displacement of the center of gravity out of the BOS. A downward response of the legs is seen at 4 months. Protective extension of the upper extremities becomes evident when the infant begins to sit with support. Displacement in sitting results in her brisk extension of the arm to catch and protect against falling. The infant can prop forward on extended arms if placed around the same time. Upper extremity protective reactions begin at 6 months in sitting and develop sequentially forward, sideways, and backward. Haley[16] found that this order

of acquisition is not always followed. Protective reactions are generally completely developed by 10 months of age. These reactions become our backup system if we fail to regain our balance by the use of an equilibrium reaction. Unfortunately, the use of these automatic responses can result in unintentional injury, as when an older adult sustains a Colles fracture from falling on an outstretched arm.

Righting reactions begin at birth and exhibit peak occurrence at 10 to 12 months. These reactions can be elicited by any one of a number of sensory stimuli: vestibular, proprioceptive, visual, or tactile. Righting reactions become incorporated into equilibrium reactions and therefore persist as part of our automatic balance mechanism (Table 12-1).

Table **12-1**

Automatic Postural Reactions

Reaction	Age at Onset	Age at Integration
Head-Righting		
Neck (immature)	34 wk of gestation	4-6 mo
Labyrinthine	Birth-2 mo	Persists
Optical	Birth-2 mo	Persists
Neck (mature)	4-6 mo	5 yr
Trunk-Righting		
Body (immature)	34 wk of gestation	4-6 mo
Body (mature)	4-6 mo	5 yr
Landau	3-4 mo	1-2 yr
Protective		
Downward lower extremity	4 mo	Persists
Forward upper extremity	6-7 mo	Persists
Sideways upper extremity	7-8 mo	Persists
Backward upper extremity	9 mo	Persists
Stepping lower extremity	15-17 mo	Persists
Equilibrium		
Prone	6 mo	Persists
Supine	7-8 mo	Persists
Sitting	7-8 mo	Persists
Quadruped	9-12 mo	Persists
Standing	12-24 mo	Persists

Data from Barnes MR, Crutchfield CA, Heriza CB: *The neurophysiological basis of patient treatment*, vol 2, Atlanta, 1982, Stokesville.

Righting is defined as maintenance or restoration of the proper alignment of the head or trunk in space. One category of righting reactions produces movement in one plane; these movements are described as anterior, posterior, or lateral head-righting or trunk-righting. When held upright in vertical and tilted in any direction, the head and trunk right or tilt in the opposite direction. Likewise, when we are in side-lying position, the somatosensory cue of the trunk on the supporting surface cues lateral head-lifting (righting). Head-righting develops during the first several months in response to gravity's effect on the vestibular system and through the body's contact (somatosensation) with the supporting surface.

A second category of righting reactions produces rotation around the body axis, as in rolling to maintain alignment of body segments. These righting reactions of the head and trunk function to produce rotation around the long axis of the body and are an integral part of producing a smooth movement transition from one posture to another. Mature neck- and body-righting allow for the developmental change from log rolling to segmental rolling seen in the 4- to 6-month-old infant.

Equilibrium reactions are more sophisticated than righting reactions and involve a total body response to a slow shift of the center of gravity outside the BOS. In a lateral sitting equilibrium reaction, the head and trunk right, and the arm and leg abduct opposite the weight shift, followed by head and trunk rotation toward the abducted extremities (Figure 12-5). Equilibrium reactions begin to appear at 6 months of age in the prone position, even as the infant is experiencing supported sitting. The remaining equilibrium reactions appear in an orderly sequence: prone, supine, sitting, quadruped, and standing. The maturation of the reactions in these postures lags behind the attainment of movement in the next higher developmental posture. For example, equilibrium reactions mature in the sitting position when the child is creeping and mature in the quadruped position when the child is walking.

The various protective, righting, and equilibrium reactions are triggered by sensory cues such as visual recognition of a changing horizon. Vestibular or somatosensory cues are also used to perceive that a postural response is needed. Head-righting occurs before trunk-righting. Postural control is mastered in developmental positions sequentially but with some overlap. For example, equilibrium reactions may mature in a lower developmental position such as sitting as the child moves around in quadruped. In summary, the common concept of posture has two facets: the idea of balance, or preserving alignment, and the function of righting, or moving from one posture to another to attain erect standing posture.

Systems Model

A fundamental concept in the systems perspective is that postural adjustments precede most functional movement. That is, posture is adjusted before the performance of an overt action or movement. For example, if we stand flush against a wall, it is impossible to lean forward and pick up an object on the floor directly in front of our feet. We will fall. To lean forward, weight must be shifted back onto the heels. In the latter description, this shift is prevented from occurring because the wall is in the way. Lee and colleagues[17] looked at the postural adjustments required to abduct one leg while in a standing position. The COP moves over the leg to be stood on even before the ankle rises. In fact, the shoulder and

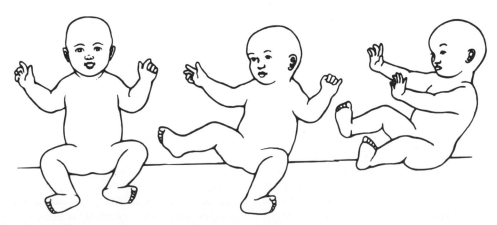

Figure 12-5 Sitting equilibrium reaction in response to lateral weight shift. Equilibrium reactions in sitting mature when the infant begins creeping.

hip movements that counteract the change in COP also occur before the rise of the ankle.

Anticipatory responses depend on feedforward or anticipatory control (defined in Chapter 4). These responses change over time and appear to depend on age, musculoskeletal maturity, context, and cognitive abilities. Anticipatory control develops along with reactive postural control.[7] The ability to anticipate changes in COP before movement comes from experiences in responding to perturbations of the COP within and out of the BOS. Sensory-motor information about position of the head precedes that of the trunk. The COM is higher in children because of their larger heads and shorter legs, resulting in a greater rate of postural sway. As strategies are acquired, picking the most favorable one within a given context becomes more challenging. Within the context of a task, posture supports movement. The standing posture we would assume while stirring a pot on the stove is different from the standing posture we would assume while playing tennis.

Postural control can be changed through learning and experience. One of the most basic premises of a systems perspective is that with practice and repetition, motor behavior can change. The more a pattern of movement, in this case, a postural adjustment, is repeated, the more adaptable it becomes. Practice and experience allow the organization of postural responses to accomplish a functional end such as support of movement. Learning requires that all perceptual systems contribute useful information to the control of posture. Infants are capable of using perceptual information from many different senses after 6 months of age. Therefore, the development of postural control as viewed within a systems model is also suggestive of mapping or associating sensory input from a sensory systems to a particular action, such as head lifting. Experience influences "the strength of the connections between sensory and motor pathways controlling balance.[7]" When learning is compromised, as in persons with mental disabilities, it may be possible to make postural adjustments but not in a timely manner. The implementation of the muscular response is slower due to nervous system immaturity. Also, anticipatory postural control, which requires experiential learning, appears to be inadequate or delayed in children with Down syndrome.[18]

Although the reflex/hierarchical model of postural control is central nervous system dependent and focused on reactive balance, the systems model encompasses the maturation of the musculoskeletal system as well as the central nervous system and focuses on all aspects of balance: reactive, anticipatory, and adaptive. Two systems models of the control of standing balance have been proposed.

Nashner Model of Postural Control of Stance

Nashner formulated a model for the control of standing balance over the course of some 20 years.[19] His model describes three common sway strategies seen in steady-state standing: the ankle strategy, the hip strategy, and the stepping strategy. Depending on the characteristics of the support surface, the speed of perturbation, and the degree of displacement, different strategies emerge.

An adult sways about the ankle when the foot is fully supported during quiet stance (Figure 12-6, *A*). This strategy depends on solid contact under the foot to provide a resistive force, enabling the ankle muscles to exert their effect through "reverse action." With the foot fixed on the ground, either the plantar flexors or the dorsiflexors contract to pull the leg backward and forward with respect to the foot, keeping the COM within the BOS. If we sway backward, the anterior tibialis fires to bring us forward; if we sway forward, the gastrocnemius fires to bring us back to the midline. This strategy depends on having a solid surface under the feet and intact vision, vestibular system, and somatosensation. The ankle strategy is used when the perturbations or disturbances to balance are small.

An adult sways about the hip when standing crosswise on a narrow balance beam, as shown in Figure 12-6, *B*. An ankle strategy cannot be used in this situation because there is no support under the toes and heels to provide a reactive force to the ankle motion. Therefore, the only

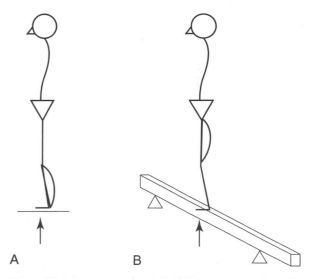

Figure 12-6 Sway strategies. **A,** Postural sway about the ankle in quiet standing, with the foot fully supported. **B,** Postural sway about the hip in standing on a balance beam, with the foot partially supported. (From Martin ST, Kessler M: *Neurologic intervention for physical therapist assistants*, Philadelphia, 2000, WB Saunders, p 38.)

successful strategy is the hip strategy, in which hip flexion and extension combine with knee extension and flexion to ensure balance. Larger perturbations elicit a hip strategy if the feet are supported, as when performing a postural stress test.

The last sway strategy, that of stepping, occurs when the speed and strength of the balance disturbance are sufficient to produce a protective step. By taking a step, the BOS is widened and balance is regained because the COM is once again within the BOS. It had been thought that the COM had to exceed the BOS for stepping to occur, but such is not the case.[20] Some researchers have found that the directions given to subjects during a balance task may constrain them from stepping.[21]

Children 18 months old are able to demonstrate an ankle strategy in quiet standing when balance is disturbed.[22] Their response time is longer than that for adults. According to Shumway-Cook and Woollacott,[23] children 4 to 6 years old displayed varying strategies to the same type of perturbations in standing; sometimes a hip strategy was used, and sometimes an ankle strategy was used. A consistent ankle strategy performed in a timely manner was not evident until 7 to 10 years of age. This coincides with the maturation of nervous system myelination of major tracts by age 10. Adult sway strategies are present in 7- to 10-year-old children.

Winter Stiffness Model of Postural Control of Stance

Research has looked at how the body's COM is controlled during quiet stance. Winter and colleagues[24] proposed a straightforward model that gives an almost immediate corrective response. "The model assumes that muscles act as springs to cause the center-of-pressure (COP) to move in phase with the center-of-mass (COM) as the body sways about some desired position.[24]" The stiffness control in the sagittal plane comes from the torque produced by the ankle plantar flexors/dorsiflexors. In the frontal plane, the stiffness comes from the hip abductor/adductor torque. The model of Winter and colleagues[24] is also an inverted pendulum. Movement of the COP under the feet regulates the body COM. The difference between the body COM and the COP are proportional to the acceleration of the body COM. The researchers showed that the torque needed to restore posture was set by the joint stiffness.

Rietdyk and co-workers[25] measured joint moments during balance recovery from a mediolateral perturbation at the trunk or pelvis. Their results validated the model of Winter and colleagues[24] and showed that the first response to the perturbation was provided by muscle stiffness, not reflex-activated muscle activity. The joint moments detected were sufficient to move the COP in appropriate directions to control the lateral collapse of the trunk. The moments at the hip and spine accounted for 85% of the recovery response, whereas the ankles contributed 15%.

In a review of proprioceptive control of posture, Allum and colleagues[26] questioned whether the proprioceptive cues from the ankles do trigger balance responses in standing and during locomotion. The research reviewed supports the idea that postural strategies other than sway strategies are possible. Input to the trunk and hip may be more important than input to the ankle in triggering balance correction in standing. This may reflect the fact that the hip is the joint in the lower extremity that is used to recover stability when posture/balance is disturbed in a mediolateral direction. Hip muscles are activated before ankle muscles when balance is disturbed mediolaterally.[27] Responses to mediolateral postural disturbances activate muscles in a proximal-to-distal order.

ASSESSMENT OF POSTURE AND BALANCE

There are many ways in which to assess balance (Clinical Implications Box 12-1: Assessment of Balance—Adults for an overview). Testing of the sensory systems that support balance can be done using the Clinical Test of Sensory Integration on Balance (CTSIB) or the Sensory Organization Test (SOT) (Figure 12-7). Essentially, these are the same test. The examiner measures how long a client can stand in six different sensory conditions; those conditions are shown in (Figure 12-7, *A*). The clinical test uses dense foam support to provide inaccurate somatosensory input and a Japanese lantern to provide inaccurate visual input. A force platform is not used. The Pediatric-CTSIP uses the same equipment as the adult test. Quiet standing in bilateral and tandem stance is tested in the six conditions.[28] In the SOT (Figure 12-7, *B*), a force platform is used. The client stands on a force platform in each of the six conditions. The platform is perturbated to provide inaccurate somatosensory input in three conditions. The apparatus moves to provide inaccurate visual information in two conditions. Children with attention deficit hyperactivity disorder have been tested using the SOT.[29] They were found to have more difficulty under all conditions than a control group. They reported that the visual system appeared to contribute more to the balance deficits than the vestibular and somatosensory systems.

Postural sway with eyes open and eyes closed can be observed under different stance configurations, such as those used in the Romberg and sharpened Romberg. The postural stress test is a way to quantify the effect

CLINICAL IMPLICATIONS Box 12-1

Assessment of Balance—Adults

There are many ways to assess postural control and balance. Thus, it is important to understand the types of assessment to differentiate the components and types of postural control. Some tests are specific to the component or type of control, whereas others are more general measures of balance. Functional scales are also available. A brief description of some of these tests is provided in the text, but an in-depth discussion of balance assessment is beyond the scope of this chapter.

Component of Postural Control	Test
• Sensory reception and organization • Musculoskeletal system	• Clinical Test of Sensory Integration on Balance (CTSIB) • Sensory Organization Test (SOT) • Manual muscle test • Range of motion

Type of Postural Control	Test
• Quiet standing	• Postural sway—Equitest • Romberg
• Reactive	• Righting and equilibrium reactions postural stress test (nudge/pull test)
• Anticipatory	• Functional reach

Functional Scales of Balance	Test
• Berg Balance Scale	• Fourteen tasks from everyday life test static and dynamic balance skills. Items use mainly steady-state and anticipatory balance. The test is able to discriminate older adults at risk for falls.
• Timed Up and Go (TUG)	• A quick measure of mobility and balance. Timed version is a good indicator of fall status in community-dwelling older adults.
• Tinetti Performance Oriented Mobility Assessment (POMA)	• Scale rates performance on 16 items involving balance and gait. Static and dynamic tasks use reactive, steady-state, and anticipatory balance. The score can be used to determine risk for falls.

of nudging or pushing someone by using a defined force to displace them backward.[30] Functional reach[31] is a quick measure of balance in standing. The subject stands with an arm outstretched and reaches as far forward as possible without losing balance (Figure 12-8). The test measures the limits of stability while performing a forward maximal reach. The test assesses dynamic balance and anticipatory control. Even though the test was originally devised for a geriatric population, norms have been established for children.[32,33] Recently, modifications have been suggested to the functional reach test that appear to improve its reliability in children and adolescents.[34] The pediatric version (PRT) includes testing reaching forward and sideways in standing and sitting. The PRT is appropriate for children 2.6 to 14 years of age.[35] See the Clinical Implications Box 12-2: Assessment of Balance—Children.

Functional scales of balance have mainly been used with the older population to screen for risk of falls and include the Berg Balance Scale,[36] the Timed Up and Go test,[37] and the Tinetti Performance Oriented Mobility Assessment[38] that includes balance and gait. The Berg is considered the gold standard in the area of functional balance in the elderly (see Clinical Implications Box 12-1: Assessment of Balance—Adults).

The Berg and the Timed Up and Go tests have been modified for use with children. Franjoine and colleagues[39] modified the Berg to use it to identify balance problems in school-age children. In previous research, Kembhavi and colleagues[40] had shown that the Berg could be used to assess balance in children with cerebral palsy. The Timed Up and Go (TUG) has also been modified to provide a measure of dynamic balance and functional mobility in the pediatric population.[41] Modification includes starting or stopping the time when the child's bottom leaves or returns to the chair. The chair height ensures that the child's feet are flat on the floor and the knees are flexed to 90 degrees. The test has been found to be reliable with children as young as 3 years of age.

POSTURE AND BALANCE ACROSS THE LIFE SPAN

For physical therapists, the study of posture and balance development is an integral part of the study of motor development. Posture, like movement, varies characteristically with age. *Balance* is a developmental characteristic related to posture. In this chapter, the specific changes in human postural function are examined from a life span perspective. A real constraint to a broad and systematic study of posture is the lack of information about posture during large periods of the human life span. Typically, research and collections of literature regarding posture, even when claiming a life span perspective, skip important life periods. We know most about the very young infant, child, and older adults. Less is known about postural development in later childhood, adolescence, and young and middle adulthood.

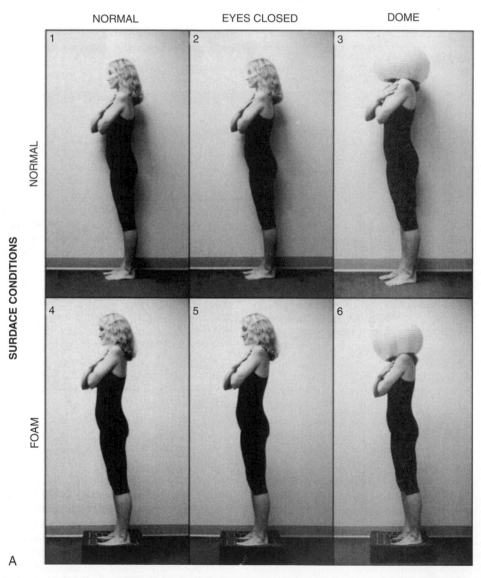

VISUAL CONDITIONS

Figure 12-7 Assessment of balance using tests of sensory reception and organization. **A,** The Clinical Test of Sensory Integration on Balance (CTSIB) uses foam and a Japanese lantern to replicate six sensory conditions.

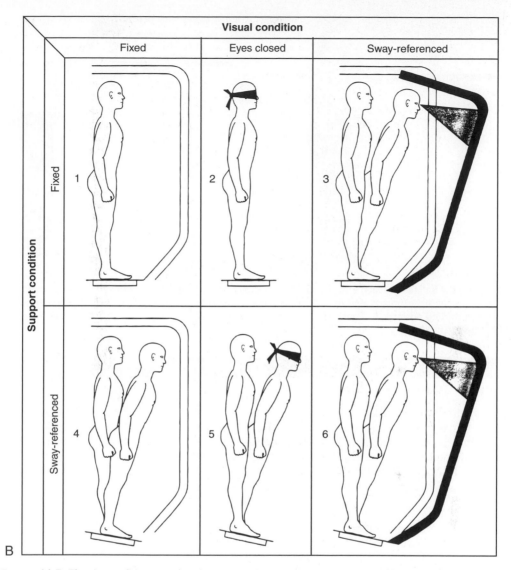

B

Figure 12-7—cont'd **B,** The six conditions used in the Sensory Organization Test (SOT). (**A** From Umphred DA: *Neurological rehabilitation*, ed 4, St Louis, 2001, Mosby, p 631; **B** From Hasson S: *Clinical exercise physiology*, St Louis, 1994, Mosby, p 216.)

Infancy and Childhood

Postural control develops in a cephalocaudal and proximal-distal sequence in infants. Head control is achieved before trunk control, shoulder control before finger control, and pelvic control before foot control. Once erect stance is achieved, the relationship with the support surface initiates a caudocephalic sequence of responses or distal to proximal as described by Nashner.[19] Postural control is essential to developing skilled actions such as locomotion and manipulation. Bertenthal and Von Hofsten[42] stated that eye, head, and trunk control are the foundation for reaching and manipulation.

Development of Spinal Curves

Static postural alignment is dependent to some extent on the spinal curves seen when viewing upright posture from the side. Everyone is familiar with the anatomical landmarks used to determine alignment. Spinal curves develop over the life span. Although the adult spine has

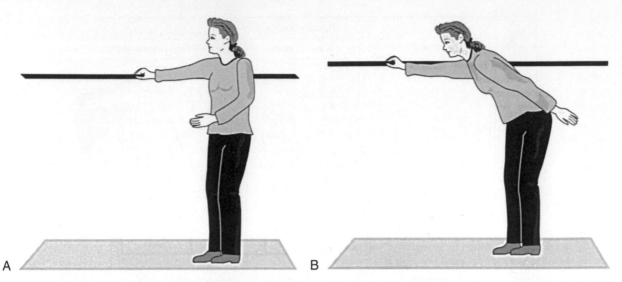

A   B

Figure 12-8 During the functional reach test, the client is asked to reach forward as far as possible from a comfortable standing posture. The excursion of the arm from start to finish is measured via a yardstick affixed to the wall at shoulder height. **A,** Functional reach-starting position. **B,** Functional reach-ending position. (From Umphred DA: *Neurological rehabilitation*, ed 4, St Louis, 2001, Mosby, p 629.)

CLINICAL IMPLICATIONS Box 12-2

Assessment of Balance—Children

Balance in children can be assessed as part of a standardized test of motor function. Several tools are available that serve this purpose, including the Alberta Infant Motor Scale (AIMS), the Peabody Developmental Motor Scales (PDMS-2), and the Bruininks Oseretsky Test of Motor Proficiency (BOT-2).

Recently, several adult balance assessment tools have been modified for use in the pediatric population. A brief description of some of these tests is provided in the text, but an in-depth discussion of balance assessment is beyond the scope of this chapter.

Component of Postural Control	Test
• Sensory reception and organization	• Pediatric Clinical Test of Sensory Integration for Balance (P-CTSIB)
• Musculoskeletal system	• Manual muscle test
	• Range of motion

Type of Postural Control	Test
• Quiet standing	• Eyes open versus eyes closed
	Vision should not be occluded between birth and 3 years.
	• Postural sway
	• Single limb stance time
	• Various arm positions
• Reactive	• Righting and equilibrium reactions
• Anticipatory	• Pediatric functional reach
	Forward and sideways in standing and sitting

Functional Scales of Balance	Test
• Pediatric Berg Balance Scale Children 5-15 years of age	• Fourteen tasks from everyday life test static and dynamic balance skills. Items use mainly steady-state and anticipatory balance. The original test was modified to match a functional developmental sequence.
• Pediatric Timed Up and Go Children 2.6-14 years of age	• A quick measure of mobility and balance Reliable with children as young as 3 years of age

sagittal curves in the cervical, thoracic, lumbar, and pelvic regions, the infant has only two curves. The flexed posture of the newborn is the result of physiological flexor tone and the need to conform to the mother's uterus. The infant's two curves are concave forward: one in the thoracic region and the other in the pelvic region. The latter is formed by the curve of the sacrum, which is composed of separate vertebral components at this stage of development.

As the infant grows and develops sufficient strength to lift the head, the cervical curve develops and is convex forward. This curve becomes more noticeable as the infant holds the head up at 3 to 4 months. The lumbar curve is also convex forward and develops when the baby begins to sit up. The curves could fail to develop if the child is unable to develop head control and sitting.

Development of Postural Control

Postural development proceeds from head control to trunk control. The infant assumes a prone on elbows posture at approximately 3 months when the head and upper back are extended sufficiently to allow the freeing of the arms from under the infant. Weight bearing in the posture is important for developing proximal shoulder girdle stabilization. The prone progression of developmental postures consists of achieving a prone on elbows position and then moving to prone on extended arms and finally moving up to quadruped or all fours. From a hands and knees posture, the infant pulls to stand and achieves upright posture. Initially, support of hands or tummy may be required.

With the achievement of upright stance, erect posture is precarious. Because the newly erect infant's center of gravity is relatively high (T12 compared with L5-S1 in an adult), the BOS is widened. The center of gravity is also forward due to a large liver. For the upper trunk to achieve a vertical position, the lumbar lordosis is increased, and the arms are brought into a high guard position (see Figure 3-18).

Sensory Contributions to Balance in Infants Jouen and colleagues[6] showed that 3-day-old infants made postural adjustments of the head in response to optical flow patterns. These are patterns of light associated with movement. The brain uses this information to know where the head and the body are relative to the surrounding environment. Spontaneous head control is noted in infants at 10 weeks of age when electromyographic responses can be recorded in reaction to being tilted.[43] Bertenthal and associates[44] investigated the developmental changes in postural control of 5-, 7-, 9-, and 13-month-old infants in response to optical flow. The infants were able to scale their postural responses to the visual information. The scaling was even possible in presitters but improved with practice and the development of sitting. The ability to use visual information for postural responses increased from 5 to 9 months of age. Vestibular and somatosensory systems can also trigger balance responses in infants and toddlers in sitting.[45]

Sitting Sitting is a new posture in which the COM is suspended above the BOS. Fairly rapid postural adjustments are needed to resist or to compensate for sudden losses of balance. Even infants who were unable to sit alone were able to integrate visual information and make a motor response (postural adjustment) without having the strength and coordination to maintain a sitting posture independently. Improvement in muscle activation patterns is a function of experience with perceptual modulation of posture.[46]

Balance Strategies in Sitting Infants develop directionally specific postural responses before being able to sit.[47] These responses appear to be innate and are guided by an internal representation of the limits of stability, such as orientation of the vertical axis and relationship of COM to BOS. This is consistent with the hypothesis of a central pattern generator being the source of initial postural responses.[45] This circuitry determines the spatial characteristics of muscle activation that is triggered by afferent information. During this period of time, the infant demonstrates a large number of responses. With further development, the circuitry matures, and with experience, the initial variability is reduced. The temporal and spatial features of responses are fine-tuned to match task-specific demands. According to the neuronal group selection theory, experience continues to shape postural networks by changing the synaptic strength of intergroup and intragroup connections.[26] Multisensory afferent input is used to shape these adaptive responses.

Most studies of the development of anticipatory postural control have been conducted in sitting, using reaching as the task. Postural activity in the trunk was measured while an infant reached from a seated posture.[48] Trunk muscles were activated before muscles used for reaching. Researchers concluded that anticipatory postural control occurs before voluntary movements and is present in infants by 9 months of age.[49] Children appear to tolerate more imbalance as they grow up.[50] Anticipatory control of posture increases from 3 to 8 years of age, with older children demonstrating more refined scaling of responses. In other words, children become better at matching the amount of postural preparation needed for a specific task. Less postural activation is needed when picking up a light object versus picking up a heavy object.

Recently, the development of sitting postural control has been studied using COP data. By using a force platform, Harbourne and Stergiou[51] longitudinally assessed the postural sway of infants at three stages of sitting. The first stage begins when the infant holds the head and upper trunk up but does not sit alone. The second stage involves the infant sitting alone briefly and is followed by the third stage of the infant being able to sit alone. Nonlinear measurement showed significant changes in center of pressure distribution over time. This method has been shown to be a reliable way to assess the development of sitting postural control in typically developmentally delayed infants.[52,53] Nonlinear dynamics provides an alternate explanation for the development of postural control. Rather than being the result of a central pattern being generated and subsequently modulated, the infant's ability to control the body's degrees of freedom to master postural control in sitting is a result of a dynamic process.[54]

Sit to Stand Transition   Moving from sitting to standing is an everyday occurrence and a necessary prerequisite for walking. Cahill and colleagues[55] studied three age groups of children on a sit to stand task. The children were grouped as follows: 12 to 18 months, 4 to 5 years, and 9 to 10 years. The movement became more coordinated as measured by the smoothness of phase-plane plots. The youngest group could perform the movement but could not cease moving once a standing posture was attained and either took steps or raised onto their toes. The oldest group generated a pattern of vertical ground reaction force like that of adults when coming to stand but could not do so consistently. Differences in performance were attributed to developmental differences in the children's ability to control horizontal momentum of the body mass, use sensory input for balance, and understand the task.

Standing Posture in Childhood   Children 2 to 3 years of age exhibit a characteristic lumbar lordosis that ranges between 30 and 40 degrees.[56] When infants begin to stand and walk, their feet are flat and they begin to exhibit a longitudinal arch only as the fat pad in the foot diminishes. Changes in lower extremity alignment in the stance posture occur over a 6-year period. The 18-month-old child stands with bow legs (genu varum), but by 3 years of age the legs may exhibit genu valgus or knock knees. The legs straighten out by 6 years.[57]

Balance on two feet increases as independent locomotion is achieved (see Chapter 13). Once double limb support is mastered in standing, the next challenge is to develop balance while standing on one foot. Unilateral support begins at approximately age 3 years with

Table 12-2

Age-Related Expectations for One-Foot Standing Balance

Age (yr)	Time
3	Momentary to 3 sec
4	4-6 sec
5	8-10 sec
6	10+ sec eyes open and eyes closed

momentary to 3 seconds and progresses sequentially to 10-plus seconds at 6 years (Table 12-2). Momentary to 3-second one-foot standing balance is needed to ascend a step or to step over an object. Longer unilateral standing balance is a prerequisite for motor skills, such as hopping, galloping, and skipping.

Sensory Contributions to Standing Balance   The maturation of the sensory systems and their relative contribution to balance have been extensively studied with some conflicting findings. As children master independent walking, the primacy of vision for postural control lessens gradually. Balance control changes from being primarily visual-vestibular to being somatosensory-vestibular by age 3.[58]

Proprioception function is mature by 3 to 4 years of age.[9] Therefore, within the 4- to 6-year-old range, vision is still important for balance, but proprioception and touch are being used more.

In normal support conditions, children 6 to 10 years old are more stable with vision.[59] For 8-year-olds, central vision produced greater postural stability than peripheral vision. Peripheral visual cues were more important for postural stabilization in children 11 to 13 years old.[60] When studying one-foot standing balance, static balance was dependent on visual information. However, dynamic destabilization in a medial-lateral direction was linked to motor response speed.

Postural sway in standing on a moveable platform under normal vestibular and somatosensory conditions is greater for children 4 to 6 years of age than for children 7 to 10 years of age.[23] By 7 to 10 years of age, an adult sway strategy is demonstrated wherein the child has been thought to depend primarily on somatosensory information. Vestibular information is also being used, but the system is not yet mature. Interestingly, children with visual impairments are not able to minimize postural sway to the same extent as nonvisually impaired children.[61] This may be related to the child's inability to fully use either somatosensory or vestibular information during this age period.

Research supports that there is a transition period around 7 to 8 years that can be explained by the use of the head stabilization in space strategy.[62] By 7 years of age, children are able to make effective use of HSSS that depends on dynamic vestibular cues.[4] However, the transition to adult postural responses in standing is not complete by 12 years of age. Children at 12 to 14 years of age are still not able to handle misleading visual information to make appropriate adult balance responses.[63] These researchers found that although the somatosensory inputs and scores in the 6- to 14-year-old subjects were as good as the young adults studied, their sensory organization was different. They concluded that children prefer visual input to vestibular input for determining balance responses and that vestibular information is the least effective for postural control.

It is generally accepted that visual, vestibular, and somatosensory information must be integrated to control standing balance; however, there are conflicting findings about their relative contributions to balance. In a large study using the SOT, Steindl and colleagues[64] tried to shed light on some of the conflicting data on the effect of age and maturation of sensory systems on balance. They reconfirmed that the proprioceptive system is fully developed in 3- to 4-year-olds and that visual input appears to be more crucial to balance under conditions of support surface instability. Visual afference of postural control is mature at approximately 15 or 16 years of age. Vestibular maturation occurs in adolescence and is the last sensory system involved with postural control to mature. The ability to solve intersensory conflicts requires that all three sensory systems be mature, and one can assume this happens in adolescence.

In summary, visual input dominates posture and balance during the first 3 years of life. The 4- to 6-year-old child is able to make more use of proprioceptive information, but the balance responses in standing are highly variable. By 7 to 10 years of age, the child is able to demonstrate adultlike strategies in response to perturbations in standing, such as swaying over the ankles like an inverted pendulum. Balance responses are not completely mature, however, until 15 to 16 years.

Anticipatory Control

Donahoe and associates[32] tested children between 5 and 15 years of age using the functional reach test. Balance was seen to improve with age up to the 11- to 12-year-old age category and then appeared to stabilize. The ability to anticipate the postural adjustments needed to allow for reaching forward is used on a daily basis in childhood activities. The task is an example of feed-forward control of balance and is a test of anticipatory control.

Adolescence and Transitional Movements

Lebiedowska and Syczewska[65] looked at the relationship between body size and its effect on postural sway in children 7 to 18 years of age. They wanted to know if the structural changes in body height and mass affected spontaneous sway parameters. They found no significant correlations between the parameter and developmental factors of age, body height, and body mass. However, there was a decrease in sway parameter when values were normalized to body height that indicated a small improvement in static equilibrium with taller children. COP was used as a measure of the movement of the center of gravity. As such, COP motion did not change in the children studied.

A study of rising from the floor movements in teenagers revealed what appears to be a peak in incidence of symmetrical movement patterns around the age of 15 years.[66] Younger and older teens were found to exhibit more asymmetry while rising than did middle teens. This is particularly true for lower limb movements. It may be that peak performance in a task occurs when most individuals demonstrate the greatest ability to control force within this task. Although children seem to have difficulty controlling force production in this task, and as a result demonstrate asymmetry in their rising actions, teens exhibit a refined competence in simultaneously controlling the upper limb, trunk, and lower limb movements. They move from recumbency by flexing the trunk and moving the feet directly in front of their buttocks while balancing in a sitting position, and then they transfer weight from the buttocks to the feet with ease. Control of the force and direction of movement in the righting task is impressive at this age.

Adulthood and Transitional Movements

The midteen peak in symmetrical performance is diminished slightly during the late-teen period and in the early 20s. Although symmetrical performance is the most common form of rising, it is the mode of action of approximately one-fourth of young adults. The remainder demonstrate asymmetry in at least one component of body action, be it the upper limbs, the trunk, or the lower limbs. This is when individuals are making the transition from high school to college or the workforce. Compared with the high school years, young adulthood presents fewer formalized opportunities to participate in physical activity. Green and Williams[67] found that activity level is related to performance in the rising from the floor task during the middle adult years. More active adults are more likely to use symmetrical patterns.

Patterns of movement change with age, and movement patterns used by older adults are highly variable.[68] Posture and balance may decline as an individual ages because of changes in static posture, loss of flexibility and muscle strength, vestibular impairments affecting postural awareness and head stabilization, tone changes resulting from medications or pathologies, changes in sensorimotor input and integration, and visual changes. Many of the changes in movement patterns seen in an older adult are the result of inactivity and the lack of motor practice.[69]

Balance in Older Adults

Posture

The ability to maintain an erect aligned posture decreases with advanced age. Figure 12-9 depicts the general postural differences that can be anticipated to occur as a result of typical aging. The secondary spinal curves that developed in infancy begin to be modified. The cervical curve decreases. The lumbar curve usually flattens. Decreased movement can accentuate age-related postural changes. The older adult who sits most of the day may be at greater risk for a flattened lumbar area. The thoracic spine becomes more kyphotic. Aging alters the properties and relative amount of connective tissue in the interior of the disc.[70,71] The discs lose water, and initially flexible connective tissue stiffens, causing older adults to lose spinal flexibility. In general, there is

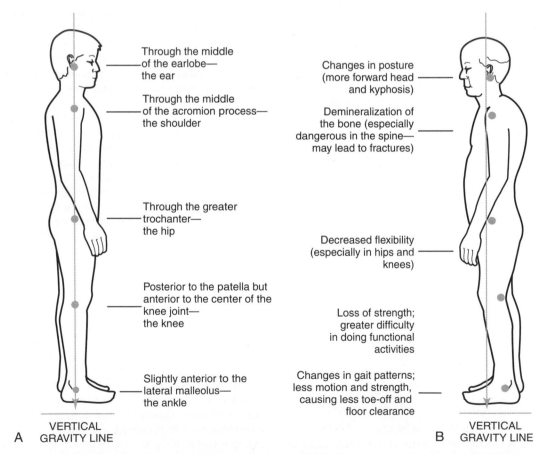

Figure 12-9 Comparison of standing posture: changes associated with age. **A,** Young adult. **B,** Older adult. (Adapted from Lewis C, editor: *Aging: the health care challenge*, ed 2, Philadelphia, 1990, FA Davis.)

a decrease in connective tissue flexibility. The strength of the muscles declines with age and could contribute to a decline in the ability of the older adult to maintain postural alignment.

Postural changes seen with aging can include forward head, kyphosis of the thoracic spine, loss of lumbar lordosis, loss of hip and knee flexion, and loss of ankle mobility. All of these changes shift the center of gravity forward and create instability during standing and walking. A loss of flexibility and diminished postural responses lead to less-organized motor patterns, further leading to destabilization and diminished motor coordination. Postural, somatosensory, and vestibular changes diminish an older adult's ability to accommodate to loss of balance, to environmental changes, and to other concurrent tasks often involved in functional activities.

Effect of Sensory Changes with Age

Sensory input for balance changes with advancing age. The three sensory systems (visual, vestibular, and somatosensory) responsible for posture undergo age-related changes. The visual system is less able to pick up contours and depth cues because of a decline in contrast sensitivity. Both of these losses can impair postural control. The problems can be intensified if there are cataracts or macular degeneration. The vestibular system loses hair cells that detect changes in the direction of flow of the endolymph within the semicircular canals and saccule and utricle. The eighth cranial nerve (vestibulocochlear) may show a reduction of number of nerve fibers. Both of these changes can affect otolith function and result in positional vertigo. Vibratory sense in the lower extremities declines and could contribute to a decrease in somatosensory input from the support surface and awareness of the degree of postural sway. Older adults exhibit an increased postural sway when standing on a foam surface. The researchers associated the increased sway with a decline in visual contrast sensitivity and visual acuity in older adults because they could not compensate for decreased somatosensation with vision.[72] Scovil, Zettel, and Maki[73] found that stored visuospatial information from the environment is needed for planning and executing a stepping reaction. These and other findings demonstrate the importance of vision for maintaining balance under challenging conditions.[74]

Older adults appear to have more difficulty using the built-in redundancy of the sensory systems linked to postural responsiveness.[75] Under typical circumstances, an adult will use vestibular input to resolve a conflict situation in which somatosensory cues indicate the body is moving and the visual cues do not indicate movement or vice versa. The vestibular system acts as the deciding vote

as to whether we need to respond. Hay and colleagues[75] found that older adults were less stable in standing than were younger adults when visual cues were removed. Both groups had difficulty when a vibratory stimulus was applied at the ankle, thus altering proprioceptive input. However, the older adults responded less well to having normal proprioceptive input restored than did the younger adults. It appears that in addition to age-related changes in sensory receptors producing peripheral deficits, there also may be a slowing of central control mechanisms responsible for postural regulation. Conflicting sensory inputs were presented to the older adults to test the hypothesis that central processing is also involved in age-related changes of postural responsiveness. The older adults were much more affected by a combined conflicting situation that involved proprioceptive and visual information than were young adults.

Standing Balance

Humans exhibit a degree of spontaneous postural activity or sway when "standing still." Typically, this sway is considered as an ongoing adjustment to or compensation for the effects of gravity and other subtle movements such as breathing, looking, and those associated with maintaining comfort through modulating weight bearing beneath the feet. Alternatively, this spontaneous sway may not be so spontaneous at all. If postural activity is an emergent feature imposed by the constraints of the individual and the environment, it may be that the variable sway serves an informational role as a search strategy providing postural control mechanisms in the CNS with continuous information about the individual's location in space via the stimulation of sensory systems.[76] In this case, spontaneous sway provides information in an a priori fashion rather than being something that is completely compensatory in nature.

Older adults have more spontaneous sway than younger persons.[5,77] This is a common finding in the research literature. However, it is important to understand that sway can be measured in a variety of ways. Most appropriately, sway implies body movement. This is often represented by motion of the body's COM. However, most sway measurements capture dynamic aspects of the center of pressure. COP is the point of application of the ground reaction force. As a location, the center of pressure can be characterized by its amplitude (average position, path, and speed) or frequency (mean frequency of sway). With respect to the former, numerous studies have identified greater speed and range of COP motion in older adults as compared with younger adults.[5,78] On the other hand, frequency measures have shown mixed results.[78] Larger sway by older adults has been shown to be correlated with changes in sensory function as well as lower extremity muscle strength. However, it is unclear which is the cause and which is the effect: for example, are the changes in lower extremity muscle activity producing increased sway or is this activity in response to increased spontaneous sway?

Altering the sensory conditions during static standing affects older and younger adults differently. For example, older persons shift to a more asymmetrical standing posture when their eyes are closed than younger persons.[79] There are numerous studies that have identified increases in postural instability as a result of decreasing vision during standing. Interestingly, at least two studies have identified that the increase in sway in older persons is smaller than the increase in sway in younger persons when the eyes are closed or when the support surface is made narrow.[80,81] In this connection, a very interesting conclusion was drawn by Benjuya and colleagues.[80] They found that both young and older adults increased body sway when vision was eliminated. However, the younger adults' sway was disproportionately greater than the older adults' sway under this condition. They also found that when vision was eliminated, the amount of cocontraction about the ankle joints increased in the older adults. They concluded that the strategy for managing postural control by older adults shifts from a sensory input to a muscular stiffening response. Where younger adults increased sway when vision was eliminated by using other sensory inputs (proprioceptive, vestibular), older adults' sway increased to a lesser degree as a consequence of adjusting the motor response toward a stiffening strategy.

Medial-lateral sway is increasingly being used as a predictor of fall status in older adults. Maki and colleagues[82] found that lateral spontaneous sway under an eyes-closed condition was the single best predictor of falls in older persons when compared with a variety of postural control measures. Interestingly, lateral sway in older adults with a history of falling is more pronounced than in age-matched adults without a history of falling.[5] Standing in a near-tandem stance is particularly challenging to lateral balance, and older adults with a history of falling have difficulty with this task. Impaired lower extremity proprioception, decreased quadriceps strength, and slow reaction time are the best predictors of increased sway in this posture.[83]

Dynamic Balance

The interaction between posture and voluntary movement is what delineates dynamic standing balance from static standing balance. Internally generated, voluntary movements are perturbations to posture. That is, a self-generated, voluntary movement such as raising one's arm may be destabilizing. So-called anticipatory postural adjustments before or concomitant with an arm raise are necessary to prevent postural instability. In contrast, a voluntary movement of the lower extremity, such as during the process of standing on one foot, requires a lateral shift of the body's COM to unweight the stepping limb to achieve a new unipedal posture without a loss of balance. Evidence exists that for both arm and leg movements, older adults exhibit differences in postural control compared with younger adults.

Compared with movements of the arm, voluntary movements of the lower extremity pose additional and greater balance challenges to older persons. Gait initiation, stepping on or over an object, or sport-related actions such as kicking all require the transition from a bipedal to a unipedal stance configuration. The requisite postural adjustment in these examples is a lateral weight transfer before limb liftoff. Additionally, forward-oriented actions such as gait initiation also include an anterior-posterior postural adjustment.

Older adults are known to exhibit both delays in reaction time of the prime mover and longer onset latencies of responses in the postural muscles necessary for stabilizing balance.[84] Rogers, Kukulka, and Soderberg[85] examined self-initiated and reaction time arm movements in older and younger adults. They found that when older adults were asked to raise an arm at their own pace they were less likely to demonstrate the necessary lower extremity postural muscle activity before activating the shoulder prime mover. Moreover, older adults exhibited a significantly shorter interval between contraction of the postural muscles and those responsible for the focal shoulder movement. Collectively, this suggests that aging may alter necessary anticipatory postural adjustments and affect the timing between postural and focal movement elements during voluntary arm movements.

Besides prolonged reaction time to initiating the focal movement, older adults exhibit a prolonged weight transfer time. Weight transfer is the postural adjustment, and weight transfer time represents the time to complete the postural adjustment. It has been determined that the prolonged time taken to transfer body weight off the stepping foot is actually of greater importance than the delays seen in reaction time for initiating the task itself.[86-88]

It is unclear why older adults generally take longer to perform the postural adjustment for lateral weight transfer during tasks such as step initiation. It may be partially attributable to changes in the torque-generating capacity of muscles important in accelerating the body's COM laterally, namely the hip abductors.[89] However, Jonsson, Henriksson, and Herschfeld[90] suggest alterations in weight transfer is a function of the sequencing of forces during this phase as compared with the ability to generate absolute force. This suggests that problems of coordination between posture and movement may lie at the heart of the age-related changes in postural adjustments associated with leg movements. Data from a rhythmic stepping in place task appears to support the contention that older persons adapt coordination to maintain balance and step performance during time-critical stepping.[91]

There is evidence that changes in step performance with age may be dependent on the type of step executed and the specific step-related conditions. Older adults take smaller steps than younger adults under voluntary step initiation conditions[92,93] but apparently do not take smaller steps during self-paced rhythmical stepping in place.[94] Additionally, protective steps induced by a large external perturbation also appear not to exhibit an age-related difference in step length.[95]

Step direction affects the amount of lateral weight transfer necessary to step or initiate gait. The COM does not need to be shifted as far for a lateral step versus a forward step. Therefore, a side step requires less postural adjustment, that is step limb vertical ground reaction force, than a forward step.[86] Older adults, however, produce a greater peak vertical ground reaction force for lateral stepping than younger adults. This greater force results in a greater shift of the COM towards the stance limb. Older adults shift their weight toward the support limb more than younger adults. Collectively, a greater force combined with a longer time to produce the weight shift may be reflective of a safer, more conservative strategy being opted for by older persons. It is safer because the weight shift is greater and more conservative because the time taken to accomplish the postural adjustment is longer.

Previous and present level of activity or function also affects the postural adjustment necessary for step initiation in older persons. Physically active older adults exhibit postural and balance changes when initiating a step. Henriksson and Hirschfeld[96] found that older persons stand more asymmetrically than younger adults before initiating gait. The asymmetry may be an active compensation for the prolonged weight transfer times in older persons. Being more asymmetrical so that the stepping limb is relatively unloaded before a step requires less weight transfer during step initiation. Not surprisingly, weight transfer time is also prolonged during step initiation for lower-functioning older persons.[97]

As a response to an external perturbation, stepping was once thought to be a balance strategy of last resort.[98,99] This is no longer the case. Rogers, Hain, Hanke, and Janssen[100] found that stepping is a common balance strategy and this response is conditioned by the context of the perturbation parameters applied to the subject. That is, the combination of perturbation direction, displacement, direction, and speed influences whether or not a stepping response occurs. However, instruction is also very important. Too often, research studies have instructed subjects to try not to step. Instructing a person to either "react naturally" or "try not to step" will elicit very different responses. A person is far more likely to step when given the instruction "react naturally.[101]"

Pai and colleagues[102] and Pai and associates[103] evaluated a dynamic mechanical model of the COM-BOS relationship and found that externally induced, protective stepping frequently occurred before the COM reached the limits of the BOS. Evidently, protective stepping does not depend solely on the mechanical constraint of the position of the COM exceeding the BOS. Stepping can no longer be considered a balance strategy of last resort, and it may actually be a preferred response under real world conditions.[101] Therefore, clinical physical therapists should strongly consider focusing efforts toward the evaluation and treatment of stepping strategies over so-called ankle and hip strategies typically observed during very small perturbations or when the BOS is altered in an artificial manner such as standing perpendicular on a balance beam.

Older adults respond differently to external perturbations than do younger adults. Older persons tend to step more frequently, step to lower perturbation magnitudes, take multiple steps in response to larger perturbations, and often take a more laterally directed forward step than do younger adults given the same perturbation amplitude.[95,101,102,104–106] Importantly, the later second step, often laterally, is made because of a primary problem in arresting the COM velocity or terminating the step to regain a stable stance position.[95,107] The more laterally directed step is particularly evident for those older persons with a history of falling.

The timing of a protective step is also affected by age and fall status. Older persons tend to step as fast as younger persons when given an external perturbation.[88,108] However, older adult fallers have been shown to step *earlier* than older adults without a history of falling. This may be due to older adult fallers preplanning a step or, on the other hand, willingness by younger persons and older persons without a history of falling to be displaced further before initiating a step under similar conditions.

Lateral stability in the face of a lateral perturbation has received a great deal of attention recently.[109-112] As with anterior-posterior perturbations, older adults are more likely to step and take multiple steps to a lateral perturbation.[109] When younger adults step, they typically respond with a side step of the limb in the direction of the perturbation. Older adults exhibited more crossover steps and limb collisions during these crossover steps.[111] There does appear to be a difference in response when the perturbation is oriented at the floor (moveable platform) or waist (waist pull perturbation).[109,111] Regardless, limb collisions during crossover stepping are a common finding in older persons and should be identified as such in any clinical balance examination by a physical therapist. Finally, for medial-lateral balance performance, taking multiple steps along with hip abductor strength and functional axial mobility are predictive of falls in older persons.[112]

SUMMARY

Posture and balance rely on the sensory and motor subsystems of the central nervous system and the musculoskeletal system to influence age-related changes in the various types of postural control. In addition, the somatosensory, visual, and vestibular systems play a pivotal role in organizing responses to external disturbances of posture. It is important to recognize that many types of balance (static, dynamic, and reactive), as well as anticipatory and adaptive postural control, can be exhibited within a task-specific context. The ability to maintain a posture, whether standing still or while moving, is an ongoing challenge. Balance requires reacting to challenges appropriately and generating an anticipatory posture before the onset of overt movement. Lastly, adaptive postural control allows us to adapt to changing task and environmental conditions, including gravity, which protects us from losing balance.

Postural networks evolve during the course of early development. Changes in synaptic strength within the nervous system occur at a relatively rapid rate early and later in the human life span. These changes, which seem influenced by use, contribute to both the acquisition of postural abilities and their decline. The neural control of posture varies with age, and the acquisition and modulation of posture are dynamic processes that involve more than just the nervous system.

The effects of the musculoskeletal system on posture are related to physical growth. We grow when we are young. We get bigger and taller, and our body proportions change. These physical changes challenge the postural systems across the growing years. The anatomical structures of bone and muscle also change with age. These changes contribute to our ability to generate force, to be flexible, and to attain a certain stature. The acquisition and loss of spinal curves provide a perfect example of age-related change. The ability of the body to control the degrees of freedom of its segments changes over time as has been demonstrated in the development of postural control in sitting and standing.

During adulthood, activity level and experiences with different movements influence our weight and body dimensions, which then affect postural control. Physical dimensions vary with age, not only because of internally mediated growth processes but also because of psychological and sociocultural factors related to work, lifestyle, mental status, and activity level.

The factors that contribute to age-related change in posture and balance are widely and richly varied. Understanding these various factors and their relationships leads to increased understanding not only of postural development but also of all motor development throughout the human life span.

REFERENCES

 1. Thomas CL, editor: *Taber's cyclopedic medical dictionary*, ed 18, Philadelphia, 1997, FA Davis.
 2. Forssberg H: Neural control of human motor development, *Curr Opin Neurobiol* 9:676–682, 1999.
 3. Massion J: Postural control systems in developmental perspective, *Neurosci Biobehav Rev* 22:465–472, 1998.
 4. Assaiante C, Amblard B: An ontogenetic model of the sensorimotor organization of balance control in humans, *Hum Mov Sci* 14:13–43, 1995.
 5. Maki BE, McIlroy WE: Postural control in the older adult, *Clin Geriatr Med* 12:635–658, 1996.
 6. Jouen F, Lepecq JC, Gapenne O, et al: Optic flow sensitivity in neonates, *Infant Behav Dev* 23:2761–2784, 2000.
 7. Shumway-Cook A, Woollacott MH: *Motor control: translating research into clinical practice*, ed 3, Philadelphia, 2007, Lippincott, Williams & Wilkins.
 8. Jouen F: Visual-vestibular interactions in infancy, *Infant Behav Dev* 7:135–145, 1984.
 9. Hirabayashi S, Iwasaki Y: Developmental perspective of sensory organization on postural control, *Brain Dev* 17:111–113, 1995.
10. Assaiante C, Amblard B: Ontogenesis of head stabilization in space during locomotion in children: influence of visual cues, *Exp Brain Res* 93:499–515, 1993.
11. DiFabio RP, Emasithi A: Aging and the mechanisms underlying head and postural control during voluntary action, *Phys Ther* 77:458–475, 1997.
12. Lundy-Ekman L: *Neuroscience: fundamentals for rehabilitation*, ed 3, Philadelphia, 2007, WB Saunders.
13. Basmajian JV, DeLuca CJ: *Muscles alive: their function revealed by electromyography*, ed 5, Baltimore, 1985, Williams & Wilkins.

14. Bobath B: *Adult hemiplegia: evaluation and treatment*, London, 1978, William Heinemann Medical Books.
15. Iyer MB, Mitz AR, Winstein C: Motor 1: lower centers. In Cohen H, editor: *Neuroscience for rehabilitation*, ed 2, Philadelphia, 1999, Lippincott, Williams & Wilkins, pp 209–242.
16. Haley SM: Sequential analysis of postural reactions in non-handicapped infants, *Phys Ther* 66:531–536, 1986.
17. Lee RG, Tonolli E, Viallet F, et al: Preparatory postural adjustments in parkinsonism patients with postural instability, *Can J Neurol Sci* 22:126–135, 1995.
18. Virji-Babul N, Latash ML: Postural control in children with Down syndrome. In Hadders-Algra M, Carlberg EB, editors: *Postural control: a key issue in developmental disorders*, London, 2008, Mac Keith Press, pp 131–147.
19. Nashner LM: Sensory, neuromuscular and biomechanical contributions to human balance. In Duncan P, editor: *Balance: proceedings of the APTA forum*, Alexandria, Va, 1990, American Physical Therapy Association, pp 5–12.
20. Brown AL, Shumway-Cook A, Woollacott MH: Attentional demands and postural recovery: the effects of aging, *J Gerontol A Biol Sci Med Sci* 54:M165–M171, 1999.
21. McIlroy WE, Maki BE: Changes in early "automatic" postural responses associated with the prior planning and execution of a compensatory step, *Brain Res* 63:203–211, 1993.
22. Forssberg H, Nashner LM: Ontogenic development of postural control in man: adaptation to altered support and visual conditions during stance, *J Neurosci* 2:545–552, 1982.
23. Shumway-Cook A, Woollacott MH: The growth of stability: postural control from a developmental perspective, *J Mot Behav* 17:131–147, 1985.
24. Winter DA, Patla AE, Prince F, et al: Stiffness control of balance in quiet standing, *J Neurophysiol* 80:2111–2121, 1998.
25. Rietdyk S, Patla AR, Winter DA, et al: NACOB presentation CSB New Investigator Award. Balance recovery from medio-lateral perturbations of the upper body during standing. North American Congress on Biomechanics, *J Biomech* 32:1149–1158, 1999.
26. Allum JH, Bloem BR, Carpenter MG, et al: Proprioceptive control of posture: a review of new concepts, *Gait Posture* 8:214–242, 1998.
27. Horak FB, Moore S: Lateral postural responses: the effect of stance width and perturbation amplitude, *Phys Ther* 69:363, 1989.
28. Crowe TK, Deitz JC, Richardson PK, et al: Interrater reliability of the Clinical Test of Sensory Interaction for Balance, *Phys Occup Ther Pediatr* 10:1–27, 1990.
29. Shum SB, Pang MY: Children with attention deficit hyperactivity disorder have impaired balance function: involvement of somatosensory, visual and vestibular systems, *J Pediatr* 155(2):245–249, 2009.
30. Whipple R, Wolfson LI: Abnormalities of balance, gait and sensorimotor function in the elderly population. In Duncan P, editor: *Balance: proceedings of the APTA forum*, Alexandria, Va, 1990, American Physical Therapy Association.
31. Duncan PW, Weiner DK, Chandler J, et al: Functional reach: a new clinical measure of balance, *J Gerontol* 45:M192–M197, 1990.
32. Donahoe B, Turner D, Worrell T: The use of functional reach as a measurement of balance in boys and girls without disabilities ages 5–15 years, *Pediatr Phys Ther* 6:189–193, 1994.
33. Norris RA, Wilder E, Norton J: The functional reach test in 3-5 year-old children without disabilities, *Pediatr Phys Ther* 19:20–27, 2008.
34. Volkman KG, Stergiou N, Stuberg W, et al: Methods to improve the reliability of the functional reach test in children and adolescents with typical development, *Pediatr Phys Ther* 19:20–27, 2007.
35. Bartlett D, Birmingham T: Validity and reliability of a pediatric reach test, *Pediatr Phys Ther* 15:84–92, 2003.
36. Berg K: *Measuring balance in the elderly: validation of an instrument*, Dissertation. Montreal, 1993, McGill University.
37. Podsiadlo D, Richardson S: The timed "Up & Go": a test of basic functional mobility for frail elderly persons, *J Am Geriatr Soc* 39:142–148, 1991.
38. Tinetti ME: Performance-oriented assessment of mobility problems in elderly patients, *J Am Geriatr Soc* 34:119–126, 1986.
39. Franjoine MR, Gunther JS, Taylor MJ: Pediatric Balance Scale: a modified version of the Berg Balance Scale for the school-age child with mild to moderate motor impairment, *Pediatr Phys Ther* 15:114–128, 2003.
40. Kembhavi G, Darrah J, Magill-Evans J, et al: Using the Berg Balance Scale to distinguish balance abilities in children with cerebral palsy, *Pediatr Phys Ther* 14:92–99, 2002.
41. Williams EN, Carroll SG, Reddihough DS, et al: Investigation of the timed "Up and Go" test in children, *Dev Med Child Neurol* 47:518–524, 2005.
42. Bertenthal B, Von Hofsten C: Eye, head and trunk control: the foundation for manual development, *Neurosci Biobehav Rev* 22:515–520, 1998.
43. Prechtl HFR, Hopkins B: Developmental transformations of spontaneous movements in early infancy, *Early Hum Dev* 14:233–238, 1986.
44. Bertenthal B, Rose JL, Bai DL: Perception-action coupling in the development of visual control of posture, *J Exp Psychol Hum Percept Perform* 23:1631–1643, 1997.
45. Hirschfeld H, Forssberg H: Epigenetic development of postural responses for sitting during infancy, *Exp Brain Res* 97:528–540, 1994.
46. Hadders-Algra M, Brogren E, Forssberg H: Training affects the development of postural adjustments in sitting infants, *J Physiol* 493:289–298, 1996.
47. Hadders-Algra M: Development of postural control. In Hadders-Algra M, Carlberg EB, editors: *Postural control: a key issue in developmental disorders*, London, 2008, Mac Keith Press, pp 22–73.
48. Riach CL, Hayes KC: Anticipatory control in children, *J Mot Behav* 22:25–26, 1990.

49. Hadders-Algra M, Brogren E, Forssberg H: Ontogeny of postural adjustments during sitting in infancy: variation, selection and modulation, *J Physiol* 493:287–288, 1996.

50. Hay L, Redon C: Feedforward versus feedback control in children and adults subjected to a postural disturbance, *Exp Brain Res* 125:153–162, 1999.

51. Harbourne RT, Stergiou N: Nonlinear analysis of the development of sitting postural control, *Dev Psychobiol* 42:368–377, 2003.

52. Kyvelidou A, Harbourne RT, Stuberg WA, et al: Reliability of center of pressure measures for assessing the development of sitting postural control, *Arch Phys Med Rehabil* 90:1176–1184, 2009.

53. Deffeyes JE, Harbourne RT, Lyvelidous A, et al: Nonlinear analysis of sitting postural sway indicates developmental delay in infants, *Clin Biomech* 24(7):564–570, 2009.

54. Kyvelidou A, Stuberg WA, Harbourne RT, et al: Development of upper body coordination during sitting in typically developing infants, *Pediatr Res* 65(5):553–558, 2009.

55. Cahill BM, Carr JH, Adams R: Inter-segmental co-ordination in sit-to-stand: an age cross-sectional study, *Physiother Res Int* 4:12–27, 1999.

56. Asher C: *Postural variations in childhood*, Boston, 1975, Butterworths.

57. Staheli L: *Pediatric orthopedic secrets*, Philadelphia, 1998, Hanley and Belfus.

58. Foudriat BA, DiFabio RP, Anderson JH: Sensory organization of balance responses in children 3-6 years of age: a normative study with diagnostic implications, *Int J Pediatr Otorhinolaryngol* 27:255–271, 1993.

59. Nougier V, Bard C, Fleury M, et al: Contribution of central and peripheral vision to the regulation of stance: developmental aspects, *J Exp Child Psychol* 68:202–215, 1998.

60. Hatzitaki V, Zisi V, Kollias I, et al: Perceptual-motor contributions to static and dynamic balance control in children, *J Mot Behav* 34(2):161–170, 2002.

61. Portfors-Yeomans CV, Riach CL: Frequency characteristics of postural control of children with and without visual impairment, *Dev Med Child Neurol* 37:456–463, 1995.

62. Rival C, Ceyte H, Olivier I: Development changes of static standing balance children, *Neurosci Lett* 376:133–136, 2005.

63. Ferber-Viart C, Ionescu E, Morlet T, et al: Balance in healthy individuals assessed with Equitest: maturation and normative data for children and young adults, *Int J Pediatr Otorhinolaryngol* 71:1041–1046, 2007.

64. Steindl R, Kunz K, Schrott-Fischer A, et al: Effect of age and sex on maturation of sensory systems and balance control, *Dev Med Child Neurol* 48:477–482, 2006.

65. Lebiedowska MK, Syczewska M: Invariant sway properties in children, *Gait Posture* 12:200–204, 2000.

66. Sabourin P: *Rising from supine to standing: a study of adolescents*, Thesis, 1989, Virginia Commonwealth University.

67. Green LN, Williams K: Differences in developmental movement patterns used by active versus sedentary middle-aged adults coming from a supine position to erect stance, *Phys Ther* 72:560B–568B, 1992.

68. Thomas RL Jr, Williams AK, Lundy-Ekman L: Supine to stand in elderly persons: relationship to age, activity level, strength, and range of motion, *Issues Aging* 21:9–18, 1998.

69. Woollacott MH, Tang PF: Balance control during walking in the older adult: research and its implications, *Phys Ther* 77:646–660, 1997.

70. Moncur C: Posture in the older adult. In Guccione AA, editor: *Geriatric physical therapy*, ed 2, Philadelphia, 2000, Mosby, pp 265–279.

71. Zhao CQ, Wang LM, Jiang LS, et al: The cell biology of intervertebral disc aging and degeneration, *Ageing Res Rev* 6(3):247–261, 2007.

72. Lord SR, Clark RD, Webster IW: Visual acuity and contrast sensitivity in relation to falls in an elderly population, *Age Ageing* 20:175–181, 1991.

73. Scovil CY, Zettel JL, Maki BE: Stepping to recover balance in complex environments: is online visual control of the foot motion necessary or sufficient? *Neurosci Lett* 445:108–112, 2008.

74. Lord SR, Menz HB: Visual contributions to postural stability in older adults, *Gerontology* 46:302–310, 2000.

75. Hay L, Bard C, Fleury M, et al: Availability of visual and proprioceptive afferent messages and postural control in elderly adults, *Exp Brain Res* 108:129–139, 1996.

76. Riccio GE: Information in movement variability about the qualitative dynamics of posture and orientation. In Newell KM, Corcos DM, editors: *Variability and motor control*, Champaign, Ill, 1993, Human Kinetics, pp 317–358.

77. Sturnieks DL, St George R, Lord SR: Balance disorders in the elderly, *Clin Neurophysiol* 38:467–478, 2008.

78. Maki BE, Holliday PJ, Fernie GR: Aging and postural control: a comparison of spontaneous- and induced-sway balance tests, *J Am Geriatr Soc* 38:1–9, 1990.

79. Blaszcyk JW, Prince F, Raiche M, et al: Effect of ageing and vision on limb load asymmetry during quiet stance, *J Biomech* 33:1243–1248, 2000.

80. Benjuya N, Melzer I, Kaplanski J: Aging-induced shift from reliance on sensory input to muscle cocontraction during balanced standing, *J Gerontol A Biol Sci Med Sci* 59(2):166–171, 2004.

81. Koceja DM, Allway D, Earles DR: Age differences in postural sway during volitional head movement, *Arch Phys Med Rehabil* 80:1537–1541, 1999.

82. Maki BE, Holliday PJ, Topper AK: A prospective study of postural balance and risk of falling in an ambulatory and independent elderly population, *J Gerontol A Biol Sci Med Sci* 49:M72–M84, 1994.

83. Lord SR, Rogers MW, Howland A, et al: Lateral stability, sensorimotor function and falls in older people, *J Am Geriatr Soc* 47(9):1077–1081, 1999.

84. Inglin B, Woollacott MH: Age-related changes in anticipatory postural adjustments associated with arm movements, *J Gerontol A Biol Sci Med Sci* 43:M109–M110, 1998.

85. Rogers MW, Kukulka CG, Soderberg GL: Age-related changes in postural responses preceding rapid self-paced and reaction time arm movements, *J Gerontol A Biol Sci Med Sci* 47:M159–M165, 1992.

86. Patla AE, et al: Age-related changes in balance control system: initiation of stepping, *Clin Biomech* 8:179–184, 1993.
87. Stemmons Mercer V, Sahrmann SA, Diggles-Buckles V, et al: Age group differences in postural adjustments associated with a stepping task, *J Mot Behav* 29(3):243–253, 1997.
88. Rogers MW, Kukulka CG, Brunt D, et al: The influence of stimulus cue on the initiation of stepping in young and older adults, *Arch Phys Med Rehabil* 82:619–624, 2001.
89. Johnson ME, Mille ML, Martinez KM, et al: Age-related changes in hip abductor and adductor joint torques, *Arch Phys Med Rehabil* 85:593–597, 2004.
90. Jonsson E, Henriksson M, Herschfeld H: Age-related differences in postural adjustments in connection with different tasks involving weight transfer while standing, *Gait Posture* 26:508–515, 2007.
91. Hanke TA, Kay BA, Maresh C, et al: Age-related changes in posture-leg movement coordination during rhythmic unipedal stepping, *Motor Control* 11(Suppl):104, 2007.
92. Halliday SE, Winter DA, Frank JS, et al: The initiation of gait in young, elderly, and Parkinson's disease subjects, *Gait Posture* 8:8–14, 1998.
93. Medell JL, Alexander NB: A clinical measure of maximal and rapid stepping in older women, *J Gerontol A Biol Sci Med Sci* 55A:M429–M433, 2000.
94. Hanke TA, Tiberio D: Lateral rhythmic unipedal stepping in younger, middle-aged, and older adults, *J Geriatr Phys Ther* 29(1):20–25, 2006.
95. Rogers MW, Hedman LD, Johnson ME, et al: Lateral stability during forward-induced stepping for dynamic balance recovery in young and older adults, *J Gerontol A Biol Sci Med Sci* 56A(9):M589–M594, 2001.
96. Henricksson M, Hirschfeld H: Physically active older adults display alterations in gait initiation, *Gait Posture* 21:289–296, 2005.
97. Mbourou GA, Lajoie Y, Teasdale N: Step length variability at gait initiation in elderly fallers and non-fallers, and young adults, *Gerontology* 49:21–26, 2003.
98. Nashner LM, McCollum G: The organization of human postural movements: a formal basis and experimental synthesis, *Behav Brain Sci* 8:135–172, 1985.
99. Horak FB, Nashner LM: Central programming of postural movements: adaptations to altered support-surface configurations, *J Neurophysiol* 55:1369–1381, 1986.
100. Rogers MW, Hain TC, Hanke TA, et al: Stimulus parameters and inertial load: effects on the incidence of protective stepping responses in healthy human subjects, *Arch Phys Med Rehabil* 77(4):363–368, 1996.
101. Maki BE, McIlroy WE: The role of limb movements in maintaining upright stance: the "change-in support" strategy, *Phys Ther* 77:488–507, 1997.
102. Pai YC, Rogers MW, Patton J, et al: Static versus dynamic predictions of protective stepping following waist-pull perturbations in young and older adults, *J Biomech* 31:1111–1118, 1998.
103. Pai YC, Maki BE, Iqbal K, et al: Thresholds for step initiation induced by support-surface translation: a dynamic center-of-mass model provides much better prediction than a static model, *J Biomech* 33:387–392, 2000.
104. Rogers MW: Disorders of posture, balance and gait in Parkinson's disease, *Clin Geriatr Med* 12(4):825–845, 1996.
105. Jensen JL, Brown LA, Woollacott MH: Compensatory stepping: the biomechanics of a preferred response among older adults, *Exp Ageing Res* 27:361–376, 2001.
106. Luchies CW, Alexander NB, Schultz AB, et al: Stepping responses of young and old adults to postural disturbances: kinematics, *J Am Geratr Soc* 42:506–512, 1994.
107. McIlroy WE, Maki BE: Age-related changes in compensatory stepping in response to unpredictable perturbations, *J Gerontol* 51A:M289–M296, 1996.
108. Luchies CW, Wallace D, Pazdur R, et al: Effects of age on balance assessment using voluntary and involuntary step tasks, *J Gerontol A Biol Sci Med Sci* 54:M140–M144, 1999.
109. Maki BE, Edmondstone MA, McIlroy WE: Age-related differences in laterally directed compensatory stepping behavior, *J Gerontol A Biol Sci Med Sci* 55:M270–M277, 2000.
110. Rogers MW, Mille ML: Lateral stability and falls in older people, *Exerc Sport Sci Rev* 31:182–187, 2003.
111. Mille ML, Johnson ME, Martinez KM, et al: Age-dependent differences in lateral balance recovery through protective stepping, *Clin Biomech* 20:607–616, 2005.
112. Hilliard MJ, Martinez KM, Janssen I, et al: Lateral balance factors predict future falls in community-living older adults, *Arch Phys Med Rehabil* 89(9):1708–1713, 2008.

13

Locomotion

OBJECTIVES

After studying this chapter, the reader will be able to:

1. Describe the development of locomotion across the life span.
2. Define several locomotion patterns and describe how each pattern evolves across the life span, including rolling, crawling and creeping, erect walking, running, galloping, hopping, and skipping.

3. Explain how our body systems, the environment, and the task to be accomplished interact to produce locomotion from one point to another.
4. Understand the contribution of locomotion to participation in meaningful activities.

Locomotion is defined as the process of moving from one place to another.[1] It is a task critical to independent function, reflecting our ability to move safely and efficiently from one place to another. Locomotion contributes to the ability to participate in meaningful work, leisure, and community activities. The essential elements of locomotion include progression, stability, and adaptation. We must have the strength and control necessary to progress toward a location, sufficient dynamic balance to maintain our posture and to overcome the force of gravity or other external forces, and the ability to adapt the locomotor pattern to meet our needs and the demands of the environment.[2]

Exactly how we accomplish the task of getting from point A to point B depends on many factors: the exact task to be done, the interaction of our body systems that will perform the task, and the environment in which the task is to take place. For example, walking uphill, walking downhill, and walking in water are very different tasks than walking on a level, firm surface. Children, young adults, and older adults will all perform these tasks differently, depending on their size, strength, and balance. We will discuss the development of locomotion across the life span, including its various forms: rolling, crawling, skipping, and walking. Further, we will examine the interrelationships between the body systems of the organism, the environment, and the specific task. All three are equally important to an individual's ability to accomplish the desired movement.

CLINICAL RESEARCH ON LOCOMOTION

The task of independently moving from one place to another can be accomplished using any one of a variety of motor patterns: rolling, crawling, creeping, walking, running, galloping, hopping, and skipping. The work of Shirley,[3] McGraw,[4] and Whitall[5] reveals that independent locomotion progresses from birth to childhood and develops from rolling to crawling to creeping to walking, the first form of erect locomotion. After walking, the locomotion patterns that develop are the upright patterns of running, galloping, hopping, and skipping.

Researchers, such as McGraw,[4] studied motor development by dividing the development of a particular pattern into phases (e.g., the four phases of rolling, the nine phases of prone progression, and the seven phases of erect locomotion). McGraw also studied transitional patterns—those patterns used to move between postures, such as moving from supine to sitting position or moving from sitting to standing position.

Another way in which researchers of motor development used descriptive analysis to study locomotion patterns was to divide a particular pattern into its component parts, that is, movement of the head and neck, the trunk, the upper extremities, and the lower extremities. The research of Roberton and Halverson[6,7] was instrumental in this concept. These researchers identified a developmental progression for the hopping patterns of children.

Exactly how a researcher investigating motor pattern development decided to study a particular motor pattern depended most often on the underlying theory chosen by the researcher. McGraw[4] was guided in her thinking by the neuromaturational theory, which posits that the motor patterns of infants and young children are the result of the developing central nervous system (see Chapters 2, 3, and 4). Roberton and Roberton thought that the changes in motor patterns over time were partly due to physical development.[8] From a systems perspective, it is important to remember that an infant's or child's locomotor patterns evolve as the child acquires sufficient strength to support the body, the ability to balance against gravity, and the coordination of different body parts.[9] Body and limb size also play a role.

Another way of studying developing motor patterns has been to describe the pattern and the changes that occur over time by using some type of biomechanical analysis. Inman and colleagues,[10] Murray,[11] Sutherland and co-workers,[12] and Winter[13] have given the most comprehensive biomechanical analyses of the locomotion patterns for upright walking. There is little biomechanical information available on most other locomotion patterns, except for running.

A biomechanical analysis usually includes a description of the kinematics, kinetics, and the electromyographic (EMG) characteristics of the movement pattern. *Kinematics* refers to the study of motion without regard for the forces. Important kinematic variables include the displacements, velocities, and accelerations of segments involved in the task. *Kinetics* refers to the study of forces and torque without regard for the motion. Kinetic analysis includes an examination of the external loads acting on the system, such as body weight and ground reaction forces. Ground reaction forces are of particular importance because the ground reaction force acts on the body center of mass to propel it in the intended direction. Using a methodological technique called inverse dynamics, the muscular torque can be evaluated when kinetic and kinematic procedures are used simultaneously. Finally, EMG activity of important muscles involved in walking can be examined. Electromyographic activity analysis is useful because it provides a window into central nervous system functioning. This is typically accomplished using surface rather than needle electromyography during gait.

Many variables are used in a biomechanical analysis of a locomotion pattern. Walking, the most common of locomotion patterns, is usually described by the variables of step length, step width, stride length, cycle time, velocity, and cadence—variables that involve distance or time.

Most forms of locomotion involve some aspect of reciprocal movements of the extremities. Reciprocal movements of the extremities were once linked conceptually by describing stance time and swing time of a particular limb. Now the extremities are linked through the ideas of interlimb and intralimb phasing. Phasing relationships are used to describe the coordination of the movement pattern.[14] *Temporal phasing* refers to the proportion of time of the stride of one limb before the contralateral limb starts its stride. *Distance* or *amplitude phasing* is defined as the proportion of the distance covered in the stride of one limb when the contralateral limb starts its stride. A *stride* is defined as the time or distance from the heel strike of one foot to the next heel strike of that same foot. In the locomotion pattern of erect walking, temporal and distance phasing are considered to be at 50%; that is, the contralateral limb starts its cycle when the other limb has completed 50% of its cycle.

The traditional method used to describe the development of locomotion patterns has been to divide the particular pattern into specific phases or component parts. Although the descriptive method of analysis has been beneficial, biomechanical analysis has provided a more in-depth and objective method for analyzing movements. Another consideration in recognizing the variety of movement patterns used by infants and children, as well as the rapid acquisition of new locomotor skills, takes into account the role of experience and practice on acquisition of efficient locomotor patterns.

LOCOMOTION PATTERNS ACROSS THE LIFE SPAN

Rolling

Rolling is the earliest pattern used for locomotion. *Rolling* is defined as moving from supine to prone or from prone to supine position, and it involves some aspect of axial rotation.

Rotation has been described as a righting reaction because, as the head rotates, the remainder of the body twists or rotates to become realigned with the head. The earliest spontaneous axial rotation is seen in the fetus at about 10 weeks of gestation.[15] Rotation around the longitudinal axis can result from rotation of the head followed by trunk rotation or from rotation of the leg or lower extremity followed by trunk rotation. In either instance, one part of the body initiates the movement, and the other parts of the body follow, which is called *segmental rotation*. Researchers believe that the functional significance of these movements is for the fetus to become repositioned from time to time to prevent adhesions and stasis.[16]

McGraw[4] provided the most detailed account of how rolling progresses from infancy to the toddler stage. Figure 13-1 provides a modified version of those four phases of rolling. The first phase is the *newborn phase,* phase A. In this phase, the newborn infant is predominantly in a posture of flexion and is unable to produce the movements that would create the activity of rolling. Infants first begin to roll spontaneously from a side-lying position to supine position; this pattern, phase B, *spinal extension,* is seen at about 1 to 2 months of age. Rolling from side-lying to prone position is observed at about 4 to 5 months of age. These movements are initially performed with the body moving as a unit; the movement is described as "log rolling," a movement performed without segmental rotation.

Why is the infant unable to roll segmentally at 1 to 2 months of age when the infant was capable of segmental rotations in utero? The answer to this question is best sought from a biomechanical perspective. The infant at 1 to 2 months of age does not have the necessary strength to overcome gravity for rolling supine to prone or for rolling segmentally. Muscle strength was not as critical in utero to produce movement because gravity for the most part was eliminated in the fluid-filled environment. According to McGraw,[4] infantile rolling is complete but has no purpose; that is, the movement is not performed to accomplish some other

function, such as to obtain a toy or to achieve a sitting posture.

At about 4 months of age, infants begin to roll from the prone to supine position more deliberately; by 6 to 8 months, such deliberate action involves segmental rotations of the body. This pattern is referred to as phase C, or *automatic rolling.* It is most often initiated by the upper extremities, followed by the trunk and lower extremities; the pattern can also be initiated by the lower extremities, followed by the trunk and the upper extremities. Performance of the movement with more segmentation and with more deliberation is described by McGraw as phase D, *deliberation.* Rolling from supine to prone is also seen at 6 to 8 months of age.

Adult rolling patterns have been described by Richter and colleagues,[17] who studied young adults, aged 20 to 29 (Figures 13-2 and 13-3). The most important finding was that normal adults used a variety of movement patterns to roll. Most likely, the variety of the patterns was related to flexibility and muscle strength of the individual performing the movement.

Crawling and Creeping

Crawling and creeping are terms that are frequently used interchangeably. For the purpose of this text, *crawling* is defined as prone progression in which the belly remains

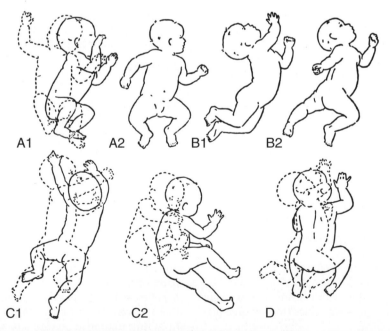

Figure 13-1 Four positions (A-D) in the pattern of an infant rolling from supine to prone position. (From McGraw MB: *The neuromuscular maturation of the human infant,* New York, 1945, Columbia University Press, reprinted by permission of the publisher.)

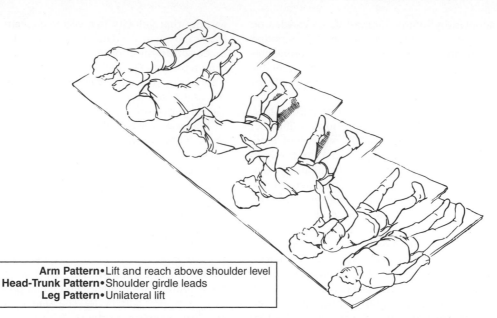

Arm Pattern	•Lift and reach above shoulder level
Head-Trunk Pattern	•Shoulder girdle leads
Leg Pattern	•Unilateral lift

Figure 13-2 A common form of rolling in adults, as shown from the lower right-hand corner to the upper left-hand corner. (From Richter RR, VanSant AF, Newton RA: Description of adult rolling movements and hypotheses of developmental sequence, *Phys Ther* 69:63-71, 1989.)

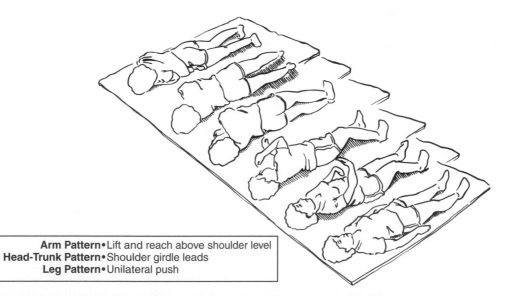

Arm Pattern	•Lift and reach above shoulder level
Head-Trunk Pattern	•Shoulder girdle leads
Leg Pattern	•Unilateral push

Figure 13-3 A second common pattern of rolling in adults, as shown from the lower right-hand corner to the upper left-hand corner. (From Richter RR, VanSant AF, Newton RA: Description of adult rolling movements and hypotheses of developmental sequence, *Phys Ther* 69:63-71, 1989.)

on the supporting surface as the arms and legs move in a reciprocal pattern to propel the body forward or backward. *Creeping* is defined as a prone progression in which the abdomen is lifted off the supporting surface while the arms and legs move reciprocally to propel the body forward or backward.

According to McGraw,[4] the prone progression of crawling and creeping is a nine-phase sequence. McGraw further indicated that she had not observed a movement sequence with more individual variation than this progression. Adolph and colleagues[18] also report significant variability in the prone progression patterns adopted by infants. Some infants crawled on their bellies; others skipped this mode of locomotion totally and no strict stagelike progression of prone progression was noted. The majority of infants are able to perform a reciprocal creeping pattern (belly off the floor) by 10 months of age.

McGraw[4] attributed the progression to cortical maturation, which results in effective inhibition of earlier components of reflexive control of the movement. From a biomechanical perspective, muscle strength is important in getting the belly up off the ground and propelling the body forward or backward. Limb length should also be considered in that children may not creep on hands and knees until their arms are long enough and strong enough to support them off the ground. Most likely, the truth behind this or any motor pattern progression is a combination of cortical development, musculoskeletal development, and the environment in which the progression is taking place.

Adult patterns of crawling and creeping have not been studied extensively. The literature indicates that the reciprocal pattern used in early childhood is the adult pattern of this movement behavior. How this pattern of locomotion evolves with aging has not yet been studied. This is not surprising given that this is not a preferred pattern of locomotion for most older adults. We can assume, however, that the patterns of creeping and crawling for older adults remain very similar to the patterns that young adults display. The parameters that would change the progression of creeping in older adults most likely are biomechanical, such as muscle strength and joint flexibility.

Erect Walking

Walking is the act of moving on foot. *Ambulation* is another term that is used synonymously with walking. A third term, *gait,* refers to the manner in which a person walks.[1] Gait can be described by several parameters of time and distance, including stride length, step length, cadence, and velocity. A complete *gait cycle* is defined as one complete stride of one limb. *Stride length* is the distance from heel strike of one foot to heel strike of that same foot. *Step length* is the distance from heel strike of one foot to heel strike of the other foot. *Cadence* or step frequency refers to the number of steps taken per a unit of time and is usually reported as the number of steps per minute. *Walking velocity* is the measurement of distance per unit of time. It can be measured several ways, for example, velocity in m/sec = stride length (m/step) × cadence (steps/sec) × 0.5. In the clinic, the term walking (gait) speed is used synonymously with walking velocity, but it is important to note that velocity is a vector quantity while speed is a scalar quantity. This means that all measurements made within the clinic expressed in distance per unit of time represent gait speed. It is simply the time taken to walk a known distance. Dividing the known distance by the time taken to traverse that distance gives a value in meters per second or sometimes feet per minute.

Walking is a complex task, where we must use all parts of the body in a coordinated manner. The muscular and skeletal systems provide the support and mechanical mechanisms to move, whereas the nervous system assists in controlling the walking pattern. Sensory information from the visual, proprioceptive, and vestibular systems allows us to navigate through an environment.

The erect walking pattern is defined as a two-phase pattern of movement in the upright position: the *stance phase,* which is approximately 60% of a complete gait cycle, and the *swing phase,* which is approximately 40% of a complete gait cycle. The stance phase provides stability, maintaining the body in an upright position against the force of gravity, whereas the swing phase is responsible for progressing the body forward through space. At the beginning and end of the stance phase, both lower extremities are in contact with the floor, referred to as *double limb support.* In a mature gait pattern, double limb support occurs in the first and last 10% of the stance phase.[2] The percent of time spent in double limb support varies as we walk slowly or quickly and at various times across the life span.

The upper and lower extremities move in a reciprocal, contralateral pattern during walking and help to propel the body forward or backward in space. A 50% temporal and distance-phasing relationship exists between the lower limbs. As stated earlier, 50% phasing between the limbs indicates that when one limb is 50% completed with its cycle, the contralateral limb starts its cycle. According to Clark and Whitall,[19] newly walking infants coordinate their limbs in a 50% temporal phasing relationship, just like adults. These researchers revealed, however, that the young walkers exhibited significantly increased variability compared with infants who had been walking for 3 to 6 months. Once toddlers have a few months of walking experience, variability in their walking pattern decreases, and gait pattern characteristics, such as step length (normalized for limb length), step width, and walking skill begin to resemble gait of an older child or adult.[20]

Body System Impact on Walking Control

How do we control the act of walking? Arm, leg, trunk, and head movements all work together to maintain balance as our center of gravity moves outside of the base of support (BOS), but how do we organize and control this finely coordinated movement?

The nervous system plays a key role in the control of walking. Early stepping movements and locomotor patterns are controlled by pattern generators in the spinal cord or the brain stem.[21,22] Initially stepping, controlled only by these pattern generators, is stereotypic. The early stepping pattern that is produced is related to the pattern seen in reflex stepping and kicking in the infant.[23] Descending nervous system influences from the cerebellum contribute to modulation of the gait pattern and error correction. This level of control helps fine tune the gait pattern and assists us in walking over uneven terrain. The cortex also assists in the development of spatially directed movement. The visual cortex processes information from the environment so that perception and action can be linked.[2]

Sensory information is also critical to control of locomotion, assisting in the adaptation of the gait pattern to the environment in which it is occurring. Visual information is an important stimulus for locomotion. The infant is first enticed to move and to explore by seeing something or someone to move toward. Visual orientation also is important in aligning the body with the support surface. Visual flow information helps align the body in reference to the environment and helps in assessment of walking speed.

The somatosensory system contributes to the control of walking. Information from the muscle spindles and joint receptors contributes to the rhythm of walking, whereas the Golgi tendon organ influences timing of the transition from stance to swing phase of the gait cycle. Information from cutaneous receptors may also contribute to the ability to negotiate over obstacles. The vestibular system assists in alignment of the head in relationship to gravity, and the vestibulo-ocular reflex is important for head stabilization in space. The vestibular system does not appear to contribute to head stabilization during walking until age 7 years. Children up to age 6 depend primarily on visual and somatosensory information to organize and control walking. This sensory information allows them to use an ascending temporal organization of balance control (feet/pelvis to head). As the visual and vestibular systems become more functional in modulating ambulation, descending temporal organization of balance control (from head to toe) is seen in the walking child.[24] Temporal organization of balance control is described in more detail in Chapter 12.

In summary, the collective interactive effects of the neuromusculoskeletal system reveals a set of essential factors or requirements for safe and successful walking. These requirements include progression, stability, adaptability, long-term viability, and long-distance navigation.[25,26] Progression, the ability to walk from point A to point B, includes the generation of a locomotor rhythm and the ability to produce sufficient joint torque and ground reaction forces to propel the body forward. Therefore, stride characteristics and force or torque production are all relevant outcome variables associated with progression.

The center of mass is outside of the base of support during 80% of the walking cycle. Therefore stability is a major requirement for walking. Stability in walking implies an ability to proactively coordinate the body center of mass motion with stepping, adjust posture to environmental demands, and reactively adjust step length, height, and/or width to perturbations from the environment. The sensory system is integral to successful gait stability as are ongoing and rapid motor responses.

Adaptability is needed to take walking into real world, functional contexts. Adjustments to the locomotor pattern are needed to accommodate to and interact with the spaces, places, structures, and surfaces in the environment. Obstacles, stairs, ramps, curbs, grass, gravel, or other terrains all require an adaptable locomotor pattern. Vision is the primary sensory modality for the adjustment of the walking path and pattern when obstacles are present or terrain changes.[26,27]

Progression, stability, and adaptability are important for the short-term success of walking. To walk successfully for longer periods requires long-term viability. Long-term viability implies the minimization of stress on tissue and the minimization of energy expenditure. Stress on tissue is a factor when the musculoskeletal changes affect the gait pattern, as is sometimes the case when pain accompanies osteoarthritic changes to load bearing lower extremity joints. Cardiovascular and strength changes also impact one's ability to maintain energy cost within a reasonable range. The use of assistive devices, more common with increased age, may also impact energy expenditure. Energy expenditure, more formally the metabolic cost of walking, is greater in older adults than younger adults. This difference appears at approximately the seventh decade.[28] Why older persons exhibit greater metabolic cost of walking remains unclear. Irrespective of the origin, increased cost and increased stress on tissue can limit an older adult's mobility.

Finally, to possess a truly successful gait pattern, one must be able to walk to locations where the destination is not seen at the outset. This ability to navigate long distances to unseen locations is not possible without adequate perception, memory, judgment, and cognitive spatial mapping.[26]

Developmental Stages

Infants and Toddlers Independent ambulation is attained by 11.5 months of age in 50% of infants.[29] Until this point, the infant does not have sufficient strength or balance control of the head and trunk for independent walking. Extensor muscle strength is thought to be the critical variable in the development of independent locomotion.[23] Until sufficient strength is present, the stability component necessary for upright locomotion is absent. Infants also need to be able to coordinate their limb segments and adaptively deal with the challenges of environmental changes before they have sufficient control for the progression and adaptability components needed to walk.

The gait pattern of toddlers and children changes rapidly over the first months of walking and then continues to mature into childhood. The initial gait pattern is characterized by a wide BOS, arms held in a high guard position, short swing phase, lack of heel strike or push-off, and a need for the infant to propel themselves forward by leaning forward at the trunk. In addition, the new walker demonstrates less knee flexion in stance than an experienced walker and keeps the legs externally rotated during the swing phase. As the new walker gains balance and control of the upright position during movement, the gait pattern changes slowly into the mature gait pattern of the adult. At 2 to 3 years of age, the child walks with a reciprocal arm swing and demonstrates a heel strike. By approximately 3 to 4 years of age, the child's base of support has decreased to levels seen in mature walking and time spent in single limb stance during walking increases.[2,30,31] According to Sutherland and co-workers,[12] 98% of toddlers have a mature gait pattern by age 4. The gait pattern continues to be refined through 7 years of age. As previously described, the child initially uses somatosensory information and an ascending temporal organization of balance control during walking; then after age 7, a descending organization of balance is seen.[24]

The gait parameters of time and distance—step length and width, stride length, cadence, and walking velocity—all change as the physical characteristics of the child change. Step length increases as there is growth in stature and leg length. The taller and longer-legged a person, the bigger is the step length. Cadence of the infant is much greater than that of the adult. The number of steps taken per minute decreases gradually throughout childhood, with the biggest reduction seen during the first year of walking. Walking velocity increases with age in a linear manner from 1 to 3 years of age. From age 4 to 7, the rate of change of walking velocity diminishes, but the relationship to age remains linear.[12] Changes in walking speed, cadence, and stride length from ages 1 to 12 years of age are found in Table 13-1.

McGraw's[4] early observations and definitions of the development of erect locomotion reflect the gait changes discussed previously. She defined seven phases for the development of erect locomotion, which are

Table **13-1**

Gait Parameters of Children from 1 to 12 Years of Age

Age (yr)	Cadence (steps/min)	Cycle Time (s)	Stride Length (m)	Speed (m/sec)
1	127-223	0.54-0.94	0.29-0.58	0.32-0.96
1.5	126-212	0.57-0.95	0.33-0.66	0.39-1.03
2	125-201	0.60-0.96	0.37-0.73	0.45-1.09
2.5	124-190	0.63-0.97	0.42-0.81	0.52-1.16
3	123-188	0.64-0.98	0.46-0.89	0.58-1.22
3.5	122-186	0.65-0.98	0.50-0.96	0.65-1.29
4	121-184	0.65-0.99	0.54-1.04	0.67-1.32
5	119-180	0.67-1.01	0.59-1.10	0.71-1.37
6	117-176	0.68-1.03	0.64-1.16	0.75-1.43
7	115-172	0.70-1.04	0.69-1.22	0.80-1.48
8	113-169	0.71-1.06	0.75-1.30	0.82-1.50
9	111-166	0.72-1.08	0.82-1.37	0.83-1.53
10	109-162	0.74-1.10	0.89-1.45	0.85-1.55
11	107-159	0.75-1.12	0.92-1.49	0.86-1.57
12	105-156	0.77-1.14	0.96-1.54	0.88-1.60

From Whittle MW: *Gait analysis: an introduction*, ed 4, Philadelphia, 2007, Butterworth Heinemann Elsevier.

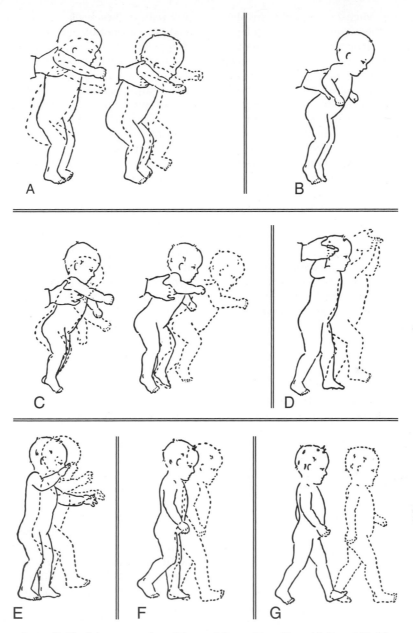

Figure 13-4 The seven phases (A-G) of the assumption of the upright position. (From McGraw MB: *The neuromuscular maturation of the human infant,* New York, 1945, Hafner Press, reprinted by permission of the publisher.)

illustrated in Figure 13-4, using a neurohierarchical, reflex theoretical framework of motor control. In phase A, the *newborn* or *reflex stepping,* the infant is in a flexed posture when held upright, and attempts to step are the result of elicitation of the stepping reflex, a primitive reflex movement pattern. In phase B, *inhibition,* or the *static phase,* elicitation of the stepping reflex is not

readily observed. As seen in the development of creeping, the infant can maintain a supported upright posture that includes active cervical and spinal extension. The infant moves the body up and down, holding the feet in position, in phase C, *transition.* The infant may stand in position and stamp the feet, but there is no progression forward. In phase D, *deliberate stepping,* the infant attempts to step when held upright. In phase E, *independent stepping,* the infant takes steps independently. During this phase, the early walker uses a wide BOS; feet are flat, and the upper extremities are maintained in a high guard position (arms held high with the shoulders in external rotation and abducted, the elbows flexed, and the wrist and fingers extended). The early walker maintains hips and knees in slight flexion to bring the COM closer to the ground. At about 12 to 13 months of age, infants are learning to walk alone. The later, more mature walker ambulates with a narrower BOS. Feet are closer together and show a heel-toe progression. The upper extremities are in low guard (shoulders in more of a neutral position with the elbows in extension), and the hips and knees are extended more. McGraw[4] called this pattern phase F, or *heel-toe progression.* Phase G, *integration,* or *maturity of erect locomotion,* finds the arms down and moving reciprocally, synchronous with the movements of the lower extremities; out-toeing has been reduced, and pelvic rotation is present, along with the double knee lock pattern. In the double knee lock pattern, there is knee extension just before heel contact, but at the moment of heel contact, there is knee flexion to help absorb impact shock; then, as the body moves forward over the foot, the knee returns to extension for weight bearing during the stance cycle. These characteristics indicate a mature gait pattern and usually have developed by age 3 or 4.

In addition to development of the nervous system, other factors such as strength and balance impact motor control and contribute to the development of walking in the infant and toddler. Biomechanical factors influence the infant's acquisition of upright locomotion. Infants must have sufficient strength of the lower limbs and trunk to support themselves upright against gravity and sufficient balance control and coordination to maintain the upright body position. Early reflex stepping behaviors demonstrated by the newborn and young infant are limited by the increased weight of the 2- to 3-month-old infant and relative lack of muscle strength to move the legs in a stepping pattern against the force of gravity. Because of the physical dimensions of the beginning walker, the COM is at the lower thoracic level, which makes balance control more difficult. By 18 to 24 months, the COM has descended, and as the COM moves closer to the BOS, the body becomes more stable. The new walker attempts to improve balance control by using a wide BOS, with the hips abducted and externally rotated. This provides medial lateral stability, but if the new walker's head moves out of the BOS in an anteroposterior direction, loss of balance occurs. There is more mediolateral movement than anteroposterior movement in the gait pattern of new walkers. New walkers, not only demonstrate more mediolateral motion but also demonstrate more of a "stepping in place" pattern of movement, with more hip flexion than is seen in mature walking.[32,33] This pattern helps the new walker safely clear the foot during gait. With experience, the walker's BOS narrows, and forward progression over a planted foot is possible. The new walker also stabilizes herself in an upright position by using coactivation of muscles to decrease the degrees of freedom that have to be controlled. The gait pattern becomes more fluid and reciprocal as this muscle coactivation is released. Within a few months of walking, toddlers use the more mature model of walking, in which they efficiently and synchronously control posture over the stance leg as they swing the other leg forward. The pendulum action of the lower extremities in this more mature walking pattern is related to limb length but also depends on strength and intersegmental coordination of the limbs.[33] Reciprocal muscle action begins at approximately 18 months of age.

From a cognitive, motor learning perspective, experience and learning also make a significant contribution to the development of locomotor patterns. The infant demonstrates the ability to modify her locomotor patterns as body size and body weight increase. With practice, the infant gains better control of intersegmental coordination of the limbs and body, making walking against the force of gravity more efficient.[33] The infant also must learn to adapt locomotor patterns when changing from quadruped patterns (creeping and plantigrade) to bipedal walking. In addition, the infant must adapt walking and locomotor skills to meet the challenges of a variety of support surfaces (tile, wood, carpet, grass, etc.), to adjust to obstacles in her path, and to meet challenges such as ascending/descending a sloped surface, uneven terrain, etc. This learning is supported by the infant's development of information processing strategies and by spending vast amounts of time practicing skills. Infants have demonstrated that they practice walking an accumulated 6 hours per day, taking approximately 9000 steps over the length of approximately 29 football fields.[20] These infants use a distributed practice model interspersing short bursts of walking with rest periods.[20] The infant also practices over approximately a dozen different types of surfaces in a day, which introduces the model of variable and random practice schedules into the learning of walking.[20] Infant experience with locomotion does not appear to totally transfer from creeping to walking behavior, but in both situations, the infants learn from their experiences to adapt to challenging situations. Experience helps infants adapt to situations and safely move through their environment.[9]

Children A child demonstrates a mature gait pattern between 3 to 4 years of age and continues to use an ascending organization of postural control with somatosensory information. On level surfaces, some influence of vestibular control is noted as the child begins to use a head stabilization in space strategy.[34] Consistent heel strike and knee flexion in early stance are present. A mature muscle activation pattern is also exhibited on electromyography. Further refinements in the temporal and spatial aspects of the gait pattern occur between 5 and 6 years of age and continue to change with child growth until adult values are reached at approximately 15 years of age.[31] Step speed and step length are greater in the 6-year-old than the 5-year-old. The 5-year-old also spends more time in double limb support than the older child. By the age of 7 years, the time spent in single limb stance during gait is nearly that seen in the adult.[2] Ground reaction forces generated during gait may also continue to increase into the sixth year.[35]

By 7 years of age, the child's COM has descended to the level of the L3 vertebra.[36] The head stabilization in space strategy is used in a variety of walking environments by age 7 years.[34] The gain of the vestibular ocular reflex does not reach adult levels until at least 7 years of age.[37] With this level of visual and vestibular maturation, the child is now able to stabilize herself using a descending temporal organization of postural control.

Adults The gait pattern of the adult was presented earlier in this chapter when erect walking was introduced. The adult can efficiently use walking as a primary means of locomotion to carry out daily tasks. An adult is able to vary gait velocity as she dashes across a busy street, adjusts to the need to walk up or down hill, and walks for long distances. While maintaining an erect posture and when normal muscle strength and endurance are present, the adult easily performs walking. In adulthood, the COM has descended to the sacral level, improving the stability of gait. The adult easily changes pace, starts and stops, and changes direction.

Older Adults Does the gait pattern change as we age? It is commonly considered that the gait pattern of older adults differs from that of younger individuals in several areas. Some of these common changes are listed in Table 13-2. Are similar gait pattern changes seen in all older adults? Although many of the body systems that support walking change with age (see Chapters 6 to 10), it should also be noted that psychosocial factors such as ageism can also contribute to changes in gait pattern. Stereotypical concepts of aging can influence an older individual's self-perception, alter gait speed, and increase time spent in the double limb support phase of gait.[38]

Table **13-2**

Gait Pattern Changes in the Older Adult

Gait Changes	Characteristics
Associated with normal aging	Decreased gait velocity
	Decreased stride length
	Decreased peak knee extension range of motion
	Decreased peak knee flexion in swing
	Slightly increased ankle dorsiflexion
	Decreased ankle plantar flexion power
Associated with decreased strength	Increased pelvic tilt, may be related to decreased abdominal muscle strength
	Decreased vertical displacement of body during gait
	Decreased gait velocity
	Decreased cadence, may be related to decreased dorsiflexion strength
Associated with decreased balance	Increased base of support
	Decreased gait velocity
	Increased time in double limb support
	Increased use of visual scanning

Data from Ostrosky KM, VanSwearingen JM, Burdett RG, et al: A comparison of gait characteristics in young and old subjects, *Phys Ther* 74:637-646, 1994; Judge JO, Ounpuu S, Davis RB: Effects of age on the biomechanics and physiology of gait, *Clin Geriatr Med* 12:659-678, 1996; Bohannon RW: Comfortable and maximum walking speed of adults aged 20-79 years: reference values and determinants, *Age Ageing* 26:15-19, 1997.

It must be understood that within the older adult population, much variation exists. Healthy, active older adults in their 60s to 70s may walk using the same pattern as a younger population. Other older adults who have a chronic illness, such as arthritis, diabetes, or heart disease, may demonstrate pathological gait deviations or exaggerated gait changes. The pain of arthritis, the sensory loss accompanying diabetes, and the lack of endurance seen in patients with cardiac disease will all affect the gait pattern. Falling becomes more of a problem as adults continue to age, becoming a health problem for the older adult population (Clinical Implications Box 13-1: Falling in Older Adults and Its Prevention). Attempts to clarify the relationship between aging and

---

CLINICAL IMPLICATIONS Box 13-1
Falling in Older Adults and Its Prevention

Falling is a common problem in older adults, often resulting in injury and hospitalization. Older adults with a history of falling exhibit some differences in their gait pattern when compared with older adults without a history of falling. These gait pattern differences can be exacerbated because after a fall, the older adult may become less active, fearing and trying to prevent another fall. Further changes in the gait pattern may be made in an attempt to increase safety during ambulation. Decreased activity levels may eventually lead to decreased levels of functional independence, and limited mobility may negatively affect quality of life.

Several factors have been identified that contribute to the increased incidence of falling in older adults, some of which are summarized here. There are also several strategies that can help in the prevention of falls in the older adult, improving functional independence and health status.

Characteristics of Gait Pattern in Older Adults Who Have Fallen
- Decreased stride length compared with nonfallers[95,96]
- Decreased walking speed compared with nonfallers[95,96]
- Decreased walking speed and cadence with increased double support time, especially when the person is concerned about a fall[97] and under dual task (e.g., walking when talking) conditions[98]
- A conservative approach (i.e., taking numerous small steps) when approaching an obstacle[96]
- Mediolateral instability in standing (more predictive of falls than anteroposterior instability)[99]
- Greater stride frequency across a range of imposed gait speeds and an inability to obtain the highest imposed gait speed[100]
- Increased stride to stride variability[64,100,101]

Kinematics
- Reduced hip extension[59,100]
- Reduced plantar flexion[100]
- Decreased trunk rotation and increased knee flexion[96]

Kinetics
- Increased hip flexion moment in stance; decreased hip extension moment in stance; decreased knee flexion moment in preswing; decreased knee power absorption in preswing[102]

Possible Factors Contributing to Falls in Older Adults
- Difficulty corralling the body center of mass in response to a perturbation requiring multiple steps[103]
- Disproportionately greater medial-lateral instability compared with nonfallers[104,105]
- Difficulty modulating step length quickly enough to avoid an obstacle[25]
- Speed and length of the step are less than they are in younger adults[106]
- Slower rate of ankle torque development in response to a trip, making it more difficult to regain balance[107]
- Increased difficulty performing another task while walking[98,108]
- Impairments in hip abductor torque generating capacity and decreased trunk axial rotation[105]

Intervention Strategies for Fall Prevention
- Reduce risk factors for falls[109]
- Multifactorial fall risk assessment and management program[110]
- Physical activity and specific exercise programs that include a balance training component[111,112]
- For the individual at high risk for falls, it may be beneficial to include a home hazard assessment and modification[112]
- Shoes with low heels and firm slip-resistant soles should be worn both inside and outside the home[113]
- Therapeutic exercise and balance training for positive outcomes of increased balance, increased lower extremity strength and balance, increased safety, increased physical and functional capacity, and increased ability to perform instrumental and basic activities of daily living[1]

walking date back to at least the early 1940s and continue today. Research provides conflicting information about exactly how the gait of older adults changes with age. It is necessary to carefully study healthy older adults and to try to separate out the gait pattern changes that are related solely to increasing age.

Progression   The most commonly reported finding when studying the gait of older persons is a slower walking speed compared with younger adults.[39-49] Recalling that gait velocity is the product of stride length and cadence, it is important to evaluate all three gait parameters of progression together. Coinciding with a slower walking velocity is a shorter step length, longer stance phase, and shorter swing time than younger adults.[50-53] At self-selected walking speeds, the stride of the older adults is typically shorter than that of the younger adults. Cadence, on the other hand, has not always demonstrated a significant change with age in healthy older persons.[39,54] It remains unclear if older adults choose to walk slower for stability purposes or if there are fundamental changes in the neuromusculoskeletal system causing the slower speed. Slowed progression is likely a combination of changes at the level of the sensorimotor systems and in some cases adaptations for stability.

The decline in gait velocity at comfortable walking speeds is not the same across decades. Persons in their 60s and 70s generally maintain a stable gait speed[44,45] but then show more marked decline in their 80s and 90s. Maximum walking speed declines more steadily throughout adulthood.[44]

Kinematics   Changes in gait speed and stride length are associated with reductions in joint motion. Changes in ankle range of motion and pelvic obliquity have been noted in older adults.[51] Ankle plantar flexion at terminal stance can be decreased and the anterior pelvic tilt increased.[55,56] Peak knee extension range of motion is also significantly decreased in the older adult compared with the younger adult.[55,57]

A significant reduction in hip extension motion is seen even during faster walking in healthy older persons.[58,59] This is an important finding because it implies that the reduced range of motion is not simply a function of walking slower. An even greater reduction in hip extension is associated with older persons who have a history of falls. In both cases, this reduction in hip extension has been attributed to hip joint tightness.[59,60] However, simply stating it is a problem of static tightness at the hip is an insufficient explanation because this tightness is not manifested in the standing position. That is, the reduced hip extension is observed only during gait.[56]

Kinetics   Reductions in gait speed and stride length are associated with reductions in joint torque and ground reaction forces. However, it is unclear which finding is

the cause and which is the effect. The difficulty with maintaining maximum walking speed appears to be related to an older adult's inability to generate as great a peak ankle plantar flexor moment as a younger adult.[55] Winter and colleagues[54] found that even fit, healthy older persons exhibit a decreased plantar-flexor push-off power burst. Power is simply force times velocity. They also found a reduction in knee absorption power. No differences were noted for hip kinetics. Judge and colleagues[55] also found reduced ankle plantar-flexor power. After adjusting for step length differences between older and younger adult groups, Judge and colleagues[55] found that older adults tend to rely instead on increasing hip flexion power in late stance to increase speed.[55] Interestingly, the age-related differences in ankle kinetics disappeared when the step length was accounted for. It appears that older persons may increase hip kinetics as a compensation for reductions in distal joint kinetic function.[61,62]

Stability   The balance capabilities of older persons have been extensively studied and there are numerous studies that suggest many of the gait adaptations observed during progression (e.g., reduced speed and stride length) are manifested to maintain balance or stability. For example, Shkuratova and associates[63] had a small group of healthy older adults change speed and walk in a figure eight pattern and assessed walking stability via temporal gait parameters. A major finding was that older persons did not adjust their maximal walking speed to the same extent as younger persons. Older persons were able to walk faster than their comfortable gait speed, but speed and stride length were reduced compared with younger adults. There were nonsignificant reductions in speed and stride length by older persons compared with younger persons during turns within the figure eight walking task. Collectively, these adaptations were seen as modifications to gait to maintain stability. Given that Maki[64] has shown a significant relationship between slower gait and smaller steps and fear of falling in older persons, it is reasonable to argue that these temporal and spatial gait changes are adaptive in order to maintain stability.

Menz and colleagues[65] also suggested that reductions in gait speed and step length (along with an increased step timing variability) by older persons is representative of a more conservative gait pattern. Stability was thought to be preserved because such a pattern reduces the magnitude of accelerations at the head and pelvis. Accelerations of major body segments near the body center of mass (pelvis) and segments containing important sensors for the successful maintenance of the gait pattern (vision and vestibular apparatus within the head segment) could be potentially destabilizing to an older person. Anterior-posterior trunk accelerations at push-off have also been observed to be lower in older persons.[66] As such, reductions in gait speed and step length may be a compensatory mechanism to preserve stability.

Mazza and colleagues[67] used upper body accelerations and the analysis of harmonic ratio as a means to understand how younger and older persons stabilize the head during walking. It is likely that younger persons synchronize accelerations in the upper body and attenuate these accelerations to maintain a stable head and thus a stable gaze during walking. A stable gaze is clearly an important feature of a stable gait because it enables the effective use of vision to adjust the gait pattern. Older adult women in the Mazza and colleagues[67] study did not attenuate head accelerations to the same extent as younger adult women.

Pavol and colleagues[68,69] used an innovative research paradigm to investigate the nature of balance during walking in older adults. They induced a trip during mid to late swing using a concealed, mechanical obstacle that rose from the floor 5.1 cm. Those older adult subjects who walked faster and/or had less response time to recover were more likely to trip than those who walked slower. This was true irrespective of the effectiveness of the reactive stepping response elicited as a result of the trip. Pavol and colleagues[68,69] concluded that not hurrying reduced the likelihood of falling as a result of a trip. In a follow-up study using modeling techniques, van der Bogert and colleagues[70] contended that there is a critical body lean angle (26 degrees) beyond which recovery from a trip is not possible. That is, the tripped foot must contact the ground before this forward body tilt is reached. Moreover, response time is an important determinant in the potential for a recovery from a trip. It is important to note that response time is made up of a number of neuromuscular processes such as detection of the perturbation via sensory channels, reflexes in the lower extremities, and the actual execution of the protective stepping response.[70]

The findings highlighted here imply that with respect to the requirements of walking, stability is a key requirement for successful walking in older persons. It is likely that the neuromusculoskeletal system is marshaled in such a way as to preserve stability during gait for older persons. Walking slower may be an adaptive strategy for the preservation of stability in older adults. However, much remains to be evaluated with respect to the assessment of balance control during walking in older adults. Specifically, much more needs to be done to assess both the proactive and reactive balance mechanisms necessary for a safe and efficient walking pattern.[71]

Adaptability Adaptability of gait is important when encountering varying terrains or surfaces in the environment and/or when encountering obstacles in the walking path. Several studies have identified differences in the adaptability of gait in older persons. For example, in one of the first studies on this subject, Chen and colleagues[72] had subjects step over obstacles ranging up to 152 mm in height. Swing foot clearance was the same for older and younger adults. Older adults were observed to exhibit what Chen and colleagues[72] called a more conservative strategy to obstacle clearance. This strategy included slower speed, shorter steps, and a shorter obstacle-heel strike distance. No subject tripped on any of the obstacles, suggesting for at least this sample of subjects that aging alone does not lead to difficulty managing obstacles of this height.

McFadyen and Prince[73] examined the kinematics and kinetics of older and younger adults avoiding an 11.75 cm high obstacle during walking and accommodating an 11.75 cm change in floor height. Although the general anterior-posterior plane kinematics were similar between groups, the older adults did exhibit a decreased toe clearance of the lead foot. Limited frontal plane pelvic motion and shorter strides may have been the reason for the decreased toe clearance. However, decreased toe clearance is not an ubiquitous finding in the literature on adapting the gait pattern to avoid an obstacle. More recently, Lu and colleagues[74] found that older adults increase joint kinematics to increased obstacle height (10%, 20%, 30% of leg length). Older adults appear to use a leading swing leg hip flexion strategy to maintain a safe distance between the foot and the obstacle. Differences in findings between these studies may be related to the nature and form of the to-be-avoided obstacle.

A number of studies have been conducted since this early work on gait adaptability in older adults. A recent systematic review of this line of research has been conducted.[75] This review concluded that although older adults adopt a more conservative strategy (see previous discussion) when given enough time, their ability to adapt the gait pattern to obstacles is not different than younger adults. However, when time is a factor, older adults are at greater risk of contacting an obstacle and thus put themselves at risk for tripping or falling.

Long-Term Viability It has been consistently observed that older adults exhibit an increased energy cost of walking.[76,77] In this connection it is reasonable to hypothesize that there is an interaction between the need for stability and energy cost. That is, maintaining stability requires greater energy cost in older adults. This hypothesis was examined by Malatesta and colleagues.[78] They measured energy cost and gait instability (stride time variability) in healthy older adults and younger adults when walking on a treadmill. While increased energy cost was again confirmed for the older adults, there was no correlation between gait instability and energy cost. Therefore, these authors concluded that the increased energy cost observed in older adults is not solely due to gait instability and that it is likely due to numerous neuromuscular factors. It is important to note that studies of overground walking may provide different results than those studies that use a treadmill. It is possible that gait on a treadmill is less automatic[78] than overground walking because of the forced mechanical pacing of the treadmill belt, which changes the stride variability in complex ways.[79]

Long-Distance Navigation Recall that long-distance navigation refers to the ability to navigate to an unseen destination. This requirement for successful walking is not related to energy expenditure but to the development and maintenance of cognitive spatial maps for navigating through realistic environments. While cognitive and perceptual motor abilities decrease with age,[80] it is unclear to what extent healthy aging affects long-distance navigation compared to pathological states such as cognitive impairment and Alzheimer disease. Clearly, such pathological states can adversely impact long-distance navigation, placing the person at risk for injury.[81]

Running, Galloping, Hopping, and Skipping

The locomotion patterns that evolve after upright walking are the patterns of running, galloping, hopping, and skipping.[19] Most literature on the development of these patterns has been descriptive research focusing on the head and neck, the trunk, and the extremities and on how these components relate to each other as a particular pattern evolves. Accomplishment of these locomotor skills is a good indicator of the development of balance.[2]

The contemporary theory of dynamic systems explains these subsequent patterns of locomotion as examples of different coordinative structures. A *coordinative structure* is defined as the coordination of the movement—how the muscles within a limb (intralimb) and between limbs (interlimb) are constrained to act as a unit. Dynamic action theory defines *coordination of a movement pattern* as the distance and temporal phasing relationships of the limbs, the stance swing relationships of the limbs, or some combination of time, distance, and velocity, which are collective variables that distinguish between different patterns of upright locomotion.

Running

Running is defined as a pattern of movement that has a stance phase and a swing phase but, more importantly, a flight phase, a period of nonsupport. The stance phase

of running is 40% of the gait cycle, whereas the swing phase is 60%. When running, a longer time is spent in the swing phase than in walking—when 60% of the gait cycle was spent in stance phase and 40% was spent in swing phase. As with walking, the temporal phasing of running is such that halfway through the cycle of one limb, the other limb begins its cycle—50% phasing.[19]

In the transition from walking to running, we have to produce sufficient force to project the body into the air for the flight phase of running. The toddler, for instance, can run only when there are sufficient vertical ground reaction forces. These forces most likely result from increases in muscle mass, changes in anthropometric measurements, improved motor neuron recruitment, improved postural system, or some combination of these parameters and others not yet defined. Footwork of the beginning runner recalls the early footflat pattern of walking. The early runner returns the arms to a high guard position. Initially, there is no reciprocal arm swing or the forward-and-back driving swing of the arms. The arms are thought to be used more for balance. Until approximately 2 years of age, the runner does not exhibit a flight stage in the running pattern.[2] Stride length of the more advanced runner is longer because more force can be generated in the lower extremity during push-off. This ability to increase force also allows for a longer flight phase and heel strike. The more advanced runner demonstrates an increase in trunk rotation and arm swing. These patterns have been documented by descriptive studies of children aged 18 months to 10 years.[82] The developmental levels of running are outlined below; these levels are adapted from the developmental levels of running defined by Roberton and Halverson.[6]

Level 1 *Upper extremities*—the arms are held in high guard to assist balance control and are otherwise not active.

Lower extremities—the feet are flat, there is minimal flight, and the swing leg is slightly abducted.

Level 2 *Upper extremities*—the arms begin to swing as spinal rotation counterbalances the rotation of the pelvis; the arms may give the appearance of "flailing."

Lower extremities—the feet may remain flat and may support knee flexes more during weight transfer; there is more flight time.

Level 3 *Upper extremities*—the arm swing increases because of the spinal rotation.

Lower extremities—heel contact is made at foot strike; the swing leg is in the sagittal plane; and at toe-off, the support leg reaches full extension.

Level 4 *Upper extremities*—the arm swing becomes independent of spinal rotation; the arms move in opposition to each other and contralateral to the leg swing.

Lower extremities—the level is similar to that of level 3.

Running in the older adult is defined according to the abilities of the adult being assessed. However, it has been determined that aging affects running speed, even in competitive sprinters,[83] and running as a physical activity has no positive effect on the redistribution of joint torque during walking in older adults.[47] Using a cross-sectional study approach of runners aged 17 to 82 years, Korhonen and colleagues[83] identified that decreased running speed is progressive with age. Reduced speed was attributed to reduced stride length and increased contact time. Swing time remained unchanged. Not surprisingly, ground reaction forces decrease over time as does more basic components of the muscular system, such as muscle thickness, type II fiber area, and the ability to rapidly generate force within a muscle.

Galloping

Galloping is defined as the first asymmetric gait mode in the young child—a walk on the leading leg followed by a running step on the rear leg. There is an asymmetrical phasing of approximately 65%/35%.[84] Clark and Whitall[19] state that galloping can be seen 20 months after a toddler begins to walk; by 4 years of age, 43% of children can gallop; and by 6.5 years, children are proficient at galloping. The phasing modes are variable but predominantly consist of two distance phasing modes: 66%/33% and 75%/25%. The variability of temporal phasing was also found to be low across subjects who ranged in age from 2 years to adulthood.

In early attempts at galloping, the arms are stiff and rarely become involved in projecting the body off the floor. They are usually held in the high guard position or out to the side to assist in balance, as was seen in the early form of running. During the early experiences of galloping, the stride is short, landings are flat-footed, and there is little trunk rotation. In addition, the tailing limb may land ahead of the lead limb. In contrast, the more advanced gallop appears more rhythmic and relaxed. The arms are no longer needed for balance and come into a low guard position or swing rhythmically in opposition to the movements of the lower extremities. These changes are accompanied by an increase in trunk rotation, which allows for more reciprocal arm movements. Research related to adults and galloping is not available.

Hopping

Hopping (one-footed hopping) is an asymmetric pattern of locomotion. Clark and Whitall[19] found that 33% of 4-year-old children could hop and that by 6.5 years of age, children were proficient at hopping. Halverson and Williams[85] studied a group of children longitudinally and presented developmental levels for the upper and lower extremities for the hop. The developmental levels of hopping as defined by Roberton and Halverson[6] are outlined here.

Level 1 *Upper extremities*—the arms are held in high guard, out to the side, and not very active.

Lower extremities—hip and knee quickly flex, pulling the body toward the floor more than lifting the body off the floor; the flight is momentary, only one or two hops; and the swing leg is inactive.

Level 2 *Upper extremities*—the arms swing upward together, perhaps to assist in balance.

Lower extremities—body lean allows extension of the knee and ankle to lift the body off the floor; there are repeated hops, but the swing leg is mostly inactive.

Level 3 *Upper extremities*—the arms are active together, pumping the body to help lift the body.

Lower extremities—there is better coordination among the hip, knee, and ankle for functional takeoff and landing, and the swing leg now assists in the movement by pumping up and down; however, the swing leg remains down and behind the support leg.

Level 4 *Upper extremities*—the arm in opposition to the swing leg is moving forward with the swing leg, assisting in the movement (to a minimal degree); the other arm is in the front or to the side.

Lower extremities—the ball of the foot is now used for the landing; the support leg has good extension at takeoff; the swing leg helps in the upward and forward movement at takeoff; and the increase in the swing leg's range of movement assists with the movement.

Level 5 *Upper extremities*—the arms work in coordination with the swing leg to assist the movement.

Lower extremities—the level is similar to that of level 4.

The swing leg is inactive in the earliest form of the one-leg hop. It is not until about 4 years of age that the swing leg begins to move in the hop, helping to propel the body forward. Ultimately, it is the swing leg that pumps up and down to assist in projection; the range of the swing leg increases so that it passes behind the support leg when viewed from the side. The arms follow a similar pattern. Initially, the arms are inactive, held in high guard. As the pattern progresses, the arms become more active, swinging in opposition to the legs. Specifically, the arm opposite the swing leg moves forward and upward in a pumping action to assist the propulsion of the body forward; the other arm moves in the direction opposite the action of the swing leg. In the adult form of hopping, the arms and legs are active, swinging in opposition as just described. The interlimb phasing patterns are probably 50% temporal and distance phasing. What should be remembered for this pattern of locomotion, as with all such patterns, is that children progress at different rates; the rate of progression can be attributed to many different parameters, including muscle strength and balance.

Skipping

Skipping is defined as an alternating gait, a step, then a hop on one leg, followed by a step, then a hop on the other leg. Clark and Whitall[19] found that only 14% of children could skip at 4 years of age. The developmental levels for skipping as defined by Roberton and Halverson[6] are outlined here.

Level 1 *Upper extremities*—the arms move bilaterally to assist as the weight is transferred from foot to foot.

Lower extremities—One foot completes the step-and-hop sequence before weight is transferred to the other foot.

Level 2 *Upper extremities*—the arms begin to oppose each other, but they mostly work together.

Lower extremities—the child continues to complete one step-and-hop sequence before transferring the weight; the feet are flat during the movement.

Level 3 *Upper extremities*—the arms are in opposition to each other.

Lower extremities—action is completely on the ball of the foot; weight transfer is more smooth between the hop-and-step sequences.

The arms are initially held in high guard. The advanced pattern ultimately involves a swinging of the arms in opposition to the moving lower extremities. It has been suggested that interlimb phasing of this locomotion pattern is most likely 50%.[19]

BODY SYSTEM INTERACTIONS RELATED TO LOCOMOTION

Structural and functional changes occur in all of the body systems with aging (see Chapters 6 to 10). The musculoskeletal, cardiovascular, pulmonary, neurological, and sensory systems contribute most to walking. Changes in these systems, seen from infancy through older adulthood, affect the development and refinement of the gait pattern.

Musculoskeletal System

Infants cannot support themselves in a standing position or walk because of insufficient strength to support the body against gravity and insufficient range of motion to fully extend their hips in the standing position. Through infancy, muscle mass increases and the child gains controlled mobility through a full range of motion to allow standing and then walking. Changes from lower extremity varus in the beginning walker to a more valgus posture in the 3-year-old influence heel and foot position during gait. In children, the gait pattern changes with increasing length of the limbs and increasing muscle strength. With increasing lower extremity length, the stride length increases. Increasing strength allows the child to exert greater forces when pushing off from the support surface. As the toddler gains more strength for push-off, she is able to take longer steps and walk faster.[86] Running cannot occur until the child can generate sufficient force to push into a flight phase.

Changes in the musculoskeletal system with aging are described in detail in Chapter 6. Some of the most specific changes within muscle tissue that may have an impact on walking include a decrease in type II muscle fibers, a decrease in the number of functional motor units, and changes in the muscle tissue with increased fat content and fibrin within the muscle fibers. Muscle strength loss is one of the main causes of a decline in activities of daily living in the older adult population.[87] It has been suggested that the changes observed in the locomotion patterns and reduced gait velocity of older adults are most likely the result of decreases in muscular strength.[51,55,58,88] Wilder[89] identified that 64% of the variation seen in the gait characteristics, such as step length and time in double support of older adults, was accounted for by the variable of muscle strength. Small differences in ankle muscle strength and significant differences in hip muscle strength resulted in significant differences in certain gait pattern parameters of older adult women.[89] Strengthening exercise programs have been shown to increase walking speed, cadence, and stride length of older adults. Increased cadence was found to be related to increased ankle dorsiflexion strength, whereas increased stride was found to be related to increased hip extension strength.[90] Decreased plantar flexion strength has also been thought to reduce step length and increase time in double limb support.[13] Decreased knee extension strength affects maximum walking speed, whereas hip abductor strength affects comfortable walking speed.[44]

However, in addition to simple changes in the force-generating capacity of muscle with age, there appears to be a redistribution of joint torque during walking in older adults[61] to a more proximal control via increased hip extensor torque and decreased knee extensor and plantar-flexor torque. This is suggestive of a potential adaptive change in coordination within the locomotor pattern itself. Therefore, aging should be evaluated both at the component level of walking (e.g., individual muscle activity) and at the locomotor pattern level. This level of control is clearly influenced by changes in sensory and motor systems but also possesses its own unique dynamic properties with respect to coordination among the segments within the lower extremity (intralimb coordination) and between limbs (interlimb coordination). Age-related changes have been observed in interlimb coordination.[91]

Cardiovascular and Pulmonary Systems

The cardiovascular and pulmonary systems are important for providing fuel to the body tissues active in walking. Under normal conditions, cardiovascular and pulmonary function should be adequate to support walking. Maximal walking speed has been associated with cardiac output and levels of fitness in older men. In general, physically active and fit individuals of any age should be able to easily walk and complete their daily activities. In deconditioned individuals, walking uses a much higher proportion of the energy reserve than when we are conditioned, and everyday functional activities and walking may become too strenuous for someone with severe deconditioning.

Nervous System

The nervous system is important in the process of motor control and provision of sensory information needed for walking. Children begin to walk at approximately 1 year of age, but their gait pattern becomes more refined and coordinated over the next 6 years. Factors such as myelination of the nervous system, dendritic formation, and the number of functional motor units contribute to the development and quality of walking. Through infancy and young childhood, these factors develop and increase in number. In older adulthood, the number of dendrites and functional motor units decreases, as does nerve conduction velocity as a result of changes in myelination and the motor unit itself. These changes with age can contribute to increased reaction time and changes in the gait pattern.

The ability to perceive and use sensory input is critical to functional gait. In older adults, cutaneous receptors are not as efficient as in younger adults. Diminished proprioception is seen, especially at the ankles. Visual and vestibular function also decreases. It may also be more difficult for older adults to integrate multiple sources of sensory input because of changes in central processing ability. These factors are thought to contribute to decreased gait velocity and increased balance difficulty. Yet while reduced plantar sensation can make an individual walk more cautiously regardless of age,[92] slight reductions in gait speed should be delineated from a "cautious" gait observed in some older adults. Cautious gait in this context is defined as mild to moderate slowing, reduced stride length, and widening of the base of support[93] and is not associated with any specific neuromuscular or sensory deficit. Herman and colleagues[94] found that older individuals with a cautious gait had a significantly increased gait variability compared with age-matched older adults without a cautious gait pattern. However, the cautious gait variability was not associated with age, muscle strength, or balance. Variability was associated with scores on the Geriatric Depression Scale and a measure of fear of falling. Herman and associates[94] concluded that this type of gait pattern appears to be an appropriate response to unsteadiness and may represent an underlying pathology. Importantly, this pattern is not due to typical sensory or motor changes as a function of so-called normal aging.

SUMMARY

Locomotion is a functional necessity of our lifestyle as humans. Parents celebrate and remember the first time their baby rolls, crawls, creeps, and takes a step, marking this function as a sociocultural milestone. The ability to move independently from one place to another is important to our independence and identity. In a rehabilitation setting, the first question a patient or her family often asks is, "When will I [she] walk again?" For some, the answer is that the important function of locomotion will be achieved using a wheelchair.

Locomotion develops across the life span from rolling to crawling and creeping to erect walking to running, galloping, hopping, and skipping. The transition from one form of locomotion to another depends on a number of factors: the interactions of the tasks to be accomplished, body systems function, and the environment in which the behavior is to be produced. The change in locomotor patterns across the life span charts a bell curve, first becoming more efficient and then potentially becoming less efficient and safe. The challenges to locomotion for the older adult may include falling, which presents health risk and negatively impacts quality of life. Therapists can better help patients improve their functional independence and quality of life when they appreciate factors that contribute to efficient ambulation.

REFERENCES

1. American Physical Therapy Association: *Guide to physical therapist practice*, ed 2, *Phys Ther*, 81: 9–744, 2001.
2. Shumway-Cook A, Woollacott MH: *Motor control: translating research into clinical practice*, ed 3, Philadelphia, 2007, Lippincott, Williams & Wilkins.
3. Shirley MM: *The first two years: a study of twenty-five babies, vol 1: postural and locomotor development*, Minneapolis, 1931, University of Minnesota Press.
4. McGraw MB: *The neuromuscular maturation of the human infant*, New York, 1945, Hafner Press.
5. Whitall J: A developmental study of the inter-limb coordination in running and galloping, *J Mot Behav* 21:409–428, 1989.
6. Roberton MA, Halverson LE: *Developing children–their changing movement: a guide for teachers*, Philadelphia, 1984, Lea & Febiger.
7. Roberton MA, Halverson LE: The development of locomotor coordination: longitudinal change and invariance, *J Mot Behav* 20:197–241, 1988.
8. Getchell N, Roberton MA: Whole body stiffness as a function of developmental level in children's hopping, *Dev Psychol* 25:920–928, 1989.
9. Adolph DE: Learning to move, *Curr Dir Psychol Sci* 17(3):213–218, 2008.
10. Inman VT, Ralston HJ, Todd F: *Human walking*, Baltimore, 1981, Williams & Wilkins.
11. Murray MP: Gait as a total pattern of movement, *Am J Phys Med* 46:290–333, 1967.
12. Sutherland DH, Olshen RA, Biden EN, et al: *The development of mature walking*, (From the Clinics in Developmental Medicine series, No. 104/105), London, 1988, Mac Keith Press .
13. Winter DA: *The biomechanics and motor control of human gait: normal, elderly, and pathological*, ed 2, Waterloo, Canada, 1991, Waterloo Press.
14. Clark JE, Whitall J, Phillips SJ: Human inter-limb coordination and control: the first 6 months of independent walking, *Dev Psychobiol* 21:445–456, 1988.
15. deVries JIP, Visser GHA, Prechtl HFR: Fetal motility in the first half of pregnancy. In Prechtl HFR, editor: *Continuity of neural functions from prenatal to postnatal life*, Philadelphia, 1984, JB Lippincott, pp 46–64.
16. Prechtl HFR: Prenatal motor development. In Wade MG, Whiting HTA, editors: *Motor development in children: aspects of coordination and control*, Dordrecht, Netherlands, 1986, Martinus Nijhoff.
17. Richter RR, VanSant AF, Newton RA: Description of adult rolling movements and hypothesis of developmental sequences, *Phys Ther* 69:63–71, 1989.
18. Adolph KE, Vereijken B, Denny MA: Learning to crawl, *Child Dev* 69(5):1299–1312, 1998.
19. Clark JE, Whitall J: Changing patterns of locomotion: from walking to skipping. In Woollacott M, Shumway-Cook A, editors: *Development of posture and gait across the life span*, Columbia, SC, 1989, University of South Carolina Press, pp 128–151.
20. Adolph KE, Vereijken B, Shjrout PE: What changes in infant walking and why, *Child Dev* 72(2):475–497, 2003.
21. Connolly KJ, Forssberg H: *Neurophysiology and neuropsychology of motor development*, London, 1997, Mac Keith Press.
22. Grillner S: Control of locomotion in bipeds, tetrapods, and fish. In Geiger SR, editor: *Handbook of physiology*, vol 2, Bethesda, Md, 1981, American Psychological Society, pp 1179–1236.
23. Thelen E, Ulrich BD, Jensen JL: The developmental origins of locomotion. In Woollacott MH, Shumway-Cook A, editors: *Development of posture and gait across the life span*, Columbia, SC, 1989, University of South Carolina, pp 25–47.
24. Assaiante C: Development of locomotor balance control in healthy children, *Neurosci Biobehav Rev* 22:527–532, 1998.
25. Patla AE, Prentice SD, Martin C, et al: The bases of selection of alternate foot placement during locomotion in humans. In Woollacott MH, Horak F, editors: *Posture and gait: control mechanisms*, Eugene, Ore, 1992, University of Oregon Press, pp 226–229.
26. Patla AE: A framework for understanding mobility problems in the elderly. In Craik RL, Oatis CA, editors: *Gait analysis: theory and application*, St Louis, 1995, Mosby, pp 437–449.
27. Simoneau GG, Cavanagh PR, Ulbrecht JS, et al: The influence of visual factors on fall-related kinematic variables during stair descent by older women, *J Gerontol A Biol Sci Med Sci* 46(6):M188–M195, 1991.
28. Waters RL, Lunsford BR, Perry J, et al: Energy – speed relationship of walking: standard tables, *J Orthop Res* 6:215–222, 1988.
29. Piper MC, Darrah J: *Motor assessment of the developing infant*, Philadelphia, 1994, WB Saunders.
30. Chambers HG: Pediatric gait analysis. In Perry J, Burnfield JM, editors: *Gait analysis: normal and pathological function*, ed 2, Thorofare, NJ, 2010, Slack Inc, pp 341–364.
31. Whittle MW: *Gait analysis: an introduction*, ed 4, Philadelphia, 2007, Butterworth Heinemann Elsevier.
32. Dominici N, Ivanenko YP, Lacquaniti F: Control of foot trajectory in walking toddlers: adaptation to load changes, *J Neurophysiol* 97:2790–2801, 2007.
33. Ivanenko YP, Dominici N, Lacquaniti F: Development of independent walking in toddlers, *Exerc Sport Sci Rev* 35(2):67–73, 2007.
34. Assaiante C, Amblard B: Ontogenesis of head stabilization in space during locomotion in children: influence of visual cues, *Exp Brain Res* 93:499–515, 1993.
35. Pellico LG, Torres RR, Mora CD: Changes in walking pattern between five and six years of age, *Dev Med Child Neurol* 37:800–806, 1995.
36. Palmer CE: Studies of the center of gravity in the human body, *Child Dev* 15:99–180, 1944.
37. Assaiante C, Amblard B: Visual factors in the child's gait: effects on locomotor skills, *Percept Mot Skills* 83:1019–1041, 1996.

38. Hausdorff JM, Levy BR, Wei JY: The power of ageism on physical function of older persons: reversibility of age-related gait changes, *J Am Geriatr Soc* 47:1346–1349, 1999.

39. Oberg T, Karsznia A, Oberg K: Joint angle parameters in gait: reference data for normal subjects, 10-79 years of age, *J Rehabil Res Dev* 30:210–233, 1993.

40. Herann JE, Cunningham DA, Rechnitzer PA, et al: Age-related changes in speed of walking, *Med Sci Sports Exerc* 20:161–166, 1988.

41. McGibbon CA: Toward a better understanding of gait changes with age and disablement: neuromuscular adaptation, *Exerc Sport Sci Rev* 31(2):102–108, 2003.

42. Murray MP, Kory RC, Clarkson BH: Walking patterns in healthy old men, *J Gerontol* 24:169–178, 1969.

43. Alexander NB: Gait disorders in older adults, *J Am Geriatr Soc* 44(4):434–451, 1996.

44. Bohannon RW: Comfortable and maximum walking speed of adults aged 20-79 years: reference values and determinants, *Age Ageing* 26:15–19, 1997.

45. Lusardi MM, Pellecchia GL, Schulman M: Functional performance in community-living older adults, *J Geriatr Phys Ther* 26(3):14–22, 2003.

46. Abellan van kan G, Rolland Y, Andrieu S, et al: Gait speed at usual pace as a predictor of adverse outcomes in community-dwelling older people: an International Academy on Nutrition and Aging (IANA) task force, *J Nutr Health Aging* 13(10):881–889, 2009.

47. Savelberg HH, Verdijk LB, Willems PJ, et al: The robustness of age-related gait adaptations: can running counterbalance the consequences of ageing? *Gait Posture* 25(2):259–266, 2007.

48. Craik R: Changes in locomotion in the aging adult. In Woollacott M, Shumway-Cook A, editors: *Development of posture and gait across the life span*, Columbia SC, 1989, University of South Carolina, pp 177–201.

49. Prince F, Corriveau H, Hebert R, et al: Gait in the elderly, *Gait Posture* 5:128–135, 1997.

50. Crowinshield RD, Brand RA, Johnston RC: The effects of walking velocity and age on hip kinematics and kinetics, *Clin Orthop* 132:140–144, 1978.

51. Hageman PA, Blanke DJ: Comparison of gait of young women and elderly women, *Phys Ther* 66:1382–1387, 1986.

52. Lord SR, Lloyd DG, Li SK: Sensori-motor function, gait patterns and falls in community-dwelling women, *Age Ageing* 25:292–299, 1996.

53. Murray MP, Kory RC, Sepic SB: Walking patterns of normal women, *Arch Phys Med Rehabil* 51:637–650, 1970.

54. Winter DA, Patla AE, Frank JS, et al: Biomechanical walking pattern changes in the fit and healthy elderly, *Phys Ther* 70:340–347, 1990.

55. Judge JO, Ounpuu S, Davis RB: Effects of age on the biomechanics and physiology of gait, *Clin Geriatr Med* 12:659–678, 1996.

56. Lee LW, Zavarei K, Evans J, et al: Reduced hip extension in the elderly: dynamic or postural? *Arch Phys Med Rehabil* 86:1851–1854, 2005.

57. Ostrosky KM, VanSwearingen JM, Burdett RG, et al: A comparison of gait characteristics in young and old subjects, *Phys Ther* 74:637–646, 1994.

58. Kerrigan DC, Todd MK, Della Croce U, et al: Biomechanical gait alterations independent of speed in the healthy elderly: evidence for specific limiting impairments, *Arch Phys Med Rehabil* 79:317–322, 1998.

59. Kerrigan DC, Lee LW, Collins JJ, et al: Reduced hip extension during walking: healthy elderly and fallers versus young adults, *Arch Phys Med Rehabil* 82:26–30, 2001.

60. Kerrigan DC, Xenopoulos-Oddsson A, Sullivan MJ, et al: Effect of a hip flexor-stretching program on gait in the elderly, *Arch Phys Med Rehabil* 84:1–6, 2003.

61. DeVita P, Hortobagyi T: Age causes a redistribution of joint torques and powers during gait, *J Appl Physiol* 88:1804–1811, 2000.

62. Riley PO, Della Croce U, Kerrigan DC: Effect of age on lower extremity joint moment contributions to gait speed, *Gait Posture* 14:264–270, 2001.

63. Shkuratova N, Morris ME, Huxham F: Effects of age on balance control during walking, *Arch Phys Med Rehabil* 85:582–588, 2004.

64. Maki BE: Gait changes in older adults: predictors of falls or indicators of fear? *J Am Geriatr Soc* 45(3):313–320, 1997.

65. Menz HB, Lord SR, Fitzpatrick RC: Age-related differences in walking stability, *Age Ageing* 32:137–142, 2003.

66. Kavanagh JJ, Barrett RS, Morrison S: Upper body accelerations during walking in healthy young and elderly men, *Gait Posture* 20:291–298, 2004.

67. Mazza C, Iosa M, Pecoraro F, et al: Control of the upper body accelerations in young and elderly women during level walking, *J Neuroeng Rehabil* 5:30–39, 2008.

68. Pavol MJ, Owings TM, Foley KT, et al: Gait characteristics as risk factors of falling from trips induced in older adults, *J Gerontol A Biol Sci Med Sci* 54A(11):M583–M590, 1999.

69. Pavol MJ, Owings TM, Foley KT, et al: Mechanisms leading to a fall from an induced trip in healthy older adults, *J Gerontol A Biol Sci Med Sci* 56A(7):M428–M437, 2001.

70. van den Bogert AJ, Pavol MJ, Grabiner MD: Response time is more important than walking speed for the ability of older adults to avoid a fall after a trip, *J Biomech* 35:199–205, 2002.

71. Woollacott MH, Tang PF: Balance control during walking in the older adult: research and its implications, *Phys Ther* 77:646–660, 1997.

72. Chen HC, Ashton-Miller JA, Alexander NB, et al: Stepping over obstacles: gait patterns of healthy young and old adults, *J Gerontol A Biol Sci Med Sci* 46(6):M196–M203, 1991.

73. McFadyen BJ, Prince F: Avoidance and accommodation of surface height changes by healthy, community-dwelling, young, and elderly men, *J Gerontol A Biol Sci Med Sci* 57(4):B166–B174, 2002.

74. Lu TW, Chen HL, Chen SC: Comparisons of the lower limb kinematics between young and older adults when crossing obstacles of different heights, *Gait Posture* 23:471–479, 2006.

75. Galna B, Peters A, Murphy AT, et al: Obstacle crossing deficits in older adults: a systematic review, *Gait Posture* 30:270–275, 2009.

76. Larish DD, Martin PE, Mungiole M: Characteristic patterns of gait in the healthy old, *Ann N Y Acad Sci* 515:18–33, 1988.

77. Martin PE, Rothstein DE, Larish DD: Effects of age and physical activity status on the speed-aerobic demand relationship of walking, *J Appl Physiol* 73:200–206, 1992.

78. Malatesta D, Simar D, Dauvilliers Y, et al: Energy cost of walking and gait instability in healthy 65- and 80-yr-olds, *J Appl Physiol* 95:2248–2256, 2003.

79. Hausdorff JM, Peng CK, Wei JY, et al: Fractal analysis of walking. In Winters JM, Crago PE, editors: *Biomechanics and neural control of posture and movement*, New York, 2000, Springer-Verlag, pp 253–264.

80. Kirasic KC: Acquisition and utilization of spatial information by elderly adults: implications for day-to-day situations. In Poon LW, Rubin DC, Wilson BA, editors: *Everyday cognition in adulthood and late life*, New York, 1989, Cambridge University Press, pp 265–283.

81. Leon de MJ, Potegal M, Gurland B: Wandering and parietal signs in senile dementia of Alzheimer's type, *Neuropsychobiology* 11:155–157, 1984.

82. Woodward KM: *Life span motor development*, Champaign, Ill, 1986, Human Kinetics.

83. Korhonen MT, Mero AA, Alen M, et al: Biomechanical and skeletal muscle determinants of maximum running speed with aging, *Med Sci Sports Exerc* 41(4):844–856, 2009.

84. Whitall J, Clark JE: *The development of interlimb coordination in galloping: theory and data*. Presented at the North American Society for the Psychology of Sport and Physical Activity, Scottsdale, Ariz, June 1986.

85. Halverson LE, Williams K: Developmental sequences for hopping over distance: a prelongitudinal screening, *Res Q Exerc Sport* 56:37–44, 1985.

86. Badaly D, Adolph KE: Beyond the average: walking infants take steps longer than their leg length, *Infant Behav Dev* 31(3):554–558, 2008.

87. Aniansson A, Grimby G, Hedberg M, et al: Muscle function of old age, *Scand J Rehabil Med* 43(Suppl 6):43–49, 1978.

88. Elbe RJ: Changes in gait with normal aging. In Masdeu JC, Sudarsky L, Wolfson L, editors: *Gait disorders of aging: falls and therapeutic strategies*, Philadelphia, 1997, Lippincott-Raven, pp 93–105.

89. Wilder PA: *Developmental changes in the gait patterns of women: a search for control parameters*, PhD Thesis, Madison, Wis, 1992, University of Wisconsin.

90. Lord SR, Lloyd DG, Nirui M, et al: The effect of exercise on gait patterns in older women: a randomized controlled trial, *J Gerontol A Biol Sci Med Sci* 51:M64–M70, 1996.

91. Wishart LR, Lee TD, Murdoch JE, et al: Effects of aging on automatic and effortful processes in bimanual coordination, *J Gerontol B Psychol Sci Soc Sci* 55B(2):P85–P94, 2000.

92. Eils E, Behrens S, Mers O, et al: Reduced plantar sensation causes a cautious walking pattern, *Gait Posture* 20:54–60, 2004.

93. Nutt JG: Classification of gait and balance disorders, *Adv Neurol* 87:135–141, 2001.

94. Herman T, Giladi N, Gurevich T, et al: Gait instability and fractal dynamics of older adults with a "cautious" gait: why do certain older adults walk fearfully? *Gait Posture* 21:178–185, 2005.

95. Wolfson L, Judge J, Whipple R, et al: Strength is a major factor in balance, gait and the occurrence of falls, *J Gerontol* 50A:64–67, 1995.

96. Newstead AH, Walden JG, Gitter AJ: Gait variables differentiating fallers from nonfallers, *J Geriatr Phys Ther* 30(3):93–101, 2007.

97. Delbaere K, Sturnieks DL, Crombez C, et al: Concern about falls elicits changes in gait parameters in conditions of postural threat in older people, *J Gerontol A Biol Sci Med Sci* 64A(2):237–242, 2009.

98. Beauchet O, Annweiler C, Dubost V, et al: Stops walking when talking: a predictor of falls in older adults? *Eur J Neurol* 16(7):786–795, 2009.

99. Maki BE, Perry SD, Norrie RG, et al: Effect of facilitation of sensation from plantar foot-surface boundaries on postural stabilization in young and older adults, *J Gerontol A Biol Sci Med Sci* 54:M281–M287, 1999.

100. Barak Y, Wagenaar RC, Holt KG: Gait characteristics of elderly people with a history of falls: a dynamic approach, *Phys Ther* 86(11):1501–1510, 2006.

101. Hausdorff JM, Edelberg HK, Mitchell SL, et al: Increased gait unsteadiness in community-dwelling elderly fallers, *Arch Phys Med Rehabil* 78:278–283, 1997.

102. Kerrigan DC, Lee LW, Nieto TJ, et al: Kinetic alterations independent of walking speed in elderly fallers, *Arch Phys Med Rehabil* 81:730–735, 2000.

103. Rogers MW, Hedman LD, Johnson ME, et al: Lateral stability during forward-induced stepping for dynamic balance recovery in young and older adults, *J Gerontol A Biol Sci Med Sci* 56A(9):M589–M594, 2001.

104. Maki BE, McIlroy WE: Postural control in the older adult, *Clin Geriatr Med* 12(4):635–658, 1996.

105. Hilliard MJ, Martinez KM, Janssen I, et al: Lateral balance factors predict future falls in community-living older adults, *Arch Phys Med Rehabil* 89(9):1708–1713, 2008.

106. Medell JS, Alexander NB: A clinical measure of maximal and rapid stepping of older women, *J Gerontol A Biol Sci Med Sci* 55:M429–M433, 2000.

107. Thelen DG, Ashton Miller JA, Schultz AB, et al: Do neural factors underlie age differences in rapid ankle torque development? *J Am Geriatr Soc* 44:804–808, 1996.

108. Toulotte C, Thevenon A, Watelain E, et al: Identification of healthy elderly fallers and non-fallers by gait analysis under dual-task conditions, *Clin Rehabil* 20(3):269–276, 2006.

109. Rubenstein LZ: Falls in older people: epidemiology, risk factors and strategies for prevention, *Age Ageing* 35(S2):ii37–ii41, 2006.

110. Chang JT, Morton SC, Rubenstein LZ, et al: Interventions for the prevention of falls in older adults: systematic review and meta-analysis of randomized clinical trials, *BMJ* 328:680–686, 2004.

111. Sherrington C, Whitney JC, Lord SR, et al: Effective exercise for the prevention of falls: a systematic review and meta-analysis, *J Am Geriatr Soc* 56:2234–2243, 2008.

112. Costello E, Edelstein JE: Update on falls prevention for community-dwelling older adults: review of single and multifactorial intervention programs, *J Rehabil Res Dev* 45(8):1135–1152, 2008.

113. Menant JC, Steele JR, Menz HB, et al: Optimizing footwear for older people at risk of falls, *J Rehabil Res Dev* 45(8):1167–1181, 2008.

CHAPTER 14

Prehension

OBJECTIVES

After studying this chapter, the reader will be able to:

1. Delineate the components and systems involved in a prehensile act.
2. Identify classic prehension patterns observed in a typical adult.
3. Describe prehensile skill as it develops and changes across the life span.
4. Demonstrate an awareness of the functional adaptations needed for prehension when underlying systems have been altered.

The human hand enhances our life through its dexterity and serves to express our intelligence, as well as our emotions, through gesture. *Prehension,* or the ability to use our hands and upper limbs effectively, can be a strong determinant of functional independence. Upper limb dysfunction limits the degree to which we use our prehensile skills even during simple tasks. To understand dysfunction, it is important to first review normal capabilities and explore prehension at different phases of the life span.

COMPONENTS OF PREHENSION

Imagine yourself supported in a chair, gazing at a cup of tea resting in front of you. Reach for the cup and secure the handle. As you drink the tea, adjust the handle within your hand. Now set the cup down on the table and let go of the handle. This simple task of drinking tea exemplifies the primary components of prehension: visual regard, reach, grasp, manipulation, and release. *Regard* is the visual attention held on an object; you perceive the location, size, and shape of the cup of tea and the handle. *Reach,* or transport, incorporates directing and grading arm position and preshaping the hand to match the location, size, and shape of an object, such as the handle of the cup. *Grasp* involves the act of closing and stabilizing the hand on an object; you secure the cup handle in your hand. *Manipulation* incorporates movement of an object while it is being held, as noted by the adjustment of the handle within your hand. *Release* is the manner in which an object leaves the hand; you let go of the cup handle. If necessary, you may also lift and carry an object, such as the cup, with both hands. The cooperative effort of both hands is termed *bimanual coordination.* The act of drinking a cup of tea, like other prehensile tasks, reflects the interaction between goal-directed movement and environmental constraints.

Prehension uses anticipatory or feedforward control and feedback allowing us to prepare the hand, arm, and body in advance of intended movement or to respond to perturbations. Other inherent features of prehension are postural control and biomechanical components.[1]

Postural Control

Visual exploration and functional reaching are closely linked to postural control. Under *feedforward* or *proactive control,* stabilizing muscle contractions or anticipatory postural adjustments (APAs) are elicited in anticipation of upcoming disturbances in equilibrium.[1] APAs prevent undesired movement and allow for adjustment in our center of gravity before the upper limb moves in space. Under *reactive control,*[1] muscle responses are also elicited after perturbations induced by a prehensile act such as reaching to a distant target.

Core stability is the ability to control the trunk's position and motion over the pelvis to optimize force control and motion in distal segments as needed for athletics and other tasks.[2] Although core stability is essential for efficient distal coordination, it is possible to have good fine-motor control despite insufficient proximal control or shoulder stability. For example, we find that children who have sustained injuries to the upper brachial plexus at birth (Erb palsy, C5-C6 spinal nerves) often have shoulder weakness and instability, yet despite some residual hand weakness have good distal coordination.

The extent of proximal and distal muscle activation is task dependent.[3,4] Typically, the joint to be stabilized is determined by the goal of the activity. Proximal trunk muscles stabilize the body during reach to grasp movements, whereas sustained pinch and grip provide distal stabilization that frees the proximal joints to move. For example, when we hold a toothbrush, the wrist, forearm, and elbow are free to move while the fingers and thumb stabilize the toothbrush for use. Thus, the goal and constraints of the task dictate which muscles serve as stabilizers.

Biomechanics

Flexible postural control that adheres to select biomechanical principles allows us to use prehensile skills effectively. Certain biomechanical principles are inherent components of efficient muscle function, including length-tension relationships and related active and passive insufficiency of muscle-tendon units. The length-tension curve compares the tension produced in a muscle with its resting length at the time of contraction (Figure 14-1). *Resting muscle length* is the length of the resting muscle when it is measured from attachment to attachment. Peak tension, which is necessary for a strong contraction, can be developed when the muscle is within 70% to 105% of its resting length, termed the *useful range*.[5] A contracting muscle or agonist demonstrates active insufficiency when its attachments are too close together, limiting tension development. Passive insufficiency results when the attachments of the agonist are too far apart for the muscle to generate adequate tension for effective contraction.

Based on these principles, many manipulative tasks are best performed with the wrist stabilized in approximately 20 to 30 degrees of extension and 10 degrees of ulnar deviation.[6] Wrist extension keeps the finger flexors within the useful range of the length-tension curve, allowing for adequate tension development during grip and pinch activities. When the wrist is extended, the thumb can move into a plane of opposition in relation to the other digits, and the fingers can achieve full flexion. These and other biomechanical principles play a significant role in manual acts.

Friction at the digit-object interface helps to maintain a secure grip on objects.[7] If the friction and fingertip forces are insufficient, objects will slip and may be dropped. To prevent object drops, feedback obtained from tactile receptors causes an increase in grip force at the fingertips. Any deficiency in tactile feedback will alter the response to slips.

Visual Regard

Visual regard and perception prompt us to reach for and grasp objects. These functions depend on the strength of our attention, visual acuity, and ocular control, including accommodation and convergence (see Chapter 10).

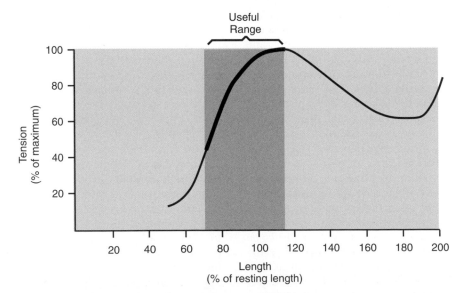

Figure 14-1 Length-tension diagram for isometrically stimulated muscle fiber, including extreme shortened and stretched states of fiber. (Redrawn from Smith LK, Weiss EL, Lehmkuhl LD: *Brunnstrom's clinical kinesiology*, ed 5, Philadelphia, 1996, FA Davis, p 140; modified from Ramsey RW, Street SF: Isometric length-tension diagram of isolated muscle fibers of the frog, *Cell Comp Physiol* 15:11, 1940. Reprinted by permission of John Wiley & Sons.)

Visual perception is the ability to use visual information to recognize, recall, discriminate, and understand what we see. As infants and children gain experience through play involving various systems, perceptual constructs are developed. Visual memory is established and complex processes develop with exposure to and interaction with different environments. Visual regard and perception also guide reach and refine manipulation skills in terms of accuracy and control. Selected visuoperceptual constructs, such as depth perception, figure ground, and visuoconstruction, play key roles in reach, grasp, and manipulation. Depth perception allows us to localize objects in space and to estimate size and distance. For example, we can discriminate how far an object is out of reach before retrieving it. Figure-ground refers to the ability to visually focus on specific details in the foreground by selectively screening out competing background stimuli. And visuoconstruction is related to the spatial planning process involved in building up and breaking down two- and three-dimensional objects. This skill is used in putting together a puzzle or copying a three-dimensional design.

Visual-motor control, or *eye-hand coordination*, is the ability of an individual to use visual information for precise guidance of movement. Visual information is used to amend an internal representation or model of an object's physical properties and location before reaching for it and to enhance accuracy before object contact during an unfolding reach. It has been postulated that *peripheral* vision aids reaching because it provides cues about object distance and direction along with object or limb motion.[8] Conversely, *central* vision supports grasp and manipulation because it provides information about object size and shape required for grip calibration and dexterous hand movement. Sighted individuals use vision to guide reaching in many everyday tasks, such as retrieving a specific shirt hanging in the closet. When our vision is compromised, we rely on proprioceptive and tactile cues or visual memory to guide reach to grasp movements.

Reach and Grip Formation

The entire upper extremity is involved in the act of reaching and grasping an object. During reach to grasp movements, the shoulder moves the hand in space over a wide area, and the elbow places it closer to or further away from the body. The forearm and wrist position the hand before grasp of an object or receipt of a weight-bearing surface. The fingers and thumb adjust their position to accommodate the perceived spatial properties of an object during grip formation, such as its size and shape. This can be exemplified when reaching for a cup visualized at chest level. There are many ways to

perform the task as exemplified below. To approach the cup, the shoulder may flex to about 80 degrees, while the scapula rotates up and protracts, and the elbow extends. As the cup handle is approached, the wrist may extend and the forearm may rotate into neutral. As the handle is approximated, the fingers may extend and the thumb may abduct in preparation. The fingers may close in on the handle by flexing, and the thumb may adduct. When the reach requires greater than 90 degrees of shoulder flexion, the trunk and neck may rotate or laterally flex and the ipsilateral pelvis may elevate.[9]

The *trajectory* of a reaching movement can be defined by the extent, orientation, and speed of the hand path as it moves the hand to a new position.[10] In adults, reaching behaviors include smooth bell-shaped velocity profiles and relatively continuous, straight hand paths with and without visual feedback (Figure 14-2).[11] Conversely, during early reaching the hand paths are characterized by accelerations and decelerations resulting in indirect hand paths until about 2 years of age.[12]

Studies examining reaching differences between the dominant and nondominant arm reveal distinct neural control mechanisms for each arm.[13] For example, during planar reaching movements, the dominant arm typically displays a straighter hand path to the target than the nondominant arm. Furthermore, the dominant arm seems to employ anticipatory strategies during arm movements, while the nondominant arm seems to rely more on feedback.

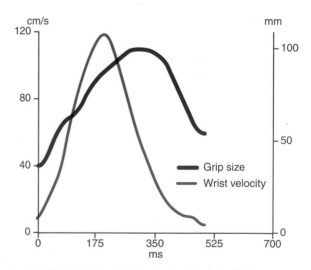

Figure 14-2 Sample velocity profile with imbedded grip aperture. (Redrawn from Paulignan Y, Jeannerod M: Visuomotor channels in prehension. In Wing AM, Haggard P, Flanagan JR, editors: *Hand and brain: the neurophysiology and psychology of hand movements*, New York, 1996, Academic Press, p 268.)

Reach and grasp are associated with two hypothesized visuomotor channels activated in parallel.[14] One channel pertains to an object's extrinsic properties, such as location, and activates proximal shoulder musculature used in the reach. The second channel is related to preshaping the grip and provides intrinsic information about the object such as its location and contour. This information activates distal finger musculature.

Preshaping of the hand, termed *grip formation,* can be divided into finger opening and finger closure or aperture. Maximum finger opening adjusts in anticipation of the size and shape of an object, based on an internal representation of the object's physical properties. As a reach to grasp movement unfolds, previous information is retrieved from memory, and the internal representation is updated via current sensory information. In typical adults, peak aperture occurs within 70% to 75% of total movement time at the point of peak deceleration (see Figure 14-2).[11,15] Inadequate timing between reach and grasp may extend the movement time and alter the path of the reach, compromising appropriate grip formation. In essence, the timing and size of peak aperture within a reach to grasp movement indicate whether it is planned for the expected target object's location and spatial properties. Furthermore, the speed of a reach and the shape of the hand as it grasps an object is dependent on the end-goal or what will be done after the object is grasped.[16]

Impairments in central vision clearly impede grip formation. Studies of transport and grasp have reported maximal finger aperture and velocity of finger aperture to be greater when the vision of healthy subjects was restricted.[17] Without a clear idea of the size or shape of an object, individuals overestimated grip aperture to ensure successful grasp. From his work on transport and grasp, Jeannerod[18] provided evidence that grip accuracy improved given visual feedback and degraded in those with visual impairment.

Grasp

Classification of Adult Grasp Patterns

Once an object is approached, one of a variety of grip patterns will be used to secure it. The location, size, and shape of an object determine the type of pattern used. Traditionally, adult prehension patterns have been classified according to the work of Napier[19] and Landsmeer.[20] Napier[19] described two types of grip: power and precision. *Power grips* are defined as forcible activities of the fingers and thumb that act against the palm to transmit a force to an object. Examples include the cylindrical, spherical, and hook grip (Figure 14-3). During *precision grip* and *pinch* activities, forces are directed between the

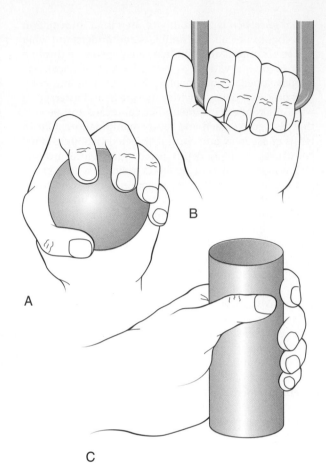

Figure 14-3 Three varieties of power grip. **A,** Spherical grip. **B,** Hook grip. **C,** Cylindrical grip. (Redrawn from Norkin CC, Levangie PK: *Joint structure and function: a comprehensive analysis*, Philadelphia, 1983, FA Davis.)

thumb and fingers, not against the palm. Examples of precision grip or pinch include pad-to-pad prehension, tip-to-tip prehension, and pad-to-side, or lateral, prehension (Figure 14-4). Sustained hold of power and precision grips require isometric muscular contractions. Typical grip and pinch patterns and the joints and muscles involved are listed in Table 14-1.

Despite their wide acceptance, the classic prehension patterns continue to be challenged and further examined. In his classification scheme, Landsmeer[20] kept the expression power grip but used the phrase "precision handling" to describe the manipulative quality of prehensile function. *Precision handling* requires changes in position of the handled object, either in space or about its own axes, as well as exact control of finger and thumb position. Muscular contractions will vary between isometric and isotonic. Precision grip and

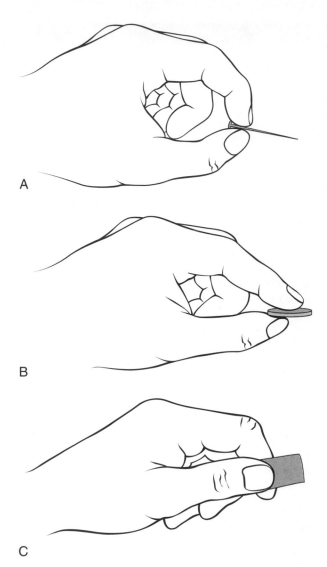

Figure 14-4 Three varieties of precision pinch and handling. **A,** Tip-to-tip. **B,** Pad-to-pad. **C,** Pad-to-side (lateral). (Redrawn from Norkin CC, Levangie PK: *Joint structure and function: a comprehensive analysis*, Philadelphia, 1983, FA Davis.)

handling exemplifies the strong connection present between the motor cortex and the pyramidal tract. Wong and Whishaw[21] examined the precision grip in terms of the high degree of variability in contact strategies of the digits, purchase patterns, and the digits used between and within individuals. They provided further support that innate or adaptive neural factors make important contributions to the grasping patterns used.

After an extensive survey of the literature, Casanova and Grunert[22] introduced their own classification system based on anatomical nomenclature and contact

surfaces. They proposed the use of the terms "static" and "dynamic prehension." *Static prehension* refers to any form of prehension in which the object does not move within the hand, although proximal joint movement may occur. An example of static prehension is isometrically holding a key using a lateral pinch. *Dynamic prehension* resembles Landsmeer's term of precision handling[20] because it is associated with positional changes of an object that occur within the hand rather than at the proximal joints. This is exemplified when a needle is rolled between the fingers to visualize its eye before threading it. The force used during static or dynamic prehension may be strong or light in magnitude. For example, during precise static prehension, as in turning a key in a tough lock, a strong steady force is needed, whereas a light force is sufficient to secure a cotton ball.

We usually grade the fingertip forces we use during prehension. This ability to grade forces is based on previous learning and memory of the weight, texture, and other properties of the object.[23] Sensorimotor memories help form internal representations of the physical properties of objects and are used to scale the grip (squeeze) and load (vertical) forces in advance. This ability to scale fingertip forces in advance of object contact is a form of *anticipatory control*.

Significance of Thumb Opposition

Although prehension is evident in many forms of animal life, it attains maximum function in humans given the addition of thumb opposition. *Opposition* involves rotation at the carpometacarpal joint of the thumb to place the thumb pad diametrically opposite to the pad of one or all of the other digits (see Figure 14-4). The thumb, because of its unique ability to oppose, is a common feature in most grip classifications, contributing 40% to 70% of total hand function.[24] The comparative length of the index finger to the thumb is a major factor when attempting opposition or pad-to-pad contact. A reduction in thumb length, seen in an individual whose distal thumb phalanx has been amputated, limits the ability to fully rotate the thumb to the index pad. Thumb opposition in conjunction with movement at other digits is used to execute functional prehension, such as turning a doorknob or buttoning a shirt.

Significance of Other Digits

The index finger is considered the most important digit after the thumb because of its mobility and independent muscle attachments. It has been found to be the most dominant of the four fingers and accounts for 20% of lateral pinch, 20% of power grip from a

Table 14-1

Classification of Prehension Patterns

Patterns	Joint Motion	Muscles Used	Function
Cylindrical grasp	Thumb opposition, finger adduction and flexion	FPL and thenar group, AdP, select interossei (task dependent), fourth lumbrical and FDP (FDS for more power)	Holding onto a cylindrically shaped object such as a soda can
Spherical grasp	Thumb opposition, finger flexion and abduction	FPL and thenar group, AdP, FDP (FDS for more power), fourth lumbrical interossei (except second)	Holding onto a round object such as a baseball
Hook grasp	MCPs neutral, finger flexion at PIPs and DIPs, thumb extension	Finger FDS and FDP, thumb, EPL and EPB, EDC, fourth lumbrical and fourth dorsal interossei	Holding onto a brief case handle
Pad-to-pad prehension	Thumb opposition and slight flexion of all thumb joints; finger flexion at MCP and PIP; flexion or extension of DIP of involved fingers	Thenar group, FPL, select interossei and FDS of involved fingers (FDP if DIP flexion is present)	Holding onto a coin
Tip-to-tip prehension	As in pad-to-pad prehension, with greater thumb and finger flexion, including DIP flexion	As in pad-to-pad prehension, with greater FDP force FDP secondary to DIP flexion, interossei of involved fingers	Holding a needle
Pad-to-pad prehension (lateral)	Thumb adduction with IP flexion, index finger flexion, and abduction	Thumb, FPL, FPB, and AdP; involved fingers; FDS and FDP; reduced interossei and lumbricals except first dorsal interossei	Holding a key

FPL, flexor pollicis longus; *AdP,* adductor pollicis; *FDP,* flexor digitorum profundus; *FDS,* flexor digitorum superficialis; *MCP,* metacarpophalangeal; *PIP,* proximal interphalangeal; *DIP,* distal interphalangeal; *EPL,* extensor pollicis longus; *EPB,* extensor pollicis brevis; *EDC,* extensor digitorum communis; *IP,* interphalangeal; *FPB,* flexor pollicis brevis.
Data from Landsmeer JMF: Power grip and precision handling, *Ann Rheum Dis* 21:164-169, 1962; Long C, Conrad PW, Hall EA et al: Intrinsic-extrinsic muscle control of the hand in power grip and precision handling, *J Bone Joint Surg* 52(5):853-867, 1970; Napier JR: The prehensile movement of the human hand, *J Bone Joint Surg* 38:902-913, 1956; Napier JR: Function of the hand. In Napier JR, editor: *Hands,* New York, 1980, Pantheon Books, pp 68-83.

supinated position of the forearm, and 50% of power grip from a pronated forearm position.[25,26] The long finger is the strongest and longest and has significant functional value. In some individuals, it replaces the index as the dominant finger and is used for pointing and manipulating small objects.[25] The index and long fingers are considered the prehensile digits and are the most anatomically stable. The small and ring fingers are recruited for power grip prehension. Although they are considered the most anatomically mobile, they also are the weakest digits.[26] Both the index and small fingers can produce isolated extension via the extensor indicis and the extensor digiti minimi, respectively. Because all of the digits are important in prehension, the loss of any one of them will limit prehensile ability to some degree.

Manipulation

Manipulation involves a series of tasks used to achieve a specific goal. Once we pick up an object through grasp, we may either sustain a hold on it or manipulate it with one or both hands to accomplish a task. All forms of manipulation demand the use of the small intrinsic and extrinsic muscles of the fingers or thumb.

Sustained Grip and Pinch

Once the index finger and thumb contact a target object with a stable grip, the goal is to generate sufficient fingertip forces to lift it. Sustaining a grip or pinch on an object or tool is done primarily with isometric contractions and intermittent isotonic contractions, as when writing with a pencil over a long period.

During object manipulation, a dynamic lift is generally combined with static hold and release of an object. The sequential tasks involved in grasping and lifting an object are triggered by discrete mechanical events that relay information from somatosensory receptors.[23] Experience aids in the development of internal representations of object properties. This information is used for anticipatory control or planning before lifting and manipulating an object. Without anticipatory control or scaling of fingertip forces, objects may slip from grasp or be squeezed too tightly because the feedback mechanisms are too slow to upgrade or to downgrade forces quickly.

In-Hand Manipulation

The ability to move objects within one hand, termed *in-hand manipulation*, is divided into three components, called shift, rotation, and translation.[27] *Shift* refers to the movement of an object on the finger pads or between the fingers. *Rotation* is the movement of an object around its axis using the fingers. *Translation* is the movement of an object from fingers to palm or from palm to fingers.

To translate objects such as a raisin from the palm to the fingertips, finger flexion and extension are used. Shift incorporates the pads of the fingers with thumb opposition as when turning thin pages in a book. Simple rotation involves turning an object on its axis 90 degrees, such as when turning a pencil to write. Complex rotation is defined as 180 to 360 degrees of object rotation, as when using the pencil eraser (Figure 14-5, *A*). In-hand manipulation skills can also incorporate stabilization of one object or part of an object within the hand while another object or object part is simultaneously being manipulated within the same hand.[27] Typically, if two objects are held in the same hand, the ring and small (ulnar) fingers stabilize one object while the index and long (radial) fingers manipulate the other object or part. Shift with stabilization is used to separate a group of keys from a single key when opening a lock (Figure 14-5, *B*). All three forms of in-hand manipulation can be exemplified with the use of a penny. For example, a penny

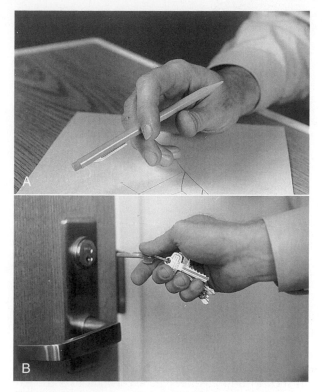

Figure 14-5 Examples of in-hand manipulation: **A,** Rotation component used to access the eraser of a pencil. **B,** Shift component with ulnar stabilization used to manipulate a key when opening a lock.

can be translated from the palm up to the fingertips and then shifted across the finger pads to end with a hold between the index finger and the thumb. If you turned the penny over from heads to tails with your fingertips, that would be considered a rotation.

Stereognosis

Haptic perceptual exploration, or *stereognosis,* is the ability to recognize the names and properties of objects without vision through sensory cues and in-hand manipulation. Manipulation abilities, as well as sensibility, foster object identification, yet it is the memory of an object that makes it recognizable. Reach into your purse or pocket and retrieve a quarter. How did you know it was a quarter and not a nickel? You probably used tactile cues and proprioceptive-kinesthetic input to judge the size and weight of the coin, based on memory of a previous visual or other sensory experience. Although visual memory is a strong component of stereognosis, individuals without sight can develop this ability once they are taught, demonstrating that memory based on haptic exploration also plays a significant role in object recognition.

The vast number of receptors in our fingertips, muscles, joints, and skin provide the tactile and proprioceptive cues used to identify characteristics of an object. The slow and fast adapting mechanoreceptors in the fat pads and ridges of our fingers supply varied tactile information.[28] Proprioception conveys information regarding muscle force, limb movement, and changes in limb position. Afferent input contributing to proprioception includes information from muscle spindles, Golgi tendon organs, joint receptors, and cutaneous mechanoreceptors.[29] All of the receptors contribute to stereognosis. Without sensory input, the ability of humans to identify objects without vision is significantly impaired.

Release

Release is the process of letting go of a held object or taking pressure off an object. Release can be crude, as when we drop the hot handle of a frying pan, or it can be graded and controlled, as when we set a crystal glass onto a counter. Graded release is mastered and refined individually through the practice of specific tasks. Playing a musical instrument is a beautiful demonstration of how graded release is achieved. A master jazz pianist is able to hold and release pressure on the keys in such a controlled and graded fashion that the end result is a varied sound combination of loud or soft, sustained or short-lasting tones. A novice player may not exhibit the same degree of finesse with regard to holding or releasing the pressure on the piano keys, perhaps making all the tones loud and sustained. Tool use also demonstrates graded release. When using a screwdriver to drive in screws, a series of quick, graded grasps and releases are used to turn the handle effectively without engaging the whole shoulder girdle. Imagine a 5-year-old performing the same task. She would probably display an alternating lateral trunk tilt or engage the shoulder girdle in the movement. This may be due to weakness, reduced ability to supinate the forearm, or insufficiently graded grasp and release. As control of release improves, our repertoire of fine-motor activities grows.

Bimanual Coordination

Bimanual coordination requires the spatial and temporal cooperation of both hands. Bimanual skills can be separated into *symmetrical* tasks in which there is a strong coupling between limbs, as when we throw a ball with two hands, and *asymmetrical* tasks or differentiation, as when one hand stabilizes an object while the other manipulates it. Examples of asymmetrical bimanual tasks include opening small containers (Figure 14-6)

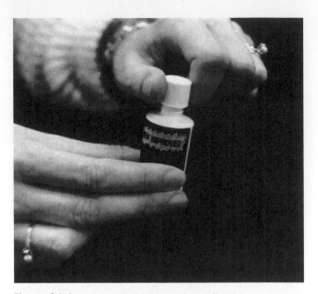

Figure 14-6 Asymmetrical bimanual coordination demonstrating two prehension patterns: three-fingered palmar pinch (three-jaw chuck) to hold the base and dynamic lateral pinch to turn off the top.

or playing musical instruments, such as the guitar or violin. The neural organization associated with these two types of bimanual tasks varies depending on task goals and constraints.[30]

Wiesendanger and colleagues[31] described motor control principles that affect bimanual coordination: (1) the assimilation effect, (2) neural division of labor, and (3) hierarchical organization. The *assimilation effect* refers to the temporal coupling and synchronization of two hands during movement initiation. It is possible that coupling of bimanual actions occurs at the level of bilaterally linked central pattern generators or neuronal ensembles. The *neural division of labor* refers to the asymmetric roles taken by the two hands, which reflects a specialization of brain function. For example, in right-handed individuals, the left or dominant hemisphere may strongly influence the roles assumed by each hand during asymmetrical bimanual tasks. *Hierarchical organization* incorporates the concepts of goal invariance and motor equivalence in which the goal of a task remains intact yet can be accomplished by variable means. Research has shown that even when task conditions are altered (visual occluded, unilateral pull load varied, anesthetized unilateral thumb and index), the goal of a task remains intact, thus maintaining a motor equivalence.[32] Any or all of the three principles described may be involved in specific bimanual activities depending on individual capabilities, task goals, and environmental and task conditions.

PREHENSION DEVELOPMENT ACROSS THE LIFE SPAN

Prenatal Period

Growth of the Upper Limb

The limb buds, which represent the earliest form of the upper limb, begin to appear between the 26th and 27th days of gestation. By the end of the seventh week, the fingers are defined and the upper limb has rotated medially to its typical position at birth. Table 14-2 describes and illustrates upper limb growth until the seventh week of gestation. The dermatomes of the skin, which influence both the tactile and proprioceptive systems, begin to develop as early as 7 weeks of gestation. The classic proprioceptive system also begins to develop in utero with the differentiation of the articular skeleton and muscular systems around the seventh week of gestation.[33] The prenatal period ends with full development of the upper limbs.

Prenatal Action Development

Upper limb actions do not develop in isolation from the environment in which they occur. Therefore, the uterine environment plays a significant role in early prehension development. Sparling and colleagues[34] used ultrasound imaging to examine fetal movements and found that although limb movements are variable, they are not random. Instead, they found movements were directed toward specific targets, as seen in the thumb-to-mouth activity of an 18-week-old fetus. This thumb-to-mouth action may have been facilitated by the ease of movement available within the amniotic fluid and sac. McCartney and Hepper[35] provided evidence for the expression of preferred hand use prenatally, reporting that in utero 83% of arm movements were exhibited with the right versus the left arm. They hypothesized that lateralized motor behavior may play a causative role in asymmetric brain development and postnatal lateralized behavior.

Infancy

Upper limb and hand movements are present at birth, yet continued development is strongly influenced by neuromaturation, task goals, and the ever-changing interaction between the environment and the characteristics of an individual infant.[36,37] All components of prehension undergo a great deal of development during infancy.

Visual Regard

At birth, vision is limited. Newborns seem to have 20/800 vision, a fixed gaze of 7.8 inches (20 cm), and little accommodation.[38] Because vision needs the stimulation of light to develop, it is not until the second month of life that the structures associated with accommodation, oculomotor function, and convergence are established. Despite having low vision, newborns can fixate or sustain their gaze for brief periods and follow or track a moving target through a small range. As the newborn follows moving visual information (visual flow) from birth to 1 month of age, visual gaze typically lags behind a moving stimulus. Rosander and von Hofsten[39] have provided evidence that vestibular control over smooth gaze stabilization and adjustment, while the head and body are moving, functions earlier than visual control. This is not surprising, because ocular movements induced by vestibular input in the fetus occur several months earlier than do ocular movements stimulated by light postnatally. By 2 to 3 months of age, visual control improves as convergence and accommodation enable the infant to fixate for sustained periods and to follow a moving target through a wider range.[39] At approximately 3 months of age, the initial visual lag to a moving stimulus is diminished, and by about 5 months of age, the infant begins to demonstrate anticipatory tracking and can project her gaze ahead of a moving object.[40] By 4 to 5 months of age, the infant can usually reach for objects in her visual field. As visual memory develops, between 6 and 7 months, the infant may realize that an object still exists even if it falls out of the visual field, and by 8 months, she will search for it. Binocular vision, accommodation, and acuity progress over an infant's second year of life, strengthening eye-hand coordination. It is not until 2 years of age that the infant can attend to stimuli presented in two visual fields, simultaneously demonstrating interhemispheric coordination.[41]

Reaching

The nerves to the proximal joint musculature myelinate approximately 1 month ahead of the small hand muscles, which may be one reason why reaching behaviors precede the development of grasp patterns.[42] Although reaching behaviors in young infants are quite variable, they become more refined and consistent with age and experience.

Early reaching is described as a fling or thrust and is considered a ballistic, preprogrammed, and inaccurate movement. Visually guided, anticipatory reaching behaviors begin to emerge about 4 months of age. von Hofsten and Lindhagen[43] confirmed that 18-week-old (4-month-old) infants could visually catch a ball moving at 15.4 inches/sec (39 cm/sec). Thus, they could predict the future position of the moving ball and direct the reach toward the point of contact between the hand

Table 14-2

Development of the Upper Limb in the Embryonic Period

Age of Embryo	Upper Limb Development	Illustration
28-30 days	Upper limb buds "flipper-like" Lower limb buds appear	
31-32 days	Upper limb buds "paddle-like"	
33-36 days	Hard plates formed	
41-43 days	Digital or finger rays appear	
44-46 days	Elbow region visible, notches appear between finger rays	
47-48 days	All limb buds extend ventrally	
49-51 days	Upper limb longer and bent at elbow Fingers distinct but webbed	
52-53 days	Hands and feet approach each other Fingers are free and longer	
7th week	Upper limb rotates 90° laterally in longitudinal axis (elbows face posterior) Lower limb rotates 90° medially (knees face anterior) Tissue breaks down between digits from the circumference inward, producing fingers and toes	

Adapted from Moore KL, Persund TVN: *The developing human: clinically oriented embryology*, ed 6, Philadelphia, 1998, WB Saunders.

and the moving object. Although vision provides a stimulus to reach forward, Clifton and colleagues[44] found infants as young as 15 weeks were able to reach for glowing or sounding objects without the use of guided vision. Despite the ability of infants to reach by 3 or 4 months of age, it is not until 2 years of age that more stereotypic adultlike reaching patterns are displayed (see Figure 4-1).[45] With experience and gains in motor control, reaching behaviors become less variable.

Factors that are likely to influence the type of reach an infant performs include the degree of postural control, the location of the target object, and task goals, motivation, and cognition. Rochat[46] reported that when infants initially began to reach, even if they could not sit independently, they tended to do so with two hands. Older infants who sit independently often display unimanual reaches. Halverson[47,48] documented that practically all reaches in the 9-month-old infant were unilateral and directed straight at the target. These findings infer a strong connection between postural control and reaching. Changing coordination in other behaviors, however, may also influence how reaching movements are executed. Corbetta and Thelen[49] found unimanual and bimanual reaching to fluctuate during the first year. During periods of strong bimanual reach, nonreaching interlimb activity tended to be synchronous. Yet, no specific form of interlimb coordination was observed during periods of unimanual reach. The authors postulated that changing coordination tendencies seem to influence the organization of goal-oriented reaching behaviors during the first year of life.

Grip Formation

As reviewed earlier, we preshape our hand to the contour and size of target objects during reaching. Crude preshaping of the hand or anticipatory grip formation has been documented in infants as young as 18 weeks.[50] von Hofsten and Ronnqvist[51] later examined grip formation during reaching in older infants 5 to 6, 9, and 13 months of age. They found that although the 5- to 9-month-old infants began to close their hands near the time of target contact, the 13-month-old infants initiated closure well before object contact. Opening aperture was adjusted to target size in the 9- to 13-month-old infants but not in the 5- to 6-month-old infants. In addition, finger opening was initiated earlier in the reach in 13-month-olds than in 9-month-olds, yet the timing did not vary for different-sized objects. Adults showed an earlier onset of opening for larger objects, or greater anticipatory grip formation. The progression in anticipatory grip formation or preshaping of the hand develops in infancy yet does not become adultlike until late childhood.[52]

Grasp and Manipulation

Within the first 6 months of life, early random responses and reflexes develop into voluntary prehension. In the first few months, tactile and proprioceptive reflexes control finger closure via palmar stimulation and opening of the fingers via dorsal stimulation (Table 14-3). Mass movement patterns are exemplified through elicitation of a traction response, in which stretching of one of the flexor muscle groups induces flexion of the entire upper limb.

When the newborn enters infancy, the hand reflexes are gradually integrated and progress into voluntary prehensile patterns. As the motor cortex develops, prenatally and postnatally, independent finger movements, or fractionation, emerges. Initial grasp patterns typically involve the fingers only, leaving the thumb passive. Thumb function, including opposition, progressively develops between 3 and 12 months and is responsible for the development of varied prehensile patterns. During the first 5 months, infants display an array of patterns including the following: fists, preprecision grips associated with numerous digit postures, precision grips including the pincer grasp, and self-directed grasps.[53] Direct connections from the pyramidal tract that are functioning early may be responsible for the expression of these sophisticated prehension patterns.

Index isolation typically begins around 10 months of age, and by the end of the first year, the infant is able to isolate the index finger as a dominant pointer. Sometime around 11 months of age, the infant demonstrates pad-to-pad opposition of the thumb to the index finger to grasp small objects. Prehension patterns become more adultlike as the infant approaches 1 year of age. Further development and experience with objects allow the infant's repertoire of grasp patterns to expand and adapt to functional need.

Table 14-4 depicts a historical sequence of prehension development. Some researchers have begun to view this sequence as conservative and inflexible because it does not accurately reflect the functionally adaptive prehension seen in infants given various task constraints.[54-56] For example, Halverson's work[48] on prehension indicated that an ulnar grasp, elicited by tactile cues to the ulnar side of the hand, preceded a radial grasp. Forssberg and colleagues,[55,57] however, found that following palm contact, infants may reach for and grasp a dumbbell-like object without consistently using an ulnar grip. Even the young infant may use the index finger to contact and initiate the grasp first; the index finger exhibits a stronger grip force than the other fingers. Although inconsistency in the prehensile responses of normal infants makes it difficult to accurately label patterns, their prehensile responses can be grouped into three phases. During phase 1, infants use

Table 14-3

Hand Reflexes

Reflex	Appears	Disappears	Stimulus	Response
Grasp	2 wk	4-5 mo	Tactile stimulus initially; later, proprioceptive input also is needed to elicit grasp	Flexion of fingers, adduction and flexion of the thumb
Traction response	Week 28 of gestation	2-5 mo	Stretch to shoulder flexors and adductors with traction	Flexion of the wrist and fingers with synergistic flexion of elbow and shoulder
Avoidance response	Neonatal period	5-6 mo; fully integrated by 6-7 years	Light tactile stimulus along dorsum of hand to fingertips	Extension and abduction of fingers and wrist (withdraw from stimulus)
Instinctive grasp reaction	4-5 mo	Remnants persist into adult life	Stationary or moving light touch; radial palm contact; ulnar palm contact	Orienting reaction; slight supination; slight pronation
	6-7 mo		Ulnar or radial palm contact	Orienting and groping to find the object
	8-10 mo		Moving stimulus withdrawn from any part of the palm	Orienting, groping, and grasping of stimulus
Asymmetrical tonic neck reflex	Week 28 of gestation	4-5 mo	Passive rotation of head	Elbow flexion on skull side, with elbow extension on face side

Data from Ammon JE, Etzel ME: Sensorimotor organization in reach and prehension: a developmental model, *Phys Ther* 57(1):7-14, 1974; Fiorentino MR: *Normal and abnormal development: the influence of primitive reflexes on motor development*, Springfield, Ill, 1972, Charles C Thomas; Twitchell TE: Reflex mechanisms and the development of prehension. In Connelly K, editor: *Mechanisms of motor skill development*, London, 1970, Academic Press, pp 25-59.

their whole hands in a gross or unspecialized manner. In phase 2, infants use parts of their hands as they begin to develop specialization. By phase 3, infants use the pads of their distal phalanges in a precise, specialized manner.[54]

The ability to use anticipatory control to coordinate fingertip forces during grasp and manipulation of objects is not innate.[57,58] It develops gradually over the first 2 years of life, as the young child interacts with various objects. Observing the ability to grasp and lift before 2 years of age, Forssberg and colleagues[57] found that infants and toddlers increase grip and load forces sequentially, using a feedback strategy. After the second year, grip and load forces begin to be generated in parallel, demonstrating a transition to anticipatory (proactive) control. Such coordination of fingertip forces is important to smooth prehension and development of in-hand manipulation and stereognosis.

In-hand manipulation skills develop gradually from infancy to childhood. The easiest skills are those of finger to palm translation and simple rotation, seen before 2 years of age. Complex rotation is still being refined in the 6- to 7-year-old child. Stereognosis also develops gradually after birth. In early infancy, the mouth and hands are used to gain information about objects. Intramodal and intermodal exploration and integration begin to develop in infancy and continue through adolescence. Intramodal integration is the ability to recognize objects by one modality (touch) after learning about the object using the same modality (touch). This ability appears first in infants as young as 2 to 3 months of age.[59] Intermodal integration develops next and is the ability to recognize an object by a different modality (vision) from which it was first explored (touch). Infants as young as 6 months can visually recognize a

Table **14-4**

Historical Sequence of Prehension Development from Birth to 1 Year

Description	Age	Illustration	Stimulation
Recognizes hands	8 wk (2 mo)		Hand enters visual field assisted by the asymmetrical tonic neck reflex
Reflexive ulnar group	12 wk (3 mo)		Ulnar placement of objects encourages grasp; hanging toys may promote visual tracking
Retains objects placed in hand: Midline fingering; mouthing of fingers; swiping in visual field	16 wk (4 mo)		Placing objects anywhere in hand will encourage grasp; hanging toys will encourage swiping if they are within visual field and reach
Primitive squeeze grasp (wrist flexed); raking	20 wk (5 mo)		Introduction of toys of varied textures, sizes, and shapes will promote voluntary grasp and raking
Palmar grasp (no thumb participation, wrist moving into neutral)	24 wk (6 mo)		Placing toys in different positions will encourage eyes and hands to search before reach and grasp
Radial palmar grasp (thumb adduction begins); mouthing of objects	28 wk (7 mo)		Ideal toys are washable and those that can be picked up and transferred easily from one hand to the other
Scissors grasp (thumb adduction stronger)	32 wk (8 mo)		Introduction of toys with a thin circumference will strengthen thumb adductor
Radial-digital grasp (beginning opposition)	36 wk (9 mo)		Pliable materials such as clay or finger food will encourage opposition of thumb
Inferior pincer grasp (volar hold vs. pad to pad; hand supported before grasping); isolated index pointing	36-52 wk (9-12 mo)		Small objects varied in shape will promote exploration via poking, feeling, and manipulation
Pincer grasp—pad to pad (some support before grasping)	38-52 wk (10-12 mo)		Tiny objects, such as raisins, to pick up and drop will encourage development
Superior pincer grasp—tip to tip (hand unsupported before grasping)	52-56 wk (1 yr)		Thin yet safe objects the size of a pin will encourage development
Three-jaw chuck (wrist extended and ulnarly deviated); maturing release	52-56 wk (1 yr)		Toys requiring a strong radial finger hold and blocks and containers providing repeated motions will encourage strong grasp and release

shape after only tactile contact with it.[60] Recognition of common objects through haptic exploration is relatively good by 2 to 3 years of age and seems to mature around 5 years of age.[61]

Release

The ability to release objects progresses in early infancy, as voluntary control over wrist, finger, and thumb extensors emerges. Release develops off a point of stability. For example, mutual fingering in midline by the 4-month-old and transferring of objects from hand to hand in the 5- to 6-month-old infant is possible because one hand can release off the stability provided by the other hand. Voluntary release typically emerges around 7 to 9 months of age. It is initially achieved through stabilization provided by an external surface, such as the tray of a highchair or from the stable hand of someone attempting to take an object from the infant. Once a child is able to accurately release an object into a container, without external support, she is on the way to developing graded release patterns. An infant can usually release a block into a small container by 12 months and release a pellet into a small container by 15 months.[62] Ball throwing is an example of release that improves in control and accuracy as the infant moves into childhood.

Bimanual Coordination

The development of bilateral arm and hand use combines the components of prehensile function. Initially, asymmetry predominates, as seen in the 2-month-old, and antigravity control is limited. The 3-month-old displays greater symmetry, as seen during bilateral hand play on the chest in midline. The 4-month-old often displays a bilateral, or two-handed, approach to reach objects visible in midline. After 5 months of age, object presentation and size determine whether the reach will be unilateral or bilateral. The 5-month-old is able to crudely transfer objects from one hand to the other. Midline hand play away from the chest becomes more extensive as shoulder girdle strength improves. At this age, the infant can hold the bottle with two hands and displays more active object manipulation, such as banging and shaking toys. The 6- to 7-month-old displays a stronger unilateral reach and a mature hand-to-hand transfer. Despite the tendencies present in bilateral development, Corbetta and Thelen[49] found that the display of unimanual versus bimanual skill is not invariant. Most infants seem to move easily between these two patterns throughout the first year.

Differentiated bimanual movements begin at 8 to 10 months, when the two hands begin to have different roles or functions. For instance, one hand can hold the bottle while the other reaches to grasp a new toy. By 12 to 18 months of age, differentiated movements are advancing; each hand assumes either the active or stabilizing role. For example, the *active* hand may operate the dial of a toy telephone with the index finger, and the *stabilizing* hand may hold the edge of the telephone. After 2 years of age, the complexity of bimanual, or two-handed, tasks increases significantly as does capability.

Gross Motor Development and Prehension

Advances in manual performance, visuoperceptual skill, and cognition coincide with exploration of objects and the environment made available through gross motor skill development. When making gross motor transitions from one position to another, the infant strengthens and stretches various muscle groups that are later used in numerous prehensile tasks. For instance, weight bearing on extended arms in quadruped recruits shoulder and trunk musculature for stability, and weight shifting alternates pressure from the ulnar to the radial side of the hand, stretching out the intrinsic muscles.

As gross motor skill and postural control improve, the infant becomes capable of executing visuomotor acts with greater ease. Although strength and early prehensile skills naturally develop through activities executed in prone, supine, and quadruped; once postural control in sitting develops, prehensile ability improves dramatically. As trunk and upper limb strength and motor control expand, the infant is able to reach unilaterally and bilaterally with graded control. Studies examining the development of postural control in sitting reveal basic, direction-specific synergies, including anticipatory postural adjustments, adapted to task-specific conditions. von Hofsten and Woollacott[63] reported that some 9-month-old infants demonstrated proactive control by activating proximal trunk muscles before reaching.

Preschool Child

During the preschool years, prehensile patterns and eye-hand coordination skills are refined and practiced. Prehensile tasks are learned through trial and error and rehearsal from a model in collaboration with developing perceptual and cognitive processes. Often, a young child is unable to demonstrate a particular skill independently yet can do so in the presence of an adult or more capable peer. A 3-year-old child may be unable to cut paper with scissors independently yet may be successful in the presence of another capable 3-year-old by internalizing the perceptual and cognitive strategies provided. This phenomenon is known as the *Zone of*

Proximal Development.[27] Skilled hand function and the use of implements develop rapidly during this period as the preschool child expands her repertoire of play behaviors.

Reach and Grip Formation

Adultlike reaching patterns are assumed by 2 years of age yet continue to be refined through late childhood. Consistent temporal coordination across arm segments for multijoint reaches improves up until 3 years of age.[45] Kuhtz-Buschbeck and colleagues[52] compared reach and grip formation (hand preshaping) in children 4 to 12 years of age against adult behaviors. They found younger children opened their hand wider before object contact than did the older children or adults, suggesting that they grasp using a higher safety margin of error to prevent missing the target. They also reported that younger children seemed to be more dependent on vision to scale their grip aperture to the target. With increasing age, the dependence on vision decreased and reaching trajectories became straighter. These studies suggest that anticipatory reach to grasp behaviors continue to develop through the preschool years and are refined into late childhood.

Grasp and Manipulation

Preschool children gradually become more socialized and begin to engage in activities that require grasp and manipulation of various implements. Implements commonly used at this age include utensils, such as eating devices and banging instruments; tools, such as scissors or writing devices; and self-care items, such as fasteners, shoelaces, and hairbrushes.

The use of implements requires the employment of one or all three forms of manipulation: sustained grip or pinch force, in-hand manipulation, and bimanual coordination. As strength of the intrinsic muscles develops, the child usually can demonstrate *sustained pinch force* on items such as a crayon when coloring. Young children improve in the ability to coordinate fingertip forces with practice but still demonstrate inefficient control. For example, they may crush fragile objects such as paper cups or potato chips or lift light objects too quickly. This lack of anticipatory control may be due in part to insufficient internal representations for the properties of the lifted objects.

As distal control improves, crayon and pencil grips are modified. A typical sequence of pencil grip development is outlined in Table 14-5. Before in-hand manipulation skill advances, the child often adjusts the crayon position in one hand with the contralateral hand. Once fingertip force coordination improves and in-hand manipulation develops, the crayon can be translated, rotated, or shifted ipsilaterally without assistance from the opposite hand.

Bimanual coordination for symmetrical and asymmetrical tasks expands through the preschool years as children begin to incorporate anticipatory prehensile behaviors as needed for such tasks as catching a ball (Figure 14-7). Many skills develop as each hand begins to refine coordinated, asymmetrical roles. Initially, the child may need to stabilize the paper she is coloring using both elbows, but eventually just the opposite hand is needed. Other examples of bimanual skills a preschooler typically engages in are cutting paper with scissors, buttoning clothing, zipping zippers, and tying shoelaces. Motor planning, the ability to execute novel motor acts, and task-specific practice play significant roles in the acquisition of new fine-motor tasks such as those described above. Through trial and error, modeling, and practice, the preschooler expands and refines sustained pinch ability, in-hand manipulation, and bilateral hand use. By the end of this period, hand preference for specific tasks such as coloring and cutting with scissors may be demonstrated.

Hand Preference

Hand preference and hand dominance are often confused in definition. *Hand preference* refers to a *tendency* to use one hand for prehension instead of the other. *Hand dominance* is the *consistent use* of one hand over the other for such tasks as throwing a ball, writing with a pencil, and eating with a fork. Hand preference can be verified through interview and observation of performance during select tasks. Although some researchers have reported that hand preference for swiping objects can be noted within days after birth, it remains controversial.[64] The preschooler develops a hand preference as she practices skilled tasks, such as eating with utensils, coloring, and throwing a ball. By 4 to 6 years of age, hand preference is well established. Lateralization of the brain, the process by which the hemispheres become specialized for particular functions, is generally thought to be the driving force behind hand dominance.[65] Consistent use of one hand for skilled tasks promotes lateralization. Some children may not demonstrate a hand preference during the preschool years because the preferred hand is not yet sufficiently influenced by the contralateral motor cortex. However, by 6 to 7 years of age, laterality is demonstrated through the consistent and superior use of one hand to hold a pencil during writing tasks. Most agree that the dominant hand performs better than the nondominant during fine, dexterous activities. However, for some manual tasks, it is possible that by altering the context requirements such as speed and accuracy of the task, performance between hands may become more similar.[66]

Table 14-5

Sequential Acquisition of Pencil Grip

Pencil Grip	Age	Description	Illustration
Palmar-supinate	1-2 yr	Pencil or crayon is held by fisted hand; forearm slightly supinated; wrist slightly flexed; shoulder motion produces movement of pencil	
Digital-pronate	2-3 yr	Pencil or crayon is held by fingers and thumb; forearm pronated, wrist ulnarly deviated; pencil controlled by shoulder movement	
Static-tripod	3+ yr	Pencil held proximally between thumb and radial two fingers; minimal wrist mobility; pencil controlled by shoulder movement	
Dynamic-tripod	4+ yr	Pencil is held distally through thumb opposition to the index and long fingers, with the ring and small fingers stabilizing in flexion; small movements at the metacarpophalangeal and interphalangeal joints control the pencil; stabilization occurs at the shoulder, elbow, forearm, and wrist	

Data from Erhardt RP: *Developmental hand dysfunction: theory, assessment, and treatment,* Laurel, Md, 1982, RAMSCO, pp 9-3; Knobloch H, Stevens F, Malone AF: *Manual of developmental diagnosis: the administration and interpretation of the revised Gesell and Amatruda's developmental and neurological exam,* Houston, Tex, 1987, Developmental Evaluation Materials, pp 24-260; Rosenbloom L, Horton ME: The maturation of fine prehension in young children, *Dev Med Child Neurol* 13:3-8, 1971.

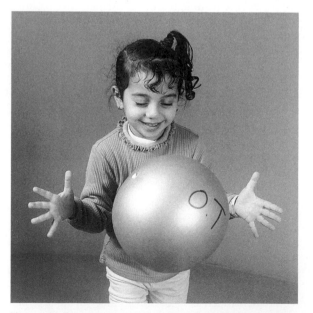

Figure 14-7 Bimanual anticipatory reach and grip formation exhibited by a 4-year-old when catching a ball.

School-Aged Child

Mastery

During this period, children often demonstrate mastery of many components of prehension. A child's knowledge and abilities for an activity are considered domain or task specific, which allows for rapid encoding and response to certain fine-motor situations. The degree to which a particular skill is mastered depends on the amount of time spent practicing specific tasks and the strength of the supporting systems.

Reach to grasp behaviors expand in the school-aged child. For instance, 6-year-olds display an exaggerated grip aperture during reaching, whereas 12-year-olds can scale the grip aperture more closely to object size.[52] Although some children between 6 and 8 years of age may demonstrate adultlike fingertip force coordination when grasping and lifting objects, some do not achieve this capacity until 11 years of age or later.[57] Reportedly by 6 years of age, most children can demonstrate adequate in-hand manipulation, which allows for the expansion of prehensile activities in which they can engage. Complex asymmetrical bimanual coordination progresses during the school-aged period. For example, building model airplanes is a complex task that requires one hand to stabilize the base and the other hand to glue small parts onto that stable base. Children of the same age demonstrate very different levels of skill at building models. As a child matures into adolescence, interest and experience further guide the refinement of prehensile skills.

School-aged children often spend a large amount of their time involved in task-specific practice. For example, the demands for written work increase by 8 to 9 years of age, necessitating skill in holding and sustaining a pencil grip while completing the complex task of handwriting. Writing requires selective attention and other cognitive processes and is affected by the state of arousal.

Handwriting

Many of the components of prehension play a role in handwriting. Visual regard of the paper and pencil and accurate perception of the workspace are needed. When copying from a chalkboard, we must shift visual gaze from the board to the paper without losing our place. The spatial relationships between the desk, the paper, and the blackboard need to be accurately perceived, as do the spatial relationships between the letters, words, and sentences on a page. Position in space and form constancy will guide recognition of letters and numbers. Grasp and manipulation, sustained grip and pinch, in-hand manipulation, and bimanual coordination contribute to handwriting and can be analyzed separately for clarity.

Pencil grip is an example of sustained pinch. Examples are shown by order of frequency in Figure 14-8. The most frequently used pencil grip is the dynamic tripod, which is demonstrated when a pencil is held between the pads of the index and thumb while it rests against the long finger. This position is considered the most efficient in terms of speed and dexterity because pencil movement is controlled distally by the fingers and thumb. Alternative pencil grips are considered efficient if the thumb and index form a circle or open web space, allowing for skillful distal manipulation. Inefficient grips limit the range, speed, and fluidity of distal movement and demand greater proximal movements of the wrist and elbow to control the pencil, reducing precision. The lateral tripod, considered a functional yet inefficient grip because the web space is closed, is used by up to 25% of nondysfunctional children and up to 10% of adults.[67] With adequate strength and somatosensory feedback, a child can sustain a hold on a pencil without the need for excess pressure. Endurance for sustained pinch, required during prolonged handwriting tasks, is gained with practice.

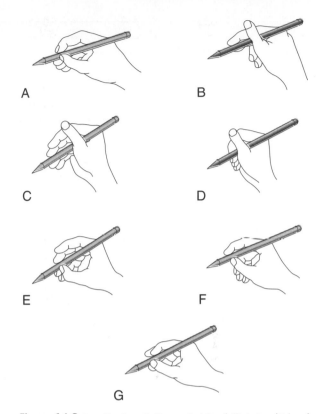

Figure 14-8 Pencil grips. **A,** Dynamic tripod. **B,** Lateral tripod. **C,** Transpalmar interdigital. **D,** Cross-thumb. **E,** Dynamic bipod. **F,** Dynamic bipod with omitted third digit. **G,** Static tripod. (Redrawn from Bergmann KP: Incidence of atypical pencil grasps among nondysfunctional adults, *Am J Occup Ther* 44:736-740, 1990.)

Grip and pinch strength increase throughout childhood and contribute to all prehensile abilities. Mathiowetz and colleagues[68] collected normative data on grip and pinch strength for children and adolescents 6 to 19 years of age, comparing males to females. Figure 14-9, *A* illustrates the increasing grip strength exhibited by these children. Pencil grip strength may be best inferred from palmar pinch and key pinch strength.

In-hand manipulation is frequently used for pencil writing. If a demand is made for quick writing and erasing, a child learns to adjust the pencil in one hand and rotate it longitudinally to use the eraser. Bimanual coordination is required for writing because one hand must stabilize the writing surface and the other hand must actively use the pencil.

Adolescence

During this phase of development, primary occupations include schoolwork, socialization, part-time employment, and prereadiness for later employment or career.

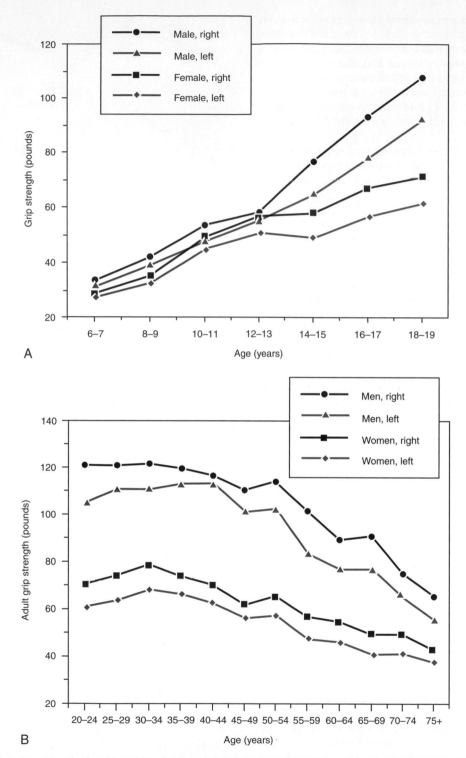

Figure 14-9 A, Grip strength of males and females from 6 to 19 years old. **B,** Grip strength of men and women. Note the downward trend from 20 to 75 years of age. (**A** Data from Mathiowetz V, Wiemer DM, Federman SM: Grip and pinch norms for 6- to 19-year-olds, *Am J Occup Ther* 40:705-711, 1986; **B** Data from Mathiowetz V, Kashman N, Volland G et al: Grip and pinch strength: normative data for adults, *Arch Phys Med Rehabil* 66:16-21, 1985.)

The prehensile demands resemble those of the school-age child, except that the skill level required is often higher. Less time is spent in trial and error and more time is spent in perfecting skill. Skills performed with the dominant hand continue to advance beyond those of the nondominant hand. Bimanual skills, including the use of a computer keyboard or sports-related activities, do play a strong role at this stage of development. Adolescents often are cognitively aware of their strengths and weaknesses in terms of coordination and skill with manipulative tasks. Success heightens interest and helps boost self-esteem; thus, motivation for a task and practice are strongly correlated. A comparison between male and female grip strength in adolescents is shown in Figure 14-9. Young adults demonstrate a significant increase in grip and pinch strength, which may correlate with the functional gains seen in prehensile tasks.

By the time we reach adolescence, adultlike coordination of fingertip forces is demonstrated. This ability allows an individual to fine-tune manual skills related to specific areas of interest.

Adulthood

Occupational Choices

Early in adulthood, most vocational and avocational choices are made. Some occupations require fine dexterity and skilled hand use. Dental hygiene, surgery, and stained glass artistry all require skill in precision handling and a strong pinch for sustained tool use. Pickleman and Schueneman[69] devised a rating form for testing proficiency in surgery and a neuropsychological test battery for assessing psychomotor, perceptual, and perceptual-motor abilities in surgical residents. For example, they found that those with demonstrated strength in the area of complex visuospatial problem-solving and manual dexterity displayed superior surgical technique. Not all researchers agree with these results. Graham and Deary[70] discussed that although spatial ability tests correlate with surgical skill ratings, manual dexterity tests do not. Harris and colleagues[71] assessed manual dexterity, eye-hand coordination, and visuospatial ability. They found that although surgical trainees performed quicker on tests of eye-hand coordination than other trainees, there were no differences between specialties or sex in terms of visuospatial ability. In all specialties, women were significantly more accurate than men on eye-hand coordination tests. They concluded that self-selection of a surgical specialty based on skill is unlikely.

Although not measured in the studies reported above, other components play a role in the fine manual dexterity needed for such occupations as dentistry and surgery. These include endurance, efficiency, and accuracy. When we enter early adulthood with strong prehensile skills, those other components may require nurturing before true mastery is achieved. Motivation, patience, and task-specific practice enhances the refinement of most prehensile skills, including proficiency of surgical technique. If skills do not improve, the individual may need to choose a profession in which exceptional prehensile ability is not required.

Strength

The magnitude of grip and pinch strength needed to perform most activities of daily living tasks and job duties varies. Available grip and pinch strength may also influence our career choice. Conversely, grip and pinch strength increase if our occupational tasks require greater hand use.[72] For example, office workers have the weakest grips, and heavy manual workers have the strongest.

Reportedly, if the right hand is dominant, the strength of the right hand is approximately 10% greater than that of the left hand, and if the left hand is dominant, the strength of the two hands are usually equal.[73] However, other studies have found that grip strength of the dominant and nondominant hands to be relatively equal regardless of handedness.[74,75] Interestingly, grip and pinch strength can vary between 14% and 24% when tested over a 2-week period for different reasons.[76] Therefore, improvements in grip strength documented as progress in rehabilitation settings may in fact just represent the day-to-day variability and should be interpreted with caution.

Mathiowetz and colleagues[75] outlined normative grip strength on people older than 20 years of age (see Figure 14-9, *B*). The 25- to 39-year-old age group exhibited the highest grip strength values. Although the values varied little between 20 to 59 years of age, a gradual decline was noted between 60 to 75-plus years of age, especially among men.

Maintenance of Prehensile Skill and Function

In middle adulthood, most of the systems involved with prehension continue to function well, as long as they are maintained and not overextended. Performance in most activities of daily living is maintained easily because such activities are practiced repeatedly over the years and are generally nonstrenuous. When dysfunction does occur, it is commonly caused by congenital or traumatic limb loss, learned nonuse, peripheral neuropathy, or cumulative trauma disorders. We discuss strategies to improve function in Clinical Implications Box 14-1: Prehensile Dysfunction Across the Life Span.

CLINICAL IMPLICATIONS Box 14-1

Prehensile Dysfunction Across the Life Span

Skilled prehension helps us perform many everyday activities. Throughout the life span, however, individuals may be faced with the challenge of completing prehensile tasks despite injury, illness, or congenital limb deficiencies. Some of the common causes of prehensile dysfunction are described here, as well as strategies that are available to enhance function.

Common Causes of Prehensile Dysfunction
• Congenital and Traumatic Upper Extremity Limb Loss

Limb deficiencies may develop in response to abnormal constraints placed on the developing upper extremity. For example, amniotic bands present in a growing hand or arm may result in partial amputations or other tissue damage in response to band-induced compression and ischemia.[86] Trauma can result in amputations or neuromuscular damage leading to a loss in upper limb function. Injury to the brachial plexus at birth or injury to cervical spinal nerves secondary to an accident can result in paralysis of one or more arm and hand muscles. Prehensile capabilities present after injury depend on the muscles that remain innervated.

• Learned nonuse

Learned nonuse[87] occurs when voluntary movement of a limb is suppressed, as seen in individuals with congenital limb deficiencies, unilateral brachial plexus injury, or hemiplegia secondary to cerebral palsy or stroke. In cases of unilateral nonuse, one limb does not develop efficient prehension secondary to neuromuscular or musculoskeletal impairments and thus is ignored while tasks are primarily performed with the intact extremity.

• Peripheral neuropathy

Carpal tunnel syndrome, diabetes mellitus, and Raynaud disease can cause peripheral neuropathies, which are pathological conditions that reduce sensibility and function.[88-90] Studies reveal that tactile deficits alone lead to incoordination during object manipulation and to targeting errors during reaching.[91,92] Proprioceptive deficits can also lead to errors in reaching and deficits in interjoint coordination as noted in those with large fiber sensory neuropathy.[93,94] Visual cues have been found to greatly improve prehensile performance in the presence of tactile and proprioceptive deficits.[95]

• Cumulative trauma disorders

Cumulative trauma disorders, such as tendinitis, can result from sustained pinch or prehensile activities performed repetitively without adequate endurance and subsequent rest to refuel energies.[96]

Cumulative trauma disorders are the most frequent cause of lost work and workers' compensation claims in certain industries.[97] For example, as many as 30% of professional musicians will develop cumulative trauma disorders.[98] The presence of tendinitis or tendinosis can lead to compensatory prehension patterns, which are often less efficient than those typically used.

Strategies to Improve Prehensile Function

Those with limited prehension have options. They could engage in training activities to enhance capabilities. Alternatively, they could use adaptive devices, take advantage of surgical reconstruction, or use a neuroprosthetic device. Before intervention, however, it is important to evaluate individual needs and long-range plans based on the current functional level.

• Adaptive devices

Most individuals adapt quite easily to subtle deficits in prehension. If the deficits make simple tasks difficult, the use of adaptive devices may improve performance. Self-care items commonly used to maximize prehensile capabilities include universal cuffs to hold various implements (e.g., an eating utensil) and button hooks to button clothing with one hand. Writing devices that place the fingers and thumb in a position resembling a tripod or lateral grip can be fabricated or obtained commercially. While adaptive devices can increase independent function, they are not always accepted.

• Surgical reconstruction

One example of surgical intervention to reduce the negative effects of congenital anomalies on limb development is fetal upper limb surgery. For example, there has been reported success with the release of amniotic bands in utero, which constrict limb development and growth.[99] If these circumferential bands are released early enough, they may prevent amputations or other limb deficits before birth.

Tendon transfers are an option available to individuals with peripheral nerve damage. The transfer of intact muscles to nonfunctional muscle-tendon units can improve motion in various conditions such as: (1) shoulder external rotation and elevation after brachial plexus birth injury (Erb palsy)[100], (2) thumb opposition after median nerve injury[101], or (3) lateral pinch and elbow extension after cervical spinal cord injury.[102–104] Research indicates that tendon transfers improve independence in everyday activities and may allow individuals to resume life roles with greater satisfaction.[105]

Pollicization is a procedure used to reconstruct an opposable digit, which may be an option for those born without a thumb or those who have sustained traumatic loss of a thumb. Typically, the index finger is rotated to oppose the remaining digits.[105,106] Transplantation of the great or second toe to replace a lost thumb can also be performed successfully. Although function after transplantation is generally good, the resultant sensibility seems to vary between adults and children and between surgical techniques performed.[107,108]

Prostheses

Prosthetic devices provide an alternative means of prehension to those with nonfunctional hands or upper limb amputation, whether congenital or traumatic. The addition of a prosthesis has the potential to enhance unilateral and bilateral function. Passive prostheses without active control can be used as a first prosthesis in infants who sit independently, or as a cosmetic prosthesis for older children or adults. Later in infancy, a terminal device that is either active opening or closing can be issued to enhance prehension. The key to acceptance of an upper limb prosthesis in cases of congenital absence is fitting before the age of 2 years and promoting parental involvement in the process.[109,110] Interestingly, while prostheses are often used for social occasions or specialized activities, they do not necessarily improve function or quality of life.[102] Adolescents and adults may be more accepting of an active prostheses if it significantly improves function. Otherwise, a cosmetic prosthesis may be used for social occasions only.

Prosthetic devices include the standard hook and harness unit, myoelectric devices, and implanted electrical stimulation, termed a *neuroprosthesis*. Standard prosthetic devices use a terminal device that resembles a hand or consists of a hook to provide a strong pinch force. Terminal devices are activated through a harness via shoulder movement. Myoelectric units use remaining arm musculature to activate the terminal device through the use of electrodes strategically placed in the socket to lie over the most active site of the muscle belly. Neuroprostheses have been implanted in those with high-level cervical spinal cord injuries without adequate transfer muscles. This system can provide lateral pinch and palmar grasp function. Research has indicated that implantation of a neuroprosthesis in adolescents with tetraplegia improves their independence in activities of daily living and ability to grasp and lift objects.[111–113] New methods for controlling the wrist and hand are being developed, including the use of implanted intracortical electrodes and wireless wearable devices.[114,115]

Training Activities

• Strategies for learned nonuse

Individuals with learned nonuse can be encouraged to use the involved extremity through constraint induced movement therapy (CIMT) or bimanual training. The CIMT approach has been used successfully in adults post-stroke[116,117] and in children with hemiplegic cerebral palsy.[118-121] Huang and colleagues[122] did a systematic literature review and found increased upper extremity use after CIMT, yet further research is needed to determine the best dosage. Bimanual training has also been found effective for adults poststroke and children with hemiplegic cerebral palsy.[123] Charles and Gordon[123,124] outlined an effective program titled Hand-Arm Bimanual Intervention (HABIT).

Coordination impairments found in those with neurological impairments can also be addressed with specific practice schedules. Duff and Gordon[125] found that extended blocked or random practice in grasping and lifting novel objects, without constraining the limb, was an effective means of promoting anticipatory scaling of fingertip forces in children with hemiplegic cerebral palsy. Improvements in anticipatory control may contribute to greater prehensile skill.

• Strategies to prevent cumulative trauma disorder

For adults, the best methods for maintaining prehensile skill without causing undue harm to neuromuscular structures require (1) the use of correct postural alignment for tasks, (2) frequent breaks during sustained pinch or grip tasks, (3) use of tools to simplify tasks, and (4) use of ergonomically redesigned tools and musical instruments to prevent undue stress on anatomic structures.[98,126,127] Given the prevalence of cumulative trauma disorders, it is important to employ these strategies not only in work-related activities but recreational tasks as well.

Maintenance of skill during the period of middle adulthood is differentiated from early adulthood in terms of performance, that is, the amount of domain-specific practice, motivation, and efficiency. When interest and motivation for activities drop, so does practice time. We may have been an expert at the piano at the age of 25 years, but by age 50, we may spend too little time at the keyboard to maintain and preserve our former skill. Conversely, concert pianists, who continue to demonstrate fine technique well into their older adult years, may be able to maintain their skills because of continued practice. Sustained practice time promotes greater endurance, yet it is demanding. It requires us to maintain a high tolerance for aerobic work to avoid fatigue of associated structures.

Older Adulthood

Manual performance and psychomotor behaviors decline as adults age.[77,78] Shiffman[79] found that hand strength, performance time, and the frequency with which prehension patterns are used are affected by age. These changes in manual skill reflect functional adaptation to changes in the visual, nervous, somatosensory, and musculoskeletal systems associated with aging.

Sensory Changes

Sensory changes have been documented through the visual and somatosensory systems. Visual acuity, imaging power of the retina, and the transparency of the lens are all reduced in older adulthood. It also takes older individuals 33% longer to process visual information than it does younger people.[80] In addition, there is a sharp decrease in depth perception from 60 to 75 years. Loss in sensibility through the arms and hands may be due to a decrease in sensory nerve conduction, alterations in mechanoreceptors, and a decline in spatial acuity of touch.[81] Furthermore, Cole and colleagues[82] reported that there is an increased threshold to touch pressure and a decreased sensitivity to vibration sense.

Musculoskeletal Changes

Musculoskeletal changes are found in both muscle performance and skeletal integrity. The decline in muscle strength with aging may be attributed to a notable loss in muscle mass and to a decrease in motor nerve conduction velocity. A decrease in the number of muscle fibers will affect muscle strength and mass. Functionally, there may be a decrease in the speed of muscle contractions and in the ability to sustain a contraction. Within the skeletal system, degeneration of the articular cartilage reduces the efficiency of joint movement and reduces shock absorption. This change may result in pain and altered hand use during manipulation.

During complex hand movements, an increase in planning time in older adults was most frequently noted.[83] The time needed to plan for precise movements of the distal extremities increases linearly from 50 to 90 years of age. Thus an older adult often cannot easily achieve the quick reaction time needed to count out change in a checkout line at a grocery store.

Adaptations to System Changes

What are some of the adaptations that older adults make in response to system changes, and what are the resultant alterations in hand function? Due to a reduction in mechanoreceptors, there may be a greater dependency on muscular feedback to enhance proprioception. If somatosensory feedback is reduced, a tighter grip may be used to provide the needed sensory input. A tighter grip may not only strain joints but also recruit more muscle fibers too because of the reduction in strength and contraction speed that occurs with aging. If muscle contraction speed is reduced, dexterity will be affected. This system change combined with reduced sensibility and greater time to plan precise distal movements may expand the time to task completion. For example, older adults may need more time to count out change at the checkout line.

Despite the system changes that occur with aging, overall eye-hand coordination and manipulative skills may be relatively maintained in older adults as long as task-specific practice is continued and the systems involved remain generally intact. For example, although a reduction in sensibility typically affects fine-motor function, it may not reduce function in all tasks.[82] Furthermore, studies have indicated that with significant practice, older adults can decrease their overall response time for select motor tasks.[84] This is beneficial because improving the speed of performance can enhance movement consistency and safety.[85] In general, motivation and arousal for specific tasks do not decline with age. Therefore, unless there are specific system deficits, prehensile skills can continue to be useful into older adulthood.

SUMMARY

During many everyday activities, the primary components of prehension are engaged: visual regard, reach, grasp, manipulation, and release. Depending on the task goal and constraints, postural control and bimanual coordination may be used. The development and maintenance of prehensile skill incorporate many interdependent systems. Indeed, strong relationships exist between prehension, postural control, cognition, and visuoperceptual skill.

Flexible prehensile skills allow us to mold actions to constraints and environmental demands while meeting task goals. When prehension is viewed across the life span, we can only marvel at its highly developed features. The prehensile abilities of someone at any age with hand dysfunction are even more amazing. Simple tasks become ambitious acts of adaptation enhanced with a touch of creativity.

REFERENCES

1. Patla AE: A framework for understanding mobility problems in the elderly. In Craik RL, Oatis CA, editors: *Gait analysis: theory and application*, St Louis, 1995, Mosby, pp 436–449.

2. Kibler WB, Press J, Sciascia A: The role of core stability in athletic function, *Sports Med* 36(3):189–198, 2006.

3. Case-Smith J, Fisher AG, Bauer D: An analysis of the relationship between proximal and distal motor control, *Am J Occup Ther* 43:657–662, 1989.

4. Schieppati M, Trompetto C, Abbruzzese G: Selective facilitation of responses to cortical stimulation of proximal and distal arm muscles by precision tasks in man, *J Physiol* 491(pt 2):551–562, 1996.

5. Smith LK, Weiss EL, Lehmkuhl LD: *Brunnstrom's clinical kinesiology*, ed 5, Philadelphia, 1996, FA Davis.

6. O'Driscoll SW, Horil E, Ness R, et al: The relationship between wrist position, grasp size, and grip strength, *J Hand Surg* 17:169–177, 1992.

7. Aoki T, Niu X, Latash ML, et al: Effects of friction at the digit-object interface on the digit forces in multi-finger prehension, *Exp Brain Res* 172(4):425–438, 2006.

8. Abahnini K, Proteau L: Evidence supporting the importance of peripheral visual information for the directional control of aiming movements, *J Mot Behav* 29:230–242, 1997.

9. Kaminski TR, Bock C, Gentile AM: The coordination between trunk and arm motion during pointing movements, *Exp Brain Res* 106:457–466, 1995.

10. Abend W, Bizzi E, Morasso P: Human arm trajectory formation, *Brain* 105:331–348, 1982.

11. Jeannerod M: The timing of natural prehension movements, *J Mot Behav* 16:235–254, 1984.

12. Konczak J, Borutta M, Topka H, et al: The development of goal-directed reaching in infants: hand trajectory formation and joint torque control, *Exp Brain Res* 106(1):156–168, 1995.

13. Duff SV, Sainburg RL: Lateralization of motor adaptation reveals independence in trajectory and steady state position, *Exp Brain Res* 179(4):551–561, 2007.

14. Jeannerod M: Intersegmental coordination during reaching at natural visual objects. In Long J, Baddeley A, editors: *Attention and performance IX*, Hillsdale, NJ, 1981, Lawrence Earlbaum.

15. Jakobson LS, Goodale MA: Factors affecting higher-order movement planning: a kinematic analysis of human prehension, *Exp Brain Res* 86:199–208, 1991.

16. Ansuini C, Santello M, Massaccesi S, et al: Effects of end-goal on hand shaping, *J Neurophysiol* 95(4):2456–2465, 2005.

17. Chieffi S, Gentilucci M: Coordination between the transport and the grasp component during prehension movements, *Exp Brain Res* 94:471–477, 1993.

18. Jeannerod M: Mechanisms of visuomotor coordination: a study in normal and brain-damaged subjects, *Neuropsychologia* 24:41–78, 1986.

19. Napier JR: The prehensile movement of the human hand, *J Bone Joint Surg* 38:902–913, 1956.

20. Landsmeer JMF: Power grip and precision handling, *Ann Rheum Dis* 21:164–169, 1962.

21. Wong YJ, Whishaw IQ: Precision grasps of children and young and old adults: individual differences in digit contact strategy, purchase pattern, and digit posture, *Behav Brain Res* 154(1):113–123, 2004.

22. Casanova JS, Grunert BK: Adult prehension: patterns and nomenclature for pinches, *J Hand Ther* 2:231–244, 1989.

23. Johansson RS, Cole KJ: Sensory-motor coordination during grasping and manipulative actions, *Curr Opin Neurobiol* 2:815–823, 1992.

24. Flatt A: The absent thumb. In Flatt A, editor: *The care of congenital hand anomalies*, St Louis, 1977, Mosby.

25. Raj R, Marquis C: Finger dominance, *J Hand Surg* 24:430, 1999.

26. Tubiana R: Architecture and functions of the hand. In Tubiana R, Thomine JM, Mackin EJ, editors: *Examination of the hand and upper limb*, Philadelphia, 1984, WB Saunders, pp 1–98.

27. Exner C: The zone of proximal development in in-hand manipulation skills of nondysfunctional 3- and 4-year-old children, *Am J Occup Ther* 44:884–891, 1990.

28. Vallbo AB, Johansson RS: Properties of cutaneous mechanoreceptors in the human hand related to touch sensation, *Hum Neurobiol* 3:3–14, 1984.

29. Edin BB, Abbs JH: Finger movement responses of cutaneous mechanoreceptors in the dorsal skin of the human hand, *J Neurophysiol* 65:657–670, 1991.

30. Kazennikov O, Wiesendanger M: Bimanual coordination of bowing and fingering in violinists: effects of position changes and string changes, *Motor Control* 13(3):297–309, 2009.

31. Wiesendanger M, Kazennikov O, Perrig S, et al: Two hands—one action: the problem of bimanual coordination. In Wing AM, Haggard P, Flanagan JR, editors: *Hand and brain: the neurophysiology and psychology of hand movements*, San Diego, 1996, Academic Press.

32. Perrig S, Kazennikov O, Wiesendanger M: Time structure of a goal-directed bimanual skill and its dependence on task constraints, *Behav Brain Res* 103:95–104, 1999.

33. Moore KL, Persaud TVN: *The developing human: clinically oriented embryology*, ed 6, Philadelphia, 1998, WB Saunders.

34. Sparling JW, Van Tol J, Chescheir NC: Fetal and neonatal hand movement, *Phys Ther* 79:24–39, 1999.

35. McCartney G, Hepper P: Development of lateralized behaviour in the human fetus from 12 to 27 weeks' gestation, *Dev Med Child Neurol* 41:83–86, 1999.

36. Thelen E: Motor development: a new synthesis, *Am Psychol* 50:79–95, 1995.

37. Auer T, Pinter S, Kovacs N, et al: Does obstetric brachial plexus injury influence speech dominance? *Ann Neural* 65(1):57–66, 2009.

38. Coren S, Ward LM, Enns JT: *Sensation and perception*, ed 5, Orlando, Fla, 1999, Harcourt Brace.

39. Rosander K, von Hofsten C: Visual-vestibular interaction in early infancy, *Exp Brain Res* 133:321–333, 2000.

40. von Hofsten C, Rosander K: Development of smooth pursuit tracking in young infants, *Vision Res* 37:1799–1810, 1997.

41. Liegeois F, Bentejec L, de Schonen S: When does inter-hemispheric integration of visual events emerge in infancy? A developmental study on 19- to 28-month-old infants, *Neuropsychologia* 38:1382–1389, 2000.

42. McBryde C, Zivani J: Proximal and distal upper limb motor development in 24-week-old infants, *Can J Occup Ther* 57:147–154, 1990.

43. von Hofsten C, Lindhagen K: Observation on the development of reaching for moving objects, *J Exp Child Psychol* 28:158–173, 1979.

44. Clifton RK, Muir DW, Ashmead DH, et al: Is visually guided reaching in early infancy a myth? *Child Dev* 64:1099–1110, 1993.

45. Konczak J, Dichgans J: The development toward stereotypic arm kinematics during reaching in the first 3 years of life, *Exp Brain Res* 117:346–354, 1997.

46. Rochat P: Self-sitting and reaching in 5- to 8-month-old infants: the impact of posture and its development on eye-hand coordination, *J Mot Behav* 24:210–220, 1992.

47. Halverson HM: An experimental study of prehension in infants by means of systematic cinema recording, *Genet Psychol Monogr* 19:107–285, 1931.

48. Halverson HM: A further study of grasping, *J Gen Psychol* 7:34–64, 1932.

49. Corbetta D, Thelen E: The developmental origins of bimanual coordination: a dynamic perspective, *J Exp Psychol Hum Percept Perform* 22:502–522, 1996.

50. von Hofsten C, Fazel-Zandy S: Development of visually guided hand orientation in reaching, *J Exp Child Psychol* 38:208–219, 1984.

51. von Hofsten C, Ronnqvist L: Preparation for grasping an object: a developmental study, *J Exp Psychol Hum Percept Perform* 14:610–621, 1988.

52. Kuhtz-Buschbeck JP, Stolze H, Joehnk M, et al: Development of prehension movements in children, *Exp Brain Res* 122:424–432, 1998.

53. Wallace PS, Whishaw IQ: Independent digit movements and precision grip patterns in 1-5-month-old human infants: hand-babbling, including vacuous then self-directed hand and digit movements, precedes targeted reaching, *Neuropsychology* 41(14):1912–1918, 2003.

54. Hohlstein RR: The development of prehension in normal infants, *Am J Occup Ther* 36:170–175, 1982.

55. Lantz C, Melen K, Forssberg H: Early infant grasping involves radial fingers, *Dev Med Child Neurol* 38:668–674, 1996.

56. Newell KM, Scully DM, McDonald PV: Task constraints and infant grip configurations, *Dev Psychobiol* 22:817–831, 1989.

57. Forssberg H, Eliasson AC, Kinoshita H, et al: Development of human precision grip. IV: tactile adaptation of isometric finger forces to the frictional condition, *Exp Brain Res* 104:323–330, 1995.

58. Pare M, Dugas C: Developmental changes in prehension during childhood, *Exp Brain Res* 125:239–247, 1999.

59. Streri A: Tactile discrimination of shape and intermodel transfer in 2- to 3-month-old infants, *Br J Dev Psychol* 5:213–220, 1987.

60. Rose SA, Gottfried A, Bridger W: Cross-modal transfer in infants: relationship to prematurity and socioeconomic background, *Dev Psychol* 14:643–652, 1978.

61. Stilwell JM, Cermak SA: Perceptual functions of the hand. In Henderson A, Pehoski C, editors: *Hand function in the child: foundations for remediation*, Philadelphia, 1995, Mosby, pp 55–80.

62. Hirschel A, Pehoski C, Coryell J: Environmental support and the development of grasp in infants, *Am J Occup Ther* 44:721–727, 1990.

63. von Hofsten C, Woollacott HM: *Postural preparations for reaching in 9-month-old infants*, 1990 Unpublished manuscript.

64. Korczyn AD, Sage JI, Karplus M: Lack of limb motor asymmetry in the neonate, *J Neurobiol* 9:483–488, 1978.

65. Sainburg RL: Handedness: differential specializations for control of trajectory and position, *Exerc Sport Sci Rev* 33(4):206–213, 2005.

66. Lewis SR, Duff SV, Gordon AM: Manual asymmetry during object release under varying task constraints, *Am J Occup Ther* 56(4):391–401, 2002.

67. Schneck CM, Henderson A: Descriptive analysis of the developmental progression of grip position for pencil and crayon control in nondysfunctional children, *Am J Occup Ther* 44:893–900, 1990.

68. Mathiowetz V, Wiemer DM, Federman SM: Grip and pinch strength norms for 6- to 19-year-olds, *Am J Occup Ther* 40:705–711, 1986.

69. Pickleman J, Schueneman AL: The use and abuse of neuropsychological tests to predict operative performance, *Am Coll Surg Bull* 72:7–11, 1987.

70. Graham KS, Deary IJ: A role for aptitude testing in surgery? *J R Coll Surg Edinb* 36:70–74, 1991.

71. Harris CJ, Herbert M, Steele RJ: Psychomotor skills of surgical trainees compared with those of different medical specialists, *Br J Surg* 81:382–383, 1994.

72. Josty IC, Tyler MP, Shewell PC, et al: Grip and pinch strength variations in different types of workers, *J Hand Surg* 22:266–269, 1997.

73. Peterson P, Petrick M, Connor H, et al: Grip strength and hand dominance: challenging the 10% rule, *Am J Occup Ther* 43:444–447, 1989.

74. Armstrong CA, Oldman JA: A comparison of dominant and non-dominant hand strengths, *J Hand Surg* 24:421–425, 1999.

75. Mathiowetz V, Kashman N, Volland G, et al: Grip and pinch strength: normative data for adults, *Arch Phys Med Rehabil* 66:16–21, 1985.

76. Young VL, Pin P, Kraemer BA, et al: Fluctuation in grip and pinch strength among normal subjects, *J Hand Surg* 14:125–129, 1989.

77. Hughes S, Gibbs H, Dunlop D, et al: Predictors of decline in manual performance in older adults, *J Am Geriatr Soc* 45:905–910, 1997.

78. Weir PL, MacDonald JR, Mallat BJ, et al: Age-related differences in prehension: the influence of task goals, *J Mot Behav* 30:79–80, 1998.

79. Shiffman LM: Effects of aging on adult hand function, *Am J Occup Ther* 46:785–792, 1992.

80. Kline D, Schieber F, Coyne A: Aging, the eye and visual channels: contrast sensitivity and response speed, *J Gerontol* 33:211–216, 1983.

81. Stevens JC, Cruz LA: Spatial acuity of touch: ubiquitous decline with aging revealed by repeated threshold testing, *Somatosens Mot Res* 13:1–10, 1996.

82. Cole KJ, Rotella DL, Harper JG: Tactile impairments cannot explain the effect of age on a grasp and lift task, *Exp Brain Res* 121:263–269, 1998.

83. Williams HG: Aging and eye-hand coordination. In Bard C, Fleury M, Hay L, editors: *Development of eye-hand coordination across the life span*, Columbia, SC, 1990, University of South Carolina Press, pp 327–357.

84. Falduto L, Baron A: Age-related changes and effects of practice and task complexity on card sorting, *J Gerontol* 41:659–661, 1960.

85. Light KE: Information processing for motor performance in aging adults, *Phys Ther* 70:820–826, 1990.

86. Light TR, Ogden JA: Congenital constriction band syndrome: pathophysiology and treatment, *Yale J Biol Med* 66:143–155, 1993.

87. Taub E, Goldberg IA, Taub P: Deafferentation in monkeys: pointing at a target without visual feedback, *Exp Neurol* 46:176–186, 1975.

88. Casanova JE, Casanova JS, Young MJ: Hand function in patients with diabetes mellitus, *South Med J* 84:1111–1113, 1991.

89. Lowe BD, Freivalds A: Effect of carpal tunnel syndrome on grip force coordination on hand tools, *Ergonomics* 42:550–564, 1999.

90. Patri B, Gatto A: Raynaud's syndrome, Dupuytren's disease, force of prehension and sensitivity of the hand: study of age-related changes, *Ann Chir Main* 5:144–147, 1986.

91. Gentilucci M, Toni I, Daprati E, et al: Tactile input of the hand and the control of reaching to grasp movements, *Exp Brain Res* 114:130–137, 1997.

92. Westling G, Johansson RS: Factors influencing the force control during precision grip, *Exp Brain Res* 53:277–284, 1984.

93. Gordon J, Ghilardi MF, Ghez C: Impairments of reaching movements in patients without proprioception. 1. Spatial errors, *J Neurophysiol* 73:347–360, 1995.

94. Sainburg RL, Poizner H, Ghez C: Loss of proprioception produces deficits in interjoint coordination, *J Neurophysiol* 70:2136–2147, 1993.

95. Ghez C, Gordon J, Ghilardi MF: Impairments of reaching in patients without proprioception. II. Effects of visual information on accuracy, *J Neurophysiol* 73:361–372, 1995.

96. Duff SV: Neuromuscular conditions. In Sanders MJ, editor: *Management of cumulative trauma disorders*, Boston, 1997, Butterworth-Heinemann, pp 41–103.

97. Barr AE, Barbe MF, Clark BD: Work-related musculoskeletal disorders of the hand and wrist: epidemiology, pathophysiology, and sensorimotor changes, *J Orthop Sports Phys Ther* 34(10):610–627, 2004.

98. Markison RE: Treatment of musical hands: redesign the interface in hand injuries, *Sports Performing Arts Hand Clin* 6:525–544, 1990.

99. Quintero RA, Morales WJ, Phillips J, et al: In utero lysis of amniotic bands, *Ultrasound Obstet Gynecol* 10:316–320, 1997.

100. Waters PM: Obstetric brachial plexus injuries: evaluation and management, *J Am Acad Orthop Surg* 5:205–214, 1997.

101. Brand PW: *Drag in clinical mechanics of the hand*, St Louis, 1985, Mosby, pp 166–191.

102. James MA, Bagley AM, Brasington K, et al: Impact of prostheses on function and quality of life for children with unilateral congenital below-the-elbow deficiency, *J Bone Joint Surg Am* 88(11):2356–2365, 2006.

103. Kutz JE, Van Heest AE, House JH: Biceps-to-triceps transfer in tetraplegic patients: report of the medial routing technique and follow-up of three cases, *J Hand Surg* 24:161–172, 1999.

104. Weiss AA: Tendon transfers in tetraplegia: surgical technique. In Betz RR, Mucahey MJ, editors: *The child with a spinal cord injury*, Rosemont, Ill, 1996, American Academy of Orthopaedic Surgeons, pp 405–418.

105. Mulcahey MJ, Betz RR, Smith BT, et al: A prospective evaluation of upper extremity tendon transfers in children with cervical spinal cord injury, *J Pediatr Orthop* 19:319–326, 1999.

106. Manske PR, Rotman MB, Dailey LA: Long-term functional results after pollicization for the congenitally deficient thumb, *J Hand Surg* 17:1064–1072, 1992.

107. Cheng GL, Pan DD, Zhang NP, et al: Digital replantation in children: a long term follow-up study, *J Hand Surg* 23:635–646, 1998.

108. Songcharoen P, Thanapipatsiri S, Mahaisavariya B, et al: Thumb reconstruction with a big toe microvascular wrap-around flap: a report of fifteen cases, *Ann Acad Med Singapore* 24(Suppl 4):46–50, 1995.

109. Datta D, Ibbotson V: Powered prosthetic hands in very young children, *Prosthet Orthot Int* 22:150–154, 1998.

110. Postema K, van der Donk V, van Limbeek J, et al: Prosthesis rejection in children with unilateral congenital arm defect, *Clin Rehabil* 13:243–249, 1999.

111. Duff SV, Mulcahey MJ, Betz RR: Adaptation in sensorimotor control after restoration of grip and pinch in children with spinal cord injury, *Top Spinal Cord Inj Rehabil* 13(4):54–71, 2008.

112. Kilgore KL, Peckham PH, Keith MW, et al: An implanted upper-extremity neuroprosthesis: follow-up of five patients, *J Bone Joint Surg* 79:533–541, 1997.

113. Mulcahey MJ, Betz RR, Smith BT, et al: Implanted functional electrical stimulation hand system in adolescents with spinal cord injuries: an evaluation, *Arch Phys Med Rehabil* 78:597–607, 1997.

114. Lauer RT, Peckham PH, Kilgore KL: EEG-based control of a hand grasp neuroprosthesis, *NeuroReport* 10:1767–1771, 1999.

115. Wheeler CA, Peckham PH: Wireless wearable controller for upper-limb neuroprosthesis, *J Rehabil Res Dev* 46(2):243–256, 2009.

116. Ostendorf CG, Wolf SL: Effect of forced use of the upper extremity of a hemiplegic patient on changes in function, *Phys Ther* 61:1022–1027, 1981.

117. Taub E, Miller NE, Novack TA, et al: Technique to improve chronic motor deficit after stroke, *Arch Phys Med Rehabil* 74:347–354, 1993.

118. Charles J, Lavinder G, Gordon AM: Constraint-induced therapy in children with hemiplegic CP, *Pediatr Phys Ther* 13(2):68–76, 2001.

119. Charles JR, Wolf SL, Schneider JA, et al: Efficacy of a child-friendly form of constraint-induced movement therapy in hemiplegic cerebral palsy: a randomized control trial, *Dev Med Child Neurol* 48(8):635–642, 2006.

120. Crocker MD, MacKay-Lyons M, McDonnell E: Forced use of the upper extremity in cerebral palsy: a single-case design, *Am J Occup Ther* 51:824–833, 1997.

121. Gordon AM, Charles J, Wolf SL: Efficacy of constraint-induced movement therapy on involved upper-extremity use in children with hemiplegic cerebral palsy is not age-dependent, *Pediatrics* 117(3):363–373, 2006.

122. Huang HH, Fetters L, Hale J, et al: Bound for success: a systematic review of constraint-induced movement therapy in children with cerebral palsy supports improved arm and hand use, *Phys Ther* 89(11):1126–1141, 2009.

123. Gordon AM, Schneider JA, Chinnan A, et al: Efficacy of a hand-arm bimanual intensive therapy (HABIT) in children with hemiplegic cerebral palsy: a randomized control trial, *Dev Med Child Neurol* 49(11):830–838, 2007.

124. Charles J, Gordon AM: Development of hand-arm bimanual intensive training (HABIT) for improving bimanual coordination in children with hemiplegic cerebral palsy, *Dev Med Child Neurol* 48(11):931–936, 2006 (review).

125. Duff SV, Gordon AM: Learning of grasp control in children with cerebral palsy, *Dev Med Child Neurol* 45(11):746–757, 2003.

126. Blair SJ, Bear-Lehman J: Editorial comment: prevention of upper extremity occupational disorders, *J Hand Surg* 12:821–822, 1987.

127. Meagher SW: Tool design for prevention of hand and wrist injuries, *J Hand Surg* 12:855–857, 1987.

128. Kozin SH, Weiss AA, Webber JB, et al: Index finger pollicization for congenital aplasia or hypoplasia of the thumb, *J Hand Surg Am* 17:880–884, 1992.

15

Health and Fitness

OBJECTIVES

After studying this chapter, the reader will be able to:

1. Discuss the relationships between health, fitness, and physical activity.
2. Describe the contributions of health, fitness, and physical activity to level of participation and quality of life.
3. Understand the integrated role of all body systems in the development and maintenance of fitness.
4. Identify the effects of exercise and training on the body systems.
5. Identify age-related considerations in developing exercise, training, and fitness programs.

Earlier units in this textbook discussed theories of development, motor control, and motor learning, as well as the roles of various body systems in relation to participation in meaningful functional physical activity. The ability to function at our best in all activities throughout the life span is a goal shared by everyone.

Physical activity is an important component of fitness and health. Health, fitness, and participation in meaningful activities help define each person's quality of life. In this chapter the relationships between physical activity, fitness, and health will be explored. Lifestyle changes, including decreasing amounts of time spent in physical activity and increased time spent in sedentary activity, are apparent across the globe.[1-6] Decreases in physical activity seem to be related to a variety of negative health factors, such as obesity and cardiovascular disease.[1,2,7-11] It is important for health care providers to appreciate the interactions of physical activity and fitness in maintaining optimal levels of physical functioning and health throughout the life span. Health care providers are uniquely qualified to assist clients in reaching the goals of lifelong fitness, enhancing participation in meaningful life activity and overall quality of life.

HEALTH AND FITNESS

Health

Since the 1940s, the World Health Organization has defined *health* as "a state of complete physical, mental, and social well-being, and not merely the absence of disease or infirmity.[12]" In reality, health is a condition of the human body and mind. As a condition, health is represented on a continuum from good health to poor health. Good health reflects the ability to enjoy life and to withstand challenges, with the highest level of functional capability. Poor health reflects morbidity and ultimately mortality. Diseases such as arthritis, heart disease, and diabetes have the potential to diminish functional capacity. These limitations in physical function can also interfere with the ability to actively meet social demands and to participate in leisure-time activities. A person's health is measured at a specific point of time and may fall any place in the continuum from good to poor health. Individuals may strive to live a healthier lifestyle and improve their health, often making lifestyle changes in diet, exercise, and tobacco use. As health is optimized in all three domains (physical, social, and mental), a person is best able to participate in life activities.[7]

The term *wellness,* which comprises biological and psychological well-being, is also used to denote a state of positive health.[13] This term reflects a holistic concept of health. The second edition of the *Guide to Physical Therapist Practice* defines wellness as "concepts that embrace positive health behaviors that promote a state of physical and mental balance and fitness.[14]" A more comprehensive definition of wellness might incorporate promotion of physical, mental, and social health. Wellness is multidimensional and incorporates an understanding of the cognitive components of wellness and a commitment to a lifestyle including wellness behaviors and practices.[15]

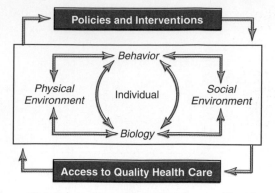

Figure 15-1 Schematic model of determinants of health. (Redrawn from US Department of Health and Human Services: *Healthy People 2010: understanding and improving health,* ed 2, Washington, DC, 2000, US Government Printing Office.)

Each person, along with society, contributes to individual health and wellness (Figure 15-1). Society contributes to the health of a community through policies such as laws mandating the use of seat belts, childhood immunization policies, and clean air regulations. Access to health care is also important, and social policies can assist in making health care available to all individuals. Communities sponsor health promotion efforts aimed at the prevention of smoking or drug abuse, hoping to improve the health of their citizens. Communities can also develop and provide walking or bike paths to encourage physical activity among residents. The social and physical environment in which we live contributes to the choices we make about following healthy lifestyles.[16] Each individual has both genetic and medical profiles that may increase risk for specific diseases such as diabetes or heart disease. Each individual also makes choices about level of physical activity, smoking habits, and diet, which when paired with her health profile defines her level of health and wellness.

Fitness

Some general definitions describe *fitness* as a state of optimal well-being and the capacity to successfully meet the present and potential physical challenges of life. To be fit is to be adapted, adjusted, qualified, or suited to some purpose, function, or aim. The term *fit* is also used to describe a person who is in good physical condition, someone who is healthy. The second edition of the *Guide to Physical Therapist Practice* defines fitness as "a dynamic physical state, comprising cardiovascular/pulmonary endurance; muscle strength, power, endurance, and flexibility; relaxation; and body composition, that allows optimal and efficient performance of daily and leisure activities.[14]" More specifically, *physical fitness* is related to our ability to perform physical activity.[16,17] And as defined by the World Health Organization, it is our ability to perform muscular work satisfactorily. Physical fitness is determined by habitual activity level, diet, and heredity.[13]

Current models of physical fitness describe three components that make up physical fitness: physiological fitness, health-related fitness, and skill-related fitness (Box 15-1). *Physiological fitness* is the fitness of the biological systems and is influenced by physical activity. Blood pressure, glucose tolerance, blood lipid levels, and body composition are markers of physiological fitness.[13] These biological markers are influenced by a person's level of physical activity.[18] *Health-related fitness,* reflected by cardiovascular and respiratory endurance, muscular strength and endurance, flexibility and body composition, reflects

---

Box 15-1

Common Physical Fitness and Fitness-Related Terms

Physical Fitness
Physiological
Metabolic
Morphological
Bone integrity

Health-Related
Body composition
Cardiovascular fitness
Flexibility
Muscular endurance
Muscle strength

Skill-Related
Agility
Balance
Coordination
Power
Speed
Reaction time

Skills
Sports
Team
Individual
Lifetime

Adapted from President's Council on Physical Fitness and Sport Research Digest. http://www.fitness.gov/digest_mar2000.htm.

a person's level of health. *Skill-related fitness* reflects the level of skill and efficiency with which a person can perform movement skills. Components of skill-related fitness include agility, balance, coordination, power, speed, and reaction time.[18] These components are very similar to the dimensions discussed in Chapter 1 that contributed to the quality of physical function. Within this model of physical fitness, it is evident that components of health-related fitness contribute to skill-related fitness characteristics of agility, power, balance, coordination, and speed during physical activity.

COMPONENTS OF HEALTH-RELATED FITNESS

Cardiovascular and *respiratory endurance* reflect the ability of the heart, vasculature, and lungs to provide oxygen to working muscle during physical activity. *Muscular strength* is the force that can be generated in a muscle, whereas *muscular endurance* reflects the ability of the muscle to complete many repetitions of muscle contraction before fatiguing. *Flexibility,* the ability to move without restriction, depends on adequate muscle length and appropriate mobility within the joints of the body. Good flexibility improves efficiency of movement and decreases the potential for injury. *Body composition* refers to the amount of lean body mass (fat-free mass) and fat mass. Lean body mass includes muscle, bone, other nonfat substances (e.g., water, minerals), and a small amount of fat stored in the nervous system, bone marrow, and other body organs.[17] Because in most physical activity we must support and carry the body weight, our active lean body mass should preferably be greater than nonactive fat mass.

FACTORS INFLUENCING HEALTH AND FITNESS

Individual factors such as heredity, age, sex, physical activity, lifestyle, and environment contribute to one's level of physical fitness. A model of the interactions between exercise, health, and fitness was developed by Bouchard and colleagues in 1990 (Figure 15-2).[13] Personal attributes as defined for this diagram are age, sex, socioeconomic status, personality, and motivation.

Physical Factors

Age, growth, and sex can influence fitness. The ability to perform physical activities with physiological efficiency improves through childhood, adolescence, and young adulthood. Performance is often maintained in adulthood but then declines in older adulthood. Some of this decline may be related to physical changes, such as loss of strength and muscle mass in older adults. Social and environmental factors also influence health and fitness. Functional losses in physical fitness may be due to decreased activity level in adulthood and older adulthood, rather than solely a result of aging. Maintaining an active lifestyle appears to moderate physical changes related to aging within the various body systems and to contribute to overall fitness.[19-22]

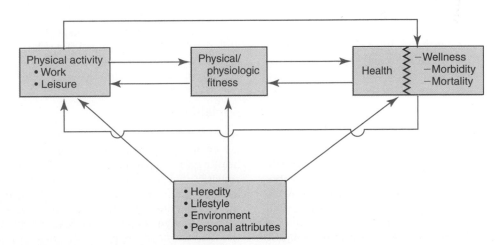

Figure 15-2 Schematic model of the complex relationships between habitual physical activity, fitness, and health. (Redrawn from Bouchard C, Shepard RJ, Stephens T, et al: *Exercise, fitness and health: a consensus of current knowledge*, Champaign, Ill, 1990, Human Kinetics.)

Physiological improvements through training occur at a similar rate and magnitude in all individuals, regardless of age.[17,23,24]

Growth is most often recognized as the changes in height and weight measured through childhood. Loss of height in older adults also reflects a change. Individual organs such as the heart and lungs also change in size over the life span. In childhood, the developmental changes in aerobic capacity, muscular strength and endurance, and power are similar to the growth changes in height and weight.[25] Increase in stature gradually slows and ceases after adolescence, whereas weight increases into the mid-20s.[25] Bone growth continues through the life span, but peak bone mass is attained by the mid-20s. After age 35, body weight continues to slowly increase, reflecting an increase in body fat. In older adulthood both bone and muscle mass decrease, resulting in a decrease in lean body mass.[26] Loss in bone mass begins at about 50 years of age in both men and women, with rate of loss accelerating immediately after menopause for women. Both trabecular and cortical bone are lost, with women losing more bone density than men.[24] Men appear to lose more muscle mass than women, with 0.5% to 1.0% loss in muscle mass per year through young and middle adulthood. In older adulthood, loss of muscle mass is more significant.[24,27]

Before puberty, gender does not appear to greatly affect fitness. Maximal aerobic capacity is slightly higher in boys than in girls through childhood.[28] After puberty, differences in maximal aerobic capacity between males and females become more dramatic. This change reflects the increased percentage of body fat seen in females, increased oxygen-carrying capacity of males compared with females because of increased levels of blood hemoglobin, and larger muscle fiber area in males compared with females.[28] Strength also increases more dramatically in males than females during puberty and young adulthood.[24] In older adulthood, loss of muscle mass and muscle strength has been shown to be greater for men than women.[27]

Heredity

Heredity influences several factors that contribute to fitness, such as body size and muscle fiber composition. Whether we are tall or short is determined by heredity. The percentage of slow-twitch and fast-twitch muscle fibers found in skeletal muscle is determined genetically.[17,29] Genetics is also a factor in determining maximal aerobic capacity, blood pressure, and heart rate.[30] Inherited factors may influence our selection of physical activities, such as choosing to be a sprinter rather than a marathon runner, or impose limits on the possible level of fitness we may achieve.

Environmental Factors

Environmental factors such as climate, oxygen pressure, and air quality can affect exercise performance. Extreme hot or cold climates stress the exercising individual trying to maintain internal body temperature. This is especially true for children and older adults. Children have a high ratio of surface area to body weight, allowing a greater rate of heat exchange with the environment. Children are also less able to sweat, making it more difficult to dissipate heat.[31] People who live and exercise in regions of high altitude must adjust to low oxygen pressures. Indoor air contaminants, such as cigarette smoke, radon, and wood smoke, may diminish air quality. Environmental air quality consists of by-products of industry and engine exhaust. Specific pollutants such as ozone and sulfur dioxide affect lung function.[32]

Physical Activity

Participation in regular physical activity contributes positively to both health and fitness. Physical activity, which is defined as body movement that results in greater than resting levels of energy expenditure, can include leisure-time physical activity, housework, job-related physical tasks, exercise, and sport.[33] Physical activity has been demonstrated to improve muscle strength, cardiorespiratory endurance, bone mineral density, and physical function in older adults.[21,24,26,34–36] Through adulthood, levels of fitness are influenced by exercise habits and body composition.[20] Obesity, which has become a global concern, is often related to low levels of physical activity.[2,9,10,37] Regular physical activity and increased fitness diminish the risk for cardiovascular disease, Type II diabetes mellitus, osteoporosis, cancer, and metabolic syndrome decrease.[10,38,39]

Social Factors

Social factors play a role in determining an individual's involvement in physical activity and fitness, influencing health. Over the past decades, participation in sedentary activities such as television watching and computer use has increased, which seems to be related to increased incidence of obesity and development of health risk factors in children.[2,6,9,37] Children walk or ride their bikes less than they used to, more often being transported to activities by car.[5] As individuals of all ages spend more time in these sedentary activities, the amount of leisure time spent in physical activity is reduced.

Toddlers and preschoolers are very active. Their "job" is to learn new skills and to explore their environment through movement. Parents may influence this level of activity by guiding the child's choice of movement experiences and minimizing more sedentary activities such as television watching. By school age, children become more competitive, and achieving an adequate level of skill in sports and games is important for the child's social acceptance. Children who function well motorically are encouraged to continue with physical activities, whereas children who are less skilled may become frustrated and less active. Successful motor performance is a positive reinforcer for increasing levels of physical activity. Physical activity decreases for both boys and girls in late adolescence. At age 10, almost 80% of youth in the United States report participating in physical activity at least 3 days per week, but by 15 to 17 years of age, less than 65% of youth reported this level of physical activity.[40] This reduction may be influenced by social models, peer pressure, and the need to enter the work force.[25] Adults report that job and family demands frequently do not allow time for exercise programs.[41]

Society influences the awareness of and participation in fitness programs. With increased public awareness of the benefits of fitness, fitness centers and aerobic exercise programs have become more available in the United States. Community agencies sponsor fitness-related activities for individuals of all ages. Corporations also provide fitness programs for their employees, seeking to improve health and productivity. As the communities we live and work in provide social and physical environments that foster increased levels of physical activity, individuals are encouraged to make positive choices regarding physical activity and fitness.

PERCEPTION: HOW FIT ARE WE?

Fitness has been associated with increased health and well-being. Improved quality of life and preventive health maintenance are valuable benefits of fitness. The U.S. Department of Health and Human Services has promoted a public health agenda focusing on health promotion and disease prevention. This agenda has been promoted in the Healthy People 2000, Healthy People 2010, and drafts of Healthy People 2020.[16] Healthy People 2010 included physical activity and fitness objectives,[16] with goals to increase public awareness of appropriate levels of exercise, promote cardiovascular fitness, and increase participation in physical activity programs. Drafts of Healthy People 2020 continue to include objectives that emphasize good nutrition, weight status, physical activity, and fitness. New focus areas, such as the needs of older adults, quality of life, and well-being, are included in the draft. The vision of the Healthy People agendas has been to help members of society live long, healthy lives.

Over the past 20 years, positive changes have been seen in areas such as decreasing the rates of infant mortality; improving cancer screening methods and cancer survival rates; and decreasing the number of deaths related to cardiac disease, stroke, and diabetes.[42] On a less positive note, low levels of physical activity and increasing rates of overweight/obesity are global health concerns (Box 15-2). Several organizations in the United States and other countries have published recommendations for daily physical activity and reduction of sedentary activity, such as television and computer time.[10,16,43-45] Even with these guidelines, minimal change has been seen in level of physical activity.[3]

Box 15-2

Obesity—A Global Health Concern

Obesity has increased over the past 2 to 3 decades in many countries around the globe. The World Health Report[83] indicates that more than 1 billion adults are overweight globally and 300 million are obese. In the United States, the prevalence of obesity has more than doubled in the last 30 years.[84] Figure 15-3 shows the increase from 2000-2009 in the percent of the population in the United States who present with obesity. No states have attained the reduction in the prevalence of obesity of 15%, which was a goal of Healthy People 2010. In 2009[84] the adult obesity prevalence was less than 20% in only Colorado and the District of Columbia. In 9 states the prevalence of adult obesity was less than 30%. Thirty-two percent of U.S. youth between 12 to 19 years of age had a body mass index (BMI) greater than the 85th percentile for their age. Fifteen percent were overweight (BMI >85th percentile) and 12% obese (BMI >95th percentile).[84]

Overweight and obesity are defined in terms of body mass index (BMI), which is calculated from a person's weight and height data using the formula (weight [kg]/height [m²]).

(Continued)

Box 15-2

Obesity—A Global Health Concern—Cont'd

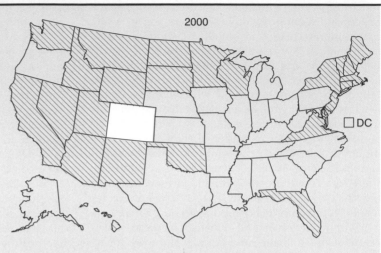

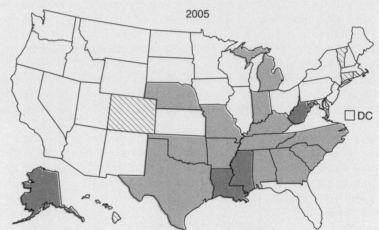

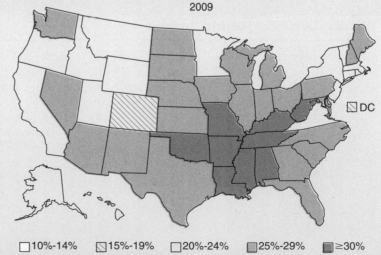

Figure 15-3 Self-reported prevalence of obesity* among adults—Behavioral Risk Factor Surveillance System, United States, 2000, 2005, and 2009. This figure compares the prevalence of state-specific obesity in 2009 with 2005 and 2000. A total of 33 states had obesity prevalences greater than 25% in 2009, and 9 of those states had prevalences of 30%. In contrast, 28 states had prevalences less than 20% in 2000, and no state had a prevalence of 30%.*Body mass index (BMI) =30.0; BMI was calculated from self-reported weight and height (weight [kg]/height [m]²). (From CDC: Vital signs: state-specific obesity prevalence among adults—United States, 2009, *MMWR Morb Mortal Wkly Rep* 59:1-5, 2010.)

☐10%-14%   ⊠15%-19%   ☐20%-24%   ▨25%-29%   ■≥30%

Box 15-2

Obesity—A Global Health Concern—Cont'd

With pediatric and adolescent populations, BMI percentiles, based on growth charts specific to age group and sex, are used to indicate weight status.

85th to 94th percentile = overweight
Greater than or equal to 95th percentile = obesity
In adult populations (20 years of age and older):
Overweight = BMI of 25 to 29.9
Obesity = BMI equal or greater than 30
Extreme obesity BMI equal or greater than 40

Obesity is considered a health problem because it appears to be related to:

- Increased health care costs
- Decreased quality of life
- Increased risk for premature death
- Increased risk for development of:
  - Metabolic syndrome
  - Cardiovascular disease
  - Type II diabetes
  - Stroke
  - Hypertension
  - Some cancers

Obesity has been linked to:

- Race
  - Both black and Hispanic adults have a higher prevalence for being overweight and obese than adults in other racial groups. Reports vary as to which of these two groups has the highest prevalence for being overweight.[84]

- Hispanic children are more likely to become overweight and obese than other racial groups[11,43]
- Gender
- African American and Hispanic women have the highest prevalence of obesity[84]
- Educational level—prevalence of obesity inversely related to educational level of adult or parent

Interventions/Prevention to Decrease Prevalence of Obesity in Children and Adults

- Health care professionals should:
- Include measurement of body mass index into the patient/client examination
- Educate patients/clients as to risks associated with being overweight and obese as well as prevention strategies
- Provide ongoing support/coaching

Adults

- Make dietary changes
- Seek diet and nutritional counseling to assist in weight management
- Increase level of physical activity

Children

- Make health dietary choices
- Increase level of physical activity
- Decrease screen time with computers and television

Significant numbers of individuals, of all ages, fail to meet the recommended levels of physical activity. A progressive and predictable decline in regular physical activity participation with age has been reported (Figure 15-4).[17,41,46–48] Although levels of physical activity are high in children, activity rates decline from childhood to adolescence and then decline further through adulthood. A longitudinal study of children from 9 years of age to 15 years of age showed that almost all children participated in physical activity for the recommended 60 minutes per day, but by 15 years of age, only 32% of children met the requirement on weekdays and 18% on weekends. In this study, the amount of time spent in moderately vigorous physical activity decreased by 35 to 40 minutes per year over the 6 years of the study.[49] Another cross-sectional study in the United States of 4- to 12-year-olds showed that 37% of children had low levels of activity play, 65% had high levels of sedentary activity ("screen time"), and

26% had both low levels of active play and high screen time. The children in this last category tended to be older, female, and had higher body mass index (BMI > 95% for age matched growth curves).[2] Less than 50% of adults in the United States reported participating in the recommended 30 minutes of moderately vigorous physical activity at least 5 days a week, and of adults over the age of 65 years, less than 40% reported meeting the activity recommendations.[3] Participation in regular physical activity is influenced by other factors, and levels of participation decrease as education and income levels decrease.[3,43,47]

As obesity and low levels of physical activity increase health risks for individuals around the world, efforts by government agencies, public entities, and private groups are attempting to improve access and adherence to healthy lifestyle activities. Public education programs have incorporated fitness programs into physical education and are increasing the time spent in

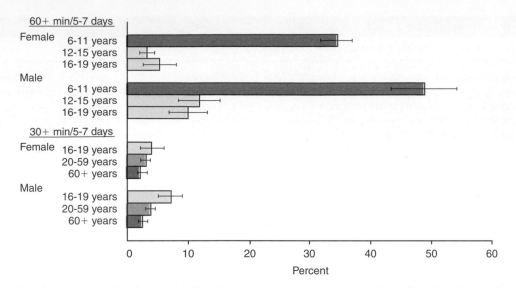

Figure 15-4 Regular physical activity throughout life is important for maintaining a healthy body, enhancing psychological well-being, and preventing premature death. This graph shows the percentage of children, adolescents, and adults who achieved recommended levels of physical activity (as measured by accelerometer) in the United States in 2003-2004. Data from National Health and Nutrition Examination Survey (NHANS, NCHS, CDC). (From Troiano RP, et al: Physical activity in the United States measured by accelerometer, *Med Sci Sports Exerc* 40(1):181-188, 2008.)

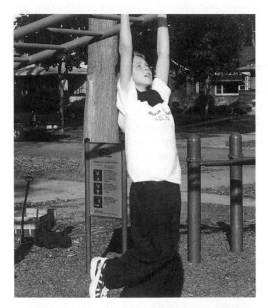

Figure 15-5 Schools and communities work together to provide fitness equipment and programs for children. This fitness court was designed to be used with six individualized activity stations at an elementary school. A local community hospital donated the funds to build the court, which is enhanced by signs that describe the preferred regimens to be used for each activity.

promoting lifetime physical activities.[40] Some schools, with local grants and support, are providing fitness equipment in their playgrounds (Figure 15-5). To meet the needs of adults, increasing numbers of employers are providing workplace fitness programs. These programs benefit both the employee and the employer because there are fewer employee absences and less sick time. Community agencies also strive to provide physical activity programs for older adults. Older adults living in senior communities also take advantage of multiple opportunities for activities such as tennis, swimming, and offerings at fitness club facilities (Figure 15-6). Communities are also developing walking and bike paths and creating local playgrounds.

Individuals in any age group participate in leisure-time physical activity to varying degrees, with the most active tending to be the most fit. Significant efforts are being made to increase the public's awareness of the importance of physical activity and fitness. Public awareness of the importance of fitness may be increasing, but even though many individuals start exercise programs, often they will stop within a short period of time. Among the barriers to adhering to physical activity programs are time constraints and financial concerns. Making a behavioral change is challenging and complex. Providing information about the importance of physical activity for health promotion may help people be

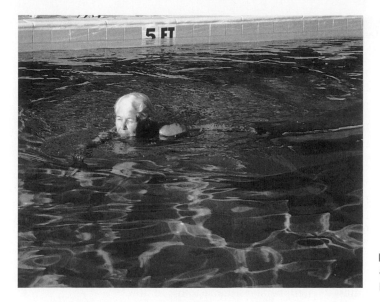

Figure 15-6 Older adults can stay active by taking advantage of community facilities such as swimming pools.

aware of a need for change but not the support to make the health behavior changes. Health care providers can play an important role in supporting individuals as they strive to make changes. Health care providers can provide individualized education and evaluate an individual's motivation to make a change. As an individual feels confident and capable of making the change, the health care provide can provide coaching and follow-up to help sustain the individual's efforts.[50]

BODY SYSTEMS INVOLVED IN FITNESS

Physical fitness is achieved when several body systems—the cardiovascular, pulmonary, musculoskeletal, nervous, and endocrine systems—interact optimally and efficiently. In the course of development, changes in the body systems affect the way in which the body delivers fuel and produces energy for movement. Capacity for physical activity may vary throughout development as a result. In children it is difficult to separate development of the body systems from development of physical fitness. Growth and maturation of the cardiovascular, pulmonary, musculoskeletal, and nervous systems contribute to the child's and adolescent's ability to move efficiently and effectively. Similarly, physical activity supports development of these systems.

Exercise and training have been found to improve body system function and levels of fitness. *Exercise* is defined as leisure-time physical activity[13] that is planned, repetitive, and purposeful.[17] Exercise includes participation in physical activity for the purpose of improving

fitness and health.[39] *Training* is regular and repeated exercise, carried out over several weeks or months, with the intention of developing physical or physiological fitness.[13] *Trainability* reflects the ability of different body systems to adapt to repeated exercise stimuli.[51]

Exercise and training affect an adult's body systems in different ways, and the endocrine system plays a special role in exercise and training. The effects of exercise and training on the body system's and endocrine system's contributions to exercise and training discussed later focus on the response in adults. When available, information specific to children and adolescents is also provided. For additional information, the reader is referred to the specific system chapters in Unit II.

Effects of Exercise and Training on the Cardiovascular System

During exercise, the cardiovascular system must carry large amounts of oxygen to the muscle tissue and remove waste products associated with energy production.

Cardiovascular responses to exercise and training are summarized in Table 15-1.

Short-Term Adaptation

During aerobic exercise, skeletal muscle demand for oxygen increases, resulting in increased cardiac output. Heart rate increases in proportion to the intensity of the exercise for 3 to 5 minutes. A steady state is then attained and maintained for short periods of exercise. After 15 to 30 minutes, heart rate again begins to rise because of fatigue and increased body temperature.

Table 15-1

Cardiovascular Adaptation to Exercise and Training

Exercise	Training
Increased cardiac output	Increased heart weight
Increased heart rate	Increased heart volume
Increased blood flow to working muscles	Increased plasma volume
Increased systolic blood pressure	Increased hemoglobin
Increased cardiac contractility	Decreased resting heart rate
Decreased peripheral resistance	Increased maximum cardiac output and stroke volume
Increased venous return	Increased arterial-to-venous oxygen difference
	Decreased systolic and diastolic blood pressure
	Improve lipid profile (increase HDL, decrease LDL)

Vasodilation occurs, helping shunt blood flow away from the viscera to the working skeletal and heart muscles. Muscle contraction squeezes nearby veins, facilitating venous return. Systolic blood pressure increases in proportion to exercise intensity and theoretically is related to the increased cardiac output. Diastolic blood pressure increases only slightly. In general, dynamic, aerobic exercise results in increased cardiac contractility, decreased peripheral resistance, and increased venous return.[17,52]

Long-Term Adaptation

Heart weight and volume, plasma volume, and hemoglobin levels increase with training.[17,53] Ventricular filling, stroke volume, and cardiac output also increase.[54] Therefore, more blood can be pumped per heartbeat, and necessary circulation is delivered to body tissues at a lower heart rate. Increased blood volume improves removal of waste products and heat, dilution of hormones, and perfusion of the kidneys while decreasing resistance to capillary flow. In prepubescent children, stroke volume increases, and an increase in cardiac size occurs in response to endurance training.[55]

Resting heart rate decreases, an effect that appears to be related to decreased sympathetic input. Maximum heart rate remains relatively stable, whereas maximum cardiac output and stroke volume increase. Maximum heart rate also remains stable for children after endurance training.[55] Stroke volume increases because of greater end-diastolic volume of the left ventricle and more forceful contraction of strengthened cardiac muscle.[17,52]

Both systolic and diastolic blood pressures decrease with training.[17] In older adults, decreases in resting systolic blood pressure are seen, but no change is seen in diastolic BP.[56] Decreases in blood pressure may be related

to autonomic nervous system control, which decreases peripheral resistance to blood flow.[52]

Exercise also appears to have a positive impact on the lipid levels circulating in the blood and the ability of the muscle to extract oxygen from the blood. With exercise, the levels of high-density lipoproteins (HDL) are increased and the levels of low-density lipoproteins (LDL) are decreased.[57] When our body is physiologically trained, we are better able to extract oxygen from the blood, as reflected by a widening of the arterial-to-venous oxygen difference (A-Vo$_2$ difference).[17] Increased capillary and mitochondrial capacities are seen in working muscle, improving the ability of the muscle to extract oxygen from the capillaries.[17] In children, no change in A-Vo$_2$ difference is seen.[55] In the older adult, even with exercise training, the ability to extract oxygen at the muscle cell level is diminished because of changes in both the muscle tissue and circulation; therefore, dramatic changes are not seen in oxygen extraction.

Effects of Exercise and Training on the Pulmonary System

During exercise, greater airflow is required to meet the oxygen demands of the body. Airflow is increased by taking deeper breaths and increasing the respiratory rate.

Adaptations of the pulmonary system to exercise and training are summarized in Table 15-2.

Short-Term Adaptation

At the onset of exercise, ventilation increases rapidly and reaches a steady state.[17] The amount of air exchanged with the atmosphere per minute (*minute ventilation*) is increased as more air is moved in each breath (*tidal volume*) and as breathing frequency increases. At

Table 15-2

Pulmonary Adaptation to Exercise and Training

Exercise	Training
Increased minute ventilation	Increased vital capacity
Increased tidal volume	Increased tidal volume
Increased breathing frequency	Decreased respiratory rate at submaximal exercise
Decreased inspiratory/expiratory reserve	

low-intensity exercise, changes in tidal volume are sufficient to maintain adequate minute ventilation. Greater tidal volume allows inspired air to perfuse more lung tissue, opening more alveoli and maximizing the ability for gas exchange between the capillaries and the alveoli. As exercise intensity becomes greater and tidal volume is 50% to 60% of vital capacity, breathing rate increases.[19]

The breathing rate at rest is approximately 14 breaths per minute. During exercise, the respiratory rate may rise up to 40 breaths per minute. Even at these higher rates, there is enough time for alveolar gas exchange to occur because alveolar ventilation increases more than does pulmonary capillary blood flow. This process works until fatigue or cardiac function limits the exercise.

During light to moderate exercise, ventilation increases linearly with levels of oxygen consumption and carbon dioxide production. At higher exercise levels, ventilation increases in relation to increased carbon dioxide concentrations produced by anaerobic metabolism. For example, blood lactate levels increase during anaerobic metabolism and must be buffered to prevent acidosis. The end product of this buffering is carbon dioxide. As the carbon dioxide levels in the blood increase, chemoreceptors in the aortic and carotid bodies, as well as in the medulla, cue the system to increase ventilation.[17]

Long-Term Adaptation

After training, resting lung volumes show little change. Strength and endurance of respiratory muscles are improved.[58] During submaximal exercise, the respiratory rate decreases and the tidal volume increases. Air stays in the lungs longer, allowing more oxygen to be extracted.[17] The amount of air that must be breathed in to deliver adequate oxygen to the tissues is decreased, requiring less work by the respiratory system. Conclusive studies of the effects of training on the ventilatory system of children have not been done.[59]

Effects of Exercise and Training on the Musculoskeletal System

The muscular and skeletal systems form the mechanical basis for human movement. Muscle cells also contain energy stores necessary for movement. Within skeletal muscle, three types of muscle fibers (type I, type IIa, and type IIb) are found, and they are used differently to produce energy. Oxygen provided during respiration activates metabolic pathways that convert carbohydrates, fats, and proteins into stored energy sources in muscle. Type I and type IIa muscle fibers effectively work in these aerobic metabolic pathways. Type IIb muscle fibers assist in the production of energy via anaerobic pathways.

Adaptations of the musculoskeletal system to exercise and training are summarized in Table 15-3. Depending on the type of activity, type I, type IIa, and type IIb muscle fibers are affected differently.

Short-Term Adaptation

At the onset of exercise, blood flow to exercising muscle increases. Increased blood flow delivers more oxygen to the muscle and helps to dissipate heat, which results from muscular work. With exercise at less than 60% to 70% of maximum aerobic power, first type I and then type IIa muscle fibers are recruited.

Long-Term Adaptation

Training affects all components of the musculoskeletal system. Both weight-bearing and the mechanical forces exerted by the muscles during activity contribute to musculoskeletal changes. Exercise increases the bone density[57,60-63] and strengthens the bone architecture. Ligaments become stronger, thicker, and more flexible. Articular cartilage also becomes thicker and more resistant to compression. Muscle tissue undergoes significant change, which varies with the type of exercise performed.

Resistance training increases muscle strength via hypertrophy of muscle fibers or neural recruitment of

Table 15-3

Musculoskeletal Adaptation to Exercise and Training

Exercise	Training
Increased blood flow to working muscle	Increased bone mineral density
	Increased strength, flexibility, and thickness of ligaments
	Increased thickness of articular cartilage
	Increased muscle strength
	Increased fat-free body mass
	Improved lipid profile (increase HDL, decrease LDL)
	Increased glucose tolerance
	Increased oxidative capacity
	Increased number of type I fibers
	Increased oxidative enzymes
	Increased mitochondria
	Onset of blood lactate accumulation at higher percent of maximum oxygen uptake

motor units. Children increase strength primarily via increased neural recruitment.[57,62,64] Neural recruitment also plays a major role in strength gains of older adults. In older adults, increases in strength also have been related to reversal of fast-twitch fiber atrophy.[65] Muscle hypertrophy occurs after puberty, when increased levels of hormones such as testosterone, growth hormone, and other growth factors are present.[62] Muscle hypertrophy is seen in adults when high levels of resistance are used. Anaerobic metabolic pathways are used primarily in this type of exercise, resulting in increased anaerobic enzyme levels in type II muscle fibers.

With endurance training, oxidative capacity of the muscle is maximized, increasing the number of type I muscle fibers.[66] Levels of enzymes used by oxidative metabolic pathways increase, especially in oxidative type I and type IIa muscle fibers. The size and number of mitochondria increase with training,[17,65] as does capillarization.[17,53] These changes all contribute to the efficient use of oxygen by muscle tissue, fueling the oxidative metabolic pathway. Aerobic exercise also improves the ability of the skeletal muscle to use glucose, improving glucose tolerance.[67]

High-intensity training increases the number of type II fibers active in anaerobic metabolism.[66] Anaerobic threshold increases during submaximal exercise as a result of increased mechanical efficiency and muscle strengthening. Blood lactate accumulation begins at 50% to 55% of maximal oxygen uptake in the untrained individual and at approximately 80% to 90% of maximal oxygen uptake in the trained individual.[17] Prepubertal children are less able to use anaerobic metabolism

because of lower muscle glycogen levels. Limited muscle mass in children also limits anaerobic metabolism.[17]

Metabolic, Endocrine, and Hormonal Contributions to Fitness and Training

The endocrine system (see Chapter 11) allows the body to adapt to vigorous physical activity and ensures that fuel is delivered to working muscles. Fuel can be supplied aerobically or anaerobically, through metabolism of carbohydrates or fats. Several endocrine organs are activated during exercise. The hormones they secrete play a role in the use of carbohydrates and fatty acids, maintenance of fluid volume, contractility of the heart, and distribution of blood within the vascular system (Table 15-4). Responses of children differ from adults in that children metabolize fats during exercise, rather than carbohydrates.[68] Certain hormones make specific contributions to fitness and wellness.

Growth hormone, secreted by the anterior pituitary gland, decreases the use of carbohydrates and increases the use of fat metabolism for energy production. By maintaining glucose levels, growth hormone increases endurance. Growth hormone also promotes protein synthesis, cartilage formation, and skeletal growth. Intensity and duration of exercise affect the secretion of growth hormone. The mechanism for control of growth hormone secretion during exercise is not known, but it is probably related to neural mechanisms. There does not appear to be a training effect that raises the levels of growth hormone in adults.[17] In prepubescent children, no change in growth hormone levels is noted during bouts of exercise.[68]

Table **15-4**		

Hormonal Activity Related to Physical Activity

Hormone	Secreted by	During Exercise
Growth hormone	Anterior pituitary gland	Decreased carbohydrate use Increased fat use
Corticotropin	Anterior pituitary gland	Increased fat use Increased protein use; stimulates secretion of cortisol
Antidiuretic hormone	Posterior pituitary gland	Increased water retention

Norepinephrine/
epinephrine
	Adrenal medulla	Affects cardiac contractibility and distribution of blood in vascular system
		    Fat—fatty acid
		    Glycogen—glucose

Cortisol	Adrenal cortex	Protein—glucose Fatty acid—glucose
Insulin	Pancreas	Decreased secretion during exercise; inhibits epinephrine and glucagon
Glucagon	Pancreas	Increased secretion during exercise; forms glucose from liver, glycogen, and amino acids; breaks down fat

Corticotropin (ACTH), also secreted by the anterior pituitary gland, improves the mobilization of fat as an energy source, increases the rate of glucose formation, and stimulates the breakdown of proteins. ACTH also controls the secretion of hormones from the adrenal cortex, including cortisol, which is important during intense exercise. After training, ACTH levels are slightly elevated during exercise.[17]

Antidiuretic hormone secretion is controlled by the posterior pituitary gland. During exercise, this gland increases water retention by the kidneys, maintaining fluid volume.[17]

Norepinephrine and epinephrine secretion, by the adrenal medulla, is stimulated by exercise and increases as the intensity of the exercise increases. A greater response to exercise is seen in older rather than younger individuals and in men rather than in women. Also known as catecholamines, these hormones are related to activity of the sympathetic branch of the autonomic nervous system. They increase cardiac contractility, heart rate, distribution of blood within the vascular system, and so forth. They are also active in the breakdown of stored fat into free fatty acids and of glycogen into glucose.[17]

Cortisol is secreted by the adrenal cortex. It promotes the formation of glucose from proteins and fatty acids during intense exercise. ACTH stimulates the release of cortisol. After training, levels of cortisol are slightly increased with exercise.

Insulin is secreted by the pancreas when blood glucose levels are too high. It inhibits the effects of epinephrine and glucagon on fat metabolism and facilitates glucose uptake by the muscle cells. Insulin secretion is usually decreased during prolonged exercise.[17,69] Insulin levels appear to increase during exercise in prepubertal children and remain stable in exercising pubescent children.[68] After training, levels of insulin are maintained at closer to resting levels during exercise.[17]

Glucagon also is secreted by the pancreas when blood glucose falls below a threshold. It stimulates the formation of glucose from liver glycogen stores and amino acids. It can also stimulate the breakdown of fat stores. Glucagon acts in opposition to insulin, functioning to raise blood glucose levels.[17] Similar to insulin, after training, glucagon levels remain closer to resting level during exercise.

Maximal Aerobic Capacity and Maximal Oxygen Uptake

All of the systems discussed here work together to allow our bodies to efficiently use their energy stores and to produce the mechanical work necessary for physical activity. A measure of how efficiently the body can perform this task is the maximal aerobic capacity, or maximal oxygen uptake (VO_{2max}), which reflects the maximal rate at which oxygen can be used by the tissues during exercise. Both how well the cardiovascular and pulmonary systems deliver oxygen to the tissues and the ability of the tissues to use the oxygen contribute to VO_{2max}. Maximal aerobic capacity measures the maximum level of work an individual can perform. It is a major determinant of overall functional ability and a good measure of aerobic fitness. Aerobic fitness has also been related to levels of health risk.

Maximal aerobic capacity appears to be closely related to our level of activity and body composition. This measure improves as our level of fitness improves and decreases with inactivity. Aerobic capacity decreases as the percent of body fat increases and is improved in individuals with lower percentages of body fat. Indeed, our habitual level of physical activity is thought to be more of a determinant of aerobic capacity than chronological age.

Age does affect maximal aerobic capacity. Maximal aerobic capacity appears to be lower in children than in adults, but it increases through childhood as size increases. Cardiac size and pulmonary capacity increase through childhood and limit the child's aerobic capacity. The child's higher heart rate does not appear to totally compensate for decreased stroke volume, because the cardiac output of children is smaller than that of adults.[70] Other differences are seen in the cardiovascular system of children compared with adults. Blood volume and hemoglobin levels increase through childhood and are correlated with the peak VO_2 that can be attained.[28] Because children have less hemoglobin than adults, they have less oxygen-carrying capacity than adults. Their ability to extract oxygen from the blood at the tissue level (A-VO_2 difference) has been reported to increase slightly with age, especially after puberty, and reaches adult levels by late adolescence. This change may be related to the growing child's increased muscle mass, changes in muscle enzyme perfusion, and changes in the ratio of capillary to muscle fiber.[28,71]

Training effects, specifically improvements in maximal aerobic power, in prepubescent children have been demonstrated, but the improvements in children are less than those seen in adults.[72–74] Increases in maximal aerobic power appear to be related to improvements in the child's stroke volume during maximal exercise.[55] High levels of habitual activity, mechanical inefficiency in performing physical activity, and body size limitations affect the maximal aerobic capacity of children.[75]

Through childhood and adolescence, a child's level of physical activity is slightly to moderately related to her aerobic fitness.[76]

Through childhood, peak VO_2 of boys is slightly greater than that of girls, with the difference increasing even more after puberty. Studies of children and adolescents between 12 and 19 years of age in the United States have shown that VO_{2max} increases with age in males, while VO_{2max} of females decreases with age.[77] The increased muscle mass of boys compared with girls contributes to this difference.[28] Peak VO_2 increases by 150% in boys and 80% in girls between the ages of 8 and 16 years. This increase also seems to be related to increased left ventricular size and stroke volume.[28] Higher levels of physical activity, less than 3 hours per day of sedentary leisure activity, and normal weight were also related to higher levels of VO_{2max} in 12- to 19-year-olds in the United States.[77]

Once adult levels of cardiovascular performance have been reached, some sex-related differences surface. The stroke volume of women is approximately 25% less than that of men. Men have 15 to 16 g Hb/100 mL blood, whereas women have 14 g Hb/100 mL blood; this gives men a greater oxygen-carrying capacity. Teenage and adult women have a 5% to 10% higher cardiac output during submaximal exercise than do men, possibly to compensate for their decreased oxygen-carrying capacity.[17]

Longitudinal and cross-sectional studies of adults and older adults have demonstrated that aerobic capacity decreases through adulthood.[20,21,48,78,79] The decrease is most likely related to both age-related changes in the cardiovascular and musculoskeletal systems and to the level of physical activity. Cardiorespiratory fitness decline accelerates after 45 years of age.[34]

When considering the previously discussed cardiovascular, pulmonary, and musculoskeletal system changes with age, it is understandable that the ability to transport and absorb oxygen at the tissue level would change with age. More specifically, the maximum heart rate does decrease with age regardless of training.[78] Muscle mass also decreases with age, affecting the amount of oxygen that can be used. Not all of the changes in aerobic capacity of adults can be attributed to changes in the body systems. Lifestyle factors such as an increase in percent body fat and decreased levels of physical activity are major contributors to the diminishing aerobic capacity in adults.[80] Longitudinal studies have indicated that the age-associated decrease in peak VO_2 decreases 3% to 6% per decade from ages 20 to 40 and accelerates greater than 20% per decade decline after the age of 70.[79]

DEVELOPMENTAL CONSIDERATIONS IN OTHER COMPONENTS OF PHYSIOLOGICAL FITNESS

Pulmonary System

The pulmonary system development also affects aerobic power in children. The growth of the lungs parallels the general growth of the child. Children's airways are small in diameter, resulting in higher resistance to airflow and increased work of breathing. Because children demonstrate poorer ventilatory efficiency than adults in both submaximal and maximal exercise, they must maintain a higher breathing frequency when performing similar tasks.

For the older adult, structural pulmonary system changes such as a stiffer bony thorax increase the work of breathing. Decreased compliance of the lungs and airways increases resistance to airflow. As a result of structural and functional changes, the older adult's residual lung capacity is increased with age. Vital capacity, inspiratory reserve, and expiratory reserve volumes are decreased in both resting and dynamic states. Although changes in pulmonary function are seen with aging, older adults who remain physically active demonstrate less change than sedentary older adults.[17]

Flexibility and Body Composition

Childhood and Adolescence

Especially after periods of skeletal growth, flexibility is an issue for children. Because bone growth precedes muscle growth, children should be reminded to stretch before exercising. Throughout childhood, girls are more flexible than boys.

Through infancy, the amount of fat mass increases, but then it decreases once children start increasing muscle mass. Girls' fat mass is slightly higher than that of boys in early childhood, and the difference increases with puberty. Exercise and diet are important to control increased fat mass, and with strength training, increased bone density and muscle mass contribute to increase fat-free body mass.

Flexibility and body composition change through adulthood. Body fat increases 2% to 2.5% per decade even in individuals who participate regularly in moderate- to high-intensity exercise.[78] Both longitudinal and cross-sectional studies have also found fat weight to increase per decade, even when fat-free body mass remains stable.[20] Activities to increase muscle strength and mass, and to sustain or improve bone density, assist in the maintenance of fat-free body mass.

Exercise and Training Considerations Across the Life Span

As body systems mature and develop across the life span and an individual's work and leisure habits are formed, regular participation in physical activity is important. Because of differences in the aerobic capacity and the ability of muscle tissue to respond to exercise, exercise programs must be designed for each individual based on his or her lifestyle and age. General recommendations regarding appropriate exercise for individuals of different ages are listed in Clinical Implications Box 15-1: Components of Beneficial Exercise Prescriptions.

CLINICAL IMPLICATIONS Box 15-1

Components of Beneficial Exercise Prescriptions

In general, we all benefit from maintaining a physically active lifestyle with regular exercise. Regardless of age, physical activity assists in increasing fat-free body mass and in improving cardiovascular and pulmonary endurance. Not only does this reduce the incidence of obesity, but it also decreases the risk for heart disease and osteoporosis. Exercise can increase functional capacity and minimize the decrease often experienced in older individuals; the capacity to participate in physical activity is influenced by the development of the body systems and their level of fitness.

Exercise recommendations to maximize health, fitness, and function and participation in children, adults, and older adults have been developed by several organizations and are summarized here. Expanded discussion of the recommendations for children can be found in guidelines developed by the National Strength and Conditioning Association[62], the Canadian Society for Exercise Physiology[63], and the U.S. Department of Health and Human Services (DHHS).[43] Recommendations for adults and older adults have been made by the American College of Sports Medicine/American Heart Association[44,45] and DHHS.[43]

(Continued)

CLINICAL IMPLICATIONS Box 15-1

Components of Beneficial Exercise Prescriptions—Cont'd

Children
- Encourage young children to participate in physically active play
- Structure 30 minutes of moderate intensity physical activity for children older than 6 years, preferably 7 days per week
- Include the following in moderate physical activity:
  1. Activities that use all muscle groups
  2. Activities that will go through the full range of motion
  3. Multijoint exercises
- Structure weight training with the following provisions:
  1. Include a dynamic warm-up (whole body movement activities such as skipping, jumping)
  2. Two to three weekly sessions, on nonconsecutive days
  3. Provide appropriate training and supervision to ensure use of proper technique
  4. Include a cool-down activity, which includes stretching
  5. Initially use low to moderate resistance and slowly increase as tolerated
  6. Include 8 to 12 exercises addressing upper extremity, lower extremity, and trunk strengthening
  7. Complete 1 to 2 sets of 8 to 15 repetitions
  8. Incorporate balance activities to develop better force generation, power, and coordination

Adults
- Encourage everyday physical activity, with moderate to vigorous aerobic activity most days of the week and strength training on 2 to 3 days of the week; also include flexibility and balance activity
- Include warm-up and cool-down components for both aerobic and strength training sessions
- Include endurance activities with 20 to 60 minutes of physical activity that will raise the heart rate to 70% to 85% of the maximum heart rate, 3 to 5 days per week

- Include strength training 2 to 3 times per week on nonconsecutive days
- Include flexibility and balance activities
- Structure endurance exercise to include large muscle groups (e.g., walking, running, swimming, dancing)

Older Adults
Older adults should be encouraged to participate in everyday physical activity and incorporate the following elements into their fitness program as recommended by the American College of Sports Medicine and the American Heart Association:[44]
- Moderate intensity aerobic activity 5 days per week or vigorous intensity aerobic activity for 20 minutes 3 days per week
- Strength training at least 2 days of the week
- Flexibility exercise at least 2 days per week
- Balance activity

Additional considerations for older adults are:
- Benefits of exercise are also seen with three, short, 10-minute exercise sessions per day
- Structure training to increase VO_{2max} with intensity at 50% to 85% of VO_{2max}
- Know that improvement in submaximal exercise response is seen at an exercise intensity of less than 50% VO_{2max}
- Know that activities such as walking, aquatics, and cycle ergometry minimize musculoskeletal stress
- Prevent injury in a progressive exercise program by increasing the duration of the exercise session, not the intensity of exercise

Build in precautions to include the following:
1. *Use of conservative exercise prescriptions and progression for older adults due to their varied health and fitness levels*
2. *Use of a percentage of measured peak heart rate because it is more accurate than an age-predicted maximum heart rate*
3. *Consideration of the prescription medications a client is taking because medication may influence exercise response*

---

*There are many ways to calculate maximum heart rate. An exercise physiology textbook will provide additional information about several possible methods. If an age-predicted maximum heart rate is used to recommend an exercise prescription, recognize that there is an inherent error in such a measurement. Compiled from references 43, 44, 45, 62, 63.

Childhood

It is difficult to define optimal intensity, duration, and frequency of endurance training for children. Regular physical activity should be encouraged to promote optimal physiological fitness and to establish health behavior patterns for the child to carry into adulthood. Children are learning and perfecting motor skills that promote agility, balance, coordination, speed, and power. Fitness evaluations and programs for children should include a motor skills component.[25] Endurance activities that require anaerobic metabolism should be thoroughly evaluated for appropriateness. Children may have difficulty participating in strenuous activity that lasts more than 15 to 30 seconds because of immaturity of the glycolytic metabolism and decreased sympathetic nervous system activation.[68] Participation in events such as middle or long-distance running should be monitored very closely with prepubescent children.

Older Adulthood

Older adults are generally happy with their level of fitness but underestimate their ability to exercise.[41] As maximal exercise capacity decreases with age, it begins to affect the intensity of exercise that can be considered submaximal work. For example, activities of daily living are considered submaximal work. The energy required to perform these activities remains constant, but the percentage of maximal capacity they require increases as the maximal exercise capacity decreases. In older adults, activities such as walking or housework may be considered high-intensity exercise; in younger adults, these same activities offer a low-intensity exercise. For the older adult, these activities may become more stressful. If the individual can no longer complete activities of daily living because of the level of physiological stress, functional independence is decreased. Therefore, it is very important for older adults to maintain aerobic capacity and to maximize their functional independence. Studies have shown that regular exercise, even in older adults, can increase maximal aerobic capacity and submaximal work capacity (Figure 15-7).[21,23,36,81]

Exercise programming for the older adult should emphasize the functional needs of the individual. A person's level of fitness and interests must be kept in mind. Aerobic exercise, resistance training flexibility, and balance exercises should be included in the older adult physical activity program to improve cardiovascular endurance, improve or maintain muscle strength, control weight and loss of bone mineral, and improve flexibility. It has been found that even older adults who exercise at less than 50% aerobic capacity show an improvement in submaximal exercise response.[82] To increase VO_{2max}, exercise intensity should be at 50% to 85% of VO_{2max}.

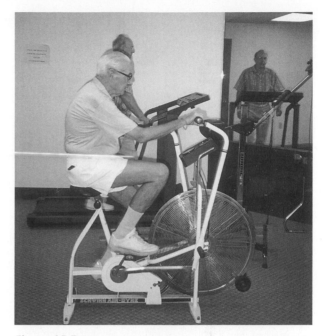

Figure 15-7 Maintaining an active exercise program through older adulthood improves physical function.

SUMMARY

We continue to emphasize a premise that is discussed throughout this book: exercise and training programs can improve our health, fitness, quality of life, and level of participation. Quality of life is improved when we feel better, do more, and develop a positive self-image. Exercise helps us attain and maintain body efficiency, allowing us to function optimally within the environment. This is why health promotion and maintenance of appropriate levels of physical activity are increasingly important in today's health care arena.

Our level of health and physical fitness is related to our level of physical activity. Many body systems work together to produce efficient, effective physical activity. Each of these systems develops uniquely, and this development can be enhanced by participation in physical fitness programs.

Because optimal health and fitness reflect our ability to maintain a physically active and independent lifestyle, fitness programming is an important focus of health care. Exercise planning and programming form a complex process. Detailed assessment of a person's ability to participate in an exercise program is necessary. Exercise programs differ according to age, health, level of fitness, and interests. As health care providers, we should become familiar with the age-related aspects of exercise and training programs to help our clients attain lifelong fitness, as well as to maintain a healthy lifestyle for ourselves.

REFERENCES

1. Aires L, Silva P, Silva G, et al: Intensity of physical activity, cardiorespiratory fitness, and body mass index in youth, *J Phys Act Health* 7:54–59, 2010.
2. Anderson SE, Economos CD, Must A: Active play and screen time in US children aged 4 to 11 years in relation to sociodemographic and weight status characteristics: a nationally representative cross-sectional analysis, *BMC Public Health* 8:355, doi: 10.1186/1471-2458/8/366, 2008.
3. CDC: Prevalence of self-reported physically active adults–United States, 2007, *MMWR Morb Mortal Wkly Rep* 57(48):1297–1300, 2008.
4. Janz KF, Dawson JD, Mahoney LT: Tracking physical fitness and physical activity from childhood to adolescence: the Muscatine study, *Med Sci Sports Exerc* 32(7):1250–1257, 2000.
5. Mackett RL, Paskins J: Children's physical activity: the contribution of playing and walking, *Child Soc* 22:345–357, 2008.
6. Nelson MC, Neumark-Stzainer Hannan PJ, Sirary JR, et al: Longitudinal and secular trends in physical activity and sedentary behavior during adolescence, *Pediatrics* 118:e1627–e1634, 2006.
7. Dean E: Physical therapy in the 21st century (part I): toward practice informed by epidemiology and the crisis of lifestyle conditions, *Physiother Theory Pract* 25(5):330–353, 2009.
8. Hallal PC, Victora CG, Azevedo MR, et al: Adolescent physical activity and health: a systematic review, *Sports Med* 36(12):1019–1030, 2006.
9. Mitchell JA, Mattocks C, Ness AR, et al: Sedentary behavior and obesity in a large cohort of children, *Obesity* 17(8):1596–1602, 2009.
10. Strong WB, Malina RM, Blimkie CJR, et al: Evidence based physical activity for school-age youth, *J Pediatr* 146:732–737, 2005.
11. Whitaker RC, Orzol SM: Obesity among US urban preschool children: relationships to race, ethnicity, and socioeconomic status, *Arch Pediatr Adolesc Med* 160:578–584, 2006.
12. World Health Organization: *The first ten years of the World Health Organization*, Geneva, 1958, World Health Organization.
13. Bouchard C, Shepard RJ, Stephens T, et al, editors: *Exercise fitness and health: a consensus of current knowledge*, Champaign, Ill, 1990, Human Kinetics.
14. American Physical Therapy Association: *Guide to physical therapist practice*, ed 2, *Phys Ther* 81(1):14–747, 2001.
15. Fair SE: *Wellness and physical therapy*, Boston, 2011, Jones and Bartlett.
16. US Department of Health and Human Services: *Healthy People 2010: understanding and improving health*, ed 2, Washington, DC, 2000, US Government Printing Office.
17. McArdle WD, Katch FI, Katch VL: *Exercise physiology: energy, nutrition and human performance*, ed 7, Philadelphia, 2010, Wolter Kluwer/Lippincott, Williams & Wilkins.
18. US Department of Health and Human Services: *Definitions: health, fitness, and physical activity*, 2000, The Presidents Council on Physical Fitness Research Digest. www.fitness.gov/digest_mar2000.htm Accessed July 5, 2010.
19. Frontera WR, Evans WJ: Exercise performance and endurance training in the elderly, *Top Geriatr Rehabil* 2:17–32, 1986.
20. Jackson AS, Wier LT, Ayers GW, et al: Changes in aerobic power of women, ages 20-64 years, *Med Sci Sports Exerc* 28:884–891, 1996.
21. Lemura LM, VonDuvillard SO, Mookerjee S: The effects of physical training of functional capacity in adults ages 46-90: a meta-analysis, *J Sports Med Phys Fitness* 40:1–10, 2000.
22. Sarkisian CA, Liu H, Gutierrez PR, et al: Modifiable risk factors predict functional decline among older women: a prospectively validated clinical prediction tool, *J Am Geriatr Soc* 48:170–176, 2000.
23. Green JS, Crouse SF: The effects of endurance training on functional capacity in the elderly: a meta-analysis, *Med Sci Sports Exerc* 27:920–926, 1995.
24. Suominen H: Physical activity and health: musculoskeletal issues, *Adv Physiother* 9:65–75, 2007.
25. Malina RM: Growth, exercise fitness and later outcomes. In Bouchard C, Shepard RJ, Stephens T, et al, editors: *Exercise, fitness and health: a consensus of current knowledge*, Champaign, Ill, 1990, Human Kinetics, pp 637–653.
26. Sattelmair JR, Pertman JH, Forman DE: Effects of physical activity on cardiovascular and noncardiovascular outcomes in older adults, *Clin Geriatr Med* 25:677–702, 2009.
27. Goodpaster BH, Park SW, Harris TB, et al: The loss of skeletal muscle strength, mass, and quality in older adults: the health, aging and body composition study, *J Gerontol A Biol Sci Med Sci* 61A(10):1059–1064, 2006.
28. Armstrong N, Welsman JR: Development of aerobic fitness during childhood and adolescence, *Pediatr Exerc Sci* 12:128–149, 2000.
29. Faulkner JA, White TP: Adaptation of skeletal muscle to physical activity. In Bouchard C, Shepard RJ, Stephens T, et al, editors: *Exercise, fitness and health: a consensus of current knowledge*, Champaign, Ill, 1990, Human Kinetics, pp 256–279.
30. Bouchard C, Perusse L: Heredity, activity level, fitness and health. In Bouchard C, Shephard RJ, Stephens T, editors: *Physical activity, fitness and health: international proceedings and consensus statement*, Champaign, Ill, 1994, Human Kinetics, pp 106–118.
31. Bar-Or O: The growth and development of children's physiologic and perceptional responses to exercise. In Ilmannen J, Valimaki I, editors: *Children and sport-pediatric work physiology*, New York, 1984, Springer Verlag, pp 3–17.
32. Folinsbee LJ: Discussion: exercise and environment. In Bouchard C, Shepard RJ, Stephens T, et al, editiors: *Exercise, fitness and health: a consensus of current knowledge*, Champaign, Ill, 1990, Human Kinetics, pp 179–183.
33. Bouchard C, Shephard RJ: Physical activity, fitness, and health: the model and key concepts. In Bouchard C,

Shephard RJ, Stephens T, editors: *Physical activity, fitness and health: international proceedings and consensus statement,* Champaign, Ill, 1994, Human Kinetics, pp 77–88.

34. Jackson AS, Sui X, Hebert JR, et al: Role of lifestyle and aging on the longitudinal change in cardiorespiratory fitness, *Arch Intern Med* 169(19):1781–1787, 2009.

35. Lovell DI, Cuneo R, Gass GC: Can aerobic training improve muscle strength and power in older men? *J Aging Phys Act* 18:14–26, 2010.

36. Cress ME, Buchner DM, Quiestad KA, et al: Exercise effects on physical functional performance in older adults, *J Gerontol* 54A:M242–M238, 1999.

37. Aires L, Andersen LB, Mendonca D, et al: A 3-year longitudinal analysis of changes in fitness, physical activity, fatness and screen time, *Acta Paediatr* 99:140–144, 2010.

38. Powell K, Blair S: The public health burdens of sedentary living habits: theoretical but realistic estimates, *Med Sci Sports Exerc* 26:857–865, 1994.

39. Vuori I: Physical activity and health: metabolic and cardiovascular issues, *Adv Physiother* 9:50–64, 2007.

40. US Department of Health and Human Services: *Promoting health-preventing disease: year 2000 objectives for the nation,* Washington, DC, 1990, US Public Health Services, National Institutes of Health.

41. Buskirk ER: Exercise, fitness and aging. In Bouchard C, Shepard RJ, Stephens T, et al, editors: *Exercise, fitness and health: a consensus of current knowledge,* Champaign, Ill, 1990, Human Kinetics, pp 687–697.

42. US Department of Health and Human Services: *Healthy People 2010 midcourse review, 2005,* 2010, Healthy People (website). www.healthypeople.gov/data/midcourse. Accessed July 8, 2010.

43. US Department of Health and Human Services: *2008 physical activity guidelines for Americans,* Publication #00036, Washington, DC, 2008, Office of Disease Prevention and Health Promotion.

44. Nelson ME, Rejeski WJ, Blair SN, et al: Physical activity and public health in older adults: recommendation from the American College of Sports Medicine and the American Heart Association, *Circulation* 116:1094–1105, 2007.

45. Haskell WL, Lee IM, Pate RR, et al: Physical activity and public health: updated recommendations for adults from the American College of Sports Medicine and the American Heart Association, *Med Sci Sports Exerc* 39:1423–1434, 2007.

46. Brooks CM: Leisure time physical activity assessment of American adults through an analysis of time diaries collected in 1981, *Am J Public Health* 77:455–460, 1987.

47. Caspersen CJ, Christenson GM, Pollard RA: Status of the 1990 physical fitness and exercise objectives: evidence from NHIS 1985, *Public Health Rep* 101:587–592, 1986.

48. Talbot LA, Metter EJ, Fleg JL: Leisure time physical activities and their relationship to cardiorespiratory fitness in healthy men and women, 18-95 years old, *Med Sci Sports Exerc* 32:417–425, 2000.

49. Nader PR, Bradley RH, Houts RM, et al: Moderate-to-vigorous physical activity from ages 9 to 15 years, *JAMA* 300(3):295–305, 2008.

50. Dean E: Physical therapy in the 21ˢᵗ century (part II): evidence-based practice within the context of evidence-informed practice, *Physiother Theory Pract* 25(5–6):354–368, 2008.

51. Bar-Or O: The prepubescent female. In Shangold MM, Mirken G, editors: *Women and exercise: physiology and sports medicine,* Philadelphia, 1988, FA Davis, pp 109–119.

52. Mitchell JH, Raven PB: Cardiovascular adaptation to physical activity. In Bouchard C, Shephard RJ, Stephens T, editors: *Physical activity, fitness and health: international proceedings and consensus statement,* Champaign, Ill, 1994, Human Kinetics, pp 286–301.

53. Green HJ: Discussion: adaptation of skeletal muscle to physical activity. In Bouchard C, Shepard RJ, Stephens T, et al, editors: *Exercise, fitness and health: a consensus of current knowledge,* Champaign, Ill, 1990, Human Kinetics, pp 281–291.

54. Saltin B: Cardiovascular and pulmonary adaptation to physical activity. In Bouchard C, Shepard RJ, Stephens T, et al, editors: *Exercise, fitness and health: a consensus of current knowledge,* Champaign, Ill, 1990, Human Kinetics, pp 187–203.

55. Obert P, Mandigouts S, Nottin S, et al: Cardiovascular responses to endurance training in children: effect of gender, *Eur J Clin Invest* 33(3):199–208, 2003.

56. Kelley GA, Kelley KS: Aerobic exercise and resting blood pressure in older adults: a meta-analytic review of randomized controlled trials, *J Gerontol A Biol Sci Med Sci* 56(5):M298–M303, 2001.

57. Faigenbaum AD: State of the art reviews: resistance training for children and adolescents: are there health outcomes? *Am J Lifestyle Med* 1:190–200, 2007.

58. Babcock MA, Dempsey JA: Pulmonary system adaptations: limitations to exercise. In Bouchard C, Shephard RJ, Stephens T, editors: *Physical activity, fitness and health: international proceedings and consensus statement,* Champaign, Ill, 1994, Human Kinetics, pp 320–330.

59. Mahon AD, Vaccaro T: Ventilatory threshold and VO_{2max} changes in children following endurance training, *Med Sci Sports Exerc* 21:425–431, 1989.

60. Kemper HC: Skeletal development during childhood and adolescence and the effects of physical activity, *Pediatr Exerc Sci* 12:198–216, 2000.

61. Hass CJ, Feigenbaum S, Franklin BA: Prescription of resistance training for healthy populations, *Sports Med* 31(14):953–964, 2001.

62. Faigenbaum AD, Kraemer WJ, Blimkie CJR, et al: Youth resistance training: updated position statement paper from the National Strength and Conditioning Association, *J Strength Cond Res* 23(5):s60–s79, 2009.

63. Behm DG, Faigenbaum AD, Falk B, et al: Canadian Society for Exercise Physiology position paper: resistance training in children and adolescents, *Appl Physiol Nutr Metab* 33:547–561, 2008.

64. Van Praagh E, Dore E: Short-term muscle power during growth and maturation, *Sports Med* 32(11):701–728, 2002.

65. Knortz KA: Muscle physiology applied to geriatric rehabilitation, *Top Geriatr Rehabil* 2:1–12, 1987.

66. Van Praagh E: Development of anaerobic function during childhood and adolescence, *Pediatr Exerc Sci* 12:150–173, 2000.

67. Thompson L: Physiologic changes associated with aging. In Guccione K, editor: *Geriatric physical therapy*, ed 2, St Louis, 2000, Mosby.

68. Boisseau N, Delamarche P: Metabolic and hormonal responses to exercise in children and adolescents, *Sports Med* 30(6):405–422, 2000.

69. Sutton JR, Farrell PA, Harber VJ: Hormonal adaptation to physical activity. In Bouchard C, Shepard RJ, Stephens T, et al, editors: *Exercise, fitness and health: a consensus of current knowledge*, Champaign, Ill, 1990, Human Kinetics, pp 217–257.

70. Payne VG, Isaacs LD: *Human motor development: a life span approach*, Mountain View, Calif, 1987, Mayfield.

71. Cunningham DA, Paterson DH, Blimke CJR: The development of the cardiorespiratory system with growth and physical activity. In Bouleau RA, editor: *Advances in pediatric sport science, vol 1: biological issues*, Champaign, Ill, 1984, Human Kinetics, pp 85–116.

72. Mandigout S, Lecoq AM, Courteix D, et al: Effect of gender in response to an aerobic training programme in prepubertal children, *Acta Paediatr* 90:9–15, 2001.

73. Mandigout S, Melin A, Lecoq AM, et al: Effect of two aerobic training regimens on the cardiorespiratory response of prepubertal boys and girls, *Acta Paediatr* 91:403–408, 2002.

74. Baquet G, Van Praagh E, Berthoin S: Endurance training and aerobic fitness in young people, *Sports Med* 33(15):1127–1143, 2003.

75. Bar-Or O: *Pediatric sports medicine for the practitioner*, New York, 1983, Springer Verlag.

76. Morrow JR, Freedson PS: Relationship between habitual physical activity and aerobic fitness in adolescents, *Pediatr Exerc Sci* 6:315–329, 1994.

77. Pate RR, Wang CY, Dowada M, et al: Cardiorespiratory fitness levels among US youth 12 to 19 years of age: findings from the 1999-2002 National Health and Nutrition Examination Survey, *Arch Pediatr Adolesc Med* 160:1005–1012, 2006.

78. Pollock ML, Mengelkoch LJ, Graves JE, et al: Twenty-year follow-up of aerobic power and body composition of older track athletes, *J Appl Physiol* 82:1508–1516, 1997.

79. Fleg AJ, Morrell CH, Bos AG, et al: Accelerated longitudinal decline of aerobic capacity in healthy older adults, *Circulation* 112:674–682, 2005.

80. Jackson AS, Beard EF, Wier LT, et al: Changes in aerobic power of men, ages 25-70 years, *Med Sci Sports Exerc* 27:113–120, 1995.

81. Cunningham DA, Paterson DH: Discussion: exercise, fitness and aging. In Bouchard C, Shepard RJ, Stephens T, et al, editors: *Exercise, fitness and health: a consensus of current knowledge*, Champaign, Ill, 1990, Human Kinetics, pp 699–704.

82. DeVito G, Hernandez R, Gonzalez V, et al: Low intensity physical training in older subjects, *J Sports Med Phys Fitness* 37:72–77, 1997.

83. World Health Organization: *World Health Report: Reducing Risks, Promoting Healthy Life*, Geneva, Switzerland, 2002, WHO Organization.

84. CDC: Vital signs: state-specific obesity prevalence among adults–United States, 2009, *MMWR Morb Mortal Wkly Rep* 59:1–5, 2010.

Index

Note: Page numbers followed by *b* indicates boxes, *f* indicates figures and *t* indicates tables.

A

AAP. *See* American Academy of Pediatrics
Academic skills, 179t
Accommodation, 23
Action potential, 175–176
Activity, 4. *See also* Physical activity
  in aging, 40–41
  characteristics of, 89–93
  evaluation of, 88–104
  functional, participation and, 4–5
  selection considerations, 90
Activity-dependent plasticity, 185
ADAM. *See* Androgen decline in the aging male
Adams, J.A., 76
Adaptability, 293
  in older adults gait patterns, 300
Adaptation, 19–20
  cardiovascular, to training, 344t
  dark, 227t
  environmental, 268
  light, 227t
  long-term, 344, 345
  musculoskeletal system, to training, 346t
  nervous system, 184–187
  in older adulthood, 330
  posture and, 268
  pulmonary system, to training, 345t
  short-term, 343–345
Adaptive postural control, 265
Adolescence, 15
  alcohol and, 204
  balance in, 279–280
  bone in, 120–121
  cardiovascular system in, 167
  endocrine system in, 241–242
  FAS in, 203
  flexibility in, 349
  motor control in, 75
  nervous system in, 191–192
  posture in, 279
  prehension in, 325–327
  pulmonary system in, 167
  sensory system in, 223–225
  skeletal muscle development in, 136–137, 142
  skeletal system in, 122–124
  sleep-wakefulness in, 248–249
  strength in, 142
Adulthood, 15
  alcohol and, 204
  ambulation in, 297
  balance, 279–280
    assessment in, 273b

Adulthood *(Continued)*
  bone in, 121
  cardiovascular system in, 167–170
  development, 35–36
  emerging, 35
  endocrine system, 242
  FIM for, 97–101
  grasp in, 312–313
  hypertension in, 163
  motor control in, 75
  nervous system in, 192–193
  obesity in, 341
  physical activity in, 350
  posture and, 279–280
  prehension in, 327–330
  pulmonary system in, 167–170
  sensory system in, 225–229
  skeletal muscle development in, 137–138, 142–147
  sleep-wakefulness in, 248–249
  strength in, 142
Advanced stage, 78
Affordance, 29, 213
Afterload, 157
Age-related changes, 39f, 201f
Aging. *See also* Life span changes; Older adults
  activity in, 40–41
  aldosterone in, 241t
  bone and, 114–116
  of brain, 194f
  cardiovascular system and, 167–170
  cartilage and, 107
  cognitive processing speed and, 39
  cortisol in, 241t
  epinephrine in, 241t
  estrogen in, 241t
  genetic theories, 36–37
  glucagon in, 241t
  growth hormone in, 241t
  heart, 168
  immune system in, 38
  insulin in, 241t
  intelligence and, 39
  isometric strength and, 145f
  kinesthesia and, 226t
  motor control and, 74–75
  nervous system and, 187–196
  neuroendocrine system in, 38–39
  nongenetic theories, 37–39
  norepinephrine, 241t
  pressure and, 226t
  programmed, 36–37
  proprioception and, 226t

Aging *(Continued)*
  pulmonary system and, 167–170
  respiratory system in, 170
  sarcopenia and, 139*f*
  sensory system and, 218–233
    changes in, 281
  sleep changes with, 250*b*
  sociocultural theories on, 40–41
  strength and, 137
  successful, 41
  testosterone in, 241*t*
  theories of, 36–41
    biophysical, 36–39
  thyroid hormones in, 241*t*
  touch and, 226*t*
  vascular system, 168
  vasopressin in, 241*t*
  ventilatory pump and, 169–170
  vibration and, 226*t*
  vision and, 227*t*
AIMS. *See* Alberta Infant Motor Scale
AIMS-2. *See* Arthritis Impact Measurement Scale, 2nd edition
Ainsworth, M.S., 32
Alberta Infant Motor Scale (AIMS), 276
Alcohol. *See also* Fetal alcohol spectrum disorders;
  Fetal alcohol syndrome
  adolescence and, 204
  adulthood, 204
  childhood and, 204
  development and, 204*b*
  infancy, 204
  older adults and, 204
  prenatal, 204
Aldosterone, 241*t*
Alveolar cells, 158
Alveolar sacs, 158
Alveoli, 166–167
Alzheimer disease, 203–205, 206*b*, 233
  changes in, 205*f*
Amblyopia, 229–230, 230*b*
Ambulation, 292. *See also* Walking
  in adults, 297
  in children, 297
  in infancy, 294–296
  in older adults, 297–301
  in toddlers, 294–296
America, older adults in, 16*f*
American Academy of Pediatrics (AAP), 229–230
American College of Sports Medicine, 146–147
Amplitude phasing, 289
Amsler grid, 231*f*
Androgen decline in the aging male (ADAM), 240
Andropause, 243
Angiogenesis, 160
ANS. *See* Autonomic nervous system
Anticipatory control, 70, 313
  postural, 265, 279
Anticipatory grip, 324*f*
Anticipatory postural adjustments (APAs), 309
Anticipatory reach, 324*f*
Antidiuretic hormone, physical activity and, 347*t*
Anti-gravity neck flexion, 56
APAs. *See* Anticipatory postural adjustments
Aponeurosis, 136
Apophyseal avulsion, 123, 124

Apophyses, 114
Apoptosis, 37, 185
Arnett, Jeffrey J., 35
Arteries, 155–156, 162. *See also* Vascular system
  conducting, 156
  diagram of, 155*f*
  distributing, 156
  muscular, 156
Arthritis Functional Assessment Scale, 92
Arthritis Impact Measurement Scale, 2nd edition (AIMS-2), 92
Arthrogryposis, 19–20
Articular cartilage, 106
Assessment of Life Habits (LIFE-H), 97, 101
Assimilation, 23
  effect, 316
Association areas, 178*t*
Associative phase, 78
Associative play, 33
Astrocytes, 176–177
Asymmetrical bimanual coordination, 316*f*
Asymmetrical tonic neck reflex, 55*f*, 320*t*
Attachment, 32
Attention, 197–199
  directed, 242–243
Automatic postural reactions, 269*t*
Automatic rolling, 290
Autonomic efferent system, 181
Autonomic nervous system (ANS), 181
  organization of, 182*f*
  selected effects of, 183*t*
Autonomous phase, 78
Avoidance response, 320*t*
Axon pruning, 185

B
Babinski sign, 190
BADL. *See* Basic activities of daily living
Balance, 263
  adolescence and, 279–280
  adulthood and, 279–280
  assessment of, 272–273
    in adults, 273*b*
    in children, 276*b*
  in childhood, 275–279
    assessment of, 276*b*
  dynamic, 11, 282–284
  function and, 11
  functional scales of, 273*t*, 276*t*
  hierarchical model, 268–269
  in infancy, 275–279
  life span changes in, 274–284
  neural basis for, 268–272
  in older adults, 280–284
  one-foot standing, 278*t*
  sensory contributions to, 277, 278–279
  sensory organization and, 274*f*
  sitting and, 277–278
  standing, 281–282
  static, 11
Ballistic movements, 70
Baroreceptors, 156
Barthel Index, 97, 98*t*
Basal ganglia, 179–180
Base of support (BOS), 264–265
Basic activities of daily living (BADL), 4–5, 89

Bateson, G., 33, 34*t*
Battelle Developmental Inventory Screening Test (BDIST), 96
Bayley Scales of Infant Development, 64
BDIST. *See* Battelle Developmental Inventory Screening Test
Behavioral Risk Factor Surveillance System, 340*f*
Behaviorists, 31
Berg test, 273, 273*t*
    pediatric, 276*t*
Bernstein, N., 72
Bimanual coordination, 309, 316, 323
    asymmetrical, 316*f*
    in infancy, 322
    symmetrical, 316
Biocultural influences, 17*f*
Biomechanics, 310
Biophysical domain, 7, 7*f*
    aging theories, 36–39
    in human development, 21*t*, 22
        child, 25–27
Blocked practice, 79–80, 80*f*
BMI. *See* Body mass index
Body composition, 337
Body functions, 4
Body mass index (BMI), 339, 340*f*
Body structures, 4
Bone, 107–116. *See also* Skeletal system
    in adolescence, 120–121
    in adulthood, 121
    aging and, 114–116
    cancellous, 108
    cartilage model of, 112*f*
    compact, 108
    cortical, 108
    development, 110*f*
    form, 108–111
    growth, 115*f*
        areas of, 120
        dynamic, 119–120
    lamellar, 108
    long, 109*f*
    mineral content, 119*f*
    muscular attachments to, 115*f*
    in older adulthood, 121–122
    spongy, 108
    structure, 108–111
BOS. *See* Base of support
Brain. *See also* Nervous system
    aging of, 194*f*
    metabolism, 201*f*
    in sleep-wakefulness, 245*f*
    weight, 190–191
Brainstem, 177, 180*f*
Bronchi, 157–158
    development of, 160*f*
Bronchial buds, 160–161
Bronchioles, 157–158, 166–167
Bronfenbrenner's ecological model, 25, 26*f*
Bruininks-Oseretsky Test of Motor Proficiency, 64, 276
Bundy's Test of Playfulness, 64

C

Cadence, 292
Caeyenberghs, K., 74–75
Callosum, 184
Caloric intake, skeletal muscle and, 140

Cancellous bone, 108
CAPE. *See* Children's Assessment of Participation and Enjoyment
Capillaries, 155–156
Cardiac output, 151
Cardiovascular endurance, 337
Cardiovascular system, 151–173
    adaptation to training, 344*t*
    in adolescence, 167
    in adulthood, 167–170
    aging and, 167–170
    birth adjustments, 161
    components, 151–156
    control, 156
    development of, 159–170
    in fitness, 343–344
        long-term adaptation, 344
        short-term adaptation, 343–344
    functional changes in, 169
    functional implications of changes in, 170–171
    heart
        aging, 168
        conducting system, 154*f*
        layers of, 154*f*
        rate, 151
    life span changes, 162*t*
    in locomotion, 304
    neonatal schematic, 153*f*
    prenatal development, 159–160
Career consolidation, 35
Carpal tunnel syndrome, 328
Cartilage, 105–107
    aging and, 107
    articular, 106
    bone model, 112*f*
    elastic, 105–106
    formation, 107
    hyaline, 105–106
    injury to, 124
    properties of, 106–107
    types of, 106*f*
Casby, Michael, 33
Catecholamines, 156, 169
Center of mass (COM), 264–265, 271, 272, 282, 283, 293
Center of pressure (COP), 266–267, 270–271, 272
Central nervous system (CNS), 176, 177–181
Cephalocaudal, 46
Cerebellum, 177, 180, 180*f*
Cerebrospinal fluid, 193
Cerebrovascular accident (CVA), 92–93
Chaining, 68
Chemoreceptors, 156
Childhood, 15
    alcohol and, 204
    ambulation in, 297
    balance in, 275–279
        assessment of, 276*b*
    biophysical domain in, 25–27
    cardiovascular system in, 161–165
    defecation in, 256
    development in, 25–35
        biophysical, 25–27
        psychological, 27–31
        sociocultural, 31–35
    digestion, 253–255

Childhood *(Continued)*
 FIM for, 94–95
 flexibility in, 349
 grasp in, 323
 grip in, 323
 hypertension, 163
 ingestion, 253–255
 micturition in, 257–258
 motor control in, 74–75
 motor development, 61–64
 motor learning in, 82–83
 muscle development, 142
 nervous system in, 189–191
 obesity in, 341
 physical activity in, 350, 351
 posture in, 275–279
 prehension in, 322–323, 324–325
 pulmonary system in, 165–167
 reach in, 323
 sensory system, 219–223
 skeletal system in, 119–120
  functional implications, 122–124
 sleep-wakefulness in, 248
 sociocultural domain in, 31–35
 strength in, 142
Children's Assessment of Participation and Enjoyment
  (CAPE), 97
Chondrocytes, 106
Chondromalacia, 124
Choudhury, S., 75
Circadian rhythms, 239, 249
Circular reactions
 primary, 28
 secondary, 28
 tertiary, 28
Circulation
 mechanics of, 157
Client symptoms, 3
Clinical Test of Sensory Integration on Balance (CTSIB), 272
Closed-loop control mode, 70
 model, 70*f*
Closed-loop theory, 76
CNS. *See* Central nervous system
Cognition, 197
Cognitive development, 28*t*
 styles, 179*t*
Cognitive phase, 78
Cognitive processing speed
 aging and, 39
Cognitive reserve theory, 40
Collagen, 141
Color discrimination, 228
COM. *See* Center of mass
Compact bone, 108
Concrete operational period, 29
Concurrent feedback, 81–82
Concurrent validity, 91
Conducting arteries, 156
Conducting portion, 157–158
Cone of stability, 265*f*
Constant practice, 80–81
Constraint-induced movement therapy, 79*b*, 329
Construct validity, 91
Content validity, 91
Continuity theory, 41

Contraction, 130
 properties, 137–138, 140
Cooperative play, 33
Coordination
 function and, 11
Coordinative structure, 301
COP. *See* Center of pressure
Corpus callosum, 184
Cortex, 180*f*
 functions of, 177*t*
Cortical bone, 108
Cortical development, 203*f*
Corticotropin
 physical activity and, 347*t*
Cortisol
 in aging, 241*t*
 physical activity and, 347*t*
Crawling, 292–293
Creeping, 60, 292–293
Cretinism, 188
Critical periods, 184–185
Cross-links, 38
Cruising, 60
 maneuvers, 61*f*
Crystallized intelligence, 201
CTSIB. *See* Clinical Test of Sensory Integration on Balance
Culture, 20
Cumming, E., 40
Cumulative trauma disorders, 328
 prevention of, 329
Cutaneous receptors, 215*f*
CVA. *See* Cerebrovascular accident
Cylindrical grasp, 314*t*

D
Dark adaptation, 227*t*
Declarative memory, 30
Defecation, 256
 in childhood, 256
 control mechanisms, 256
 in older adulthood, 256
Degrees of freedom, 72
Dehydroepiandrosterone (DHEA), 140
Del Rey, P., 82
Deliberate stepping, 294–296
Deliberation, 290
Dendritic growth, 183*f*
Dental development, 254–255
Depth perception, 227*t*
Dermatomes, 188
Development. *See also* specific types
 child, 25–35
  biophysical, 25–27
  psychological, 27–31
  sociocultural, 31–35
 cognitive, 28*t*
 concepts of, 16–18
 continuity of, 21
 dental, 254–255
 domains of, 14–15
 factors affecting, 20
 function and, 6–7
 individual differences in, 17–18
 life span in, 16–17
  theories, 22–25

Development *(Continued)*
  maturity in, 16
  motor learning and, 82–84
  periods of, 15, 15*t*
  physical function, 8–9
  processes, 21–22
  proximal, 32
  senescence in, 16
  stages of, 23*t*
  theories affecting, 14–44
    adult, 35–36
    assumptions, 21 22
    biophysical, 21*t*, 22
    psychological, 21*t*, 22–23
    sociocultural, 21*t*, 24–25, 31–35
DHEA. *See* Dehydroepiandrosterone
Diabetes mellitus, 328
Diaphysis, 111
Diarthrosis joints, 116
Diaschisis, 187
Diastolic blood pressure, 169
Dichgans, J., 73
Digestion, 250–259
  childhood, 253–255
  control mechanisms, 251–252
  infancy, 253–255
  life span changes, 252, 253–256
  prenatal, 253
Directed attention, 242–243
Directionality, 225
Disability, 3
Disengagement, 40
Dissolution, 69
Distance phasing, 289
Distributed control, 71–72
Distributed practice, 78–79
Distributing arteries, 156
DLPFL. *See* Dorsolateral prefrontal cortex
Doll eye phenomenon, 221
Dopamine, 195
Dorsolateral prefrontal cortex (DLPFL), 200–201
Double limb support, 292
Down syndrome, 271
Driving, 232–233, 233*t*
Dynamic balance, 11, 282–284
Dynamic bone growth, 119–120
Dynamic flexibility, 10
Dynamic prehension, 313
Dynamic stability, 47
Dynamic strength, 143
Dynamic systems model, 71
Dynamic systems theory, 22, 52*f*
  on motor control development, 49–53
  themes relative to, 49–52

E
Ear anatomy, 216*f*
Early motor program theory, 71
Ecological plasticity, 185
Ecology, 24–25, 26*f*
Egocentric, 267
Elastic cartilage, 105–106
Elasticity, lung, 170
Electron micrographs, 124*f*
Elimination, 256

Embodiment, 51
Embryo, 135*f*
Embryonic period, 15
Emergent movement pattern, 49*f*
Emerging adulthood, 35
Emotions, 179*t*
Endocardial cushions, 159–160
Endocardium, 154
Endochondral ossification, 111
Endocrine system, 240–243
  in adolescence, 241–242
  in adulthood, 242
  fitness and, 346–347
  in infancy, 241–242
  life-span changes in, 240–243
  in older adulthood, 242–243
  prenatal, 240
  training and, 346–347
Endomysium, 129–130
Endurance
  cardiovascular, 337
  function and, 11–12
  muscular, 143, 336
  respiratory, 337
Entrainment, 246
Environmental adaptation, 268
  posture and, 268
Ependymal cells, 176–177
Epicardium, 154
Epinephrine
  in aging, 241*t*
  physical activity and, 347*t*
Epiphyseal plate, 111
Epiphysis, 111, 114
Equilibrium reactions, 270
  sitting, 270*f*
Erect walking, 294–301
Erikson, EH, 23*t*, 33, 34*t*
Esophagus, 251
Estrogen, 241*t*
Evaluation
  of activity, 88–104
  characteristics, 89–93
  design, 93
  focus, 92–93
  formats
    nonstandardized, 89–90
    standardized, 89–90
  of function, 88–104
  measurement issues, 90–93
  of participation, 88–104
  selection considerations, 90
Excitation-contraction coupling, 130
Executive function, 199*f*
  development of, 200*t*
Exercise. *See* Fitness; Physical activity
Exocentric, 267
Experience-dependent, 185
Experience-expectant, 185
Expert stage, 78
Explicit memory, 30, 197–198
  development of, 198*t*
External lamina, 129
Eye-hand coordination, 311
Eye-head stabilization, 267

F

Faded feedback, 81
Falling, 298*b*
  factors, 298
  prevention, 298
Family systems, 35–36
FAS. *See* Fetal alcohol syndrome
FASD. *See* Fetal alcohol spectrum disorders
Feedback, 81, 82–83
  concurrent, 81–82
  examples, 81*t*
  faded, 81
  intermittent, 81
  summarized, 81
  terminal, 81–82
Feedback control, 69–70
Feedforward, 309
Fetal alcohol spectrum disorders (FASD), 202
Fetal alcohol syndrome (FAS), 202–203
  in adolescence, 203
  clinical features of, 202–203
Fetal period, 15
FEV. *See* Forced expiratory volume
Fibroblasts, 134
Fibrocartilage, 105–106
FIM. *See* Functional Independence Measure
Fine motor milestones, 54*t*
Firing rate, 137–138
Fitness, 197. *See also* Physical activity
  body systems involved in, 343–348
    cardiovascular, 343–344
    musculoskeletal, 345–346
    pulmonary, 344–345, 349
  common terms, 336*b*
  endocrine contributions to, 346–347
  factors influencing, 337–339
    physical, 337–338
  health and, 335–354
  health-related, 336–337
    components of, 337
  heredity and, 338
  hormonal contributions to, 346–347
  life span changes and, 349–351
  metabolic contributions to, 346–347
  physical activity and, 338
  physiological, 336–337
  pulmonary system and, 349
  skill-related, 336–337
  social factors, 338–339
Fitts' stages, 78
Flexibility
  body composition, 349
    adolescence, 349
    childhood, 349
  defined, 337
  dynamic, 10
  function and, 10–11
  static, 10
Flexion synergy, 73–74
Fluid intelligence, 201
Focus, 92–93
Fontanelles, 119
Foramen ovale, 159–160
Force control, 140–141
Forced expiratory volume (FEV), 159

Formal operational period, 29
Frailty, 37*f*
Free radical theory, 37–38
Freedom, degrees of, 72
Freud, Sigmund, 33, 34*t*
Frontal lobe, 177*t*, 178*t*
Function
  acquisition of, 5*f*
  balance and, 11
  body, 4
  characteristics of, 89–93
  client assessment, 3
  components, 9–12
  coordination and, 11
  defined, 1–7
  development and, 6–7, 8–9
  domains of, 7
    biophysical, 7, 7*f*
    psychological, 7, 7*f*
    sociocultural, 7, 7*f*
  endurance and, 11–12
  evaluation of, 88–104
  executive, 199*f*
    development of, 200*t*
  flexibility and, 10–11
  health and, 2
  life span perspective, 5–7
  lung volumes, 159*f*
  physical, 7–12
    development of, 8–9
  physical growth and, 5–6
  power and, 11
  pulmonary system, 158, 170–171
  selection considerations, 90
  sensory system, 229–233
  skeletal muscles, 142–147
  skeletal system, 122–125
  total hand, 313
  vital, 239–262
    life span changes in, 243–259
    in older adults, 242
    sleep-wakefulness, 245–246
    ventilation-respiration, 243–250
Functional activities, participation and, 4–5
Functional independence, 1–13
Functional Independence Measure (FIM), 99–101, 100*f*
  for adults, 97
  for children, 94–95
Functional limitation, 3–4
Functional lung volumes, 159*f*
Functional reach test, 276*f*
Functional scales of balance, 273*t*, 276*t*
Functional status, 3
Functions
  of cortex, 177*t*

G

Gabbard, C., 74
Galloping, 62, 302
Gap junctions, 182
Gastroesophageal reflux (GER), 251
Generativity, 24
Genetic theories of aging, 36–37
Genotype, 17
Genu valgus, 120

Geographic atrophy, 230
GER. *See* Gastroesophageal reflux
Germinal period, 15
Germinal zone, 188
Gesell, A., 22, 48
Gibson, Eleanor, 29
Glia, 176–177
Glucagon
    in aging, 241*t*
    physical activity and, 347*t*
GMFM. *See* Gross Motor Function Measure
Grasp, 312–314, 320*t*
    adult patterns, 312–313
    in childhood, 323
    classification of, 312–313
    cylindrical, 314*t*
    hook, 314*t*
    in infancy, 319–322
    inferior pincer, 321*t*
    instinctive, 320*t*
    palmar, 321*t*
    pincer, 321*t*
    primitive squeeze, 321*t*
    radial palmar, 321*t*
    radial-digital, 321*t*
    scissors, 321*t*
    spherical, 314*t*
    superior pincer, 321*t*
Grip
    anticipatory, 324*f*
    in childhood, 323
    formation, 311–312
    in infancy, 319
    pencil, 324*t*, 325*f*
    power, 312, 312*f*
    precision, 312
    strength, 138*f*, 326*f*
    sustained, 315
Gross motor development in infancy, 322
Gross Motor Function Measure (GMFM), 92–93, 95
Gross motor milestones, 54*t*
Growth, 18
    bone, 115*f*
        areas of, 120
        dynamic, 119–120
    dendritic, 183*f*
    differential rates of, 18*f*
    across life span, 19*f*
    physical, 5–6
    upper limb, 317, 318*t*
Growth hormone, 110–111, 346
    in aging, 241*t*
    physical activity and, 347*t*
Guide to Physical Therapist Practice, 3–4, 335
Gymnasts, 124

H

HABIT. *See* Hand Arm Bimanual Intervention
Hand Arm Bimanual Intervention (HABIT), 329
Hand dominance, 323
Hand function, total, 313
Hand preference, 323
Hand reflexes, 320*t*
Handicap, 3
Handwriting, 325

Haptic perception, 220, 315
Harman, D., 37–38
Haversian canals, 108
Hayflick limit theory, 36
Head control, 55*f*
Head stabilization in space strategy (HSSS), 264
Health
    defined, 335
    determinants of, 336*f*
    fitness and, 335–354
    function and, 2
    heredity and, 338
    physical activity and, 338
    social factors, 338–339
    status models, 3–4
    WHO on, 335
Health-related fitness, 336–337
    components of, 337
Hearing, 217, 219, 223
Heart
    aging, 168
    conducting system of, 154*f*
    layers of, 154*f*
    rate, 151
Heel-toe-progression, 294–296
Hemiplegia, 79*b*
Henry, W.E., 40
Heredity
    fitness and, 338
    health and, 338
Hickman, J.M., 81
Hierarchical model, 69
    balance, 268–269
Hierarchical organization, 316
Hierarchy of needs, 25*f*
High guard, 61
Hippocampus, 174, 193
Homeostatic control mechanisms, 240
Hook grasp, 314*t*
Hopping, 302–303
    lower extremities in, 302
    upper extremities in, 302
HPA. *See* Hypothalamic-pituitary-adrenal
HSSS. *See* Head stabilization in space strategy
Hyaline cartilage, 105–106
Hypertension, 157, 163*b*
    in adults, 163
    in children, 163
    diagnosis, 163–164, 165*t*
    prevention of, 164*t*
Hypothalamic-pituitary-adrenal (HPA), 38–39
Hypothalamus, 179, 239, 242

I

IADL. *See* Instrumental activities of daily living
ICF. *See* International Classification of Functioning, Disability, and Health
ICIDH. *See* International Classification of Functioning, Disability, and Health
Immediate memory, 30–31
Immune system, aging and, 38
Immunosenescence, 38
Impairments, 4
Implicit memory, 30, 197–198
    development of, 198*t*

Independent stepping, 294–296
Independent walking, 62f
Index finger, 313–314
Individuality, 51–52
Infancy, 15. *See also* Toddlers
    alcohol and, 204
    ambulation in, 294–296
    balance in, 275–279
    behavioral states in, 247t
    bimanual coordination in, 322
    cardiovascular system in, 161–165
        schematic, 153f
    digestion, 253–255
    endocrine system in, 241–242
    grasp in, 319–322
    grip in, 319
    gross motor development, 322
    ingestion, 253–255
    manipulation in, 319–322
    micturition in, 257–258
    motor development in, 53–54
    nervous system in, 189–191
    posture in, 275–279
    prehension, 317–322
    pulmonary system in, 165–167
    reach in, 317–319
    release in, 322
    sensory system, 219–223
    skeletal muscle development in, 136–137
    skeletal system in, 119–120
    sleep-wakefulness in, 247–248
    temperament in, 31t
    visual regard in, 317
Inferior pincer grasp, 321t
Inflammatory effects, 140
Information processing, 30
Ingestion, 250–259
    childhood, 253–255
    control mechanisms, 251–252
    infancy, 253–255
    life span changes, 252, 253–256
    in older adulthood, 255–256
    prenatal, 253
In-hand manipulation, 315f, 320–322
Inhibition, 294–296
Inner ear labyrinths, 216f
Instinctive grasp reaction, 320t
Instrumental activities of daily living (IADL), 4–5, 89
    limitation in, 9f
Insulin
    in aging, 241t
    physical activity and, 347t
Integration, 294–296
Intelligence, 27–29, 199–202
    aging and, 39
    crystallized, 201
    fluid, 201
Intermittent feedback, 81
International Classification of Functioning, Disability, and
        Health (ICF), 2–4, 92
    model, 2f
International Classification of Impairments, Disabilities, and
        Handicaps (ICIDH), 3–4
Interneurons, 184

Interrater reliability, 90
Intersensory integration, 217, 225
Interview assessment, 93
Intramembranous ossification, 111
Intrarater reliability, 90
Intrasensory integration, 217
Involutional osteoporosis, 125
Isometric strength, 143
    aging and, 145f

J
Joint position sense (JPS), 226
Joints, 116
    diarthrosis, 116
    synarthrosis, 116
    synovial, 116f
JPS. *See* Joint position sense

K
Kahn, R.L., 41
KAT. *See* Kinesthetic Acuity Test
Kinematics, 289, 298
    in older adults, 299
Kinesthesia, 226t
Kinesthetic Acuity Test (KAT), 220
Kinesthetic memory, 220
Kinetics, 289, 298
    in older adults, 299
Knowledge
    of performance, 81
    of results, 81–82
Knox Preschool Play Scale, 64
Konczak, J., 73
Kyphosis, 124–125

L
LAG. *See* Longevity assurance genes
Lambert canals, 158
Lamellae, 108
Lamellar bone, 108
Language acquisition, 192t
Lateral righting reaction, 57f
Lateral stability, 284
Learned nonuse, 328, 329
Learning, 19–20, 68–87, 197–199. *See also*
        Motor learning
    sequential, 83
    social, 24–25, 32
Left hemisphere, 179t
Left ventricular wall thickening, 168
Leisure, 36
Levinson, D.F., 35
Life span changes, 5–7. *See also* Aging
    in balance, 274–284
    biocultural influences on, 17f
    cardiovascular system, 162t
    in development, 16–17
        theories, 22–25
    digestion, 252, 253–256
    in endocrine system, 240–243
    in function, 5–7
    growth across, 19f
    ingestion, 252, 253–256
    in locomotion, 289–303

Life span changes *(Continued)*
  in micturition, 257–259
  motor development and, 53–65
  in posture, 274–284
  pulmonary system, 162*t*
  training and, 349–351
  in vital functions, 243–259
    sleep-wakefulness, 245–246
    ventilation-respiration, 243–250
LIFE-H. *See* Assessment of Life Habits
Light adaptation, 227*t*
Limbic lobe, 177*t*, 178*t*
Limbic system, 174, 180
  components of, 174–181
Linear rating scale, 92*f*
Lipofuscin, 38, 168, 195
Liquids, 29*f*
Locomotion
  cardiovascular system in, 304
  clinical research on, 288–289
  life span changes, 289–303
  maturity of erect, 294–296
  musculoskeletal system in, 303–304
  nervous system in, 304
  pulmonary system in, 304
Locus ceruleus, 246
Long bone, 109*f*
Long term memory, 30–31
  development of, 198*t*
Long-distance navigation, 301
Longevity, 18
Longevity assurance genes (LAG), 37
Long-term adaptation, 344, 345
Low guard, 61
Lower extremities
  alignment, 114*t*
  in hopping, 302
  in running, 301
  in skipping, 303
Lungs. *See also* Pulmonary system
  compliance, 170
  development, 160*f*
  elasticity, 170
  volumes, functional, 159*f*

M
Macroglia, 176–177
Macula, 217*f*
Macular degeneration, 230–232, 232*b*
Manipulation, 309, 314–316
  in childhood, 323
  in infancy, 319–322
  in-hand, 315*f*, 320–322
Maslow's hierarchy of needs, 25*f*
Massed practice, 78–79, 79*b*
Maturation, 19, 25–27
  motor control and, 49
  in motor development, 48–49
Maturity
  in development, 16
  in locomotion, 294–296
  skeletal system, 121
Maximal aerobic capacity, 347–348
Maximal oxygen uptake, 347–348

Mead, G.H., 33, 34*t*
Meal preparation, 92*f*
Measurement instruments, 93–101
  adult assessment tools, 97–101
  pediatric assessment tools, 94–97
    activities assessed in, 95*b*
Mechanoreceptors, 214
Medial-lateral sway, 282
Medium veins, 156
Medulla, 180
Meissner corpuscles, 214, 225
Memory, 30–31, 197
  declarative, 30
  development of, 198*t*
  explicit, 30, 197–198, 198*t*
  formation, 31*f*
  immediate, 30–31
  implicit, 30, 197–198, 198*t*
  long term, 30–31, 198*t*
  nondeclarative, 30
  preexplicit, 198*t*
  procedural, 30
  short term, 30–31
  types of, 30*t*, 197–199
  working, 31, 198*t*
Menarche, 242
Menopause, 243
Merkel discs, 214
Mesenchyme, 188
Metabolism
  brain, 201*f*
  fitness and, 346–347
  oxidative, 143
  training and, 346–347
Metacommunicative theory, 34*t*
Metaphysis, 111
Microglia, 176–177
Micturition, 256–259
  in childhood, 257–258
  control mechanisms, 257
  in infancy, 257–258
  life span changes, 257–259
  in older adults, 258–259
  prenatal, 257
Midguard, 61
Milk, 253–254
Minimal detectable change, 91
Minimally clinically important difference, 91
Minute ventilation, 159, 344–345
Mobility, 47
Modeling, 21
Motivation, 25
Motor areas, 178*f*
Motor behavior, 179*t*
  multiply determined, 50–51
  soft assembled, 50–51
Motor control, 48–49, 68–87. *See also* Nervous
    system
  in adolescents, 75
  in adults, 75
  aging and, 74–75
  in children, 74–75
  issues related to, 71–74
  maturation and, 49

Motor control *(Continued)*
  in older adults, 75
  theories, 68–69
Motor coordination, posture and, 268
Motor development, 45–67
  childhood, 61–64
  concepts, 46–47
  directional concepts, 46
  at eight months, 59–60
  fine motor milestones, 54t
  at five months, 56–57
  at four months, 56
  functional implications, 53–65
  goals, 46
  gross motor milestones, 54t
  in infancy, 53–54
  as layered system, 50f
  life span changes in, 53–65
  maturation of systems, 48–49
  at nine months, 60
  sequence, 46
  at seven months, 58–59
  at six months, 57–58
  sixteen to eighteen months, 61
  theories, 49–53
  time frames, 48
  toddler, 60–61
Motor learning, 48–49, 68–87
  in children, 82–83
  defined, 75
  developmental aspects of, 82–84
  elements of, 78–82
    practice, 78–81
  in older adults, 83–84
  stages of, 77–78, 77t
  theories of, 75–77
    closed-loop, 76
    schema theory, 76–77
Motor program models, 70–71
  theory, 71
Motor time, 196
Motor unit, 132–133
  remodeling, 139
Movement therapy, constraint-induced, 79b
Multiply determined motor behavior, 50–51
Muscle fibers
  development, 135
  migration of, 136
  primary, 134f
  secondary, 134f
  subcellular elements, 131f
  types, 130–132
    changes in, 135–136
Muscle system changes, 129–150
Muscular arteries, 156
Muscular attachments, 115f
Muscular endurance, 143, 336
Muscular strength, 337
Musculoskeletal system, 303–304. *See also* Skeletal muscle
  adaptation to training, 346t
  in fitness, 345–346
    long-term adaptation, 345–346
    short-term adaptation, 345
  in older adults, 330
  posture and, 267–268

Myelin, 176
Myelination, 192
  timetable, 191f
Myocardium, 154, 168
Myocytes, 161
Myofibers, 133–134
Myofibrils, 130, 161
Myogenic precursor cells, 133
Myotomes, 188
Myotubes, 133

N
Nagi, Saad, 3–4
Nashner model of postural control, 271–272
National Health and Nutrition Survey (NHANS), 342f
Neo-Bernsteinien model, 78
Nervous system, 174–212
  adaptation of, 184–187
  in adolescence, 191–192
  in adulthood, 192–193
  aging and, 187–196
  autonomic, 181
    organization of, 182f
    selected effects of, 183t
  central, 176, 177–181
  in childhood, 189–191
  communication within, 181–184
  functional implications, 196–205
  in infancy, 189–191
  injury response, 186–187
  in locomotion, 304
  in older adults, 193–196
  peripheral, 176, 184–187
  prenatal, 187–189
  reaction time and, 196–197
Neural division of labor, 316
Neural plasticity, 184–185
  activity-dependent, 185
  ecological, 185
  experience-dependent, 185
  experience-expectant, 185
Neural representation, 71
Neuroendocrine system, aging in, 38–39
Neurofibrillary tangles (NFTs), 195
Neuroglia, 188
Neuromuscular junction, 130, 132f
Neuron cell death, 185–186
Neuronal group selection, 52, 52f
Neuronal vulnerability, 186
Neurons, types of, 175f
Neuroprosthesis, 329
Neurotransmitters, 182–184
NFTs. *See* Neurofibrillary tangles
NHANS. *See* National Health and Nutrition Survey
Nondeclarative memory, 30
Nongenetic theories of aging, 37–39
Nonrapid eye movement (NREM), 242
Nonstandardized examination, 89–90
Norepinephrine
  in aging, 241t
  physical activity and, 347t
Novelty, 219
Novice stage, 78
NREM. *See* Nonrapid eye movement
Nutrition, 20

O

Obesity
  in adults, 341
  in children, 341
  effects of, 341
  as global concern, 339*b*
  prevalence of, 340*f*
Object permanence, 28
Occipital lobe, 177*t*
Occupational choices, 327
Ocular dominance columns, 219
Older adults. *See also* Aging
  adaptation in, 330
  alcohol and, 204
  ambulation in, 297–301
    adaptability, 300
    kinematics, 299
    kinetics, 299
    long-distance navigation, 301
    long-term viability, 300–301
    progression of, 299
    stability, 299–300
  in America, 16*f*
  balance in, 280–284
  defecation in, 256
  development in, 36
  digestion in, 255–256
  endocrine system in, 242–243
  falling in, 298*b*
  gait pattern changes in, 297*t*
  ingestion in, 255–256
  micturition in, 258–259
  motor control in, 75
  motor learning in, 83–84
  musculoskeletal changes in, 330
  nervous system in, 193–196
  in older adulthood, 121–122
  physical activity in, 343*f*, 350, 351
  posture in, 280–281
  prehension in, 330
  pulmonary system in, 169–170
  skeletal muscle development in, 138–147
  sleep-wakefulness in, 249–250
  strength in, 142, 145*t*
  vital functions in, 242
Oligodendrocytes, 176–177
One-foot standing balance, 278*t*
Ontogenetic scheme, 264*f*
Open-loop control mode, 70
  model, 70*f*
Optimization principles, 73–74
Oropharyngeal anatomy, 253*f*
Osteoarthritis, 106
Osteoporosis
  involutional, 125
  prevention, 123*b*
  senile, 125
Outcomes, 71
Overweight, 339
Oxidative damage hypothesis, 37–38
Oxidative metabolism, 143

P

PAC. *See* Preference for Activity of Children (PAC)
Pacinian corpuscles, 214, 225
Pad-to-pad prehension, 314*t*
Pain, 220
Palmar grasp, 321*t*
Papillae, 217
Paradoxical sleep, 243
Parallel play, 33
Parasympathetic stimulation, 183*t*
Parathyroid hormones, 242
Parietal lobe, 177*t*, 178*t*
Parietooccipitotemporal lobe, 178*t*
Part practice, 81
Part task training, 72
Participation
  characteristics of, 89–93
  defined, 4
  evaluation of, 88–104
  functional activities and, 4–5
  restriction, 4
  selection considerations, 90
Peabody Developmental Motor Scales, 64, 276
PEDI. *See* Pediatric Evaluation of Disability Index
Pediatric assessment tools, 94–97
  activities assessed in, 95*b*
Pediatric Evaluation of Disability Index (PEDI), 95–96
Pediatric Quality of Life Inventory (Peds QL), 97
Pencil grip, 324*t*, 325*f*
Perception, 179*t*
Perceptual trace, 76
Perceptual-cognitive theory, 29–31
Performance, rating, 91–92
Performance-based assessments, 93
Perichondrium, 106–107
Perimysium, 129–130
Peripheral nervous system (PNS), 176, 184–187
Peripheral neuropathy, 328
Phasing
  amplitude, 289
  distance, 289
  temporal, 289
Phenotype, 17
Physical activity. *See also* Fitness
  in adults, 350
  antidiuretic hormone and, 347*t*
  in childhood, 350, 351
  corticotropin and, 347*t*
  cortisol and, 347*t*
  effects of, 342*f*
  epinephrine and, 347*t*
  fitness and, 338
  glucagon and, 347*t*
  growth hormone and, 347*t*
  health and, 338
  insulin and, 347*t*
  norepinephrine and, 347*t*
  in older adults, 343*f*, 350, 351
  prescriptions, 349*b*
  regular, 342*f*
  skeletal system and, 122*t*
  in toddlers, 339
Physical fitness. *See* Fitness
Physical function, 7–12
  development, 8–9
Physical growth, 5–6
Physical manifestations, 3
Physiological fitness, 336–337

Piaget, J., 23, 33, 34t, 36
Pincer grasp, 321t
Pinch, 312, 315
  precision, 313f
Pivoting, 57f
Placode, 218
Play, 33–35
  associative, 33
  cooperative, 33
  importance of, 34t
  parallel, 33
  solitary, 33
  symbolic, 33
  types of, 34t
PNS. *See* Peripheral nervous system
POMA. *See* Tinetti Performance Oriented Mobility Assessment
Pons, 180
Pores of Kohn, 158
Positional stability, 47
Postpubescence, 15
Postural reflexes, 268–269
  automatic, 269t
Posture, 264
  in adolescence, 279
  assessment of, 272–273
  in childhood, 275–279
  control, 264–266
    adaptive, 265
    anticipatory, 279
    automatic postural adjustments, 269–270
    components of, 266–268, 266f, 273t, 276t
    conceptual model of, 266f
    development of, 277–279
    hierarchical model, 268–269
    Nashner model of, 271–272
    neural basis for, 268–272
    perturbations, 265–266
    prehension and, 309–310
    reactive, 265
    types of, 273t, 276t
    winter stiffness model, 272
  defined, 263
  environmental adaptation and, 268
  eye-head stabilization, 267
  in infancy, 275–279
  life span changes in, 274–284
  models of, 263–264
  motor coordination and, 268
  musculoskeletal system and, 267–268
  in older adults, 280–281
  ontogenetic scheme of, 264f
  predictive central set, 268
  sensory organization and, 267
  standing, 278
    comparison of, 280f
  steady-state, 264–265
  swimming, 56
Power, 143
  function and, 11
Power grip, 312, 312f
Practice, 82
  blocked, 79–80, 80f
  distributed, 78–79
  massed, 78–79, 79b
  in motor learning, 78–81

Practice *(Continued)*
  random, 79–80, 80f
  variable, 80–81
Precision, 91
  grip, 312
  handling, 312–313, 313f
  pinch, 313f
Predictive central set, 268
Preexplicit memory, development of, 198t
Preference for Activity of Children (PAC), 97
Prehension, 309–334
  in adolescence, 325–327
  in adulthood, 327–330
  biomechanics, 310
  in childhood, 322–323, 324–325
  components of, 309–316
  defined, 309
  development, 317–330
    historical sequence of, 321t
  dynamic, 313
  dysfunction, 328b
  improving, 328–329
  in infancy, 317–322
  maintenance of, 327–330
  mastery of, 324–325
  occupational choices and, 327
  in older adults, 330
  pad-to-pad, 314t
  postural control and, 309–310
  prenatal, 317
  static, 313
  surgical reconstruction and, 328–329
  tip-to-tip, 314t
Preload, 157
Premotor time, 196
Prenatal development
  action, 317
  alcohol and, 204
  cardiovascular system, 159–160
    schematic of, 152f
  digestion, 253
  endocrine system, 240
  ingestion, 253
  micturition, 257
  nervous system, 187–189
  prehension, 317
  pulmonary system, 160–161
  sensory system, 218–219
  skeletal muscle, 133–136
  skeletal system, 116–119
  sleep-wakefulness, 246–247
Preoperational period, 29
Prepubescence, 15
Presbycusis, 228
Presbyopia, 228
Pressure, age-related changes in, 226t
Primary circular reactions, 28
Primary ossification centers, 117f, 118f
Priming, 30
Primitive alveoli, 161
Primitive reflexes, 54t
Primitive squeeze grasp, 321t
Proactive control, 309
Procedural memory, 30
Progeria, 36–37

Programmed aging, 36–37
Proprioception, 214–215, 220–221
    age-related changes in, 226t
Prostheses, 329
Protective reactions, 269
Proximal development, 32
Proximal-distal, 46
Psychological domain, 7, 7f
    aging theories, 39–40
    in human development, 21t, 22–23
        childhood, 27–31
        stages of, 23–24
Pubescence, 13
Pull to sit maneuver, 59f
Pulmonary system, 151–173
    adaptation to training, 345t
    in adolescence, 167
    in adulthood, 167–170
    aging and, 167–170
    birth adjustments, 161
    childhood, 165–167
    components, 157–158
        functional, 158
    conducting portion, 157–158
    control, 158
    development of, 159–170
        respiratory system, 166–167
        ventilatory pump, 165–167
    divisions of, 157f
    in fitness, 344–345, 349
        long-term adaptation, 345
        short-term adaptation, 344–345
    functional implications of changes in, 170–171
    functional lung volumes, 159f
    infancy, 165–167
    life span changes, 162t
    in locomotion, 304
    mechanics, 158–159
    in older adults, 169–170
    prenatal development, 160–161
    regulation, 158
    respiratory portion, 158
Purkinje cells, 174–175
Purposeful events, 36–37
Pyramidal neurons, 184f

Q
QRS wave shift, 168

R
Radial palmar grasp, 321t
Radial-digital grasp, 321t
Random practice, 79–80, 80f
Raphe nuclei, 246
Rapid eye movement (REM), 242
Raynaud disease, 328
Reach, 309
    anticipatory, 324f
    in childhood, 323
    formation, 311–312
    in infancy, 317–319
Reach to grasp activity, 80f
Reaction
    automatic postural, 269t
    circular

Reaction (Continued)
    primary, 28
    secondary, 28
    tertiary, 28
    equilibrium, 270
        sitting, 270f
    instinctive grasp, 320t
    lateral righting, 57f
    postural control, 265
    protective, 269
    righting, 57, 269
    time, 196–197
Reactive control, 309
Reactive oxygen species (ROS), 37–38
Reactive postural control, 265
Recall schema, 76
Reciprocal interweaving, 22
Recognition schema, 77
Reflex model, 68
Reflex stepping, 294–296
Reflexes, 188
    asymmetrical tonic neck, 55f, 320t
    hand, 320t
    postural, 268–269
        automatic, 269t
    primitive, 54t
    spontaneous Landau, 57f
    stepping, 294–296
    vestibular ocular, 221
Reflexive stage, 23
Regard, 309
    visual, 310–311
        in infancy, 317
Release, 309, 316
    in infancy, 322
Reliability, 90
    interrater, 90
    intrarater, 90
    test-retest, 90
REM. See Rapid eye movement
Replicative senescence, 36–37
Residual volume (RV), 159
Respiratory endurance, 337
Respiratory portion, 158
Respiratory system
    aging and, 170
    development, 166–167
Responsiveness, 91
Resting muscle length, 310
Reticular activating system, 181
Rhythmic movements, 51f
Right hemisphere, 179t
Righting, 270
Righting reaction, 57, 269
    lateral, 57f
Roberton, M.A., 65–66
Rogers, W.A., 81
Role confusion, 20
Rolling, 289–290
    automatic, 290
    forms of, 291f
    patterns of, 291f
ROS. See Reactive oxygen species
Rowe, J.W., 41
Rubinstein, Arthur, 40

Ruffini endings, 214
Running, 301–303
    lower extremities in, 301
    upper extremities in, 301
RV. *See* Residual volume

S

Sabourin, P., 65
Sarcomeres, 133*f*
Sarcopenia, 138–139
    age-related, 139*f*
    factors contributing to, 139*f*
Sarcoplasmic reticulum (SR), 130, 169
Satellite cells, 134
Schema theory, 76–77
    recall, 76
    recognition, 77
Schmidt, R.A., 76–77
School Function Assessment (SFA), 96–97
Scissors grasp, 321*t*
Scurvy, 110
Sears, R.R., 32
Season's of Life, 35
Secondary circular reactions, 28
Secondary ossification centers, 117*f*
Secondary schemes, 28
Segmental rotation, 289
Self-administered assessment, 93
Self-control, 197
Self-organization, 50
Self-perception, 219–220
Semilunar valves, 151–154
Senescence, 6
    in development, 16
    replicative, 36–37
Senile osteoporosis, 125
Sensation, 47, 213–214, 217
Sensorimotor integration, 217
Sensorimotor period, 27–31
Sensory areas, 178*f*
Sensory homunculus, 179*f*
Sensory integration, 217
Sensory organization, 267
    aging and, 281
    balance and, 274*f*
    conditions used in tests of, 274*f*
Sensory Organization Test (SOT), 272
Sensory system, 213–238
    in adolescence, 223–225
    in adulthood, 225–229
    aging and, 218–233
        changes in, 281
    balance and, 277, 278–279
    characteristics of, 213–218
    functional implications, 229–233
    in infancy, 219–223
    posture and, 267
    in prenatal period, 218–219
    senses in, 214–218
    somatic, 214–215, 218, 220–221
    special, 215–219, 221–223, 224–225, 228–229
Sequential learning, 83
Serotonin, 182–184
SF-36. *See* Short Form-36

SFA. *See* School Function Assessment
Short Form-36 (SF-36), 101
Short term memory, 30–31
Short-term adaptation, 343–345
SIDS. *See* Sudden infant death syndrome
Simple response time (SRT), 196
SIS. *See* Stroke Impact Scale
Sitting, 58*f*
    balance and, 277–278
    development of, 277
Skeletal muscle. *See also* Musculoskeletal system
    caloric intake and, 140
    development, 133–142
        adolescence, 136–137, 142
        adulthood, 137–138, 142–147
        childhood, 142
        functional implications, 142–147
        infancy, 136–137
        older adulthood, 138–147
        prenatal, 133–136
    loss, 139
    organization of, 129–133
    protein synthesis, 140
    structural changes, 140
Skeletal system, 105–128. *See also* Bone
    in adolescence
        functional implications, 122–124
    in childhood, 119–120
        functional implications, 122–124
    components of, 105–116
    development, 116–122
    functional implications, 122–125
    in infancy, 119–120
    maturity, 121
    physical activity and, 122*t*
    prenatal development, 116–119
Skill-related fitness, 336–337
Skinner, B.F., 31
Skipping, 303
    lower extremities in, 303
    upper extremities in, 303
Skoura, X., 75
Sleep-wakefulness, 245–246
    in adolescence, 248–249
    in adulthood, 248–249
    aging and, 250*b*
    brain wave changes in, 245*f*
    in childhood, 248
    control mechanisms, 246
    cycles, 249*f*
    infancy, 247–248
    life span functions, 246–250
    in older adults, 249–250
    prenatal development, 246–247
Slow wave sleep (SWS), 243
Small veins, 156
Smell, 217, 219, 221–222, 228–229
Smith, L.B., 49
Social factors
    fitness and, 338–339
    health and, 338–339
Social learning, 24–25, 32
Sociocultural domain, 7, 7*f*
    in aging, 40–41

Sociocultural domain *(Continued)*
  in human development, 21*t*, 24–25
    child, 31–35
Soft assembled motor behavior, 50–51
Solitary play, 33
Somatic efferent system, 181
Somatic senses, 214–215, 218, 220–221, 224
Somatosensation, 226*t*, 267
SOT. *See* Sensory Organization Test
Space perception, 224–225
Spatial awareness, 224–225
Spatial cognition, 217
Spherical grasp, 314*t*
Spinal cord, 180*f*
Spinal curve development, 275–277
Spinal extension, 290
Spongy bone, 108
Spontaneous, 57*f*
Spontaneous Landau reflex, 57*f*
SR. *See* Sarcoplasmic reticulum
SRT. *See* Simple response time
ST segment depression, 168
Stability, 47
  cone of, 265*f*
  dynamic, 47
  lateral, 284
  limits of, 266–267
    in older adults, 299–300
  positional, 47
Stage theory, 21–22
Stance phase, 292
Stand maneuver, 59*f*
Stand transition, 278
Standardized examination, 89–90
  selection considerations, 90
Standing, 63*f*
  forms of, 66*f*
State, 219
Static balance, 11
Static flexibility, 10
Static phase, 294–296
Static prehension, 313
Steady-state posture, 264–265
Stepping, 54*f*
  deliberate, 294–296
  direction, 283
  independent, 294–296
  length, 292
  reflex, 294–296
Stereognosis, 218, 315–316
Stochastic changes, 37
Strabismus, 229
STREAM. *See* Stroke Rehabilitation Assessment of
    Movement
Strength, 327
  acquisition of, 142*b*
  in adolescents, 142
  in adulthood, 142
  age and, 137, 145*f*
  in childhood, 142
  dynamic, 143
  grip, 138*f*, 326*f*
  isometric, 143
    aging and, 145*f*

Strength *(Continued)*
  muscular, 337
    in older adults, 142, 145*t*
    training, 146–147
Stress fractures, 124
Stride, 289
  length, 292
Stroke Impact Scale (SIS), 92–93
Stroke Rehabilitation Assessment of Movement
    (STREAM), 92–93
Stroke volume, 151
Subcortical structures, 180*f*
Sudden infant death syndrome (SIDS), 247, 248*b*
Summarized feedback, 81
Superior pincer grasp, 321*t*
Surfactant, 158, 161
Sustained grip, 315
Swallowing, 250
  control mechanisms, 251–252
  phases of, 251*f*
Sway strategies, 271*f*
  medial-lateral, 282
Swimming posture, 56
Swing phase, 292
Swinnen, S.P., 82
SWS. *See* Slow wave sleep
Symbolic play, 33
Symmetrical bimanual coordination, 316
Sympathetic stimulation, 183*t*
Synarthrosis joints, 116
Synovial joints, 116*f*
Systems models, 71
Systolic blood pressure, 169

T
Taste, 217, 219, 221–222, 228–229
Temperament, 31–32
  in infants, 31*t*
Temperature, 220
Temporal lobe, 177*t*, 178*t*
Temporal phasing, 289
Tendinitis, 328
Terminal feedback, 81–82
Terminal respiratory units, 161
Terminal sacs, 161
Tertiary circular reactions, 28
Testosterone, 242
  in aging, 241*t*
Test-retest reliability, 90
Thalamus, 179
Thelen, F., 49
Thorax, 166*f*
Thought, 28–29
Three-jaw chuck, 321*t*
Thumb opposition, 313
Thyroid, 188
Thyroid hormones, 242
  in aging, 241*t*
Thyroxine, 38–39
Tidal volume, 159, 344–345
Time, 50–51
Time to task failure, 141*f*
Timed Up and Go test, 273, 273*t*
  pediatric, 276*t*

Tinetti Performance Oriented Mobility Assessment (POMA), 273*t*
Tip-to-tip prehension, 314*t*
Toddlers. *See also* Infancy
    ambulation in, 294–296
    motor development, 60–61
    physical activity in, 339
Top down control, 71–72
Total hand function, 313
Touch, 220
    age-related changes in, 226*t*
Trabeculae, 108
Traction response, 320*t*
Tracts, 181
Trainability, 343
Training, 343
    activities, 329
    cardiovascular adaptation to, 344*t*
    endocrine contributions to, 346–347
    hormonal contributions to, 346–347
    life span and, 349–351
    metabolic contributions to, 346–347
    musculoskeletal system adaptation to, 346*t*
    part task, 72
    pulmonary system adaptation to, 345*t*
    strength, 146–147
Trajectory, 311
Transition, 294–296
Transitional movements, 57–58, 279–280
Transverse tubular system, 130, 132*f*
Tropomyosin, 130
Troponin, 130
Tunica adventitia, 155–156
Tunica intima, 155–156
Tunica media, 155–156
Tunics, 154

U
Upper extremities
    growth, 317, 318*t*
    in hopping, 302
    limb loss, 328
    in running, 301
    in skipping, 303
Upright position, 295*f*
Urinary incontinence, 258*t*, 259*b*
Useful field of view (UVOF), 232–233
UVOF. *See* Useful field of view

V
VABS-C. *See* Vineland Adaptive Behavior Scales - classroom edition
Validity, 91
    concurrent, 91
    construct, 91
    content, 91
Valsalva maneuver, 256
VanSant, A.F., 65
Variable practice, 80–81
Vasa vasorum, 155–156
Vascular system, 155–156. *See also* Arteries; Cardiovascular system; Veins
    aging, 168
Vasopressin, 241*t*

VBM. *See* Voxel-based morphometry
VC. *See* Vital capacity
Veins, 156. *See also* Vascular system
    medium, 156
    small, 156
Ventilation-respiration, 243–250
    control mechanisms, 243–244
    mechanics of, 158–159
    neural system, 243–244
Ventilatory pump
    aging and, 169–170
    development, 165–166
Venules, 156
Vera, J.G., 82
Vertebral development, 113*f*
Vertical gravity line, 280*f*
Vestibular ocular reflex (VOR), 221
Vestibular sense, 215, 218, 221, 224, 227–228
Vibration, 226*t*
Vicariation, 187
Vineland Adaptive Behavior Scales - classroom edition (VABS-C), 97
Vision, 218–219, 221–222, 224, 228
    age-related changes in, 227*t*
    development of, 222*t*
Visual acuity, 227*t*
Visual information processing, 227*t*
Visual perception, 310–311
Visual regard, 310–311
    in infancy, 317
Visual-motor control, 311
Vital capacity (VC), 159
Vital functions, 239–262
    life span changes in, 243–259
        sleep-wakefulness, 245–246
        ventilation-respiration, 243–250
    in older adults, 242
Vitamin C, 110
Vitamin D, 110
VOR. *See* Vestibular ocular reflex
Voxel-based morphometry (VBM), 194
Vygotsky, Lev, 32, 33, 34*t*

W
Walking. *See also* Ambulation
    developmental stages, 294–301
    erect, 294–301
    independent, 62*f*
    parameters, 294*t*
    velocity, 292
WeeFIM, 94, 94*f*
Wellness, 335
WHO. *See* World Health Organization
Whole task training, 81
Wickstrom, R.L., 62
Winter stiffness model, 272
Wishart, L.R., 82
Wolff, J., 109–110
Working memory, 31
    development of, 198*t*
World Health Organization (WHO), 2
    on health, 335
W-sitting, 47*f*, 58